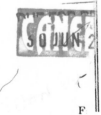

Principles of APPLIED BIOMEDICAL INSTRUMENTATION

Principles of
APPLIED BIOMEDICAL
INSTRUMENTATION

THIRD EDITION

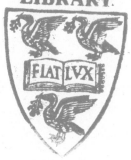
L. A. GEDDES
Purdue University

L. E. BAKER
The University of Texas at Austin

WILEY

A WILEY-INTERSCIENCE PUBLICATION

JOHN WILEY & SONS New York • Chichester • Brisbane • Toronto • Singapore

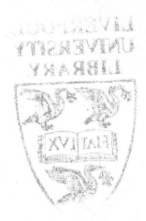

Library of Congress Cataloging in Publication Data:

Geddes, L. A. (Leslie Alexander), 1921–
    Principles of applied biomedical instrumentation / L. A. Geddes,
  L. E. Baker.—3rd ed.
      p. cm.
    "A Wiley-Interscience publication."
    Includes bibliographies and index.
    ISBN 0-471-60899-8
    1. Medical electronics. 2. Physiological apparatus. I. Baker,
  L. E. II. Title.
    [DNLM: 1. Biomedical Engineering—instrumentation. QT 34 G295p]
  R856.G4 1989
  610'.28—dc19
  DNLM/DLC
  for Library of Congress   88-27915
                                                                  CIP

The instruments change, but the
principles endure

Preface

Whereas the first two editions of the *Principles* dealt with the measurement of physiological events, this, the third edition, is much broader in scope and includes coverage of therapeutic and rehabilitative (assistive) devices. In addition to revising the earlier text, expanding it to include new applications of basic principles, four new chapters have been added.

Like its predecessors, this edition is written for both the life scientist and the physical scientist. An intimate knowledge of mathematics is not necessary to understand the principles that are presented. Many examples of the applications of each principle are given in the hope that the reader will recognize new ways of using a principle. We believe that the physical scientist will be entertained by the many ways a physical principle is used in biomedicine. It is hoped that the life scientist will develop an appreciation of how instruments work and thereby recognize their limitations. All students should find the material easy to read; the teacher will find many examples of theory to illuminate lectures. Psychophysiology, nursing, medical, and veterinary students will find that the instruments used in their fields can be reduced to simple operating principles. Physicians and veterinarians preparing for board exams will find the nonmathematical presentations of instrumentation helpful. The engineering student will find a reservoir of principles and techniques that can be used to design new instruments.

The four new chapters deal with stimulation and stimulators, radiant-energy devices, ventilators, and anesthesia. The chapter on stimulation (Chapter 10) covers the principles of excitation, which lead directly to the fundamental law embodied in the strength–duration curve. This chapter also discusses monopolar and bipolar stimulation and describes the various output circuits (constant-voltage, constant-current, and isolated-output). There are numerous examples of stimulation, such as cardiac pacing, ventricular defibrillation, and functional electrical stimulation.

Chapter 13, on radiant-energy devices, covers light-emitting diodes, blackbody radiation, gas-discharge lamps, lasers, X-rays, computerized tomography, lithotripsy, diathermy, and electrosurgery.

The various methods of providing artificial respiration are presented in Chapter 14. Coverage is given to the ways in which inspiration can be induced electrically by stimulating the nerves that innervate the inspiratory muscles.

Inhalation anesthesia and the anesthesia machine are dealt with in an elementary way in Chapter 15. The method of delivering anesthetic gases and estimating the depth of anesthesia are outlined, along with anesthesia monitoring.

To the chapter on resistive transducers (Chapter 2) have been added the thermal conductivity method for measuring cardiac output, the thermal clearance method, and the strain gauge method for measuring tissue perfusion. A new disposable pressure transducer is discussed along with its use in measuring blood pressure waveforms.

New applications of the single inductor to measure respiration and acceleration have been included in Chapter 3 on inductive transducers. The newly introduced magnetostrictive tissue fragmenter (Cavitron) is illustrated and discussed.

In Chapter 4 many new applications of capacitive transducers are presented. For example, a commercially available capacitive blood pressure transducer is described in detail, along with the method of using a differential capacitor to detect gaseous carbon dioxide. The method of detecting respiratory air flow with a low-resistance, differential capacitance pneumotachograph is also discussed.

Chapter 5, on photoelectric devices, has been expanded to include coverage of the photomultiplier and the scintillation counter. Cardiac output by the dye-dilution method, transmission, reflectance (including pulse), and fiber-optic oximetry, bilirubinometry (for jaundice detection), thermography, photoplethysmography, drop counting, and continuous noninvasive blood pressure monitoring (achieved by closed-loop control) represent new material.

In addition to expanded coverage of piezoelectric elements as detectors, more ultrasonic applications are presented in Chapter 6. For example, transcutaneous Doppler blood-flow measurement and ultrasonic imaging techniques are covered.

Thermoelectric power sources and the use of Peltier coolers have been added to Chapter 7, on thermoelectric devices. Applications of each are discussed.

An unusual amount of research has been devoted to creating chemical sensors, and Chapter 8 reflects this activity. In addition to broadened descriptions of many of the familiar transducers, attention is given to transcutaneous pO_2, pCO_2, and pH sensors. New membrane electrodes are described, and a section has been added on spectrophotometry and flame photometry. Fiber-optic and catheter-tip field-effect chemical sensors are discussed in detail, along with new types of sensors for glucose. A large section deals with measurement of the composition of respiratory gases and the mass spectrometer.

Chapter 9 has been expanded considerably to cover many new types of electrodes, such as the conducting adhesive and recessed types that are so popular in recording bioelectric events. Electrode stability is dealt with in detail. New models for the electrode–electrolyte interface and electrode–subject circuit are presented. Dry and capacitive electrodes are analyzed along with the demands that they impose on the amplifier input circuit. More coverage is given to microelectrodes including the types of amplifiers that can be used with them. There is a new section on stimulating electrodes and their properties. The current-density distribution under current-carrying electrodes is discussed along with the phenomena that occur when electrodes are operated at high current density (rectification, gas evolution, arcing, and shock-wave production).

The detection of physiological events by impedance continues to increase in popularity, and the size of Chapter 11 reflects this trend. The circuit diagram of an easily constructed constant-current, isolated, tetrapolar impedance recorder has been included. New data are presented on tissue resistivity, along with a new method of measuring blood resistivity noninvasively. The measurement of cardiac output by the saline-indicator method has been expanded and a new method for electrical calibration is included. Use of the impedance technique to measure stroke volume with a catheter electrode in the heart is discussed and is used to permit display of pressure–volume loops from which work and power can be determined. Thoracic impedance cardiography has been updated to include the use of ensemble averaging to improve the quality of the impedance signal. Venous-occlusion plethysmography and the detection of the pulse and respiration with wrist electrodes have been added.

In Chapter 12, on bioelectric events, a new section has been added on the sources of interference during recording of bioelectric events, demonstrating the need for the differential amplifier. The circuit diagram of an easily constructed isolated-input differential amplifier has been included. Measurement of the His-bundle electrogram and the measurement of sensory and motor evoked potentials have been added, along with use of the SQUID to detect the magnetic component of a bioelectric event.

In the final chapter, which is devoted to the criteria for the faithful reproduction of an event, there are new examples of the theory, along with an elementary discussion of digital techniques used in signal processing. Analog and digital tape recording are described, and an example is given of the conversion of an analog signal (the ECG) to digital form and how such a signal is displayed.

The first edition of *Principles* appeared in 1968, and the second edition seven years later. Both reflected the technologies of their times. It is hoped that the content of this third edition will not only reflect today's technology but tomorrow's. Great care has been given to retaining and selecting material of enduring value.

Just before publication of the second edition, both authors accepted new positions; Geddes at Purdue and Baker at the University of Texas. However, in the intervening years we have maintained a close liaison and continued research in our respective areas of interest. We both owe a huge debt to all of our students, technical staff, and universities, which gave us the opportunity to pursue our separate interests. We both wish to thank the National Institutes of Health for the opportunity to serve on many Study Sections, which made us aware of the emerging technologies in many fields and provided a wealth of reference literature. We are also grateful to the numerous secretaries who, over the years, transcribed almost illegible lecture notes into papers and manuscripts that ultimately became *The Principles of Applied Biomedical Instrumentation*.

L. A. GEDDES
L. E. BAKER

West Lafayette, Indiana
Austin, Texas
May 1989

Contents

Principles of APPLIED BIOMEDICAL INSTRUMENTATION

1

Biomedical Instruments and the Measurement of Physiological Events

INTRODUCTION

There are basically three types of instruments used in medicine and biology: diagnostic, therapeutic, and assistive. The diagnostic instrument acquires information for presentation to the human senses. In essence, the diagnostic or data-acquiring instrument is an extender of the human senses. It is in this area that transducers play the key role. The therapeutic instrument is used by the physician, or the physician's delegated representative, to arrest or control a physiological process that has gone awry due to disease, trauma, or some other agent. Although chemical agents (drugs) are most prominent in the therapeutic area, physical instruments, such as the high-voltage X ray (to kill cancer cells), the pacemaker (to initiate rhythmic heart beats), or the defibrillator (to arrest the lethal cardiac arrhythmia, ventricular fibrillation), are but a few prominent examples of therapeutic instruments. Assistive devices are used to make up for diminished function or to provide for a lost function, usually when a disease process has been arrested but there remains a deficit. It is in the area of rehabilitation medicine that one sees extensive application of assistive devices, which are often life-supporting or life-sustaining.

It is of particular importance to recognize that there are an increasing number of electronic implanted therapeutic devices being created. The most familiar example is the cardiac pacemaker. However, other examples are the dorsal column stimulator, the auditory prosthesis, and the bone-growth stimulator. The dorsal column stimulator is a tiny radio receiver that is connected to electrodes on the dorsal (posterior) columns of the spinal cord. Stimulation of these nerve fibers, effected by a small external transmitter, reduces or abolishes pain in a region beyond the electrodes. The auditory prosthesis is another type of implanted radio receiver having electrodes connected to an auditory nerve in a deaf person (with a functional auditory nerve). Environmental sound is detected by a microphone that delivers its signal to a speech processor, which in turn activates the transmitter that telemeters the signal to the implant. Although progress is slow in establishing communication with the deaf in this way, the initial results are very encouraging, and many auditory prostheses are used in humans today.

The implanted bone-growth stimulator is a small constant direct-current source. Electrodes applied to a fracture site promote fracture union remarkably well. The same technique can be used to stimulate bone growth in the young subject.

Perhaps the largest area of activity with implanted devices relates to the creation of drug-dispensing devices. For example, there is an implant for the slow delivery of heparin (an anticoagulant) which was reported by Blackshear et al. (1975). Implanted drug-delivery systems for insulin, antiarrhythmic drugs, and drugs to reduce blood pressure are being developed. Presently available implants permit refilling the drug reservoir from a hypodermic needle. Research is under way to set the rate of delivery of such drugs by external telemetry.

AUTOMATIC (SERVO) CONTROL DEVICES

Increasing numbers of diagnostic and therapeutic devices are being joined in closed-loop feedback systems to automatically control a body function. Surprisingly, this concept is by no means new; its first demonstration was reported by Bickford (1950, 1951), who used the electroencephalogram (EEG) to control the depth of anesthesia. Beyond a certain depth of anesthesia, the dominant frequency of the EEG decreases. Using appropriate circuitry to process the EEG, Bickford et al. created a signal that controlled the infusion of an intravenous anesthetic. However, EEG control of anesthesia is fraught with difficulties. For example, not all anesthetics affect the EEG frequency spectrum in the same way. In addition, there are other factors, such as reduced brain perfusion, that affect the EEG. For these reasons, the EEG has not been pursued as a controller of the depth of anesthesia.

Electromyographic (EMG) potentials have been used to control assistive devices in a closed-loop mode. Montgomery (1957a, b) used the EMG from residual respiratory muscles in a postpolio patient to control the cycling of a chest (cuirass) respirator. At the start of inspiration, the EMG triggered the respirator to produce inspiration. When the EMG potentials ceased, the respirator was triggered to cause expiration. If the EMG failed to occur within a preset time the respirator would cycle automatically. The modern analog for this action is in the demand cardiac pacemaker.

The EMG was also used by Geddes et al. (1959) to provide motion in paralyzed limbs of polio patients. In their device the EMG from small groups of residual muscles opened a solenoid valve to allow inflation of a McKibben artificial muscle, which is a bladder within a woven sleeve. Inflation of the bladder caused the sleeve to increase in diameter and decrease in length, and the decrease in length was used to move an arm brace on the patient. Contraction of one group of muscles triggered "contraction" of the artificial muscle; contraction of a different group of muscles triggered "relaxation" of the artificial muscle. In this way the artificial muscle could be left in any state of contraction or relaxation, as determined visually by the patient, without the need for EMG signals or inflating gas.

Gaining in importance are many applications of neuromuscular stimulation of paralyzed patients with spinal cord injuries. Already, patterned upper-extremity movement (Peckham and Mortimer, 1977), tricycle pedaling (Petrofsky et al., 1983), and the first efforts to provide walking (Vodovnik, 1977; Petrofsky et al., 1983) have been demonstrated. In Petrofsky's tricycle pedaling study, throttle information was fed to a small computer that directed the stimulation. The quadriceps muscles were stimulated from 270° to 90° of pedal rotation; the gluteus maximus muscles were stimulated from 0° to 180°, the 0° reference being for one leg at the top of the pedal position.

The first attempts to provide walking for hemiplegic patients appear to have been made about 1966 in Yugoslavia (Vodovnik et al., 1966). Vodovnik (1977) summarized these early studies and his progress. Starting with quantitative data on bone and joint motion in normal subjects, he proceeded to create a six-channel programmed stimulating system to improve the walking capabilities of 10 hemiplegic patients using skin-surface electrodes. He reported very good results in enabling these subjects to walk, but found that patient selection is a very important consideration (Vodovnik, 1977).

Having built up muscle strength in paraplegic patients using electrical stimulation, Petrofsky and Phillips (1983) developed a system designed to allow walking along a level surface. The muscle groups receiving stimuli via skin-surface electrodes were the quadriceps, iliacus, gastrocnemius, tibialis anterior, and hamstrings. Sensory input was provided by position indicators on the hip, knee, and ankle. Additional supervisory sensors were provided to limit the range of joint motion. Pressure sensors were used to report on the force under the foot. The system was activated by shoulder motion; for example, a forward thrust of the right shoulder caused the right leg to move forward.

To date, the system developed by Petrofsky et al. has been able to produce walking, but the investigators point out that much more research is needed to perfect the system. Additional sensors (e.g., body position sensed by a gyroscope) will improve the gait. Much additional research will be needed to provide a means for moving sideways and climbing stairs—activities that are an important part of the everyday life of normal subjects. Particularly important is provision of a means to regain the upright position after a fall; this has yet to be achieved.

Blood sugar was controlled automatically in humans by Kadish (1964). This system consisted of an automatic analyzer to measure the blood sugar and two motor-driven syringes, one for insulin (which reduces blood sugar) and the other for glucagon (which increases blood sugar). The control system triggered the release of insulin or glucagon when the blood sugar exceeded 150 mg % or fell below 50 mg %. The system was used on normal and diabetic human subjects.

Automatic control of blood glucose at the bedside by the controlled injection of insulin is becoming quite common. Devices for this purpose are commercially available. An excellent review of the technology was presented by Albisser (1979), one of the first creators of such a device for bedside use.

There is an important subtlety relating to the control of blood sugar by controlled insulin injection. Whereas there is a need for a basal level of insulin, there is a sudden increase in the requirement at the start of a meal when the blood sugar rises rapidly. Because existing automatic insulin-delivery systems have difficulty in accommodating this sudden requirement (owing to delays in the system), Kraegen et al. (1981) created a dual-algorithm controller that permits manual initiation of the programmed release of insulin designed to prevent the blood sugar from rising excessively. In this way, both the tonic and the phasic needs for insulin are accommodated.

Automatic control of blood pressure at the bedside was reported by Schade (1973), who used an adaptive control algorithm implemented by a digital computer located some distance from the hospital. Since then, many have researched the subject. Sheppard et al. (1980a, b), who have perhaps had the most experience with such a system, used a proportional-integral-differential (PID) algorithm to control the blood pressure in patients following cardiac surgery by the intravenous infusion of nitroprusside. The system has been used on more than 10,000 patients to date.

AUTOMATIC IMPLANTED THERAPEUTIC DEVICES

Many of the automatic (closed-loop feedback) systems just described are eligible for implementation as implanted devices. The only drawback in taking this final step is the lack of suitable long-lived implantable transducers to sense the desired physiological events. Considerable research is being undertaken in this important area.

Despite the lack of implantable transducers, a few automatic implantable therapeutic devices have been developed. Perhaps the most familiar is the demand cardiac pacemaker, which sits idle if the ventricles are beating and delivers rhythmic stimuli as needed if they are not. The transducer to detect a spontaneous (or normal) beat is the same pair of electrodes that are used for pacing. Current annual sales of pacemakers are on the order of 100,000.

Another automatic implantable therapeutic device is the automatic defibrillator. This device monitors ventricular activity continuously, and when fibrillation occurs it delivers a strong (defibrillating) shock to the ventricles. At present there are more than 500 patients with such implants.

Research is under way to create an automatic implantable blood pressure controller, because hypertension is so prevalent in western countries. It is reliably estimated that more than 10% of the U.S. population are hypertensive and only about one-quarter of these are on adequate therapy. Obviously, the creation of an implantable pressure transducer occupies the attention of many.

An area in which an automatic implantable device is obviously needed is for the treatment of diabetes. Researchers are vigorously seeking to create an implantable glucose sensor.

It is difficult to predict where the breakthroughs will occur in the creation of automatic implantable therapeutic devices. The ingenious innovator may well find unusual ways of sensing the event to be controlled or an event closely related to it.

TRANSDUCERS AND THE MEASUREMENT OF PHYSIOLOGICAL EVENTS

It is the task of the transducer to convert energy from one form to another, more useful, form. Sometimes the terms sensor or detector are used to describe a device that detects a physiological event. In biomedical applications the transducer converts a physiological event to an electrical signal. With the event available as an electrical signal, it is easy to obtain the advantages of modern computing and display equipment to present the desired information in the most useful form. With an electrical analog of a physiological event it is possible to store the event on magnetic tape or disk or in digital memory and reexamine it later. Replay and reproduction at different display rates permit examination of the data for information perhaps missed when the event was being measured. This capability provides a means of obtaining the maximum amount of information from the measurement.

Many methods are employed to convert a physiological event to an electrical signal. The event can be made to vary, directly or indirectly, electrical properties such as resistance, capacitance, inductance, or the magnetic linkage between two or more coils. The use of piezoelectric and photoelectric transducers is also common. Chemical events can be detected through potentials developed by membrane electrodes or by measurement of current flow through electrolytes. A chemically induced color change is also a useful transduction technique. Transducers for radiant energy occupy a prominent place in the detection of physiological events. Sometimes changes in the electrical properties of biological material can be employed for transduction purposes. Practical application of the principles of transduction embraces all the phenomena of the flow of electrons or ions through solids, liquids, gases, or a vacuum. In practice, however, only a few of these phenomena are convenient to use.

TRANSDUCIBLE PROPERTIES AND THE PRINCIPLE OF TRANSDUCTION

Before discussing the various methods employed to convert physiological events to electrical signals, it is important to distinguish between a transducible property and a method or principle of transduction. A transducible property is defined as a singular characteristic of a substance or event to which a principle of transduction can be applied. A principle of transduction is any one of the many methods that can be employed to convert the transducible property to an electrical signal. In essence the transducible property is the characteristic, like a fingerprint, that is singularly different from those of all the others around it; that is, it is the property that makes the event recognizable. The principle of transduction employs the device that recognizes the property and converts it to an electrical signal.

For example, if gaseous carbon dioxide is to be detected in a mixture of respiratory air (oxygen, nitrogen, and water vapor), a property that distinguishes carbon dioxide in this mixture is infrared absorption. Carbon dioxide absorbs radiation at wavelengths of 2.7, 4.3, and 14.7 micrometers (μm). Although water vapor absorbs a small amount of radiation near 2.7 μm, the use of an infrared source operating at either of the other two or all three of the principal absorption bands and a detector sensitive to the same spectrum constitutes a means for detecting carbon dioxide. Thus with the respiratory air passing between the infrared source and the detector, the output from the latter will decrease in proportion to the amount of carbon dioxide in the respiratory air. In this example the transducible property is infrared absorption, and the principle of transduction employs an infrared source and detector. Parenthetically, it is obvious that the maximum resolution attainable is intimately related to the singularity of the transducible property and the selectivity of the principle of transduction.

A transducer is in reality the sense organ for the electronic processing equipment. By its very nature it is a highly specialized device ideally possessing sensitivity to a single type of energy. For this reason it is difficult to discuss the merits of these devices in a general manner. Nonetheless, a few characteristics of high-quality transducers can be stated that will serve as a basis for their evaluation.

Irrespective of the event being measured, the transducer, insofar as possible, must obey Kelvin's first rule of instrumentation (Thompson, 1910); that is, the measuring instrument must not alter the event being measured. In biomedical studies this goal is not always realizable, and the degree of alteration must constantly be borne in mind. Frequently, indirect methods are employed that partially isolate the transducer from the event. For this reason it is essential that the transducer exhibit a high degree of selectivity for the phenomenon being measured so that it will adequately reject other events.

The transducer should also obey the three criteria for the faithful reproduction of an event: amplitude linearity, adequate frequency response, and freedom from phase distortion. Because these criteria are discussed in detail in Chapter 16 only a brief explanation of their meaning is given here.

Amplitude linearity refers to the ability of the transducer to produce an output signal that is directly proportional to the input amplitude. This requirement is presented graphically in Fig. 1 by the solid line 0–A. If the phenomenon under measurement increases in the opposite direction, the transducer must also linearly indicate this condition, as shown in Fig. 1 by the solid line 0–A'.

Although the input–output characteristic of a transducer is represented as a straight line, careful testing with known inputs usually reveals a small deviation from linearity. In high-quality transducers such a test reveals a series of values that distribute themselves on either side of a straight line. The exaggeration of a typical case is portrayed by the dashed line in Fig. 1. In such instances it is customary to describe the degree of linearity in terms of percent deviation. For example, a linearity of $\pm 1\%$ means that within the total operating range of the device, the deviation from linear response will not be greater than $\pm 1\%$.

Another quantity often related to the response of a transducer is hysteresis, which is a measure of the ability of the transducer to produce an output that follows the input independently of the direction of change in the input. In a linear system with no hysteresis, the input–output relationship is a single straight line. If hysteresis is present, an open curve is obtained, as shown in Fig. 2. It is customary to express

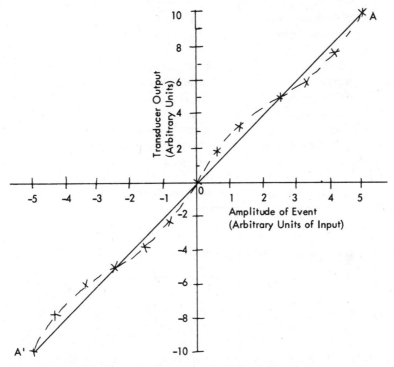

Figure 1   The meaning of amplitude linearity.

the amount of hysteresis in terms of the percentage of full-scale value. In a well-designed device this error would be less than 1%.

In connection with amplitude linearity it is pertinent to point out that the amplitude range of the event to be encountered should not exceed the physical limits of the transducer. Large inputs may permanently damage a transducer and hence decrease the linearity and increase the hysteresis error.

Frequency response and *freedom from phase distortion* refer to the ability of the transducer to provide a signal that will follow both rapid and slow changes in the event presented to it. The overall frequency response must be equal to or greater than that dictated by harmonic analysis of the waveform of the event. Freedom from phase distortion requires that the transducer maintain the time differences in

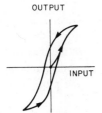

Figure 2   Hysteresis.

the sinusoidal frequency components revealed by harmonic analysis. Examples of the distortion encountered when these criteria are not fulfilled are described in Chapter 16.

Although it is highly desirable to obtain linear signals from all transducers, it is not always possible to do so. Occasionally the transducer develops a signal that is not directly proportional to the event. For example, the resistance change of thermistors is not linear with temperature. Under such circumstances linearizing networks are necessary unless the event can be tolerated with a nonlinear calibration. Sometimes the signal is nonlinear because of the nature of the physiological event itself; for example, the redness of blood, reflecting the degree of oxygen saturation, is related to a logarithmic ratio of red and infrared transmissions. Under these conditions it is necessary to employ special processing devices to develop a signal linearly related to oxygen saturation.

CALIBRATION AND STANDARDIZATION

Calibration

It is highly desirable for the output of a transducer to be linearly proportional to the amplitude of a physiological event. The act of applying a physiological event of known amplitude and measuring the transducer output is known as calibration. The transducer output may be in terms of voltage, current, or the amplitude on a meter or graphic recorder or an oscilloscope monitor. If the transducer output and display system are linear with the physiological event, a single-point calibration is sufficient. If the transducer (or display system) provides a nonlinear output, then multiple calibration points are needed to construct a calibration curve so that the amplitude of the display can be interpreted in physiological units.

A transducer that does not lend itself to calibration directly in terms of the physiological event has limited value; however, it can provide information that has meaning in the time domain. For example, waveform and time relation to another event form the basis for analyzing data that are acquired by transducers that cannot be calibrated.

Transducers can be expensive devices. For this reason selection of a particular type should be based in part on its ability to be incorporated into an existing processing or display system. Fulfilling such a requirement paves the way for the creation of a modular system that can accept a variety of transducers for many purposes.

Ultimately the transduced event is displayed by an indicating device. It is important to call attention to this fact because the type of display and use of the data frequently dictate the degree of accuracy required. Accuracy and cost are inextricably linked and often become the basis for bargaining. Perhaps the considerations in this regard were best expressed by Sir Thomas Lewis (1925), the pioneer of clinical electrocardiography, who wrote:

"Coal when weighed for sale is not thrown into a chemical balance, neither is coal placed on a coarse scale when submitted to fine analysis. Like these two machines, both classes of instruments have limitations; these should be recognized and, according to the circumstances of the case, one or the other is employed the more profitably.''

Standardization

In many instruments, a precalibration has been incorporated, a situation that is possible when the measured event obeys a known physical law. However, it is usually necessary to establish the correct operating point for the instrument each time it is turned on. This process is known as standardization and employs a variety of strategies that depend on the type of instrument. Often, setting the instrument to zero is all that is required. At other times, applying an artificial input (specified by the manufacturer) constitutes the standardizing process. Many photoelectric instruments are standardized by the application of a filter or reflector of known characteristics. Sometimes pressure transducers are standardized by the application of a signal that is equivalent to a known pressure. Note that this is standardization, not calibration.

SUMMARY

The successful transduction of a physiological event requires the selection of an appropriate transducible property to which a selective principle of transduction is applied. Sometimes there are many suitable transducible properties and principles of transduction for a particular physiological event. In selecting a principle of transduction, a good criterion to bear in mind is Rein's (Rein et al., 1940), which, although originally applied to an efficient blood pressure transducer, may be re-stated as "maximum efficiency in the transducer, and a minimum of electronics." In engineering terms the goal is to obtain the highest conversion efficiency, that is, electrical signal per unit of physiological event, while retaining all the criteria to achieve faithful conversion. Interchangeability, miniaturization, and economic compatibility with the use of the data are other obvious important considerations.

The field of electronics is replete with devices that will process and display electrical signals, but it has only a meager supply of transducers ideally suited to the measurement of physiological events. Particularly lacking at this time are rapidly responding transducers for chemical events. For this reason investigators in the biomedical sciences have often borrowed and adapted industrial transducers or devised their own. No full-scale program has yet been launched to provide transducers for the biomedical science investigator. It should not be concluded, however, that transduction of the widest variety of physiological events cannot be accomplished. Each physiological event has many transducible properties, and there are several suitable principles of transduction already in existence. That industry has recognized and solved a similar problem can be deduced from a statement made by the late Carl Berkley (1950): "In nearly twenty years of oscillography, the Allen B. Dumont Laboratories has yet to find a phenomenon which is incapable of being converted to a suitable electrical signal.''

REFERENCES

Albisser, A. M. 1979. Devices for the control of diabetes mellitus. *IEEE Proc.* **67**:1308–1320.

Berkley, C. 1950. A review of the design and application of transducers. *Oscillographer (A. B. Dumont Labs.)* **12**:9–22.

Bickford, R. C. 1950. Automatic electroencephalographic control of general anesthesia. *EEG Clin. Neurophysiol.* **2**:93–94.

Bickford, R. C. 1951. Use of frequency discrimination in automatic EEG control of anesthesia (servoanesthesia) *EEG Clin. Neurophysiol.* **3**:83–86.

Blackshear, P. J., R. L. Narco, and H. Buchwald. 1975. One year continuous heparinization in the dog using a totally implantable infusion pump. *Surg. Gynecol. Obstet.* **141**:176–186.

Geddes, L. A., A. G. Moore, W. A. Spencer, and H. E. Hoff. 1959. Electropneumatic control of the McKibben muscle. *Orthop. Prosthet. Appl. Journ.*, **13**:33–36.

Kadish, A. H. 1964. Automatic control of blood sugar. *Am. J. Med. Electron.* (Apr.–June):81–86.

Kraegen, E. W., D. J. Chisholm, and M. E. McNamara. 1981. Timing of insulin delivery with meals. *Horm. Metab. Res.* **13**(7):365–367.

Lewis, T. 1925. *The Mechanism and Graphic Registration of the Heart Beat.* Shaw & Sons, London.

Montgomery, L. H. 1957a. Electronic control of artificial respiration. *IRE Natl. Conv. Rec.* Part 4:90–93.

Montgomery, L. H. 1957b. Electronic control of artificial respiration. *Electronics* **30**:180.

Peckham, P. H., and J. T. Mortimer. 1977. Restoration of hand function in the quadriplegic through electrical stimulation. In *Functional Electrical Stimulation.* F. T. Hambrecht (ed.). Dekker, New York, 547 pp.

Petrofsky, J. S., and C. A. Phillips. 1983. Computer controlled walking in paralyzed individuals. *J. Neurol. Orthop. Surg.* **4**:153, 163.

Petrofsky, J. S., H. Heaton, and C. A. Phillips. 1983. Outdoor bicycle for exercise in paraplegics and quadriplegics. *J. Biomed. Eng.* **5**:292–298.

Rein, H., A. A. Hampel, and W. A. Heinemann. 1940. Photoelektrische Transmissionmanometer zur Blutdruckschreibung. *Pfluegers Arch. Gesamte Physiol.* **243**:329–335.

Schade, C. M. 1973. Automatic therapeutic control system for regulating blood pressure. *Proc. San Diego Biomed. Symp.* **12**:47–52.

Sheppard, L. C., N. T. Kouchoukos, J. W. Kirklin et al. 1980a. Computer controlled infusion of vasoactive agents—six year's experience. *Computers in Cardiology.* Williamsburg, VA.

Sheppard, L. C., N. T. Kouchoukos, J. W. Kirklin et al. 1980b. Computer controlled infusion of vasoactive agents—six year's experience. *Ann. Biomed. Eng.* **8**:431–444.

Thompson, S. P. 1910. *The Life of William Thomson, Baron Kelvin of Largs.* Macmillan, London.

Vodovnik, L. 1977. In *Functional Electrical Stimulation.* F. T. Hambrecht (ed.). Dekker, New York, 547 pp.

Vodovnik, L., M. Dimitrijevic, T. Prevoc, and M. Logar. 1966. Electronic walking aids for patients with peroneal palsy. *World Med. Electron.* **4**(2):58–61.

2

Resistive Transducers

INTRODUCTION

The variation of resistance has been used extensively to convert temperature and mechanical displacement to electrical signals. The resistance of a conductor, whether solid, liquid, or gas, is dependent on the material, the geometric configuration, and the temperature. Gaseous cells are used for the detection of radiant energy. Most of the transducers that operate on the resistance principle employ solids or liquids; solid conductors, however, are more common.

THERMORESISTORS

Because the resistivity of most metals exhibits a considerable degree of temperature dependence, it is relatively easy to construct a temperature transducer. A resistor designed for such purposes is called a resistance thermometer. Although almost any metallic conductor can be used, choice of the material is based on either the linearity or the sensitivity of its resistance–temperature characteristic. The variation in resistance of most metals is approximately linear over a moderate temperature range near room temperature and is given by the relationship

$$R_t = R_0 \big[1 + \alpha_0 (T_t - T_0) \big],$$

where R_t = resistance at temperature T_t (°C),
R_0 = resistance at temperature T_0 (°C), and
α_0 = temperature coefficient of resistivity at T_0.

Table 1 lists the resistivities and temperature coefficients for some of the commonly encountered metals. From these data it can be seen that most metals exhibit an increase in resistance with rising temperature (positive temperature coefficient); typical values lie in the range of a 0.3–0.5% change in resistance per degree Celsius temperature change. Platinum has a temperature coefficient of 0.37% per degree Celsius and is frequently used because of its wide linear resistance–temperature relationship.

Resistance thermometers are usually low in resistance, varying from a few ohms

TABLE 1   Resistivities and Temperature Coefficients[a]

Material	Resistivity ($\mu\Omega$-cm)	Temperature Coefficient α $[\Omega/(\Omega)(^\circ C)]$
Copper (annealed)	1.724	0.0039
Copper (hard drawn)	1.77	0.0038
Aluminum (commercial)	2.828	0.0036
Silver	1.629 (18°C)	0.0038
Platinum	10	0.00377
Nichrome	100	0.0004
Iron	10	0.005
Mercury	98.5 (50°C)	0.00089
Carbon	3,500 (0°C)	−0.0005
Silicon	85,000 (20°C)	0.005–0.007

[a]At 20°C.

Source: Handbook of Chemistry and Physics, 43rd ed. Chemical Rubber Publishing Co., Cleveland, Ohio, 1962.

to a few hundred ohms. Because of their low thermal sensitivity, it is necessary to use a Wheatstone bridge (Fig. 1a) with a sensitive indicator to show the temperature of the thermal element (R_D). The bridge can be operated from either direct or alternating current.

To minimize errors caused by changes in resistance of the wires connecting the resistance thermometer to the bridge, it is necessary to employ compensating leads. The method of obtaining temperature compensation is shown in Fig. 1b. Initially R_D and R_C are made equal at the reference temperature. When R_D is then used to measure an unknown temperature and the temperature of the wires connecting R_D to the bridge changes, an equal amount of resistance is added to R_C and R_D, thereby

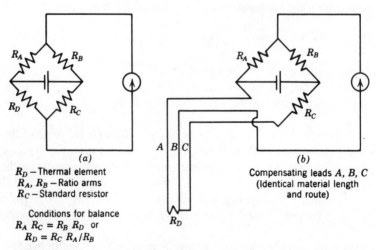

R_D – Thermal element
R_A, R_B – Ratio arms
R_C – Standard resistor

Conditions for balance
$R_A\ R_C = R_B\ R_D$ or
$R_D = R_C\ R_A/R_B$

Compensating leads *A, B, C*
(Identical material length
and route)

Figure 1   Circuits for (a) Wheatstone bridge and (b) compensated bridge.

minimizing errors caused by thermal gradients that exist along the wires. When this technique is employed, a temperature can be measured with an accuracy of a few hundredths of a degree Celsius. Miniature resistance elements that have a small thermal capacity and a short response time are available. Once calibrated, such detectors are remarkably stable.

Several precautions must be taken when using a resistance thermometer. If it is immersed in electrolytes, electrical shunting and fluid absorption must be prevented. Also, if the resistance of the thermal element is affected by magnetic fields (as is the case with some materials), its use in such environments may lead to error in temperature measurement. These effects are described in detail in this chapter. The most important precaution to be observed is to avoid heating the resistance thermometer by the current employed to measure its resistance.

THERMISTOR

Because of its high temperature coefficient, the thermistor is widely used to measure temperature. It is a hard ceramic-like device composed of a compressed and sintered mixture of metallic oxides of manganese, nickel, cobalt, copper, magnesium, titanium, and other metals. Molded into beads, rods, disks, washers, and many other forms, thermistors exhibit temperature coefficients many times larger than those of pure metals. Furthermore, the coefficient is negative; that is, with increasing temperature, the resistance of a thermistor element decreases considerably. The temperature coefficient for most thermistors approximates a 4–6% change in resistance per degree Celsius change in temperature. Figure 2 compares the variation for copper with that for a typical thermistor. The resistance–temperature relationship of the thermistor is exponential; the usual form of the relationship is given by the equation (Victory Engineering Corp., 1955)

$$R_t = R_{t_0} e^{\beta(1/T - 1/T_0)},$$

where R_t = temperature at T K,
$\quad R_{t_0}$ = temperature at T_0 K,
$\quad \beta$ = temperature coefficient (typical values 3000–4000), and
$\quad e$ = 2.71828.

Most of the thermistors used in biomedical studies are very small, thus minimizing the thermal mass and reducing the response time correspondingly. Typical resistance ranges extend from a few hundred ohms to approximately a megohm. As with the resistance thermometer, great care must be exercised to limit the current through the thermal element to reduce errors resulting from self-heating. In many of the standard units, if the power dissipation is kept to the milliwatt level, measurement of a temperature difference of 0.01 °C or smaller is easily possible. Because of the large temperature coefficient, compensating leads are not required with thermistors when making routine temperature measurements.

A survey of the characteristics of many typical thermistors was presented by

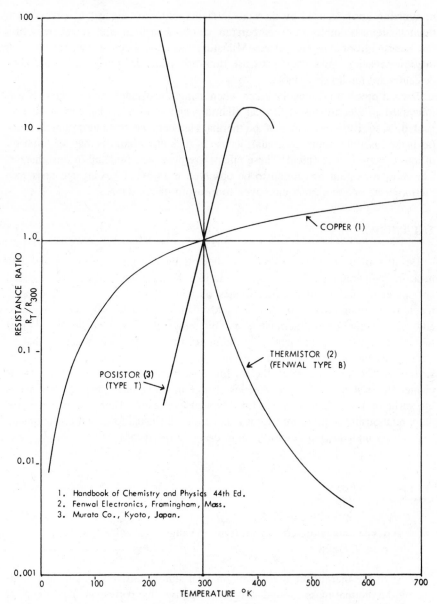

Figure 2   Resistance temperature characteristics of copper, a typical thermistor, and a posistor.

Van Dover and Bechtold (1960). In their comprehensive article they tabulated resistance range, maximum wattage dissipation, operating temperature, time constant, temperature coefficient, and dimensions of a variety of configurations.

The attractiveness of the high temperature coefficient is in part offset by the nonlinear nature of the resistance change, which becomes noticeable when large temperature changes are encountered. If a linear temperature scale is desired, it is necessary to employ linearizing techniques. One of the easiest methods for obtaining a linear scale is to connect a resistor of the appropriate value in parallel with the thermistor. A review of this technique was presented by Cornwall (1965).

One manufacturer (Yellow Springs Instrument Co., Yellow Springs, Ohio) has devised a method of overcoming the nonlinear characteristics of thermistors by developing temperature sensors that contain pairs of thermistors. With these sensors employed in the circuits shown in Fig. 3, a linear voltage–temperature or resistance–temperature characteristic can be obtained over a range of temperature change of about 100°C. With these Thermolinear® sensors the maximum departure from linearity is less than 0.2°C. Linearization can also be achieved by using the thermistor as part of the feedback circuit in an operational amplifier.

Figure 4 illustrates various thermistor configurations provided by one manufacturer (Yellow Springs Instrument Co.). In Fig. 4, (a) illustrates a catheter-tip type for rectal or esophageal use, (b) is used for air-temperature measurement, (c) is a hypodermic unit, (d) is a flexible catheter unit, (e) is for measuring surface temperature, and (f) is Pyrex-glass-covered for use in corrosive environments.

Another type of thermistor is the posistor (Murata Manufacturing Co., Kyoto, Japan). Made from barium titanate ceramic, these devices have remarkably high positive thermoresistive coefficients in the temperature range of −50 to +100°C. In one model the resistance at room temperature is multiplied tenfold by an increase of 60°C in temperature. The characteristics of the type T posistor are given in Fig. 2.

Biomedical Applications

Resistance thermometers made of pure metals and thermistors have a variety of applications in biomedical studies. Quite apart from their obvious use as electrical transducers for measuring the temperature of the skin and of many regions inside the body, they see other service. For example, because the temperature of expired

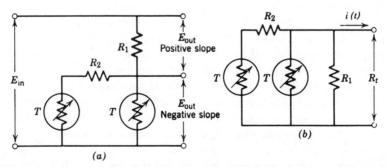

Figure 3 Circuits for obtaining linear temperature characteristics with thermolinear thermistors: (a) linear voltage versus temperature; (b) linear resistance versus temperature. (Courtesy of Yellow Springs Instrument Co., Yellow Springs, Ohio.)

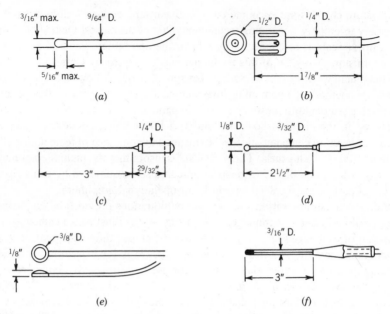

Figure 4 Thermistor probes. (*a*) Catheter type, (*b*) air-flow, (*c*) hypodermic, (*d*) semi-flexible catheter, (*e*) surface, and (*f*) Pyrex-glass-covered. (Courtesy of Yellow Springs Instrument Co., Yellow Springs, Ohio.)

air is higher than that of inspired air, a temperature sensor (usually a hermetically sealed thermistor) placed in the airway will provide a signal that allows monitoring of respiratory frequency. Simons (1962) used this technique to record the respiration of aircraft pilots. Occasionally, heated thermistors are employed as hot-wire anemometers to measure flow velocity. Heated thermistors placed in the respiratory airstream to detect respiration give a biphasic signal for a single breath, being cooled by both inspiration and expiration.

Ledig and Lyman (1927) used platinum resistance thermometers to transduce carbon dioxide and oxygen to electrical signals by measuring the thermal conductivities of these gases. By means of the same principle, Lamson and Robbins (1928) measured the amount of carbon tetrachloride in respiratory air when a small amount of this substance was injected into the lumen of the gut.

There have been several applications of the thermoresistor that demonstrate the short response time attainable. Hill (1920–1921a,b) showed that when an 11-μm heated filament was laid across the lumen of a tube connected to a conical receiver placed over a pulsating vessel, the rapid pulsations of the airstream modulated the temperature of the wire and hence its electrical resistance. The response time was short enough to show the notched transient (dicrotic wave) in the pulse curve. This pulse detector was used by Bramwell et al. (1923) in pulse-wave velocity studies. The principle was improved upon by Tucker and Paris (1921) to construct a hot-wire microphone having a resonant frequency of 200 Hz. Anrep et al. (1927) used a hot wire to show the changes in coronary blood flow during the cardiac cycle.

Blood collected in a reservoir displaced air, which passed over and cooled a heated thermal element. A somewhat different blood flow velocity transducer was described by Katsura et al. (1959); it used two thermistors, one mounted at the tip of a catheter and the other farther up the catheter. One thermistor detected the temperature of the blood, whereas the other was maintained slightly above the blood temperature. A change in flow cooled the hotter thermistor, and more current was sent through it to restore its temperature. A record of the increase in current required to maintain the temperature difference was related to blood flow. An improved isothermal blood flowmeter was described by Mellander and Rushmer (1960). The improvement consisted of a spring arrangement that held the probe in the center of the vessel.

A thermistor mounted a few centimeters from the end of a balloon-tipped (Swan–Ganz) catheter is routinely used to determine blood flow in the pulmonary artery. The technique, which is illustrated in Fig. 5, and employs injection of chilled dextrose (5%) in water (D5W) or saline into the right atrium and detection of the thermal dilution (Fig. 6) in the pulmonary artery. The inflatable balloon at the catheter tip facilitates floating the catheter tip into the pulmonary artery. When in situ, the balloon is deflated.

Right-heart output is calculated from the volume V_i and temperature T_i of the indicator, the temperature of the blood (T_b), and the area A of the dilution curve. The right-heart (cardiac) output (CO) is

$$\text{CO} = \frac{60V_i(T_b - T_i)K}{A} \quad (\text{mL}/\text{min}),$$

where V_i = the volume of indicator injected (mL),
$\quad T_i$ = the temperature of the indicator (°C),
$\quad T_b$ = the temperature of the blood (°C),

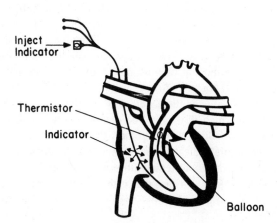

Figure 5 Method of injecting the thermal indicator into the right atrium and detecting the change in blood temperature over a period of time (thermal dilution curve) in the pulmonary artery.

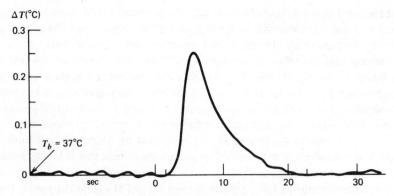

Figure 6   The thermal indicator–dilution curve.

A = the area of the dilution curve (°C-sec), and
K = a factor that depends on the ratio of the products of the specific
heat and density of the indicator and blood and the heat-loss factor
(F) through the catheter wall.

In general, $60K = 53.5$, and the dilution curve equation becomes (Geddes, 1984)

$$CO = \frac{53.5 V_i (T_b - T_i)}{A}.$$

In the curve shown in Fig. 6, the area A is 1.59 °C-sec, $T_b = 37$°C, $T_i = 0$°C, and $V_i = 5$ mL; therefore the cardiac output is 6225 mL/min.

The principle underlying the thermal dilution method was first validated by Fegler (1954). It was the development of the balloon-tipped catheter by Swan and Ganz (1970) that made the method practical for clinical use. Although soundly based on theory, the method encounters some difficulty when put into practice. Heating of the indicator by heat flow through the catheter wall is equivalent to a loss of indicator and consequent overestimation of flow. The incorporation of a constant corrects (in part) for this effect.

Taylor et al. (1982) evaluated the accuracy of the thermal dilution method using a circulatory model in which flow could be determined accurately. Using a commercially available thermodilution instrument, they compared the flow with both iced and room-temperature indicators and found that the error with iced indicator was ±16.6%; that with the room-temperature indicator was ±12.4%.

Stetz et al. (1982) pointed out that it is often necessary to obtain five thermodilution measurements and compute flow from the average of the three values that are in closest agreement.

Another problem encountered in practice is a distorted dilution curve, which occurs when the thermistor comes into contact with the vessel wall. Strategies are being developed to keep the thermistor in the axial stream.

The accuracy of the thermal dilution method in a clinical setting was investigated by Weissel et al. (1975), who found that the thermal dilution method provided values in good agreement with those obtained using dye dilution.

Thermistors are ideal for measuring tissue perfusion (milliliters per minute) of blood flow per gram of tissue). The technique involves heating a tissue bed to raise its temperature slightly. When the heating is terminated, the temperature falls exponentially. The rate of temperature decrease is proportional to local blood flow. The tissue perfusion (milliliters per minute per gram of tissue) is approximately equal to the tissue density P (grams per milliliter) divided by the thermal time constant τ (in minutes), multiplied by the ratio of the specific heats of the tissue and blood, if heat loss due to conduction is ignored (Voorhees and Babbs, 1981). Figure 7 illustrates the principle. The theory and assumptions underlying this thermal clearance method were presented by Perl (1962), Bowman et al. (1975), and Valvano et al. (1984).

The methods used to heat tissue range from inserting a tiny heating element probe into the tissue to the use of conductive electrodes to carry high-frequency current into the tissue as well as the use of capacitive and inductive diathermy or microwave energy. The induced tissue temperature rise is kept small to avoid creating heat-induced vasodilation, which would increase blood flow.

A thermal clearance probe for human muscle was described by Hensel and Ruef (1954). A single resistance-element-heated probe, 0.3 mm in diameter, was described by Chen and Holmes (1980). The element first heated the tissue locally; then the heating current was turned off and the resistance (i.e., temperature) of the probe was recorded as blood flow carried the heat away. The time constant of the exponential temperature-decay curve allowed estimation of the tissue perfusion.

Valvano et al. (1984) developed the thermal-probe method further to enable measurement of tissue properties and perfusion. After the tiny bead thermistor was

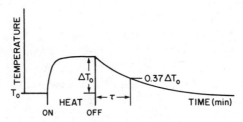

Figure 7   The thermal clearance method for determining tissue perfusion. Heat is applied to a vascular bed; then the heating is turned off. The tissue perfusion w is proportional to the reciprocal of the thermal time constant τ,

$$w = \frac{P}{\tau} \left(\frac{C_t}{C_b} \right)$$

where w = tissue perfusion [mL/(min) (g)],
P = tissue density (g/mL),
τ = thermal washout time constant (min), and
C_t and C_b = specific heats of tissue and blood, respectively.

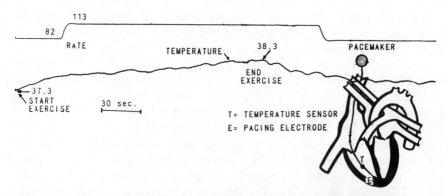

Figure 8 Pacing rate and right-ventricular blood temperature in a dog before, during, and after exercise. Note the step increase in pacing rate initiated by the increase in right-ventricular blood temperature about 40 sec after the onset of exercise.

inserted into the tissue, it was used to measure temperature. Then servo-controlled power was applied to raise the temperature a constant, but small, amount for about 30 sec. From the power–time relationship and the rate of temperature decrease, tissue properties and perfusion were calculated.

A promising skin-surface, three-thermistor, tissue-perfusion transducer was described by Valvano and Patel (1983). This device, which measured 5 mm in diameter, was fluid-coupled to the skin surface and operated under servo control for temperature elevation. The perfusion values so obtained were well within expected values.

A thermistor mounted on a cardiac pacing catheter in the right ventricle was used by Jolgren et al. (1983, 1984) to sense venous blood temperature, which increases with exercise. The increase in temperature causes a ventricular pacemaker to increase its pacing rate, thereby increasing the patient's tolerance to exercise. Figure 8 illustrates right-ventricular blood temperature and cardiac pacing rate in a dog before, during, and after exercise on a treadmill. Some seconds after the onset of exercise, the right ventricular (venous) blood temperature increased, and in about 40 sec the pacing rate switched from its resting rate of 82 B/min to 113 B/min, the exercise rate. Following cessation of exercise, the venous blood temperature started to fall, and the pacemaker reverted to its resting pacing rate of 82 B/min.

METALLIC STRAIN GAUGES

A popular use of the resistance change principle is in the detection of a small mechanical displacement from which the force producing the displacement can be determined directly. Tomlinson (1876–1877) found that when conducting wires were stretched, the length increased and the diameter decreased, and these dimensional changes were effective in increasing the resistance. The opposite situation obtains when conductors are compressed. Resistance elements constructed from specially prepared alloys that change their resistance more than an amount attributable to elongation or alteration in cross-sectional area are called strain gauges. Although virtually any metallic conductor can be used as a strain gauge, highly desirable characteristics for the material are (a) a high resistance–elongation coefficient, (b) a low value of resistance change and dimension change per unit change in temperature, and (c) a high sensitivity to strain in the direction measured and a low sensitivity to perpendicular strain.

Two types of strain gauges are in popular use: bonded and unbonded. In the bonded gauge (Fig. 9) the resistance element is cemented to a backing approximately the size of a postage stamp. The backing material is then cemented to the structure to be deformed. Via the cement bonding, the resistive element becomes an integral part of the structure. The methods of attaching strain gauges are described in Bulletin 4311A. Baldwin-Lima-Hamilton Corp., Waltham Massachusetts. The bonded gauge was patented by Simmonds (1942). In the unbonded strain gauge, the resistance wire is stretched between supporting members. With both types, the deformation to be measured is coupled to the strain gauge element, altering the length and cross-sectional area of the wire.

Strain gauges are usually made of wire approximately 0.001 in. in diameter. The term customarily employed to denote the change in resistance of the strain

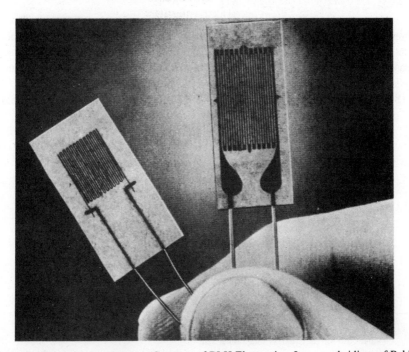

Figure 9   Bonded strain gauges. (Courtesy of BLH Electronics, Inc., a subsidiary of Baldwin-Lima-Hamilton Corporation, Waltham, Massachusetts.)

gauge material when it is stretched is the gauge factor G, defined as the fractional change in resistance divided by the fractional change in length; that is,

$$G = \frac{\Delta R/R}{\Delta L/L},$$

where R and L are the resistance and the length, respectively. Although this ratio was discussed by Tomlinson, the term gauge factor is of more recent origin.

The gauge factors of various materials appear in Table 2. These data indicate that the gauge factor of most metals is approximately 2.0, whereas that of silicon is 60 times larger. For silicon the gauge factor depends on the method of preparation and can be higher or lower than 120, and the slightly higher temperature coefficient often makes it difficult to take advantage of the high gauge factor if extremes in environmental temperature are to be encountered. In addition to the change in resistivity, Sanchez (1961) reported a slight decrease in gauge factor with increasing temperature for silicon.

In physiologic language, bonded and unbonded strain gauges are isometric devices permitting the measurement of only small displacements. The elongation permissible depends on the material and must satisfy the relationship

$$\frac{\Delta L}{L} = \frac{f}{E},$$

where f is the tensile strength of the material and E is Young's modulus. Table 3 lists typical values for Young's modulus and the tensile strengths for various materials. If large displacements are to be measured, their amplitudes must be reduced by suitable mechanical transformation.

Strain gauge elements are small and stiff; these characteristics together yield a

TABLE 2   Characteristics of Strain Gauge Materials

Material	Gauge Factor G	Temperature Coefficient[a] $[\Omega/(\Omega)(°C)]$	
Advance	2.1	0.00002	(25°C)
Constantan	2.0	0.000002	(25°C)
Isoelastic	3.5	0.00047	
Manganin	0.47	0.0000	(25°C)
Monel	1.9	0.002	
Nichrome	2.5	0.0004	
Nickel	−20 to 12.1	0.006	
Phosphor bronze	1.9	0.003	
Platinum	6.0	0.003	
Silicon	120	0.005–0.007	(25°C)

[a]Values are for 20°C unless stated otherwise.

Source: LeGette (1958), Mason and Thurston (1957), Smith (1954), and Sanchez (1961); see also Harris and Crede (1961).

TABLE 3   Mechanical Characteristics of Strain Gauge Materials

Material	Ultimate Tensile Strength f [psi $\times 10^3$]	Young's Modulus E (psi $\times 10^6$)	Information Source
Constantan	60–125	24	International Nickel Co.
Isoelastic	85–155	26	International Nickel Co.
"R" Monel	85–100	26	International Nickel Co.
Nichrome	100–200	27	Driver Harris Co.
Nickel	60–135	30	Wilbur B. Driver Co.
Phosphor bronze	130	16	International Nickel Co.
Platinum	50–100	22	Wilbur B. Driver Co.
Silicon (P)	90	27	Kulite Semiconductor Prods.
479 (Pt-Rh)	200–300	34	Sigmund Cohn

rapid response time. In practice, the speed of response is more often determined by the device to which the strain gauge is affixed. The resistance of strain gauges is relatively low, ranging from about 100 to 5000 Ω. The resistance change is small with extension. By combining the expressions for length and gauge factor we can express the change in resistance as

$$\frac{\Delta R}{R} = \frac{Gf}{E}.$$

The values for Young's modulus of elasticity E and the safe tensile stress f given in Table 3 can be used to calculate the maximum elongations and resistance change expected. In practice, however, the change in resistance produced by the maximum safe elongations is usually less than 1%.

Because temperature errors may be encountered, the use of a single strain gauge element is uncommon. To reduce temperature errors, pairs of strain gauges are usually employed in a bridge circuit, with strains in opposite directions applied to adjacent arms of the bridge, as in Fig. 10a. When strain gauges are employed in double pairs, strain in the same direction is applied to diagonal arms of the bridge, as in Fig. 10a,b. If a direct voltage is employed to energize the bridge, and an amplifier with an input resistance R_g is used (Fig. 10a), and the change in resistance ΔR is small with respect to R, where

$$R = R_A = R_B = R_C = R_D,$$

then the current through R_g for an applied strain is given by

$$I_g = \frac{\Delta R}{R}\left(\frac{E}{R + R_g}\right).$$

It is customary to use an amplifier with a high input impedance to enlarge the

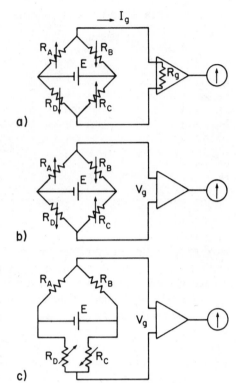

Figure 10 (*a*) A four-active-element strain gauge transducer that delivers current I_g to the input resistance R_g of an amplifier. (*b*) A four-active-element strain gauge transducer that delivers a voltage V_g to the input of an amplifier with a high input impedance. (*c*) A two-active-element strain gauge transducer that provides a voltage V_g to an amplifier with a high input impedance.

strain-induced voltage V_g appearing across the bridge. As shown in Fig. 10*b*, the voltage V_g presented to the amplifier is

$$V_g = \frac{E \, \Delta R}{R} .$$

If only two of the strain gauges are active, as shown in Fig. 10*c*, the voltage V_g presented to the amplifier is

$$V_g = \frac{E}{2}\left(\frac{\Delta R}{R}\right).$$

Both two- and four-active-element strain gauge bridges are used. The two-active-element strain gauge unit is used in catheter-tip pressure transducers. Because both active gauges are in the tip of the catheter, a change in both R_C and R_D due to temperature will not unbalance the bridge.

Biomedical Applications

One of the early biomedical applications of the strain gauge appears to have been due to Grundfest and Hay (1945), who mounted a gauge on a stiff lever to create a nearly isometric myograph. Strain gauge elements were used by Lambert and Wood (1947) to construct a transducer in which the motion of a stiff diaphragm exposed to blood pressure was detected to obtain transduction of this physiological event. Many commercially available blood pressure transducers operate on this principle.

Physiologists have long been concerned with the force of contraction of cardiac muscle. To measure this parameter of cardiac function on an excised papillary muscle, Garb (1951) developed and employed a strain gauge resistance myograph. Boniface et al. (1953) devised an ingenious strain gauge arch (Fig. 11*a*), which, when sutured to the wall of the left or right ventricle (Fig. 11*b*), provided an in situ means of continuously recording the force developed by the cardiac fibers between the "feet" of the gauge unit. Encapsulated versions of the strain gauge arch have been permanently implanted in experimental animals to study the response of the heart to imposed workloads and to drugs. A larger transducer for measurement of the same parameter of cardiac activity was described by Cotton and Maling (1957). With this device it was possible to prestress the cardiac muscle fibers to investigate the response to what is called diastolic loading (preload), that is, the effect of an increased stretch to increase the force of contraction. This response is referred to as Starling's law of the heart.

Miniature strain gauges have been bonded directly to bone to measure the strain in the bone during walking. Careful preparation of the bone surface and special adhesives and coverings are required so that the strain gauge will function in vivo for a prolonged period. Excellent reviews of the techniques have been presented by Cochran (1972), Lanyon (1976), and Wright and Hayes (1979), the latter showing that the bone preparation does not alter the bone properties.

An interesting study in which bone strain was measured in the walking dog was carried out by Cochran (1974). He bonded a strain gauge to the radius and on either side of it he placed silver–silver chloride electrodes, as shown in Fig. 12*a*. The strain gauge was connected to a Wheatstone bridge and recorder; the electrodes were connected to an amplifier and to another channel of the recorder. A 2-cm section was removed from the ulna to increase the load on the radius. Figure 12*b* shows the type of recording obtained by Cochran. The record of potential difference between the electrodes shows the piezoelectric response of bone to loading (upper), as well as the superimposed electromyographic signal. The strain record is shown in the lower recording.

As stated previously, to record strain from bone in vivo, special preparation of the bone surface is required prior to bonding of the strain gauge. Moreover, it is necessary to waterproof the leads and strain gauge, as in the case of any implant. Finally, the leads must be dressed carefully and brought to the skin surface at a distance by way of a surgically prepared tunnel. Usually the ends of the leads are

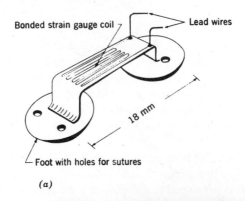

Bonded strain gauge coil

Lead wires

18 mm

Foot with holes for sutures

(a)

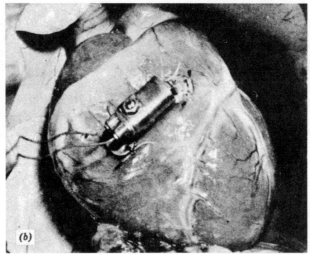

(b)

Figure 11   Strain gauge transducers for the measurement of contractile force of cardiac muscle fibers: (a) strain gauge arch; (b) encapsulated strain gauge arch attached to ventricular wall. [From J. M. Brown, *Curr. Res. Anesth. Analg.* **39**:487–488 (1960).]

left implanted subcutaneously and are retrieved surgically when the measurements are desired.

Catheter-Type Transducers

Strain gauge elements are used extensively in transducers for measuring blood pressure, Figure 13 illustrates two popular types. In these devices four strain gauge elements are arranged in a bridge circuit in which strain in the same direction is applied to opposite arms of the bridge. Because temperature changes affect resistance, all four strain gauges are affected equally and the bridge remains balanced despite variations in temperature.

Figure 13a illustrates the Statham pressure transducer. Pressure applied to the

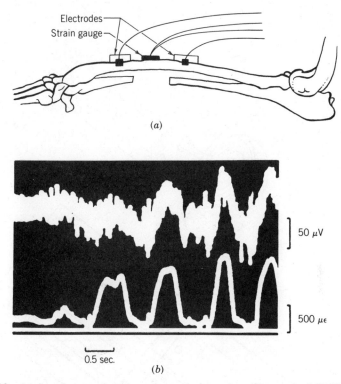

Figure 12   (a) Attachment of strain gauge and electrodes; (b) record of EMG and bone piezoelectricity (upper trace) and strain (lower trace). [Redrawn from G. Van B. Cochran, *J. Biomech.* **7**:561–565 (1974).]

corrugated diaphragm increases the tension in wires 2 and 3 and decreases it in wires 1 and 4. These tension changes produce a change in resistance that unbalances the Wheatstone bridge constituted by 1, 2, 3, and 4, thereby providing a signal proportional to pressure. A typical sensitivity is about 5 μV per volt of excitation for 1 mmHg pressure.

Figure 13b illustrates the Bell & Howell strain gauge pressure transducer. The strain gauge wires are wrapped around posts mounted on a spring member in the form of a cross. Pressure applied to the diaphragm is coupled to the center of the cross which bends, causing tension to increase in the strain gauge wires above the cross and to decrease in those below it. The strain gauge elements are arranged in a bridge circuit. The output is about 5 μV per volt of excitation per millimeter of mercury pressure.

Figure 14 illustrates a newly introduced solid-state, disposable pressure transducer (Cobe Laboratories, Denver, Colorado) consisting of a silicon diaphragm on which are deposited four strain gauge elements. The silicon diaphragm is covered with an insulating material to protect it from the fluid filling the transducer and to provide electrical insulation. The back side of the silicon diaphragm communicates

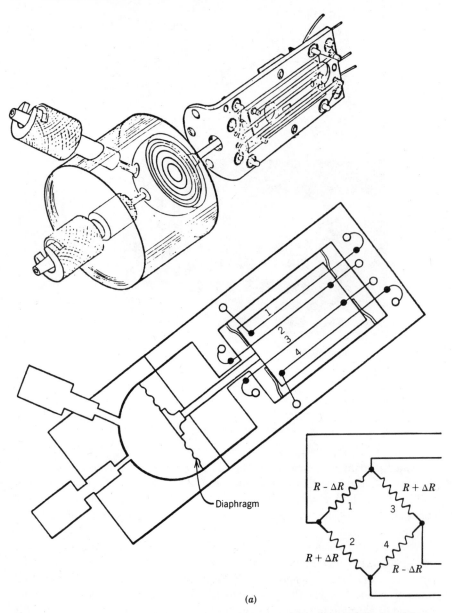

Diaphragm

$R - \Delta R$ $R + \Delta R$

1   3

2   4

$R + \Delta R$ $R - \Delta R$

(a)

Figure 13 Strain gauge pressure transducers. [(a) Courtesy of Gould (Statham) Instruments, Oxnard, California; (b) courtesy of Bell & Howell, Pasadena, California.]

with atmospheric pressure via a tube in the cable carrying the wires from the bridge to the connector. The output is typically 8 μV per volt of excitation per millimeter of mercury.

The figure of merit of a pressure transducer is its volume displacement V_d, defined as the number of cubic millimeters of fluid that must enter to produce a

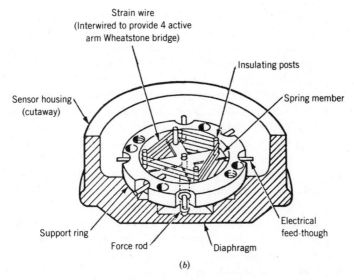

(b)

Figure 13   (*Continued*)

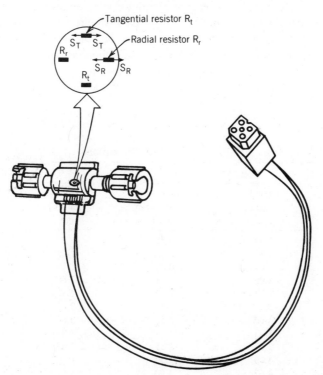

Figure 14   The Cobe Micro Switch disposable blood pressure transducer, consisting of four active piezoresistive integrated strain gauge elements on a circular silicon diaphragm (inset). Strain is applied to the radial pair and compression to the tangential pair. (Courtesy of Cobe Laboratories, Denver, Colorado, and Micro Switch Co., A Honeywell Division, Freeport, Illinois.)

pressure of 100 mmHg. Because such fluid movement into the transducer constitutes a frictional (viscous) resistance, the volume displacement along with the mass of fluid in the transducer and the moving element dictate the transducer response time. Note, however, that such transducers are connected to the pressure-measurement site by a fluid-filled catheter (Table 4 illustrates typical sizes), which also adds mass and viscous drag. These masses and the frictional forces, along with the transducer volume displacement, determine the response time and sine wave frequency response (Geddes, 1984). To obtain a high-fidelity recording of the blood pressure wave, it is highly desirable to use a transducer with a small volume displacement.

Because of the compressibility of water, which fills the transducer, it is not permissible to apply 100 mmHg of positive pressure and measure the volume of fluid entering the transducer to determine the volume displacement. To illustrate this point, the isothermal compressibility of 1 mL of water at 20°C is 0.006 mm^3 for the application of 100 mmHg. Typical transducer domes contain 0.3–1.0 mL of fluid. Therefore, the volume of fluid entering the transducer with the application of 100 mmHg positive fluid pressure represents the compressibility of the fluid and the volume displacement of the transducer.

The error produced by fluid compressibility can be eliminated by applying a negative 100 mmHg of air pressure to the back (reference side) of the elastic diaphragm, as shown in Fig. 15, and measuring the volume of fluid entering the transducer (Geddes et al., 1984). Use of this technique to measure true volume displacement requires only two simple steps. First, the pressure transducer and recording system are calibrated by the application of 100 mmHg of positive pressure

TABLE 4   Catheter Dimensions

Catheter Size	Thick-Walled Catheter		Thin-Walled Catheter	
	Outer[a] Diameter (mm)	Lumen Diameter (mm)	Outer Diameter (mm)	Lumen Diameter (mm)
3F	1.00	0.36		
4F	1.33	0.46	1.33	0.58
5F	1.67	0.66	1.67	0.86
6F	2.00	0.91	2.00	1.17
7F	2.33	1.17	2.33	1.47
8F	2.67	1.42	2.67	1.73
9F	3.00	1.63	3.00	1.98
10F	3.33	1.83	3.33	2.24
11F	3.67	2.11	3.67	2.49
12F	4.00	2.39	4.00	2.74
14F	4.67	2.90	4.67	3.25

[a]Note that the outer diameter in millimeters is the F size divided by 3.

Source: Catalog, U.S. Catheter & Instrument Co., Glens Falls, New York.

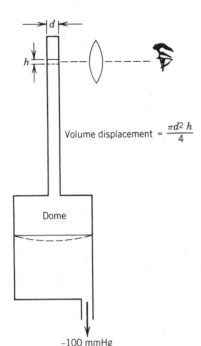

Volume displacement $= \dfrac{\pi d^2 h}{4}$

Figure 15 Method for measuring the volume displacement of a blood pressure transducer. With the application of -100 mmHg air pressure to the back of the diaphragm, the decrease in height h of the meniscus is measured and the volume displacement is $d^2 h\pi/4$. [From L. A. Geddes et al., *Med. Biol. Eng. Comput.* **22**(6):613–614 (1984).]

(air is satisfactory). The output on the pressure-indicating device is noted so that 100 mmHg can be identified later. Then the transducer is coupled to a small-bore needle (e.g., 30 gauge and clear plastic tubing, i.d. 0.28 mm). Then the transducer and catheter are carefully filled with alcohol colored with vegetable dye or any other convenient coloring agent. Great care must be taken to exclude all air bubbles. The colored meniscus in the plastic tube is transilluminated and is viewed with a calibrated microscope or an eyepiece with a graticule, so that a change in movement of the meniscus can be measured. Then an air suction pump is connected to the back (reference) side of the transducer and is adjusted until 100 mmHg pressure is indicated by the recording apparatus. The change in height h of the meniscus is measured, and the volume displacement of the transducer is calculated. A negative pressure of more than 100 mmHg can be used, and the change in height scaled to 100 mmHg.

The procedure just described was performed on several typical pressure transducers (Geddes et al., 1984). Table 5 summarizes the results.

The method just described is simple and easy to apply. While making the measurement, the volume of fluid in the dome can be determined also.

Standards are being developed by the Association for the Advancement of Medical Instrumentation for resistive strain gauge blood pressure transducers. Covered in the proposed standards are factors relative to efficacy, safety, and interchangeability. In addition to quantitative information on performance, procedures for

TABLE 5   Measured Volume Displacements

Transducer	Volume Displacement (mm^3/100 mmHg)
Statham P23Db	0.037
Statham P23ID	0.049
Statham P23-BB	0.62
Cobe disposable	0.0012

conducting the tests and for labeling are included. Although not official at this time, these proposed standards contain a wealth of useful information.

Catheter-Tip Transducers

One of the most popular high-fidelity miniature catheter-tip strain gauge transducers was described by Millar and Baker (1973) and is illustrated in Fig. 16a. Located on the side of the tip, which is 1.65 mm in diameter, is the pressure-sensitive silicone rubber diaphragm coupled to two silicon strain gauge elements

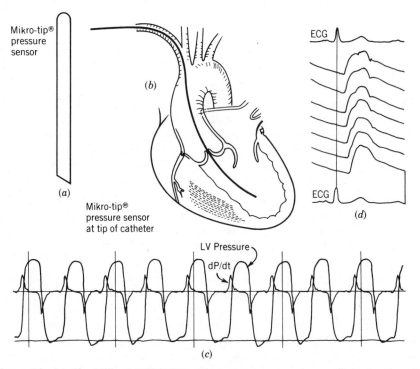

Figure 16 (a) The Millar MIKRO-TIP catheter pressure transducer, (b) its locations in the left ventricle, (c) a record of ventricular pressure and dp/dt, and (d) pressure recorded at various sites along the aorta. [Redrawn from J. P. Murgo et al., *Circulation* **62**(1):105–116 (1980) and courtesy of Millar Instruments, Houston, Texas.]

(1500 Ω each). With the application of pressure, one element is stretched and the other is compressed. The strain gauges constitute a half-bridge, the other half of which is located in the electrical connector along with a standardizing resistor that provides a signal equivalent to 100 mmHg. Freedom from drift due to temperature changes has been achieved by careful matching of the strain gauge elements for resistance and thermal coefficient. The back of the strain gauge detecting system is vented to atmospheric pressure at the connector.

The performance characteristics of the Millar MIKRO-TIP catheter transducer (Millar Instruments, Inc., Houston, Texas) are truly remarkable. For example, the typical output is 25 mV for a pressure change of 300 mmHg, either positive or negative, using 3.5 V excitation (ac or dc). The maximum excitation voltage recommended is 10 V (ac or dc). The linearity and hysteresis are within ±0.5% of any selected range from −300 to +400 mmHg. The thermal stability is equivalent to ±0.1 mmHg per degree change from 25 to 40°C. Typical overall stability is well within 1 mmHg/hr.

The dynamic response characteristics of the MIKRO-TIP transducer permit high-fidelity recording of pressure transients anywhere in the vascular system. It is particularly useful for measuring the small pressure gradients across valves and along vessels. The volume displacement is 10^{-3} mm^3/100 mmHg, and the natural resonant frequency of the pressure-sensing system is typically 35 kHz in air and 30 kHz in water, which provides a response time short enough for the detection of intravascular sounds. Electrical safety is also an important feature; the leakage current rating is less than 0.5 μA for an applied voltage of 180 V dc. Thus the insulation resistance is in excess of 360 MΩ.

The MIKRO-TIP transducer is available in a variety of configurations. Some models have a side port for withdrawal of blood or the injection of fluid at the site of pressure measurement. Models with as many as six pressure sensors and models with an electromagnetic or ultrasonic flow sensor have also been fabricated. Figure 16d illustrates typical recordings obtained simultaneously from a catheter with multiple transducers placed in the aorta. Note both the differences in waveform and the progressive delay in the arterial pulse as it travels down the aorta.

Blood Pressure Waveforms

Figure 17 illustrates a typical aortic blood pressure waveform obtained by a high-quality pressure transducer. There are three important pressures: systolic (maximum), diastolic (minimum), and mean. The difference between systolic and diastolic pressure is the pulse pressure. Mean pressure is defined as the area under one pulse wave divided by the period (base). Mean pressure is less than the average of systolic and diastolic pressure, owing to the contour of the waveform. It is often stated that mean pressure is equal to diastolic pressure plus a factor k multiplied by pulse pressure. The value for k depends on the waveform, which in turn depends on the site where the pressure is measured. For example, k for the aorta is about 0.4. For the femoral artery it is about 0.3, and for the dorsalis pedis artery it is about 0.24 (Geddes, 1984). As the pulse travels from the left ventricle to the periphery, the pulse wave becomes more peaked, as shown in Figs. 16d and 19.

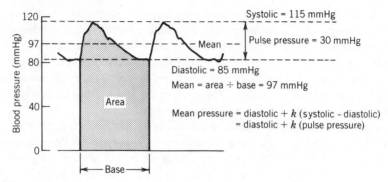

Figure 17 Diagrammatic representation and definition of systolic, diastolic, and mean pressure. Pulse pressure is the difference between systolic and diastolic pressure.

Mean pressure can be determined experimentally by reducing the bore of the catheter communicating pressure to the transducer by means of a screw clamp. Figure 18 illustrates the results of using this technique. Note that as the catheter bore is reduced, the viscous forces soon dominate, the pulse pressure becomes smaller, and the fine details of the waveform disappear. When the pulsatile oscillations were virtually abolished, mean pressure was revealed to be 120 mmHg. In this animal, systolic pressure was 182 and diastolic pressure was 105; therefore, the k value for this particular vessel is $(120 - 105)/(182 - 105) = 0.195$. Figure 19 illustrates typical pulse waves and their k values. Voelz (1981) showed that k is also dependent on pressure.

POTENTIOMETER TRANSDUCERS

Wire-wound or carbon rotary or rectilinear potentiometers can be employed as high-efficiency transducers to detect movement when the moving object can develop a moderate force. Although there are few physiological applications of this type of transducer at present, the unusually high efficiency attainable will no doubt encourage wider application. Respiration was detected by Adams (1962), who measured changes in thoracic circumference by connecting a rotary potentiometer

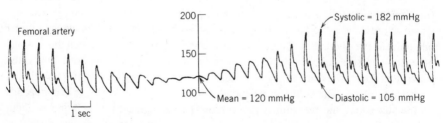

Figure 18 Mean arterial pressure recorded by gradually decreasing the diameter of the catheter leading to the transducer.

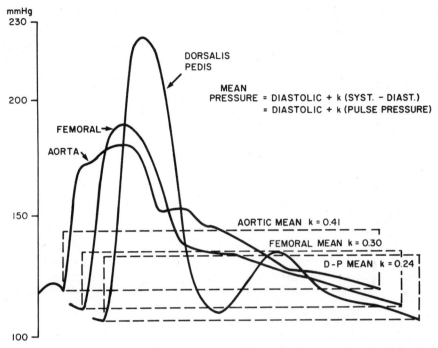

mmHg

DORSALIS
PEDIS

MEAN
PRESSURE = DIASTOLIC + k (SYST. – DIAST.)
= DIASTOLIC + k (PULSE PRESSURE)

FEMORAL

AORTA

AORTIC MEAN k = 0.41

FEMORAL MEAN k = 0.30

D-P MEAN k = 0.24

Figure 19   Aortic, femoral, and dorsalis pedis pulse waves and their *k* values.

to a chest band on a monkey. A device for recording the contraction of skeletal muscle in situ was described by Geddes et al. (1966). In this transducer (Fig. 20), a low-torque potentiometer serves as the pivot for the caliper arms, which embrace the belly of the muscle. Contraction of the muscle causes the arms to be driven apart, and their motion is measured by the potentiometer.

A miniature low-torque potentiometer transducer was used by Ackmann et al.

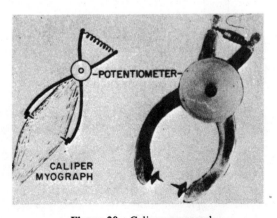

Figure 20   Caliper myograph.

(1977) to detect the tremor of Parkinson's disease. The tremor of wrist flexion and extension was detected by taping sliding rods to the dorsum of the hand and lower forearm. One rod was connected to the rotor and the other to the body of the potentiometer, which was energized by a 1.4-V mercury battery. The 0–10-degree tremor at 3–6 Hz was easily detected and recorded. The recordings were used to evaluate drug therapy.

A low-torque linear potentiometer coupled to the pulley of a spirometer (Fig. 21), described by Geddes et al. (1961), permitted recording the volume of air moved during breathing. Movement of the spirometer bell reflects the volume of each breath, which can be recorded graphically as shown in Fig. 21. When the

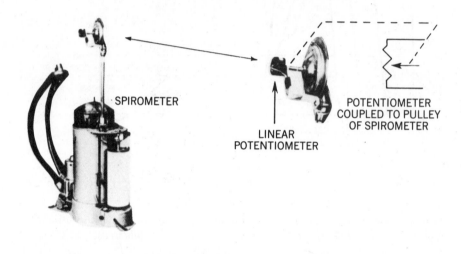

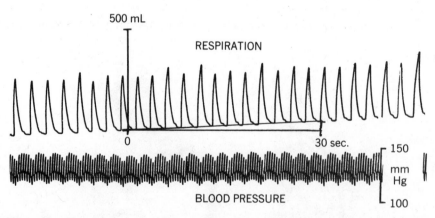

Figure 21 (Top) Method of coupling a low-torque potentiometer to permit recording respiration (and oxygen consumption) from a spirometer. (Bottom) A typical record of respiration oxygen uptake and blood pressure. During the 30 seconds shown, the oxygen uptake was 60 mL and the tidal volume was typically 250 mL.

spirometer is equipped with a carbon dioxide absorber, the baseline of the spirogram rises, indicating the oxygen consumption. The slope of the baseline is the rate of oxygen consumption.

A truly isotonic myograph for slowly contracting muscles can be constructed by passing a cord over a pulley mounted on the shaft of a low-torque potentiometer. One end of the cord is connected to the muscle, and the other to a weight. Contraction of the muscle moves the same weight through a height measured by the rotation of the pulley.

As previously stated, the unusually attractive feature of the potentiometer transducer is its high efficiency. With a large voltage applied across the potentiometer, the voltage appearing between the moving contact and one end terminal is related to the position of the moving contact. The voltage that can be applied is limited by the wattage rating of the resistance element. Potentiometers providing linear, logarithmic, sine, cosine, and other resistance changes proportional to rotation are available. Rotary units are available with 360-degree rotations, and rectilinear models can be obtained with strokes from a fraction of an inch up to almost 1 ft. With the rectilinear models a resistance–motion linearity of 1–2% is attainable. If the resistance element is a carbon film, the output is continuously related to the movement of the sliding contact. If the resistance element is wire-wound, the output versus movement is stepped; that is, the voltage changes incrementally with movement of the sliding contact as it passes from one wire to the next. With high-resistance units the number of wires is large and the increments are fine.

The force required to move the sliding contact depends on the design of the potentiometer. Between 0.2 and 0.5 oz-in. is needed to move low-torque rotary potentiometers, compared to 0.5–6 oz-in. for conventional potentiometers. The starting torque is slightly higher than the running torque.

In practical application the response time of a potentiometer transducer is difficult to describe quantitatively because it is intimately related to the mass, elasticity, and damping of the system to which the device is coupled. Nunn (1959) quoted a frequency response of up to 4 Hz for a potentiometer coupled to a Bourdon tube for pressure measurement. In the experience of the authors, potentiometric transducers can function at high efficiency for events that change at rates less than a few hertz.

MAGNETORESISTIVE TRANSDUCERS

Many substances exhibit a change in resistivity when exposed to a magnetic field. For example, the resistivity of most metals increases with increasing field strength; with ferromagnetic metals the resistivity decreases. The magnetoresistive effect is small in most metals; the resistivity of copper increases by only 0.25% when exposed to a field of 200 kilogauss (kG). When bismuth is exposed to a magnetic field, however, a considerable increase in resistivity occurs. At room temperature a field of 20 kG doubles the resistivity. If the temperature is lowered, the effect is much more pronounced. If the same field is presented to bismuth at the temperature of liquid air, the resistivity is multiplied by 250. The relationship of increase in resistivity of bismuth with increasing magnetic field strength for 0 and −50°C is plotted in Fig. 22.

The pheonomenon of resistivity change with a change in magnetic field has been employed in detectors for field strength. It was used by Hampel (1941) in a blood pressure transducer. A double resistance coil was mounted on an elastic diaphragm exposed to blood pressure; one-half of the coil entered a field while the other half moved out of the field when the diaphragm was deformed. Thus the two coils became resistors that varied in response to pressure. A record of the variation in resistance, as measured by a Wheatstone bridge and galvanometer, reproduced the blood pressure wave. A similar method was employed by Holzer (1940), who constructed a myograph in which four coils (two of copper and two of bismuth) were employed in a bridge circuit. The coils were mounted on a tube and connected so that with movement the bismuth coils were pulled out of the magnetic field. The bismuth coils constituted one diagonal pair of the bridge resistors; the copper coils, the other. The stiffness of the system and the strength of the magnetic field

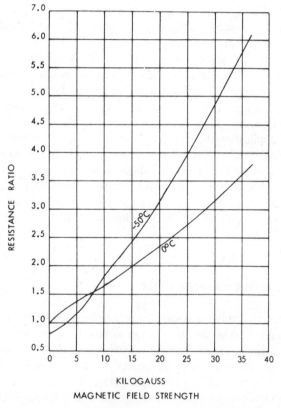

Figure 22 The effect of magnetic field intensity on the resistance of bismuth. (Redrawn from data by Graetz, *Handbuch der Elektrizität*, J. A. Barth, Leipzig, 1920.)

combined to yield a rapid response time and a high efficiency. To illustrate these characteristics, Holzer recorded the twitch of a frog gastrocnemius muscle.

The Hall Effect

The Hall effect, discovered in 1879, is an interesting phenomenon associated with a conductor that is exposed to a magnetic field. It cannot be better described than in Hall's own words: "If the current of electricity in a fixed conductor is itself attracted by a magnet, the current should be drawn to one side of the wire and therefore the resistance experienced should be increased." With this as his thesis, Hall proceeded to test the theory experimentally, using at first a thick conductor and finally a strip of gold leaf. Success rewarded his efforts, and he concluded, "It is perhaps allowable to speak of the action of the magnet as setting up in the strip of gold leaf a new electromotive force at right angles to the primary electromotive force."

To understand the nature of the Hall effect, consider a thin rectangular film of conducting material equipped with four electrodes, two at the ends (M, N) and two on the middle of the sides (P, Q). When current is led into and out of electrodes M and N, as in Fig. 23, there will be no potential E measured between the side electrodes P and Q. If a magnetic field B is caused to pass through the conducting film at right angles to the plane of the film, the moving charges will be deflected toward the top or bottom of the film, depending on the directions of the field and current. Deflection of the charge carriers causes a potential to appear across electrodes P and Q, the magnitude and polarity of which depend on the direction and intensity of the magnetic field, the current, the type of charge carrier, and the dimensions of the film. The usual form of the relationship is

$$E = KIB/t,$$

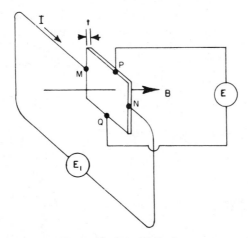

Figure 23   The Hall effect.

where E = Hall voltage,
  I = excitation current through the film (A),
  B = field strength (G), and
  t = thickness of the film (cm).

The Hall coefficient K depends on the material and temperature. It is small for most metals; the constants for bismuth, tellurium, and silicon, however, are approximately 100,000 times larger. N-Type germanium, indium antimonide, and indium arsenide Hall devices are employed to obtain high outputs (Star, 1963) and are most frequently used in Hall effect detectors for measuring ac or dc magnetic fields. The outputs available are in the range of millivolts per kilogauss for typical models with rated excitation current. Although a linear voltage–field strength relationship can be obtained, with some materials the linearity is poor when low-intensity fields are used; with other materials the reverse is true. In addition, although it would appear that with a given field B the Hall voltage can be increased by decreasing the thickness t of the film and increasing the current I, a limit is soon reached at which the current density in the film is such that excessive heat is produced and the film changes its characteristics.

The output impedance of Hall effect generators depends on the resistivity and dimensions of the film. In commercially available probe detectors for magnetic fields, it extends from a few to a few hundred ohms.

Figure 24 illustrates two typical Hall effect devices produced by one manufacturer (Bell, Inc., Columbus, Ohio). The transverse type is useful for measuring the field strength in a thin gap. The axial device finds applications in measuring the field strength inside a coil. The triaxial type contains three Hall devices mounted to be mutually perpendicular and serves for mapping magnetic fields.

Hall effect devices can be used in a variety of ways; Fig. 25 illustrates their application. In Fig. 25a(1) the Hall device occupies the null position; that is, each side is subjected to the same field intensity. Movement of either the magnets or the Hall device will produce a Hall voltage. In Fig. 25a(2) a field of varying strength exists between the magnets. The output of the Hall device is dependent on its position in this field. Thus movement along the direction of the arrow will give rise to an increase in the Hall voltage. In Figs. 25b and 25c, movement of the magnets past the Hall device produces a position-dependent voltage as shown.

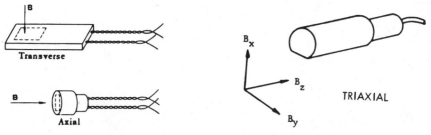

Figure 24   Typical configurations of Hall effect devices.

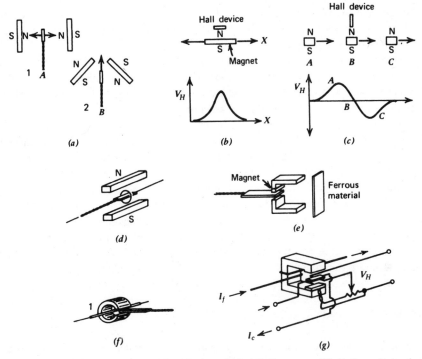

Figure 25   Applications of Hall effect devices. [(a)–(f) Courtesy of Bell, Inc., Columbus, Ohio.]

Use of the Hall device to detect rotary position is shown in Fig. 25d. Because the presence of ferromagnetic material alters the magnetic field passing through the Hall device, the assembly shown in Fig. 25e can serve as a detector for such materials. Figure 25f indicates how a Hall device can be used to measure current I by causing it to produce a magnetic field in an air gap in the magnetic circuit. The magnetic field strength is measured by the Hall effect chip as shown.

Although the technique illustrated in Fig. 25f is adequate for the measurement of direct current, difficulties are encountered when alternating current or pulsating direct current is measured. Because the Hall chip and the wires leading from it that detect the Hall voltage constitute wholly or partly a single turn in the magnetic field, a voltage is induced by the changing current that is to be measured. This transformer voltage can be demonstrated by turning off the chip excitation current and varying the current to be measured. By careful arrangement of the wires carrying the Hall voltage, this transformer voltage can often be canceled. However, a more convenient method of eliminating the undesired signal (see Fig. 25g) consists of the purposeful detection of the transformer voltage by wrapping one or two turns of wire around the core and connecting the ends to a potentiometer. The Hall voltage is then connected in series opposition with the voltage derived from the potentiometer, as in Fig. 25g. Nulling of the undesired transformer voltage is accomplished by passing alternating current I through the current winding with the Hall chip excitation current turned off and adjusting the potentiometer. Once set, this adjustment need not be altered unless the physical arrangement of the wiring is changed. After this adjustment is made, the Hall chip current is applied and the Hall effect voltage V_H accurately reflects the current I being measured, provided the rate of change of current does not exceed the rise-time limit of the Hall chip.

Figure 25g diagrams the full potential of the Hall effect device as a circuit element. In reality, two variables, current and field strength, are related in the operation of the device. The variables may be alternating current or direct current or combinations thereof. The Hall voltage is proportional to the product of the two; thus the device functions as a multiplier.

Hall effect devices have been used relatively little in biomedical studies. They have obvious application in mapping the magnetic field produced by current from externally applied electrodes in studies of electroanesthesia and ventricular defibrillation. It is expected that Hall effect devices will find use in magnetobiology studies such as those reported by Valentinuzzi (1961, 1962) and Barnothy (1964), which describe the effects of magnetic fields on living specimens.

GRANULAR STRAIN GAUGES

Another type of resistor used for transduction purposes consists of a capsule loosely packed with carbon granules. On one side of the capsule is a fixed electrode, and on the other is a movable one. When a force is applied, the granules are compacted and the resistance is reduced. Such capsules originated with the carbon-button telephone transmitter, in which the diaphragm is coupled to the moving electrode. Small movements of the diaphragm change the resistance considerably and result in a high-efficiency conversion of sound pressure to an electrical signal.

Because of its high efficiency, the carbon-granule capsule still enjoys some popularity in biomedicine for detecting changing events. Using a carbon button in contact with an artery, Waud (1924) and Turner (1928) recorded the human pulse. No amplifier was employed in either study; the carbon button served to drive a recording pen directly in the former study and a string galvanometer in the latter. Gallagher and Grimwood (1953) included it in their indirect blood-pressure measuring system to detect the pulse in the caudal artery of the rat.

A variant of the carbon-granule capsule was described by Clynes (1960). This device consisted of a distensible rubber tube filled with graphite. When it was wrapped around the chest, transduction of the respiratory movements was obtained.

Carbon-packed capsules are characterized by resistances in the hundreds of ohms and exhibit an appreciable, but inconstant, change in resistance with dimension change. High currents can be passed through them, resulting in high outputs— often sufficient to drive recorders directly. These devices, however, exhibit a poor baseline stability, and on occasion they "freeze"; that is, the granules compact and must be loosened by vibration. If a high-gain system is employed with carbon-granule capsules, the no-signal noise is quite high, a factor that caused the carbon-button microphone to be abandoned in the early days of radio broadcasting, although carbon buttons are still used in most telephones.

ELASTIC RESISTORS

By the appropriate addition of conducting material to rubber or to certain plastics, it is possible to make a resistor that increases its resistivity with strain ($\Delta L/L$), where L is the relaxed length and ΔL is the elongation. The addition of carbon to latex, which is then appropriately cured, produces a rubber with conducting properties that allows construction of elastic strain gauges. Badamo (1964) reported that one product, S-2086 electrically conducting Silastic, loaded with carbon black (Dow Corning Center for Aid to Medical Research, Midland, Michigan) has been made to have a volume resistivity ranging from 8 to 60 Ω-cm. Another manufacturer (Minor Rubber Co., Inc., Bloomfield, New Jersey) provides a standard product (UK 3032) with a resistivity of 7 Ω-cm. By varying the mixture, resistivities from 7 to 10^6 Ω-cm have been obtained. The elongation factor $(L + \Delta L)/L$ for UK 3032 is given as 2.1. The S-2086 conducting Silastic can be elongated by factors ranging from 1.4 to 2.5; the resistance of this material increases almost as an exponential function of elongation. The manufacturer reports that a 25% elongation more than triples the relaxed resistance. Figure 26 illustrates the resistance–elongation characteristic of a piece of this material measured by one of the authors. It shows that linearity is attainable only over a limited range of extension (10–20%). Although larger extensions can be tolerated by some conducting elastomers, with others elongations greater than 25–30% result in appreciable resistance hysteresis.

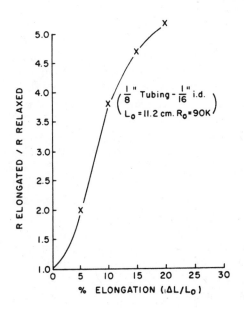

Figure 26 Elastic resistor—resistance versus elongation.

Biomedical Applications

Conducting rubber strain gauges have been used infrequently to detect force or movement; however, an application by Fromm (1967) is of more than passing interest. He fabricated an elastic strain gauge for detecting and telemetering uterine contractions in the unrestrained rabbit by using a $\frac{1}{16}$-in. diameter carbon-loaded Silastic cylinder around which he wrapped two electrodes of 35-gauge wire; the electrodes were separated by 1 mm. The elastic strain gauge was sealed in plastic tubing for waterproofing and implanted into a rabbit. This system was used to record uterine contractions for 6 weeks.

The elastic strain gauge used by Fromm exhibited a resistance of 200 Ω when relaxed. With stretch, the resistance increased by 1 Ω for 1 g of applied force, the force limit for linearity.

The attractive characteristics of elastic resistors recommended their use for the transduction of events associated with an appreciable dimension change. In practical applications, however, it is frequently difficult to establish a stable electrical contact with the material. Conducting paints, clamps, and nuts and bolts have all been employed. One of the authors has had success in making contact with conducting tubing by forcing the ends over short metal rods or tubes that served as electrodes.

ELECTROLYTIC STRAIN GAUGES

Elastic strain gauges that employ liquid conductors are used to a limited extent in biomedical studies. As far back as the turn of the century, Grunbaum (1898) described the first of such devices, an aqueous electrolytic pressure capsule 3.5 mm in diameter and 12.5 mm long mounted on the end of a catheter. On the side of the capsule was a thin rubber window carrying an electrode. The other electrode was mounted on the inside wall of the capsule, which was filled with zinc chloride. Pressure applied to the distensible window decreased the interelectrode distance, thereby reducing the resistance between the electrodes. This device was certainly one of the first catheter-tip pressure transducers and must have produced blood pressure records of high fidelity for that time. However, no such records produced by this instrument have been found.

For some reason the electrolytic strain gauge fell into disuse for many years, being revived by Müller (1942) and Dalla-Torre (1943) to record human digital volume pulses. Their strain gauges consisted of rubber tubing a fraction of a millimeter in diameter filled with an electrolyte. The ends of the tubing were plugged by the electrodes. When such tubes are stretched, the length increases and the diameter decreases, thereby raising the resistance appreciably.

Aqueous electrolyte strain gauges are lightweight, easy to make, and inexpensive. They are medium to high in resistance. Müller's units were 0.2 mm in diameter and 5–6 cm long. When filled with diluted Electroargol, the strain gauge had a resistance of 1 MΩ. After an initial elongation, the resistance increased nearly linearly with extension over a fairly wide range. Figure 27 presents the equation

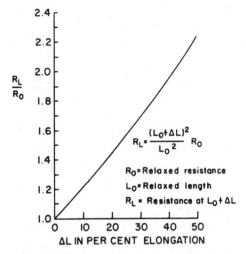

Figure 27 Electrolytic resistor—resistance versus elongation.

for the resistance increase and the degree of linearity that can be expected. Elongations to 50% of the relaxed length are often used to permit measurement of the large changes in circumference or length experienced by many organs and members. Although a large signal per unit of extension can be obtained, this advantage is partly offset by the errors introduced by temperature changes. The temperature coefficient for many aqueous electrolytes is about $-2\%/°C$. Hence temperature compensation is necessary.

In an interesting electrolytic resistor strain gauge described by Waggoner (1965), the electrolyte was an electrode paste contained in a rubber tube. Waggoner reported that the resistance of such gauges depends on the dimensions, and in practice, with tubing 0.2–3 mm in diameter, resistances varying between 1 and 400 kΩ were observed. The change in resistance varied as L^2/V, where L is the length and V the volume of the gauge. A small negative resistance–temperature coefficient was noted. Waggoner reported successful use of these strain gauges for recording respiration, cardiac contraction, kidney volume, and thumb pulse.

Aqueous electrolytic strain gauges usually have a relatively short life because electrolytic decomposition of the electrodes proceeds even when the devices are not in use. When direct current is passed through the element, the lifetime is further reduced. For maximum life, alternating current should be employed for excitation.

MERCURY STRAIN GAUGES

Whitney (1949) described strain gauges using small-bore rubber tubing filled with mercury. Like the aqueous electrolytic types, these gauges permit the measurement of small or large changes in elongation. They are lightweight, easy to construct, inexpensive, and available commercially (Parks Electronics Laboratory, Beaverton, Oregon).

Biomedical Applications

Mercury (Whitney) strain gauges are widely used in biomedical studies; for example, Whitney (1949, 1953, 1954) and Greenfield et al. (1963) employed them to measure the volume changes in body segments as blood entered and left the region encircled by the gauge. Rushmer (1955a,b, 1965) selected similar gauges to measure the changes in circumference of the rapidly beating canine left ventricle and aorta. Lawton and Collins (1959) used the mercury strain gauge to measure the pulsatile changes in aortic circumference. Maulsby and Hoff (1962) sutured similar strain gauges to the right ventricles of dogs and continuously measured the dimension changes that reflected the volume changes in that cardiac chamber. Shapiro et al. (1964) encircled the chests of human subjects with mercury-in-rubber gauges to detect the changes in thoracic circumference that accompany respiration.

The mercury-in-rubber (Whitney) strain gauge has been used extensively to measure limb blood flow by recording the increase in limb circumference when the venous outflow is suddenly arrested. Because arterial pressure is typically 120/80 mmHg and venous pressure is only a few millimeters of mercury, the sudden inflation of a cuff—say, to 50 mmHg—will arrest venous outflow while arterial inflow continues. Therefore there is a gradual increase in the circumference of the limb beyond the cuff. The increase in circumference is detected by a calibrated Whitney strain gauge.

The rate of change of volume is calculated from the initial increase in circumference following venous occlusion. Let the initial member diameter be d_0 and the increased diameter be d_1; therefore the increase in volume (ΔV) is given by

$$\Delta V = \frac{\pi}{4} (d_1^2 - d_0^2) L,$$

where L is the length of the member embraced by the strain gauge. However, it is the circumference C that is measured; therefore if C_0 is the initial circumference and C_1 is the increased circumference, the increase in volume (ΔV) is

$$\Delta V = \frac{\pi}{4} \left[\left(\frac{C_1}{\pi} \right)^2 - \left(\frac{C_0}{\pi} \right)^2 \right] L$$

$$= \frac{L}{4\pi} (C_1^2 - C_0^2).$$

Let $C_1 = C_0 + \Delta C$, where ΔC is the increase in circumference as the member swells. Then

$$\Delta V = \left[(C_0 + \Delta C)^2 - C_0^2 \right] \frac{L}{4\pi}$$

$$= \frac{L}{4\pi} (2C_0 \Delta C + \Delta C^2).$$

If ΔC^2 is small with respect to $2C_0 \Delta C$, then the volume change is

$$\Delta V = \frac{L C_0 \Delta C}{2\pi},$$

where L is the length of the member encompassed by the strain gauge, C_0 is the original circumference, and ΔC is the increase in circumference that results from venous occlusion.

Figure 28*a* illustrates an eight-strand mercury-in-rubber strain gauge wrapped around the forearm of a subject. The gauge is applied with about 30 g tension (Whitney, 1949) to ensure a good embrace. This tension can be established by first holding the gauge vertically and then hanging a 30-g weight on it and measuring the resistance. At this time, the resistance–extension relationship can be measured so that the resistance change (with the gauge on the member) can be converted to a circumference change. When the gauge is placed on the member it is stretched to achieve the same resistance as was represented by the 30-g weight.

Figure 28*b* illustrates a typical increase in forelimb circumference following sudden venous occlusion produced by quickly inflating a blood pressure cuff central to the eight-strand strain gauge encompassing 6 cm of forearm. The volume flow (in milliliters per minute) is calculated from the initial slope of the curve, which identifies the immediate postocclusion increase in forearm circumference.

It is customary to express volume flow in terms of milliliters per minute of flow

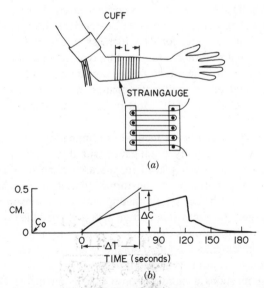

Figure 28   Eight-element mercury-in-rubber (Whitney) strain gauge applied to the forearm (*a*) to measure blood flow by venous occlusion plethysmography. (*b*) A record of circumference increase following venous occlusion caused by suddenly inflating a blood pressure cuff to occlude venous outflow but not to hinder arterial inflow.

per 100 mL of tissue. This quantity—milliliters per minute per 100 mL of tissue—is called perfusion and is the quantity that dictates tissue survival.

In Fig. 28b the venous occlusion was suddenly applied at time zero and the limb started to swell. Extrapolating the initial circumference increase, it is seen that the increase is 0.5 cm in 64 sec. The initial limb circumference C_0 was 25.3 cm, and the length L of the member under the strain gauge was 6 cm. Therefore the volume increase is 12.1 mL. This volume increase occurred in 64 sec, i.e., 1.07 min. The volume of the limb segment under the strain gauge ($LC_0^2/4\pi$) is 305.6 mL. Therefore, perfusion (mL/min per 100 mL of tissue) is 3.70.

The Whitney strain gauge and variants thereof have been used extensively to measure segmental blood flow. Whitney (1954) compared the values obtained with his strain gauge with those obtained with a water-filled, member-encircling plethysmograph. Although the correlation between the two methods was excellent, the strain gauge measurements were about 50% higher than those obtained with the water-filled plethysmograph.

When mercury is employed in small-bore (approximately 0.5 mm i.d.) elastic tubing, the resistance of typical gauges is in the vicinity of 0.02–0.20 Ω per centimeter of length. The force necessary to elongate a typical 35-mm gauge 6 mm was given by Lawton and Collins (1959) as 20 g. The force–extension curve exhibited a slight nonlinearity. Rushmer (1955a,b) noted that good linearity was obtained beyond a small initial extension. He also reported that his gauges performed satisfactorily with extensions up to 100% of the relaxed length.

The change in resistance with elongation can be determined from Fig. 27, whose values were calculated from perfect elasticity and constant-volume considerations; that is, an increase in length results in a corresponding decrease in diameter, the total volume remaining constant. For small extensions the coefficient is approximately 2% increase in resistance for a 1% increase in length. This value was quoted by Whitney, who employed rubber tubing. In a typical application, in which a low voltage was applied to a Wheatstone bridge containing a 3.5-cm gauge, a signal of 0.24 mV was obtained per millimeter change in length per volt applied to the bridge (Lawton and Collins, 1959). Most investigators employ 2–6 V to energize the bridge.

Elsner et al. (1959) described a method of eliminating many of the difficulties encountered in using the mercury strain gauge with direct current. By coupling the gauge to a step-up transformer placed in one arm of an impedance bridge and connecting balancing resistors to a transformer placed in the adjacent arm, they were able to operate the bridge on alternating current and obtain practical ease in balancing the bridge. The alternating current also permitted the use of conventional R-C coupled or carrier amplifiers to process the signal for ultimate recording. With this system these investigators reported obtaining an overall sensitivity of 1 mm of recorder deflection for 2 μm of extension of a mercury gauge 5 cm long.

In practical applications a rapid response time is attainable with the mercury strain gauge. Rushmer (1955a,b) reported a value (0–100%) of less than 0.01 sec with his 35-mm gauges, and Lawton and Collins (1959), by applying a sinusoidal stretching force, carefully measured the frequency response and phase shift of similar gauges at various elongations. They found that the sine wave frequency response curve was essentially 100% to 20 Hz, increasing to 110% at approximately 50 Hz and reaching 150% at 100 Hz. The phase shifts at these frequencies were 10, 25, and 45 degrees, respectively.

Because of its practical features, the mercury strain gauge will see continued application despite its defect. As with the aqueous electrolyte strain gauge, temperature changes constitute a source of error in many applications. Although the temperature coefficient of resistivity for mercury is considerably less than that of the copper wires employed with the gauge, Whitney described the need for compensating resistors when mercury strain gauges are employed for peripheral plethysmography on human subjects. In biothermal plethysmographic studies the thermal resistance variation becomes objectionable. Eagan (1961) reported that a 22.5°C change in temperature is equivalent to a 2% change in resistance or a 1% change in length. Honda (1962) stated that a 25°C change in temperature of the mercury is equivalent to a 1% change in length. To compensate for this change, he mounted a compensating resistor made of copper wire in a rubber tube adjacent to the mercury strain gauge element. The compensating resistor was connected to the adjacent arm of the bridge. By using alternating current on the bridge and transformer coupling to the gauge and compensating resistor, he was able to adjust the bridge for full compensation for a 25°C temperature change.

Another factor worthy of attention is the short-term creep reported by Lawton and Collins (1959). However, they felt that this was unimportant in dynamic studies.

Perhaps one of the chief drawbacks to prolonged use of mercury gauges is the corrosive nature of mercury. Some types of rubber tubing are attacked by mercury, and in nearly every case the electrodes deteriorate after a period of time. Copper, brass, and platinum electrodes have been employed with some success. All who have made mercury strain gauges have called attention to the need to use clean mercury, preferably triple distilled.

Although latex rubber tubing was employed in the early gauges, silicone rubbers are now universally used. Whitney in the United Kingdom employed No. 1 surgical drainage tubing (Dunlop Special Products, England) (0.7-mm bore, 0.7-mm wall) and latex tubing (0.5-mm bore, 0.8-mm wall). In the United States, silicone tubing can be readily obtained (Dow Corning Center for Aid to Medical Research, Midland, Michigan; Huntingdon Rubber Mills, Portland, Oregon; Becton Dickinson (Vivosil 7002-012), Rutherford, New Jersey).

HUMIDITY-SENSITIVE RESISTORS

A variety of names, including resistance or conductance hygrometer, resistance or conductance psychrometer, and humistor, have been used to describe humidity transducers. The operation of such devices relies on the moisture dependence of the resistivity of many insulators, since a change in this property is used to measure environmental humidity. In general, most materials exhibit a decrease in resistivity with increasing moisture content. However, in some materials resistivity increases with increasing moisture content. The electrical recording of relative humidity is often designated electrohygrometry.

Before describing the various humidity-sensitive resistors, it is useful to give some definitions. Humidity is a measure of the water vapor present in a gas and is expressed in either relative or absolute terms. Relative humidity is defined as the ratio of the partial pressure of the water vapor present to the water vapor pressure required for saturation at a given temperature. Percent relative humidity is this ratio multiplied by 100. Absolute humidity is the mass of water vapor contained in a volume of moist gas; the units most frequently employed are grams per cubic meter.

Traditionally the moisture content of air is determined by a psychrometer, a device containing two thermometers; the bulb of one measures the environmental temperature (dry bulb), and around the bulb of the other is a wick from which water is evaporated to produce cooling (wet bulb). The relative humidity is related to the difference in temperature between the readings on the wet- and dry-bulb thermometers. Figure 29 presents this relationship. It is perhaps unnecessary to state that the wet- and dry-bulb thermometers could be suitably waterproofed thermistors.

Relative humidity is also measured by the dew-point technique in which the temperature of a polished metal container is reduced (usually by evaporation of a volatile liquid) until there is visible condensation of water vapor. The temperature at condensation is called the dew point, and there is a relationship between the dew point, environmental temperature, and relative humidity. Figure 30 indicates this relationship.

A typical humidity-sensitive resistor consists of a dielectric film (often a plastic)

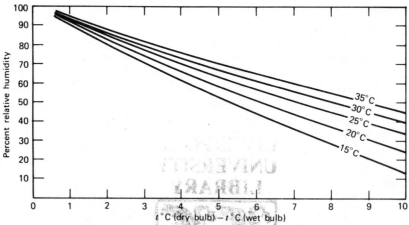

Figure 29   Percentage of relative humidity versus temperature difference between dry-bulb and wet-bulb thermometers and various environmental temperatures. (Plotted from data in *Handbook of Chemistry and Physics*, 44th ed. Chemical Rubber Publishing Co., Cleveland, Ohio, 1963.)

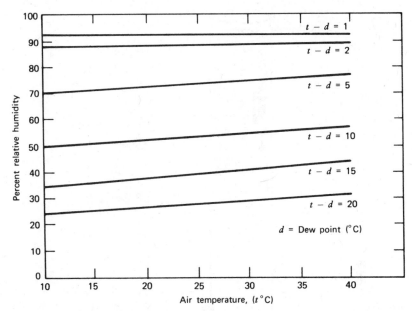

Figure 30 Relative humidity versus air temperature for various dew-point depressions ($t - d$). (Plotted from data in *Handbook of Chemistry and Physics*, 44th ed. Chemical Rubber Publishing Co., Cleveland, Ohio, 1963.)

that supports two electrodes. On the film is a hygroscopic salt such as lithium chloride, barium fluoride, potassium dihydrogen phosphate, or phosphorus pentoxide. Aluminum oxide and carbon have also been used. The resistance of such substances usually decreases nonlinearly with increasing relative humidity.

Lithium chloride is used in an interesting way to indicate humidity by one manufacturer (Yellow Springs Instruments, Yellow Springs, Ohio). The sensor (Fig. 31) consists of a cylindrical wick saturated with lithium chloride. Inside the wick is a linear thermistor temperature sensor. Wound around the wick in a spiral configuration are two electrodes, to which a constant voltage (24 V ac) is applied. The temperature of the wick increases to a value determined by its resistance, which is a function of its moisture content. An equilibrium temperature is reached when the partial pressure of the lithium chloride solution in the wick equals the water vapor pressure in the ambient air. The thermistor measures this equilibrium temperature, which is a function of the dew point. The information used to convert the equilibrium temperature to dew point is the DW10 curve available from the National Weather Service.

A simple method of measuring humidity employs organic material such as thread or hair. The shortening of human hair with increasing relative humidity is nonlinear and small in magnitude, amounting to about a 2% change in length for a change in relative humidity from 0 to 100%. Small as this change is, it is nonetheless used in a number of familiar, low-cost dial instruments that indicate relative humidity directly. Although coupling a strain gauge element to a human hair under moderate

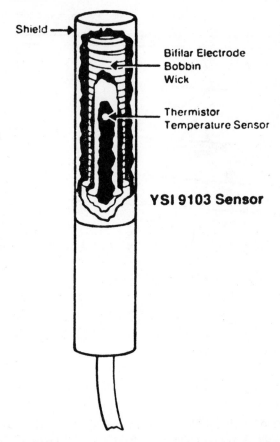

Shield

Bifilar Electrode
Bobbin
Wick

Thermistor
Temperature Sensor

YSI 9103 Sensor

Figure 31   Energy-balance dew-point hygrometer consisting of a cylindrical wick saturated with lithium chloride, inside of which is a thermistor temperature sensor. Around the wick are wound two electrodes to which a constant voltage is applied. The equilibrium temperature of the wick is a function of the dew point. (Courtesy Yellow Springs Instruments, Yellow Springs, Ohio.)

tension ought to provide an easily fabricated, low-cost electrical humidity sensor, the authors are unaware of the existence or use of such a device.

Biomedical Applications

There are several biologic applications of humidity-sensitive resistors, and in all these the presence of sweat is detected. Hemingway (1944) pointed out the interesting fact that the appearance of "cold sweat" accompanied the occurrence of motion sickness. To document the onset of motion sickness in subjects experiencing accelerative forces, Hemingway continuously recorded the resistance between two electrodes placed on the forehead. The secretion of cold sweat suddenly reduced the resistance and provided a definite index of the onset of motion sickness.

This information was used in studies of the effectiveness of drugs designed to reduce sensitivity to motion sickness. The detection of cold sweat was also described by Ackerman (1968), who developed a lithium chloride unit with a short response time. Another application of humistors is concerned with measurement of the secretion of sweat that accompanies an emotional response to a stimulus. A very obvious application of humistors is in the measurement of thermal sweating.

Humidity sensors are used to determine the rate of sweating by measurement of the relative humidity in the air passing over a circumscribed area of skin. The technique employs a small chamber applied securely to the skin where sweating is to be measured. Dry air (or air with a known moisture content) is admitted to the chamber and is moistened by the perspiration; hence there is an increase in the relative humidity of the air emerging from an exit port. Measurement of the difference in the humidity of the inlet and outlet air is accomplished by humistors. Knowledge of the rate of airflow and the difference in relative humidity between the inlet and outlet air permits calculation of the rate of sweat production.

Sulzberger and Hermann (1954) appear to have been the first to use lithium chloride as the humidity-sensitive resistance element. Nakayama and Takagi (1959) developed a device in which plant pith constituted the humidity-sensitive substance. They reported that the resistance change was linear with relative humidity in the range of 5 to 25%. Bullard (1962) employed a lithium chloride unit to record relative humidity, and Rosenberg et al. (1962) coated a plastic film with graphite to detect humidity in studies of sweating. Van Gasselt and Vierhout (1963) devised a sensor in which a layer of phosphorus pentoxide was placed between platinum wire electrodes. Najbrt et al. (1964) devised a sensor that employed a film of bentonite, glycerin, and sodium chloride. Baker and Kligman (1967) used a commercially available (Sage Instruments, Inc., White Plains, New York) humidity recorder incorporating five sensors to cover the range of 0 to 100% relative humidity. The type of sensor employed in this instrument was not identified.

Ackerman (1968) described an unusually good lithium chloride sensor that was developed to have a short response time. His construction details are presented here since the device is easy to make and is quite temperature-insensitive. The transducer consisted of two zigzag copper electrodes etched onto a circular poly-(vinyl chloride) (PVC) printed-circuit board measuring 1.5 cm in diameter (see inset, Fig. 32). The humidity-sensitive coating, which bridged the electrodes, consisted of a hygroscopic substance (a mixture of lithium chloride and aluminum chloride) dissolved in a binder to which water was added. The binder was made with 0.7 g of 98% hydrolyzed poly(vinyl alcohol) dissolved in 10 mL of distilled water under gentle heating until the solution became translucent. To this solution was added 0.1 mL of nonionic detergent (alkyl phenoxypolyethoxy ethanol) sold under the trade name Triton X-100. Ackerman's sensors were prepared by combining the desired volumes of saturated lithium chloride and aluminum chloride solutions with equal parts of binder and distilled water. The cleaned electrode assembly was then dipped into this solution, slowly withdrawn, and heat treated to 60°C for 30 min with the electrode surface in a horizontal position; then it was dried in a desiccator for at least 24 hr. Ackerman tested the performance charac-

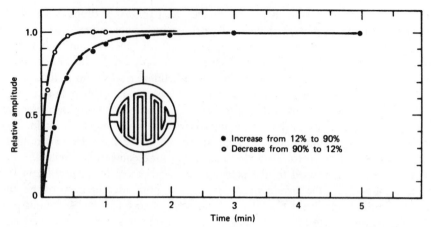

Figure 32   Response to a step change in relative humidity of a humistor consisting of a film of 0.2 vol % LiCl·H$_2$O and 0.8 vol % AlCl$_3$ applied to a zigzag electrode configuration (see inset). (Courtesy of U. Ackerman, Memorial University, St. John's, Newfoundland, 1973.)

teristics of these sensors by varying the proportions of lithium chloride in the aqueous binder. A mixture of 0.2 vol % LiCl·H$_2$O and 0.8 vol % AlCl$_3$ provided the shortest response time. Figure 32 presents typical data for such a sensor, which exhibited a resistance of about 25 Ω at 12% and 1–2 MΩ at 90% relative humidity. Ackerman used a current of 0.5 μA to measure the humidity-induced resistance change.

When sweating is measured, a skin chamber about 4 cm^2 in area is employed; the airflow rate depends on the sweat rate. In practice, a typical airflow range is 0.1–1.0 L/min. Baker and Kligman (1967) presented the following expression for the water loss W, in milligrams per square centimeter per hour, from a sweating surface area S, in square centimeters.

$$W = \frac{60DA(\Delta RH)}{100S}.$$

In this expression ΔRH is the change in relative humidity between the outflowing and inflowing air, A is the airflow (L/min), and D is the density of water (milligrams per liter of air) of saturated steam at the temperature of the flowing airstream. Values for A are obtained from standard tables.

Using the commercially available resistance hygrometer, Baker and Kligman (1967) obtained sweat-rate data for various sites on the bodies of typical human subjects. Their results are presented in Table 6 along with data obtained from their review of previous literature.

The measurement of sweat rate is not a clinical diagnostic test at present. There are, however, a variety of diseases in which sweating is enhanced or depressed. Whether the measurement of sweat rate will contribute to the early diagnosis of such diseases awaits future investigation.

TABLE 6 Rate of Sweating in Human Subjects

Authors	Site		Method	Average Value [mg/(hr)(cm^2)]
Baker and Kligman (1967)	Back	in vivo	Electrohygrometry	0.23
Baker and Kligman (1967)	Forearm	in vivo	Electrohygrometry	0.30
Baker and Kligman (1967)	Abdomen	in vivo	Electrohygrometry	0.36
Baker and Kligman (1967)	Shin	in vivo	Electrohygrometry	0.42
Burch and Winsor (1944)	Abdomen	in vivo	Gravimetric with airflow	5.8
	Abdomen	in vitro	Gravimetric with airflow	6.5
Feisher and Rothman (1945)	Abdomen	in vivo	Calcium chloride bag in closed chamber	1.1
Blank (1952)	Abdomen	in vitro	Diffusion chamber	0.1–0.2
Mali (1956)	Trunk	in vitro	Diffusion chamber	0.5–0.6
	Sole	in vitro	Diffusion chamber	3.0
Monash and Blank (1958)	Abdomen	in vivo	Calcium chloride bag in closed chamber	2.0–9.0
Rosenberg et al. (1962)	Abdomen	in vivo	Electrohygrometry, closed chamber	0.15–0.24
Onken and Moyer (1963)	Abdomen	in vitro	Diffusion chamber	0.3
Spruit and Malten (1965)	Forearm	in vivo	Electrohygrometry with airflow	0.5–1.7
Bettley and Grice (1965)	Abdomen	in vivo	Gravimetric with airflow	0.25

PHOTORESISTORS

Many materials, especially the semiconductors, exhibit a change in resistivity when exposed to radiant energy (e.g., visible, ultraviolet, and infrared light). Such devices are called photoresistors or photoconductors and are discussed in Chapter 5.

REFERENCES

Ackerman, U. 1968. A detector for the outbreak of sweating. Rept. No. 12. Institute of Biomedical Electronics. University of Toronto, 19 pp.

Ackmann, J. J., A. D. Sances, S. J. Larson, and J. B. Baker. 1977. Quantitative evaluation of long-term Parkinson tremor. *IEEE Trans. Biomed. Eng.* **BME-24**(1):49–56.

Adams, R. 1962. Personal communication. School of Aerospace Medicine, Brooks AFB, TX.

Anrep, C. V., E. W. H. Cruickshank, A. C. Downing, and A. S. Rau. 1927. The coronary circulation in relation to the cardiac cycle. *J. Physiol.* **14**:111–134.

Association for the Advancement of Medical Instrumentation (AAMI). 1985. *General Standard for Blood Pressure Transducers*. AAMI, Arlington, VA.

Badamo, D. J. 1964. The silicones as bioengineering materials. *Proc. Annu. Conf. Eng. Biol. Med.* **6**:1–129.

Baker, H., and A. M. Kligman. 1967. Measurement of transepidermal water loss by electrical hygrometry. *Arch. Dermatol.* **96**:441–452.

Barnothy, M. 1964. *Biological Effects of Magnetic Fields*. Plenum, New York, 324 pp.

Bettley, F. R., and K. A. Grice. 1965. A method for measuring the transepidermal water loss and a means of inactivating sweat glands. *Brit. J. Derm.* **77**:627.

Blank, I. H., 1956. Factors which influence the water content of the stratum corneum. *J. Invest. Derm.* **27**:451.

Boniface, K. H., D. J. Brodie, and R. P. Walton. 1953. Resistance strain gauge arches for direct measurement of heart contractile force in animals. *Proc. Soc. Exp. Biol. Med.* **84**:263–266.

Bowman, R., E. G. Cravallo, and M. Woods, III. 1975. Theory, measurement and application of thermal properties of biomaterials. *Annu. Rev. Biophys. Bioeng.* **4**:43–79.

Bramwell, J. C., A. V. Hill, and B. A. McSwinney. 1923. The velocity of the pulse wave in man. *Heart* **10**:233–256.

Brown, J. M. 1960. Anesthesia and the contractile force of the heart. *Curr. Res. Anesth. Analg.* **39**:487–498.

Bullard, R. W. 1962. Continuous recording of sweating rate by resistance hygrometry. *J. Appl. Physiol.* **17**:735–737.

Burch, G. F., and T. Winsor. 1944. Rate of insensible perspiration (diffusion of water) locally through living and through dead human skin. *Arch. Int. Med.* **74**:437.

Chen, M. M., and K. R. Holmes. 1980. The thermal pulse decay method for simultaneous measurement of thermal conductivity and local blood perfusion rate in living tissues. *Adv. Bioeng.* pp. 113–115.

Clynes, M. 1960. Respiratory control of heart rate. *IRE Trans. Med. Electron.* **ME-7**:2–14.

Cochran, G. Van B. 1972. Implantation of strain gages on bone in vivo. *J. Biomech.* **5**:119–123.

Cochran, G. Van B. 1974. A method for direct recording of electromechanical data from skeletal bone in living animals. *J. Biomech.* **7**:561–565.

Cornwall, J. B. 1965. The matching and linearising of thermistor probes. *World Med. Electron.* **3**:233–234.

Cotton, M. de V., and H. M. Maling. 1957. Relationships among stroke work, contractile force and fiber length changes in ventricular function. *Am. J. Physiol.* **189**:580–586.

Dalla-Torre, L. 1943. Utilization d'une nouvelle méthode pour l'enrégistrement du sphygmogramme des artères digitales. *Helv. Physiol. Pharmacol. Acta* **1**:C14–C15.

Eagan, C. J. 1961. The mercury gauge method of digital plethysmography. USAF Tech. Note AAL-TN-60-15 (February 1961), TN, 60–16 (March 1961), TN–60–17 (February 1961).

Elsner, R. W., C. H. Eagan, and S. Andersen. 1959. Impedance matching circuit for mercury strain gauge. *J. Appl. Physiol.* **14**:871–872.

Fegler, G. 1954. Measurement of cardiac output in anesthetized animals by a thermodilution method. *Q. J. Exp. Physiol. Cogn. Med. Sci.* **39**:153–164.

Felsher, Z., and S. Rothman. 1945. Insensible perspiration of skin in hyperkeratotic conditions. *J. Invest. Derm.* **6**:271.

Fromm, E. 1967. A miniature contractile force telemetering system. *Proc. Annu. Conf. Eng. Med. Biol.* **9**.

Gallagher, D. J. A., and L. H. Grimwood. 1953. A simple method for measuring blood pressure in the rat tail. *J. Physiol.* **121**:163–166.

Garb, S. 1951. The effects of potassium, ammonium, calcium, strontium, and magnesium on the electrogram and myogram of mammalian heart muscle. *J. Pharmacol. Exp. Ther.* **101**:317–326.

Geddes, L. A. 1984. *Cardiovascular Medical Devices*. Wiley (Interscience), New York, 392 pp.

Geddes, L. A., H. E. Hoff, and W. A. Spencer. 1961. The Center for Vital Studies—A new laboratory for the study of bodily functions in man. *IRE Trans. Bio-Med. Electron.* **BME-8:**33–45.

Geddes, L. A., H. E. Hoff, A. G. Moore, and M. Hinds. 1966. An electrical caliper myograph. *Am. J. Pharm. Educ.* **30:**209–211.

Geddes, L. A., W. Athens, and S. Aronson. 1984. Measurement of the volume displacement of blood pressure transducers. *Med. Biol. Eng. Comput.* **22**(6) (Nov.):613–614.

Greenfield, A. D. M., R. J. Whitney, and J. F. Mowbray. 1963. Methods for the investigation of peripheral blood flow. *Br. Med. Bull.* **19:**101–109.

Grunbaum, O. F. F. 1898. On a new method of recording alternations in blood pressure. *J. Physiol.* **22:**49–50.

Grundfest, H., and J. J. Hay. 1945. A strain gauge recorder for physiological volume, pressure and deformation measurements. *Science* **101:**255–256.

Hall, E. H. 1879. On a new action of the magnet on electric currents. *Am. J. Math.* **2:**287–292.

Hampel, A. 1941. Elektrisches Transmissionmanometer auf der Grundlage elektrischer Widerstandsänderungen des Wismuts Magnetfeld. *Pfluegers Arch. Gesamte Physiol.* **244:**171–175.

Harris, C. M., and C. E. Crede (eds.). 1961. *Shock and Vibration Handbook*, vol. 1. McGraw-Hill, New York, Table 16.5.

Hemingway, A. 1944. Cold sweating in motion sickness. *Am. J. Physiol.* **141:**172–175.

Hensel, H., and J. Ruef. 1954. Fortlaufende Registrieruing der Muskeldurchblutung. *Pfluegers Arch. Gesamte Physiol.* **259:**267–280.

Hill, A. V. 1920–1921a. An electrical pulse recorder. *J. Physiol.* **54:**lii–liii.

Hill, A. V. 1920–1921b. The meaning of records with the hot wire sphygmograph. *J. Physiol.* **54:**cxvii–cxix.

Holzer, W. 1940. Über die Anwendung des galvano-magnetischen Longitudinal-effektes des Wismuts zur elektrischen Fernübertragung von Bewegungsvorgängen. *Pfluegers Arch. Gesamte Physiol.* **244:**176–180.

Honda, N. 1962. Temperature compensation for mercury strain gauge used in plethysmography. *J. Appl.-Physiol.* **17:**572–574.

Jolgren, D., N. Fearnot, and L. A. Geddes. 1983. A rate-responsive pacemaker controlled by right-ventricular blood temperature. *J. Am. Coll. Cardiol.* **1**(1):720.

Jolgren, D., N. Fearnot, and A. L. Geddes. 1984. A rate responsive pacemaker controlled by right ventricular blood temperature. *Pace* **7:**794–801.

Katsura, S., R. Weiss, D. Baker, and R. F. Rushmer. 1959. Isothermal blood flow velocity probe. *IRE Trans. Med. Electron.* **ME-8:**283–285.

Lambert, E. H., and E. H. Wood. 1947. The use of resistance wire strain gauge monometer to measure intra-arterial pressure. *Proc. Soc. Exp. Biol. Med.* **64:**186–190.

Lamson, P. D., and B. H. Robbins. 1928. Thermal conductivity methods of gas analysis in the study of pharmacological problem. *J. Pharmacol. Exp. Ther.* **34:**325–331.

Lanyon, L. E. 1976. The measurement of bone strain in vivo. *Acta Orthop. Belg.* **42**(Suppl. 1):98–109.

Lawton, R. W., and C. C. Collins. 1959. Calibration of an aortic circumference gauge. *J. Appl. Physiol.* **14:**465–467.

Ledig, P. C., and R. S. Lyman, 1927. An adaptation of the thermal conductivity method to the analysis of respiratory gases. *J. Clin. Invest.* **4:**494–565.

LeGette, M. A. 1958. Strain gauge principles. *Instrum. Autom.* **31:**447–449.

Mali, J. W. H. 1956. The transport of water through the human epidermis. *J. Invest. Derm.* **27:**451.

Mason, W. P., and R. N. Thurston. 1957. Use of piezoresistive materials in the measurement of displacement, force and torque. *J. Acoust. Soc. Am.* **29:**1096–1101.

Maulsby, R. L., and H. E. Hoff. 1962. Hypotensive mechanisms of pulmonary insufflation in dogs. *Am. J. Physiol.* **202**:505–509.

Mellander, S., and R. F. Rushmer. 1960. Venous blood flow recorded with an isothermal flowmeter. *Acta Physiol. Scand.* **43**:13–19.

Millar, H. D., and L. E. Baker. 1973. A stable ultraminiature catheter-tip transducer. *Med. Biol. Eng.* **11**(1):86–89.

Monash, S., and H. Blank. 1958. Location and reformation of the epithelial barrier to water vapor. *Arch. Dermatol.* **78**:710.

Müller, A. 1942. Über die Pulsform und Wellengeschwindigkeit in den Fingeraterien. *Arch. Krieslaufforsch.* **11**:198–206.

Murgo, J. P. et al. 1980. *Circulation* **62**(1):105–116.

Najbrt, V. L., L. Rovensky, J. Pompeova, and B. Konrad. 1964. Studie o mereni dynamity bariéové funkce. *Cesk. Dermatol.* **39**(2):88–93.

Nakayama, T., and K. Takagi. 1959. Minute pattern of human perspiration observed by a continuously recording method. *Jpn. J. Physiol.* **9**:359–364.

Nunn, H. E. 1959. A guide to static pressure transducers that have a diaphragm, bellows or Bourdon pressure cell. *Prod. Eng.* **30**:48–49.

Onken, H. D., and C. A. Moyer. 1963. The water barrier in human epidermis. *Arch. Dermatol.* **87**:584.

Perl, W. 1962. Heat and matter distribution in body tissues and the determination of tissue blood flow by local clearance methods. *J. Theor. Biol.* **2**:201–235.

Rein, H., A. A. Hampel, and W. A. Heinemann. 1940. Photoelektrische Transmissionmanometer zur Blutdruckschreibung. *Pfluegers Arch. Gesamte Physiol.* **243**:329–335.

Rosenberg, E. W., H. Blank, and S. Resnik. 1962. Sweating and water loss through the skin. *JAMA* **179**:809–811.

Rushmer, R. F. 1955a. Pressure-circumference relations in the aorta. *Am. J. Physiol.* **183**:545–549.

Rushmer, R. F. 1955b. Length-circumference relations of the left ventricle. *Circ. Res.* **3**:639–644.

Rushmer, R. F. 1965. Pressure circumference relations in the left ventricle. *Am. J. Physiol.* **186**:115–121.

Sanchez, J. C. 1961. Semiconductor strain gauges—a state of the art summary. *Strain Gauge Readings* **4**:3–16.

Shapiro, A., H. D. Cohen, E. Maher, and W. J. McAveney. 1964. On-line analog computation of volume of respired air. *Proc. Annu. Conf. Eng. Med. Biol.* **6**:1–129.

Simmonds, E. E. 1942. U.S. Patent 2,292,549.

Simons, D. G. 1962. Personal communication. School of Aerospace Medicine, Brooks AFB, TX.

Smith, C. S. 1954. Piezoresistive effect of germanium and silicon. *Phys. Rev.* **94**:42–49.

Spruit, D., and K. E. Malten. 1965. Epidermal barrier formation after stripping of nerve skin. *J. Invest. Derm.* **45**:6.

Star, J. 1963. Hall effect transducers. *Instrum. Control Syst.* **36**:113–116.

Stetz, C. W., R. G. Miller, G. E. Kelley, and T. A. Raffin. 1982. Reliability of the thermodilution method in determination of cardiac output in clinical practice. *Am. Rev. Respir. Dis.* **126**:1001–1004.

Sulzberger, M. B., and F. Hermann. 1954. *The Critical Significance of Disturbances in the Delivery of Sweat.* Thomas, Springfield, IL.

Swan H., and W. Ganz. 1970. Catheterization of the heart in man with use of a flow through balloon tipped catheter. *N. Engl. J. Med.* **283**:447–451.

Swanson, C. A., and A. C. Emslie. 1954. Low temperature electronics. *Proc. IRE* **42**:402–413.

Taylor, B. D., A. P. Ormond, and D. B. Sheffer. 1982. An in-vitro evaluation of thermodilution cardiac output techniques, *Proc. AAMI Conf., 1982.*

Tomlinson, H. 1876–1877. On the increase in resistance to the passage of an electric current produced on stretching. *Proc. R. Soc. London* **25**:451–453.

Tucker, W. S., and E. T. Paris. 1921. A selective hot-wire microphone. *Philos. Trans. R. Soc. London, Ser. A* **221**:389–430.

Turner, R. H. 1928. A sphygmograph using a carbon grain microphone and the string galvanometer. *Bull. Johns Hopkins Hosp.* **43**:2–13.

Valentinuzzi, M. 1961. *Magnetobiology.* North American Aviation, Los Angeles, CA, 74 pp.

Valentinuzzi, M. 1962. *A Theory of Magnetic Growth Inhibition.* Committee on Mathematical Biology, Chicago, IL, 58 pp.

Valvano, J. W., and P. A. Patel. 1983. A non-invasive thermistor blood-flow perfusion monitor. *Proc. Annu. Conf. Eng. Med. Biol.* **25**:99.

Valvano, J. W., J. T. Allen, and H. F. Bowman. 1984. The simultaneous measurement of thermal conductivity, thermal diffusivity and perfusion in small volumes of tissue. *Trans. ASME* **106**:192–196.

Van Dover, J. and N. F. Bechtold. 1960. Survey of thermistor characteristics. *Electronics* **33**:58–60.

Van Gasselt, H. R. M., and R. R. Vierhout. 1963. Registration of the insensible perspiration and small quantities of sweat. *Dermatologica* **127**:255–257.

Victory Engineering Corp. 1955. *Thermistor Data Book.* Victory Eng. Corp., Union, NJ.

Voelz, M. 1981. Measurement of the blood pressure constant k over a pressure range in the canine radial artery. *Med. Biol. Eng. Comput.* **19**:515–517.

Voorhees, W. D., and C. F. Babbs. 1981. New method to determine the importance of blood flow in thermal clearance from deep-lying normal tissue in dogs. *Proc. 16th AAMI Annu. Meet.* p. 105.

Waggoner, W. C. 1965. High-impedance elastic force gauge. *Am. J. Med. Electron.* **4**:175–177.

Waud, R. A. 1924. An electric polygraph. *JAMA* **82**:1203.

Weissel, R. S., R. L. Berger, and H. B. Hechtman. 1975. Measurement of cardiac output by thermodilution. *N. Engl. J. Med.* **292**(73):682–684.

Whitney, R. J. 1949. The measurement of changes in human limb-volume by means of a mercury-in-rubber strain gauge. *J. Physiol.* **109**:5P–6P.

Whitney, R. J. 1953. The measurement of volume changes in human limbs. *J. Physiol.* **121**:1–27.

Whitney, R. J. 1954. Circulatory changes in the forearm and hand of man with repeated exposure to heat. *J. Physiol.* **125**:1–24.

Wright, T. M., and W. C. Hayes. 1979. Strain gage application on compact bone. *J. Biomech.* **12**:471–475.

3

Inductive Transducers

SINGLE INDUCTORS

The inductance of a coil depends on its geometry, the magnetic permeability of the medium in which it is located, and the number of turns. The approximate low-frequency inductance L in microhenries of a single-layer air-core coil can be calculated by the following formula, due to Wheeler (1928):

$$L = \frac{r^2 n^2}{9r + 10l},$$

where r and l are the radius and length in inches and n is the number of turns. This expression is accurate when the length of the coil is much greater than the diameter. Wheeler stated that the accuracy is within 1% when l is greater than 0.8 times the radius. Although there are many other expressions for the inductance of single-layer coils in which a form factor (dependent on the ratio of length to diameter) is present, the important fact is that the inductance varies with the square of the number of turns and with the geometry of the coil. Thus distortion of the coil, as by stretching or compressing, will alter its inductance. This method of inductance change is seldom used because of the small inductance and the even smaller inductance change occurring in coils that can be distorted. If a coil spring happens to be present in a system in which it is desired to detect motion, the changing dimensions of the spring can serve as an inductance transducer. If the spring is of ferromagnetic material, the inductance will be somewhat greater than that expected from calculation on the basis of coil geometry. If the coil surrounds a material having a magnetic permeability greater than that of air, its inductance is increased considerably.

Control of the inductance can be gained by altering the magnetic permeability of the medium. A considerable increase in inductance can be obtained by inserting a magnetically permeable core into the coil. Under these conditions the inductance will depend on the amount of core inside the coil, thereby affording a method of translating displacement into a change in inductance.

Biomedical Applications

Single inductors have frequently been employed to measure physiological events that can be converted to movement. One such transducer was described by Fuller and Gordon (1948), who fitted the diaphragm of a Marey tambour with a ferromagnetic ring. Inside the tambour was an iron-cored coil, the inductance of which was changed when the diaphragm was displaced by pressure. Müller et al. (1948) described a simple flowmeter consisting of a variable-inductance differential pressure transducer connected to a Pitot tube. Their transducer consisted of an iron-cored coil placed close to an elastic diaphragm that carried a small soft iron disk. Movement of the disk in response to pressure changes across the diaphragm altered the inductance and unbalanced a 5-kHz bridge circuit, thereby producing an alternating voltage proportional to pressure, which was in turn proportional to blood flow. Rushmer (1954a, b) described a remarkable application of the variable-inductance technique to measure continuously the diameter of the left ventricle of a dog as the heart was beating. He was able to suture a small coil to one ventricular wall and the core to the septum. As the diameter changed with each heart beat, the core moved within the coil, causing inductance changes that indicated, when recorded in the unanesthetized dog, alterations in the size of the ventricle during a variety of experimental conditions.

An interesting extensible inductor mounted in a neck band was patented by Sackner (1984). The device, shown in Fig. 1a, was designed for detecting the pulse and respiration. Into the distensible neck band is stitched a zigzag wire, which constitutes the inductor that determined the frequency of a resonant circuit.

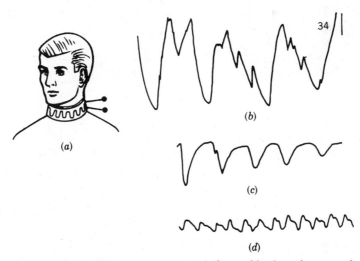

(a)

(b)

(c)

(d)

34

Figure 1 (*a*) Inductive neck-band transducer and (*b*) combined respiratory and cardiac signal. In (*c*) and (*d*), respiration and the pulse signals have been extracted by filtering. (Redrawn from M. A. Sackner, U.S. Patent 4,452,252, June 5, 1984.)

The cardiac and respiratory-induced changes in circumference altered the inductance which altered the frequency of the resonant circuit. The change in frequency was converted to an analog signal suitable for display by a stripchart recorder.

Figure 1b illustrates the combined cardiac and respiratory signal detected by the neck-band inductive transducer. Figure 1c and d illustrate the respiratory and cardiac signals separated by bandpass filters.

An interesting variable reluctance accelerometer was used by Boshes (1966) to detect the tremor of Parkinson's disease. The device (Glennite AVR 250) weighed 2.5 g and could be applied to any part of the body to sense acceleration due to muscle movement, respiration, and cardiac activity. Figure 2 illustrates the device and its application to the index finger. Also shown in Fig. 2 are recordings of tremors from the left and right index fingers. Boshes found that the tremor frequency in Parkinson's disease ranged from 6.2 to 8.8 Hz. He used such recordings to evaluate the effectiveness of drug therapy.

MUTUAL INDUCTANCE

The principle of mutual inductance, which employs two coils, is also used in the measurement of physiological events. When two coils are joined in series and their fields link, the inductance L is equal to $L_1 + L_2 \pm 2M$, where L_1 and L_2 are the inductances of the individual coils and M, the mutual inductance between them,

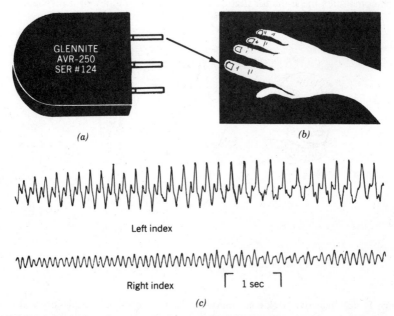

(a)   (b)

Left index

Right index   ⌐ 1 sec ⌐

(c)

Figure 2   (a) Variable reluctance accelerometer; (b) application to the index finger; and (c) a record of tremor in Parkinson's disease. [Redrawn from F. Boshes, J. Neurosurg., Suppl. 1:324–330 (1966).]

is dependent on the coupling between the coils. The positive sign applies when the fields of the two coils are additive; the negative sign applies when the fields are in opposition. The coefficient of coupling k is

$$k = M/\sqrt{L_1 L_2}$$

which can be calculated by measuring the inductance with the coils in series with the fields aiding (L_a) and opposing (L_o) each other. The value for k becomes

$$k = (L_a - L_o)/4\sqrt{L_1 L_2}.$$

The coupling can be altered by inserting a magnetically permeable core or by moving one coil with respect to the other.

If the two coils are not joined electrically and an oscillator is connected across one of them, a voltage will be induced in the other. The arrangement constitutes a transformer. The two windings are designated the primary and the secondary, the energy source being connected to the primary winding. The magnitude of the voltage appearing across the secondary coil is dependent on the coupling, which can be varied by the insertion of a magnetically permeable core or by moving one coil with respect to the other.

Biomedical Applications

There are many practical applications of two inductances connected in series opposition in which the coupling between them is altered by changing the position of a centrally mounted core. One such application is that of Gauer and Gienapp (1950), who built a unique catheter-tip blood pressure transducer. A diaphragm having the diameter of the catheter actuated a small ferromagnetic core, which, moving in response to the pressure changes, altered the coupling between the coils and produced proportional changes in inductance. This early catheter-tip pressure transducer had a resonant frequency of 1000 Hz in fluid and for a considerable time stood alone as having the highest fidelity of any blood pressure transducer.

A larger two-inductance pressure transducer, the Clark capsule, was described by Motley et al. (1947). In this device two coils were mounted on each side of a distensible, magnetically permeable, elastic diaphragm. The two coils constituted the two arms of an inductance bridge that was balanced in the absence of pressure on the diaphragm. When pressure was applied, the diaphragm was deformed and the bridge became unbalanced, producing a signal that was recorded after suitable processing. The performance was reported to be only slightly inferior to that of the Hamilton manometer, one of the highest quality optical manometers and then considered to be the standard instrument for blood pressure recording.

Scher et al. (1953) constructed an interesting inductance transducer for blood flow in which a ferromagnetic paddle in a flow tube was placed midway between two coils wrapped around the outside of the tube. The two coils formed the arms of a balanced inductance bridge. The flow of blood deflected the paddle and unbalanced the bridge. A recording of the imbalance voltage was calibrated in terms of volume flow per minute.

A pulse pickup using the two-winding variable transformer was developed by Benjamin et al. (1962). In their transducer the two coils were mounted in a small chamber, which was affixed to the skin over a pulsating artery. In the chamber facing the artery, a rubber diaphragm carried the movable coil and the frame of the capsule carried the fixed coil. The coil on the rubber membrane was energized by a 100-kHz oscillator, and its position was modulated by the pulse. Amplification, rectification, and graphic recording of the signal produced a pulse tracing of high fidelity.

Blood flow was recorded by Pieper (1958), who constructed a catheter-tip velocity flowmeter employing the variable transformer. In this device a ferromagnetic sleeve with a small flange was displaced by the velocity of the bloodstream. The displacement altered the coupling between the coils, thereby producing a recordable signal. A unique expandable, umbrella-type fixture served to maintain the transducer in the center of the vessel. Pieper reported a linear output with flow up to a velocity of 45 cm/sec and a frequency up to 25 Hz.

LINEAR VARIABLE DIFFERENTIAL TRANSFORMERS (LVDT)

When three coils are used, the device is designated a differential transformer. The most common of its many forms is an arrangement of two identical coils placed on each side of a third energizing coil (Fig. 3). This configuration was introduced by Schaevitz (1947) and is used extensively by industry (Schaevitz Engineering, Camden, New Jersey). The center coil of the LVDT is excited by alternating current, which produces a field that induces equal voltages in the two adjacent coils. The outer coils are connected in series opposition so that the voltage generated in one cancels that from the other. In practice, the residual voltage is on the order of 1% of the maximum output voltage. Insertion of a core unbalances the system so that the voltages generated in the outer coils are no longer equal. The imbalance voltage is proportional to the core position. The relationship between the output voltage and the position of core in the differential transformer is shown in Fig. 3a. In comprehensive articles, Schaevitz (1947) and Heath (1958) have further analyzed the operation of the LVDT under a variety of practical measurement conditions.

Note that an output of the same magnitude is produced if the core is displaced an equal amount in either direction from its central position. The phase of the output differs, however, by 180 degrees on either side of the neutral position. Direction sensitivity can be achieved with the LVDT with either of two techniques. In one, the core is offset and operation is centered around a position other than the one that moves the core through the central point. Thus a signal of increasing or decreasing magnitude is obtained with movement of the core. The other method of operation is illustrated in Fig. 3b. This circuit arrangement constitutes a phase-

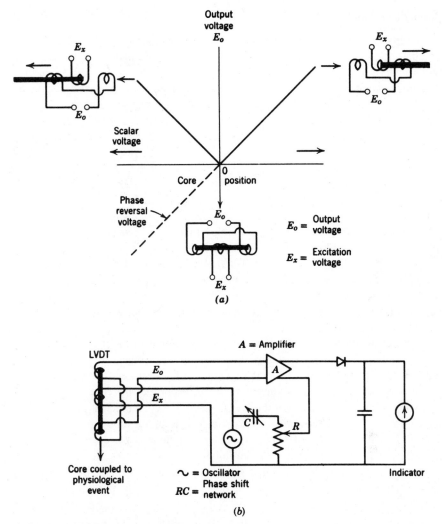

Figure 3   The linear variable differential transformer (LVDT): (*a*) output versus core position; (*b*) phase-sensitive detector for LVDT.

sensitive detector in which the oscillator voltage and that derived from the LVDT are added before rectification. With the core in its central position, the oscillator voltage, corrected for phase shifts in all of the circuitry by adjustment of C, is fed to the indicator to bring it to midscale by adjustment of R. As the core is displaced from the central position, the voltage E_o, after amplification, adds to or subtracts from the oscillator voltage, depending on the magnitude and phase of E_o, which in turn depends on the magnitude and direction of the displacement. Thus the indicator can be calibrated for the full range of core motion.

Biomedical Applications

The first catheter-tip blood pressure transducer incorporating one type of LVDT was described by Wetterer (1943). In this device the oscillator was connected to two primary coils, and the detecting system to the two secondary coils connected in series opposition. At the tip of the 3.5-mm catheter was an elastic disphragm coupled to a movable core that altered the coupling between the primary and secondary coils when pressure was applied. The small mass and high stiffness of the moving parts resulted in a high resonant frequency (515 Hz), thereby producing a rapid response time.

Small movements were detected by Tucker (1952) with a three-coil transformer transducer. His device was accurate to 0.005 cm over a 1-cm range and provided enough power to drive a pen recorder without amplification.

The relatively high efficiency of the commercially available three-coil LVDTs has stimulated many investigators to employ them for the measurement of physiological events. A blood pressure transducer featuring a differential transformer was described by Shafer and Shirer (1949). In this device the core was affixed to a small circular elastic diaphragm exposed to blood pressure, and the whole assembly was mounted in a 2-mL syringe. The natural frequency of this transducer was 600 Hz; when it was connected to a 20-gauge needle, a frequency response was obtained that was flat to 100 Hz.

Erdos et al. (1962) described an isotonic myograph incorporating the LVDT. In this device the muscle specimen under study was connected to a beam-type balance. The motion of the balancing weight, which occurred with contraction of the muscle, was measured by variations in the position of the core in the LVDT.

Figure 4 illustrates the use of the LVDT to construct an efficient pressure transducer. In this device, movement of the tip of a Bourdon tube is detected by an LVDT. Linearity, rapidity of response, and small volume displacement are achieved by means of a very stiff, short Bourdon tube.

A very interesting electric caliper incorporating the LVDT was described by Gow (1966). Employed for the continuous measurement of pulsatile arterial di-

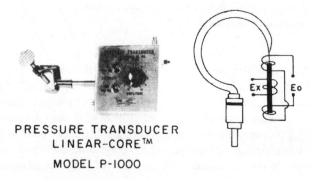

PRESSURE TRANSDUCER
LINEAR-CORE™
MODEL P-1000

Figure 4   LVDT pressure transducer, linear core model P-1000. (Courtesy of Narco Bio-Systems, Houston, Texas.)

ameter changes, this device consisted of a jeweled-bearing, scissorlike, lightweight caliper; one end embraced the artery, while the other end was affixed to the LVDT. The small pulsatile changes in the artery modulated the position of the embracing ends of the caliper to provide (after four stages of amplification) an output of 1–1.5 V for changes in the diameters of the thoracic aorta and femoral artery, amounting to 500 and 800 μm, respectively. The low mass of the instrument resulted in a sinusoidal frequency response essentially uniform to 20 Hz measured on a segment of rubber tubing. When the device was tested for transient response, the natural resonant frequency was found to be in excess of 180 Hz, dramatically illustrating the rapid response time available.

Because of the small size and low mass of the core of an LVDT, an insignificant load is imposed on the event being measured. No electromagnetic pull is imposed on the core in the null position. In practical units, very little pull is encountered when the core is displaced from the null position. Although the transduction efficiency is moderate, the differential transformer is rugged and is relatively insensitive to temperature changes, since the sensitivity alteration is due almost entirely to the resistance change of the coils. Its ability to detect rapid changes is good, being limited to the characteristics of the moving system, the frequency of the excitation voltage, and the characteristics of the magnetic material. If extremely rapid rates of change are to be measured, high-frequency excitation and powdered magnetic materials must be used in the construction of the core.

Linear variable differential transformer units are relatively low in impedance and can be constructed to have almost any dimensions. Although many component manufacturers provide a standard line, they will construct special units to meet almost any particular need. *Engineering Bulletin* A2 of the Schaevitz Co. lists transformers having linear displacement ranges of ±0.005 to ±1.000 in., with a residual output (at balance) of 0.5% of that obtained with maximum displacement. The excitation voltage of many differential transformers is 3–10 V at frequencies ranging from 60 Hz to 20 kHz. The output per unit of displacement is dependent on the excitation voltage, its frequency, and the particular differential transformer model. Typical sensitivity figures for the miniature models are approximately 0.2–5 mV per thousandth inch per volt of excitation. The higher sensitivity figures are obtained with excitation voltages in the kilohertz range.

ROTARY VARIABLE DIFFERENTIAL TRANSFORMERS

Rotary variable differential transformers are also available commercially. Although rotation through a full 360 degrees is often possible, ±1% linearity is obtained only over a range of ±40 degrees (Schaevitz R3B 1 S model). The nominal sensitivity of this particular unit is 1.8 mV per degree of rotation per volt of 2-kHz energy applied to the transformer.

Perhaps one of the most desirable characteristics of the rotary variable differential transformer is that as a transducer for rotation its output–rotation curve is smooth or stepless. In many models, however, the maximum rotation is approximately 90 degrees. When continuous rotation is possible, the output voltage varies as the sine or cosine of the angle of rotation.

ELECTROMAGNETIC FLOWMETERS

After Michael Faraday (1832) discovered the law governing magnetic induction, he speculated on the many possible ways of demonstrating this phenomenon, which, at the time his discovery was made, was evidenced by the appearance of current flow in a conductor in a changing magnetic field. Faraday was well aware of the underlying practical details. For example, he knew that the magnetic field could be stationary and the conductor could move or the conductor could be stationary and the magnetic field could change; both situations give rise to a current induced in the conductor. Faraday knew that if a conductor moved in a magnetic field, the conductor, its direction of movement, and the direction of the magnetic field had to be mutually perpendicular to maximize the induced current; this fundamental requirement is sketched in Fig. 5. Most important, Faraday discovered that the magnitude of the induced current depended on the velocity and length of conductor in the magnetic field and the strength of the magnetic field.

Faraday realized that an aqueous electrolyte flowing in a constant magnetic field should give evidence of an induced current. He set about to verify the presence of such a current by calling attention to the fact that the Thames River in England is an electrolytic conductor that moves through the earth's magnetic field; therefore, the Thames ought to sustain a current proportional to the velocity of its flow. Faraday (1832) recounted his experiment as follows:

"I made experiments therefore (by favour) at Waterloo Bridge, extending a

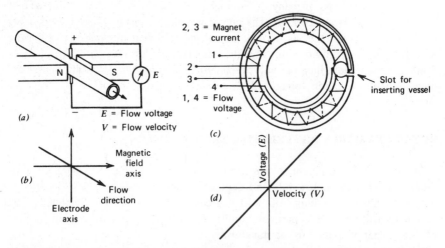

Figure 5   Basic principle of operation of an electromagnetic flowmeter: (*a*) and (*b*) direction of the electrodes and magnetic field with respect to flow; (*c*) practical arrangement for a perivascular flow probe; (*d*) linear relationship of the flow voltage E to flow velocity V.

copper wire nine hundred and sixty feet in length upon the parapet of the bridge, and dropping from its extremities other wires with extensive plates of metal attached to them to complete contact with the water. The wire therefore and the water made one conducting circuit; and as the water ebbed or flowed with the tide, I hoped to obtain currents analogous to those of the brass ball.

I constantly obtained deflections at the galvanometer, but they were very irregular, and were in succession referred to other causes than that sought for. The different condition of the water as to purity on the two sides of the river; the difference in temperature; slight differences in the plates, in the solder used, in the more or less perfect contact made by twisting or otherwise; all produced effects in turn: and though I experimented on the water passing through the middle arches only; used platina plates instead of copper; and took every other precaution, I could not after three days obtain any satisfactory results."

Undaunted by this failure, Faraday insisted that a flow-dependent current ought to exist and stated, "Theoretically it seems a necessary consequence that when water is flowing, these electric currents should be formed."

Almost a century passed before Faraday's experiment to detect the flow of fluid by induction was executed successfully. Examining the problem more carefully, Young et al. (1920), also in England, calculated that tidal water moving in the earth's magnetic field at Dartmouth ought to provide a voltage of 0.215 μV per centimeter width of stream per knot velocity of flow. Accordingly, they placed chlorided silver electrodes, 1000 yd apart, into the water at the entrance to Dartmouth Harbor. The electrodes were connected to a Paul galvanometer, and the readings obtained were plotted against time. As Faraday had predicted, the investigators obtained a slow oscillation in potential that was synchronous with the tide and had a peak-to-peak value of 18.5 μV.

It required only a decade more for application of the principle to the detection of blood flow. In 1932 Fabre and d'Arsonval (the galvanometer pioneer) constructed a glass cannula containing two diametrically opposed recessed electrodes, which were connected to a vacuum tube amplifier and an oscillograph. An artery was divided, and the cannula was inserted, allowing blood to flow through the cannula. A strong electromagnet provided a field at right angles to both the electrodes and the flow stream, and recordings of blood flow were obtained using an industrial oscillograph. Fabre and d'Arsonval then exposed a femoral artery, located it in a magnetic field, placed electrodes on its surface, and detected a weak flow-dependent voltage, thereby demonstrating that the flow signal could be detected without opening the blood vessel. Thus, in this single report, which occupies only two pages in *Comptes Rendus* (1932), Fabre and d'Arsonval described the first flow-through and perivascular electromagnetic flowmeters.

The electromagnetic blood flowmeter became a practical instrument as the result of simultaneous, but independent, studies by Kolin (1936, 1941, 1945, 1952; Kolin and Kado, 1959; Kolin et al., 1941) in the United States and Wetterer (1937, 1938) in Germany. Both men recognized that a blood vessel need not be opened to detect the flow-dependent voltage, and both placed "nonpolarizable" electrodes on the surface of the blood vessels and used strong constant-current (dc) electromagnets to obtain high-intensity magnetic fields. The voltage detected by the electrodes was found to be linearly proportional to blood flow velocity, and the polarity was dependent on the direction of flow, as predicted by theory. In their initial studies, both investigators used sensitive galvanometers to display the flow signal. With stable electrodes, high-quality recordings were obtained; an example of one of these (Fig. 6) was published by Wetterer, who placed his flow probe around the aorta of a 4.5-kg dog.

Elegantly simple as the dc electromagnetic flowmeter was, two serious problems delayed its widespread use. One problem was related to the size of the signal, which in practical situations lies in the microvolt range and demands the use of stable, high-sensitivity direct-coupled display devices. The second difficulty was related to electrode instability, manifested by slow changes in electrode–electrolyte potential with time. In addition, if current flowed through the electrodes, the electrode potential became even more unstable; in these early instruments, moreover, the indicators used to display the flow voltage were galvanometers that required current for their operation. These two problems conspired to make it difficult to specify the zero-flow point in the flow record.

When the electromagnetic flowmeter was first introduced, stable, high-gain direct-coupled (dc) voltage amplifiers were not generally available, although Wetterer had built one for use with his flowmeter. However, stable, high-gain alternating current amplifiers having a high input impedance were readily available, and Katz and Kolin (1938) connected an interrupter (driven by a 50-Hz tuning fork) to the electrode terminals of the dc electromagnetic flowmeter and amplified the resulting "chopped" flow signal using a conventional resistance–capacitance coupled ac amplifier. This technique permitted attaining high sensitivity and dramatically reduced the flow of current through the electrodes, thereby increasing stability.

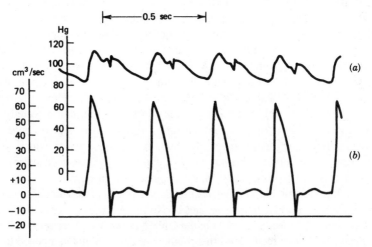

Figure 6 Recordings of (*a*) aortic blood pressure and (*b*) flow velocity in the aorta of a dog. [From E. Wetterer, *Z. Biol.* **99**:158–162 (1938). By permission.]

Sine Wave Flowmeters

A considerable advance in electromagnetic blood flowmeter technology was made by Kolin (1941), who used sinusoidal alternating current to excite the electromagnet applied to the blood vessel. The result was a mixed blessing, since now two sinusoidal voltages appeared across the electrode terminals. One voltage was large and independent of flow; the other was much smaller, and its amplitude was linearly proportional to flow velocity within the blood vessel; Fig. 7a illustrates these waveforms. Fortunately, these two voltages differ in phase by 90 degrees and can be separated. The large flow-independent signal, or "transformer voltage,"

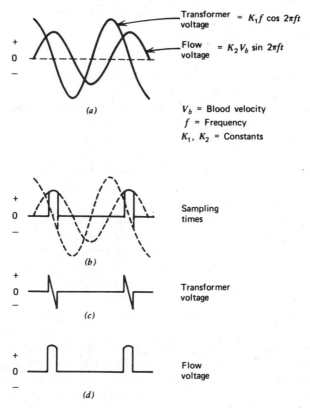

Transformer voltage $= K_1 f \cos 2\pi f t$

Flow voltage $= K_2 V_b \sin 2\pi f t$

(a)

V_b = Blood velocity
f = Frequency
K_1, K_2 = Constants

(b)   Sampling times

(c)   Transformer voltage

(d)   Flow voltage

Figure 7   Waveforms associated with the sine wave electromagnetic flowmeter. (a) Blood-flow-dependent voltage (which is in phase with the sinusoidally varying magnetic field) and the induced (transformer) voltage, which is independent of flow and 90 degrees out of phase with the flow voltage. (b) The technique of sampling the flow-dependent voltage during the period when it is maximum and while the transformer voltage is passing through zero. Over the sampling period the average value of the transformer voltage (c) is zero. The sampling technique is shown only for the positive phase of the flow signal (d); sampling could also be performed during the negative maximum of the flow signal. With this gating technique, the flow signal is recovered by synchronous detection and integration of the train of flow-dependent pulses.

results because the electrodes, the conducting path through the vessel, and the wires attached to the electrodes (Fig. 5) constitute a single-turn coil in the changing magnetic field; therefore, it has an induced voltage that is 90 degrees behind the magnetic field that produces it. The flow-dependent signal is also sinusoidal but is in phase with the magnetic field.

To remove the large flow-independent transformer voltage, Kolin (1941) developed a compensator that permitted subtraction of the transformer voltage, leaving only the flow-dependent sinusoidal voltage whose amplitude reflected the instantaneous blood flow velocity in the vessel.

The use of an alternating magnetic field yielded tremendous practical advantages. For example, since electrode–electrolyte potentials were not detected, ordinary metal electrodes could be applied directly to the unopened blood vessel, thereby reducing the overall size of the blood flow transducer. Also, because the desired flow-dependent signal was proportional to the amplitude of an alternating voltage, stable, high-gain, narrow-band ac amplifiers having a high input impedance could be used, thereby increasing the sensitivity and allowing measurement of blood flow in small vessels.

Two major improvements in the design of the sinusoidal electromagnetic flowmeter were made by Kolin and Kado (1959) and Westerstein et al. (1959). One improvement consisted of the use of higher frequency sinusoidal current (400 Hz) instead of 60 Hz to excite the electromagnet, thus providing about a 20-fold reduction in weight of the transducer and a shorter response time, which allowed faithful reproduction of phasic flow. The second improvement consisted of the use of an electronic gating technique that permitted detection of the flow-dependent signal only at the time when the transformer signal was passing through zero; this situation is diagramed in Figs. 7b–d. Thus the flow information is retrieved by continuously detecting the peak amplitude of the train of pulses, as in Fig. 7d. The amplitude of each pulse reflects blood flow velocity at that instant, and its polarity (with respect to the direction of the magnetic field) identifies forward or reverse flow.

Other improvements in the sine wave flowmeter were reported by Kolin (1945, 1952); these related to better methods of eliminating the transformer signal and improvements in the perivascular sleeve containing the electrodes. Of these many refinements it was the gating technique that permitted commercial production of the sine wave electromagnetic blood flowmeter. Most important, the problems solved during its long period of development were directly applicable to those encountered with its successors, the square wave and trapezoidal wave flowmeters.

Elimination of the bothersome large-amplitude, non-flow-related transformer voltage prompted development of the square and trapezoidal wave flowmeters. The magnitude of the transformer voltage depends on the rate of change of the magnetic field; therefore, with square wave excitation the transformer voltage is very large but lasts only a very short time (see Fig. 8); after this time only the flow-dependent voltage is present. Trapezoidal wave excitation produces a small transformer voltage, appearing only during the slopes of the trapezoid (see Fig. 10). During the flat part of the trapezoid, only the flow-dependent voltage is present. With both

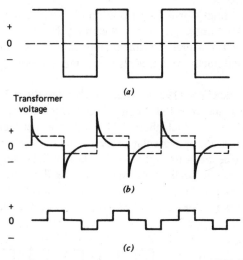

Transformer
voltage

Figure 8 Waveforms associated with the square wave electromagnetic blood flowmeter. (*a*) Magnetic field waveform. (*b*) Induced transformer voltage (produced by the reversal in direction of the magnetic field) and flow-dependent voltage (dashed), which is proportional to flow velocity and the strength of the magnetic field. By sampling the flow-dependent signal when the transformer voltage is absent, a train of pulses (*c*) is obtained; its amplitude is proportional to the flow velocity at that instant. The polarity of the pulses with respect to the direction of the magnetic field identifies with the direction of flow. Thus for unidirectional flow, a train of pulses of alternating polarity is obtained because the magnetic field alternates in direction. The flow signal is synthesized by synchronous detection of this pulse train.

the square wave and trapezoidal wave flowmeters, the flow-dependent signal is sampled only when the transformer voltage is zero.

Square Wave Flowmeters

The square wave electromagnetic flowmeter was developed by Denison et al. (1953), who employed a 30-Hz square wave to excite the magnet in the flow transducer. The flow-dependent voltage was sampled during the square wave after the transformer component had subsided, as in Fig. 8*b*. Choice of a 30-Hz frequency for magnet excitation meant that the response time was relatively long and only mean flow could be recorded. This limitation was removed by Denison and Spencer (1956), who used a square wave with a frequency of 240 Hz. These investigators made further improvements in the 240-Hz square wave flowmeter by sampling the flow signal during both the positive and negative portions of the square wave when only the flow signal was present; Fig. 8*c* illustrates the flow-dependent voltage. With this arrangement, phasic blood flow could be recorded by sampling at the rate of 480/sec, each sample lasting about 1.9 msec. Thus the blood flow velocity signal was synthesized by detecting only the flow-dependent pulses (of alternate polarity) by a demodulator that smoothed out the pulse train and inserted a small filler signal (dependent on the average flow during sampling) between the sampling times. Figure 9 reconstructs the blood flow velocity signal from the pulse train. The overall sinusoidal blood flow frequency response obtained was 0–50 Hz. Stated another way, a response time (10–90%) of about 10 msec was attained.

Moody and his associates (1972) developed an interesting version of the square wave flowmeter that incorporated automatic correction for zero flow. They employed a square wave in which there was an interval between the positive and negative phases when the perivascular probe excitation was turned off. Thus any potential appearing between the probe electrode terminals represented a no-flow signal, which was electronically subtracted from the flow signal by a high input impedance, direct-coupled, balanced amplifying system. To ensure that the zero-flow offset voltage would be as small as possible, recessed platinum black elec-

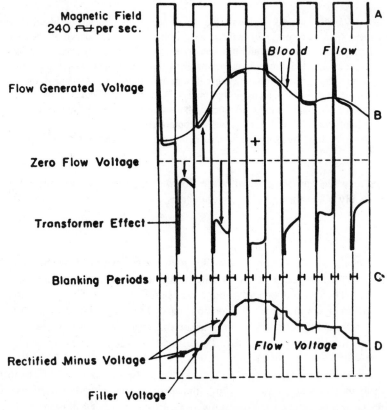

Figure 9 Synthesis of an arterial blood flow velocity wave by the square wave flowmeter. (A) The 240-Hz alternating square wave magnetic field; (B) voltage presented to the electrodes in the flow probe; (C) blanking periods (when sampling is not carried out); (D) synthesized flow signal using the timed sampling (gating) technique. [From M. P. Spencer and A. B. Denison, *IRE Trans. Med. Electron.* **ME-6:**220–227 (1959). By permission.]

trodes were coupled to the vessel by a short column of saline. The saline column could be established or flushed at any time by means of a catheter leading to a saline-filled syringe.

Single- and multiple-channel versions of this novel flowmeter were described. Because of the unique design, it is characterized by high stability and accuracy. The frequency response attainable is inversely related to the number of channels being sampled sequentially.

Trapezoidal Wave Flowmeters

The trapezoidal wave electromagnetic blood flowmeter was developed by Yanof (1961) and Yanof et al. (1963). The excitation current for its perivascular electromagnet provided a trapezoidal wave magnetic field (Fig. 10a) alternating with a frequency of 1000/sec. The transformer signal is generated only during the changing magnetic field, that is, during the sloping parts of the trapezoid, as in Fig. 10b.

During the top and bottom of the trapezoid, the magnetic field is constant and no transformer signal is induced. During this interval the voltage across the electrodes is sampled and the amplitude (Fig. 10c) is proportional to the velocity of

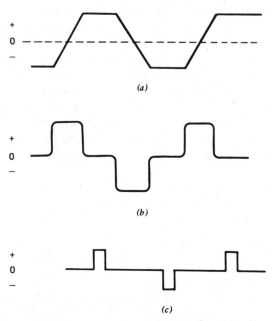

Figure 10 Waveforms associated with the trapezoidal wave flowmeter. (a) Waveform of the magnetic field; (b) curve indicating that the transformer (flow-independent) voltage occurs during the ramps of the trapezoid; (c) the sampled voltage, whose amplitude is dependent on flow velocity. The polarity of the flow voltage pulses in relation to the polarity of the magnetic field identifies the direction of flow. Synchronous detection of the pulse train provides a signal that describes the blood flow velocity.

the blood flow. In Yanof's instrument a sampling time of 0.174 msec was chosen; therefore the blood flow signal is sampled 2000 times per second with pulses 0.174 msec long. When this pulse train of alternately positive and negative pulses (for a unidirectional flow) is fed into a demodulating circuit, the peak amplitude of the train is recovered and represents the phasic blood flow in the vessel. Yanof (1961) estimated that this flowmeter had an overall sinusoidal frequency response (for blood flow) ranging from 0 to 250 Hz, which is certainly adequate to show the most rapid changes in flow encountered in the vascular systems of most mammals.

Commercially Available Electromagnetic Flowmeters

Commercially available electromagnetic blood flowmeters, almost irrespective of type, have an adequately short response time to allow faithful reproduction of the range of blood flow velocities encountered in large and small vessels in animals and humans. A study by Gessner and Bergel (1964) presented the hydraulic sinusoidal frequency response of two popular makes of flowmeters. The data indicated that the frequency response obtained hydraulically is essentially the same as that measured for the electronic amplifying channel. Bandwidths extending to beyond 15 Hz were measured.

The output voltage provided by an electromagnetic flow probe is linearly proportional to flow velocity; the actual volume flow must be computed by obtaining the average flow $\overline{V}_b$ and multiplying it by the cross-sectional area A of the flowing stream, as in Fig. 11.

Several important facts must be borne in mind in the practical application of the electromagnetic flowmeter. For example, to avoid detection of electrical interference, nearly all electromagnetic flowmeters require that the subject be grounded. It is important to recognize that there are two types of flow transducers, the flow-through and the perivascular. In the flow-through type (Fig. 12a), blood is caused to flow through a rigid plastic tube, which contains the electrodes and through which the magnetic field also passes. This type of transducer is usually employed

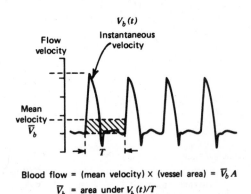

Blood flow = (mean velocity) × (vessel area) = $\overline{V}_b A$

$\overline{V}_b$ = area under $V_b(t)/T$

Figure 11   Method for computing average blood flow from a recording of instantaneous flow velocity $V_b(t)$.

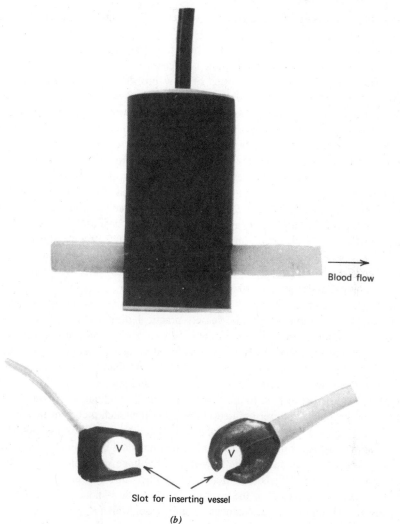

Blood flow

Slot for inserting vessel

(b)

Figure 12 Transducers (flow probes) for electromagnetic flowmeters; (a) flow-through type; (b) two perivascular probes (vessel occupies region V). (Courtesy of Carolina Medical Electronics, King, North Carolina.)

to measure large flows (e.g., the output of a heart–lung machine or cardiac bypass pump). Anticoagulants must be used because the blood comes into direct contact with plastic and metal surfaces. Since the diameter of the flow stream is known, simple processing of the transducer output voltage provides an accurate and linear display of volume flow per unit time. In addition, because the electrodes are in direct contact with the periphery of the flow stream, the flow velocity signal is immune to resistivity errors; that is, variations in hematocrit (percentage of red cells) do not alter the calibration, which is easily accomplished by pumping saline through the transducer into a graduated vessel and timing the collection with a stopwatch.

The perivascular flow probe illustrated in Fig. 12b is placed around an unopened blood vessel; therefore no anticoagulant is necessary. To measure blood flow in vessels of differing diameters, a series of flow probes must be available. With nearly all commercially available electromagnetic blood flowmeters, the electronic processing circuitry will accept the output from flow probes of all sizes, although probes are not necessarily interchangeable among instruments provided by different manufacturers. In deciding which probe size to use, the essential requirement is a snug fit with the vessel when short-term recordings are to be made; such a fit guarantees stable flow measurement. The probe size is identified by the circumference of the vessel to which the probe is to be applied. To obtain a snug fit, a probe size of about 10% less than the vessel circumference is recommended. When a flow probe is to be implanted, a slightly looser fit is desirable to allow for the tissue growth that always occurs in response to the presence of a foreign substance around the vessel. Adequacy of fit is also dependent on blood pressure. For example, with low blood pressure an artery is less distended; thus the probe fit may not be adequate, and a smaller size must be used.

Although the output voltage of a perivascular flow probe is linearly related to the flow velocity within the blood vessel, practical difficulties supervene when accurate calibration of the probe is desired. Since the electrodes are on the vessel surface, they are separated from the flow-induced voltage. Therefore, the voltage presented to the perivascular electrodes is slightly less than that developed within the vessel. Because the arterial wall consists of conducting tissue, the flow-induced voltage causes current to flow in the vessel wall and through any perivascular fluid that may be present. Wetterer pointed out in 1937 that such a current flows in the vessel wall. Figure 13a illustrates the pathways taken by these currents. Assuming either that perivascular fluid is not present or that its effect is eliminated by coating the vessel wall with mineral oil, the flow-induced voltage sends current around the vessel wall and through the bloodstream, as in Fig. 13b. The amount of current that flows depends directly on the magnitude of the flow-induced voltage E and inversely on the equivalent resistances of the vessel wall (R_V) and bloodstream (R); the latter in turn is dependent on the number of red cells in the blood, which is measured by the hematocrit (H), that is, the percentage of cells. Because the resistivity of blood increases almost exponentially with H, the voltage E' presented to the perivascular electrodes will decrease with increasing H; this is what is known as the "hematocrit error." Therefore, accurate flow calibration requires the in vivo timed collection of blood flowing through the vessel around which the flow probe is placed, or application of the flow probe to a vessel with the same dimensions and resistivity and the timed collection of flowing blood or saline with the same resistivity.

Roberts (1969) pointed out that the hematocrit error encountered with electromagnetic flowmeters is not entirely due to the conducting properties of the vessel wall. In a series of studies, using flowing blood of different hematocrits, he measured the true and indicated flows as a function of hematocrit, using several com-

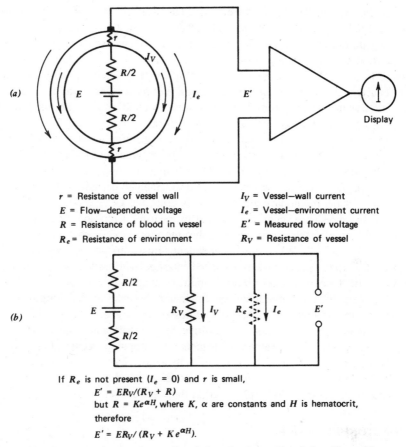

(a)

(b)

r = Resistance of vessel wall
E = Flow–dependent voltage
R = Resistance of blood in vessel
R_e = Resistance of environment

I_V = Vessel–wall current
I_e = Vessel–environment current
E' = Measured flow voltage
R_V = Resistance of vessel

Display

If R_e is not present (I_e = 0) and r is small,
$E' = ER_V/(R_V + R)$
but $R = Ke^{\alpha H}$, where K, α are constants and H is hematocrit,
therefore
$E' = ER_V/(R_V + Ke^{\alpha H})$.

Figure 13 Current pathways due to flow-induced voltage E and the effect of hematocrit H.

mercially available cannulated electromagnetic flowmeters. He found that all but one instrument tested exhibited a considerable underindication of flow with increasing hematocrit. The one that was relatively free from this error employed an amplifier input impedance of 100 MΩ; all the others had input impedances in the range of 10 to 50 kΩ. If future studies substantiate these findings, it would appear that the hematocrit error due to vessel-wall shunting may be quite small and that existing electromagnetic blood flowmeters can be improved by merely increasing the input impedance of the amplifier connected to the flow transducer.

From the foregoing discussion it can be seen that accurate calibration of perivascular flow probes is difficult. At present, a variety of techniques are used to obtain reasonably accurate flow calibrations. Some investigators perform calibrations using preserved vessels or gut with dimensions comparable to those of the blood vessel in which the in vivo measurements were carried out. Some use blood as the calibrating solution; others use saline having the same resistivity as blood at body temperature. The technique employed is dictated by the type of information required from the flow measurement. If accurate volume–flow information is desired, a calibration procedure that duplicates the in vivo situation is necessary. However, if only changes in flow are of interest, calibration is often superfluous because flow changes are linearly indicated by electromagnetic blood flowmeters.

In conclusion, one very important practical fact must be noted in using electromagnetic flowmeters—the zero flow point must be established. With many instruments this point can be obtained only by cross-clamping the vessel distal to the flow probe. In newer instruments, in which the transformer voltage has been adequately eliminated, turning off the magnetic field provides a method of establishing an output from the flowmeter that corresponds to zero flow.

Electromagnetic blood flowmeters vary considerably in design. With some, when a periaortic or peripulmonary artery probe is used, the ECG is detected. In some cases, if the impedance technique is used to measure a physiological event on a subject with an electromagnetic flow probe, the impedance carrier interferes with the blood flow signal. When two independent flowmeters are applied to a single subject, the probe excitation carriers often interfere with each other, resulting in artifacts in both flowmeter recordings. If multiple-channel flow recording is desired, it is necessary to use a multichannel flowmeter, because in the design of such instruments the interference problem is addressed and solved.

Electromagnetic flowmeters are sensitive to external radiofrequency interference. Electrosurgical and diathermy currents are particularly devastating. In fact, if such a current is applied to a subject with a flow probe, there is the risk of current flowing to ground through the electrodes in the flow probe. If the current density is high, lesions can be produced at the electrode sites.

MAGNETORHEOGRAPHY

The method of detecting blood flow within the body or an appendage by passing a strong magnetic field through the body and using surface or needle electrodes to detect the flow voltage has been designated "magnetorheography" (MRG) by Okai et al. (1967). Kolin et al. (1941) described what must be credited as the first study in this area. He applied a sleeve containing two electrodes to a blood vessel and then closed the skin and brought the leads out through a small incision. When blood flow in the vessel was to be recorded, the electrodes were connected to the amplifying-display device and a strong magnetic field was passed through the member containing the perivascular electrode assembly. The first successful demonstration of the method using body-surface electrodes was reported by Togawa et al. (1967), who passed a strong constant magnetic field [10,000 gauss (G)] through a rabbit in the chest-to-back direction and detected a blood-flow-dependent voltage with electrodes on the forelimbs (lead I). Although large-amplitude ECG artifacts were present, the flow signal was confirmed by reversal of the direction of the magnetic field. Okai et al. (1967) applied the method to the human thorax with much more success using a field strength of 7000 G and electrodes on the thorax. Later Okai et al. (1971) applied the method to the femoral region of an anesthetized dog (see Fig. 14a). Using a field strength of 10,000 G, they verified the accuracy

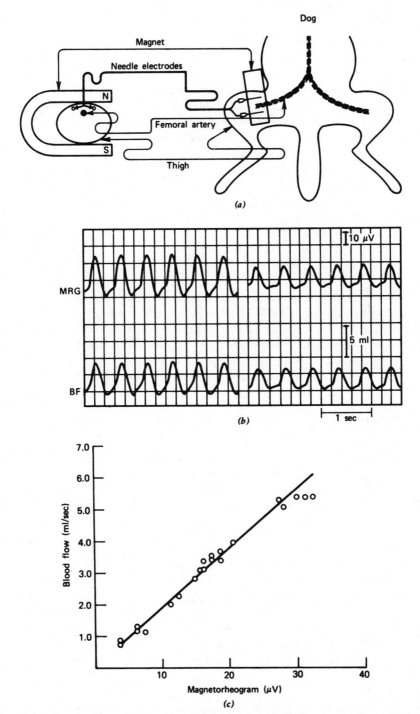

Figure 14 Magnetorheography: (*a*) application of the method to detect flow in the femoral artery of a dog; (*b*) comparison of flow signal with that obtained with an electromagnetic flowmeter; (*c*) flow-voltage relationship for this application. [From O. Okai et al., *J. Appl. Physiol.* **30**:564–566 (1971). By permission.]

of their recordings by measuring blood flow in the same artery using an electromagnetic flowmeter. Flow changes, induced by the intravenous injection of norepinephrine, were displayed equally well by the magnetorheogram and electromagnetic flowmeter recording, as in Figs. 14b and c.

There are several important considerations in the use of magnetorheography to record blood flow. For example, the electrodes detect signals due to all fluid flow in the magnetic field; that is, both venous and arterial flow components are present. By and large, arterial flow velocity is much more rapid than venous flow and therefore dominates the signal. Because the blood flow voltage is very small, the recording instruments used to date have not been direct-coupled; therefore, only pulsatile flow has been measured with resistance–capacitance coupled systems having time constants of several seconds. The small flow voltage also favors the detection of bioelectric events such as the ECG and skeletal muscle action potentials, which are difficult to eliminate by filtering because their frequency spectrum is so similar to that of the flow signal. However, cancellation by electronic subtraction may be feasible when the ECG is the interfering signal.

Many of the difficulties encountered with constant magnetic fields can be eliminated by using alternating fields; however, this technique presents problems similar to those associated with the development of the perivascular electromagnetic blood flowmeter. One difficulty—not experienced yet with electromagnetic blood flowmeters because the magnetic field intensity is so low—may arise when high-intensity alternating fields are used for magnetorheography. The alternating voltage induced in the body tissues and electrolytes will cause alternating current to flow and may cause stimulation or tissue heating, which in turn may alter local blood flow. Therefore, when alternating fields are employed, care must be exercised to choose a field intensity low enough to exclude these effects.

It is of more than passing interest to note that a high-intensity constant magnetic field is used in magnetic resonance imaging. If nonmetallic electrodes and cables are used, the aortic blood flow signal can be detected by electrodes placed to detect the ECG. To date, the optimum placement of electrodes to minimize the ECG and maximize the blood flow signal has not been ascertained.

MAGNETOSTRICTIVE TISSUE FRAGMENTER

Magnetostriction is the term used to describe the change in dimension produced by the application of a magnetic field to magnetically permeable materials. The phenomenon is important in iron, nickel, and cobalt and in many of their compounds. A typical dimension change per unit length (strain) in ferromagnetic materials is on the order of 10^{-5}, although materials are available with strains 10 to 100 times this value. The magnetostrictive strain coefficient has three-dimensional components.

The dimensional change is usually produced by a current flowing in a coil that surrounds the magnetostrictive material. A pulse of current will produce a magnetic field that induces the strain; the elastic behavior of the material results in a damped oscillation, the frequency of which depends on the mass and elasticity of the magnetostrictive material. Usually the frequency is in the low ultrasonic range. By the use of appropriate feedback and a power oscillator, sustained sinusoidal oscillations can be produced. Such magnetostrictive generators usually consist of nickel rods or tubes and are used for underwater communication and echo location.

It has been found that a probe vibrating at low ultrasonic frequencies causes fragmentation of cells with a high water content, sparing elastic and collagen fibers.

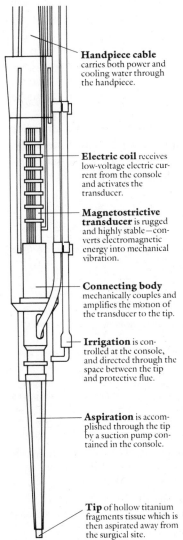

Handpiece cable carries both power and cooling water through the handpiece.

Electric coil receives low-voltage electric current from the console and activates the transducer.

Magnetostrictive transducer is rugged and highly stable—converts electromagnetic energy into mechanical vibration.

Connecting body mechanically couples and amplifies the motion of the transducer to the tip.

Irrigation is controlled at the console, and directed through the space between the tip and protective flue.

Aspiration is accomplished through the tip by a suction pump contained in the console.

Tip of hollow titanium fragments tissue which is then aspirated away from the surgical site.

Figure 15 The CUSA tissue-fragmenting ultrasonic probe. (Courtesy of Cooper Medical, Mountain View, California.)

The mechanism of destruction is believed to be produced, in part, by cavitation. Therefore, such a probe is of value in stripping the mucosal layer from internal organs such as the rectum, intestine, and bladder. A vibrating probe for this purpose is shown in Fig. 15 (CUSA, Cooper Medical, Mountain View, California). The hollow titanium tip is coupled to the magnetostrictive laminated nickel–iron element surrounded by a coil connected to a 23-kHz power supply. Irrigating fluid is forced through the hollow vibrating tube, and the tissue debris and irrigating fluid are aspirated through the tube surrounding the vibrating probe. The amplitude of motion of the probe tip is 100–300 μm, and the region of tissue fragmented is within a radius of 1–2 mm from the probe tip. Aspiratory suctions of 0–24 in. Hg are selectable. The handle, which is 2.1 cm in diameter, provides tactile feedback to aid the surgeon in controlling the rate of tissue fragmentation. Water circulates within the handle to keep the 75-W magnetostrictive element cool.

Although ultrasonic probes were first used to remove dental plaque, they see much wider use, particularly in neurosurgery for tumor destruction (Flamm et al., 1978; Hodgson, 1978). As stated previously, the ultrasonic fragmenter is used for stripping mucosal layers. It is also excellent for exposing vessels in highly vascular tissue such as the liver.

The use of controlled ultrasound for selective tissue destruction has an analog in electrosurgery, in which radiofrequency current destroys the tissue thermally. The ultrasonic probe may provide an advantage in those cases when bioelectric recordings are made, which is not possible during electrosurgery.

REFERENCES

Benjamin, F. B., E. Mastrogiovanni, and W. Helveig. 1962. Bloodless method of continuous recording of pulse pressure in man. *J. Appl. Physiol.* **17**:844.

Boshes, F. 1966. Measurement of tremor. *J. Neurosurg., Suppl.* **1**:324–330.

Denison, A. B., and M. B. Spencer. 1956. Square-wave electromagnetic flowmeter design. *Rev. Sci. Instrum.* **27**:707–711.

Denison, A. B., M. P. Spencer, and H. D. Green. 1953. Square wave electromagnetic flowmeter for application to intact blood vessels. *Circ. Res.* **3**:39–46.

Erdos, E. G., V. Jackman, and W. C. Barnes. 1962. Instrument for recording isotonic contractions of smooth muscles. *J. Appl. Physiol.* **17**:307–308.

Fabre, P., and A. d'Arsonval. 1932. Utilisation des forces électromotrices d'induction pour énregistrement des variations de vitesse des liquides conducteurs: Un nouvel hemodromographe sans palette dans le sang. *C. R. Hebd. Seances Acad. Sci.* **194**:1097–1089.

Faraday, M. 1832. Experimental researches in electricity. *Philos. Trans. R. Soc. London* **122**:125–194.

Flamm, E. S., J. Ransohoff, D. Wuchinich, and A. Broadwin. 1978. Preliminary experience with ultrasonic aspiration in neurosurgery. *Neurosurgery* **2**(3):240–245.

Fuller, J. T., and T. M. Gordon. 1948. The radio inductograph. *Science* **108**:287–288.

Gauer, O. H., and E. Gienapp. 1950. A miniature pressure-recording device. *Science* **112**:404–405.

Gessner, U., and D. Bergel. 1964. Frequency response of electromagnetic flowmeters. *J. Appl. Physiol.* **19**:1209–1211.

Gow, B. S. 1966. An electrical caliper for measurement of pulsatile arterial diameter changes *in vivo*. *J. Appl. Physiol.* **21:**1122–1126.

Heath, J. H. 1958. The differential transformer as a sensitive measuring device. *Electron. Eng.* **30:**631–633.

Hodgson, J. B. 1978. The ultrasonic scalpel. *Bull. N.Y. Acad. Med.* (Ser. 2) **65**(10):908–915.

Katz, L. N., and A. Kolin. 1938. The flow of blood in the carotid artery of the dog under various circumstances as determined with the electromagnetic flowmeter. *Am. J. Physiol.* **122:**788–804.

Kolin, A. 1936. An electromagnetic flowmeter. *Proc. Soc. Exp. Biol. Med.* **35:**53–56.

Kolin, A. 1941. An AC induction flow meter for measurement of blood flow in intact blood vessels. *Proc. Soc. Exp. Biol. Med.* **46:**235–239.

Kolin, A. 1945. An alternating field induction flow meter of high sensitivity. *Rev. Sci. Instrum.* **16:**109–116.

Kolin, A. 1952. Improved apparatus and technique for electromagnetic determination of blood flow. *Rev. Sci. Instrum.* **23:**235–243.

Kolin, A., and R. Kado. 1959. Miniaturization of the electromagnetic blood flowmeter and its use for the recording of circulatory responses of conscious animals to sensory stimuli. *Proc. Natl. Acad. Sci. U.S.A.* **45:**1312–1321.

Kolin, A., J. L. Weissberg, and L. Gerber. 1941. Electromagnetic measurement of blood flow and sphygmomanometry in the intact animal. *Proc. Soc. Exp. Biol. Med.* **47:**323–329.

Moody, N. F., D. L. Morrison, B. C. deKat, J. D. Henderson, A. M. Rappaport, and S. J. Lipton. 1972. *A Four-channel Pulsed-field Electromagnetic Blood Flowmeter System*, Dig. Pap. Canadian Medical & Biological Engineering Society, Winnipeg, Manitoba, Canada.

Motley, H. L., A. Cournand, L. Werko, D. Dresdale, A. Himmelstein, and D. W. Richards. 1947. Intravascular and intracardiac pressure recording in man: Electrical apparatus compared with the Hamilton manometer. *Proc. Soc. Exp. Biol. Med.* **64:**241–244.

Müller, A., L. Laszt, and L. Pircher. 1948. Über ein Manometer mit elektrischer Transmission zur Druck und Geschwindigkeitmessung. *Helv. Physiol. Acta* **6:**783–794.

Okai, O., T. Togawa, and M. Oshima. 1967. Magnetorheography. Observation of blood flow emf in static magnetic field by surface electrodes. *Dig. 7th Int. Conf. Med. Biol. Eng.* Paper 13-3.

Okai, O., T. Togawa, and M. Oshima. 1971. Magnetorheography: Nonbleeding measurement of blood flow. *J. Appl. Physiol.* **30:**564–566.

Pieper, H. P. 1958. Registration of phasic changes of blood flow by means of a catheter type flowmeter. *Rev. Sci. Instrum.* **29:**965–967.

Roberts, V. C. 1969. Haematocrit variations and electromagnetic flowmeter sensitivity. *Biomed. Eng.* **4:**408–412.

Rushmer, R. F. 1954a. Heart size and stroke volume. *Minn. Med.* **37:**19–29.

Rushmer, R. F. 1954b. Continuous measurements of left ventricular dimensions in intact unanesthetized dogs. *Circ. Res.* **2:**14–21.

Sackner, M. A. 1984. U.S. Patent 4,452,252, June 5.

Schaevitz, H. *Engineering Bulletin*, A2 and R38. Schaevitz Co., Camden, NJ.

Schaevitz, H. 1947. The linear variable differential transformer. *Proc. Soc. Stress Anal.* **4:**79–88.

Schafer, P. W., and H. W. Shirer. 1949. An impedance gauging system for measurement of biologic pressure variables. *Surgery* **26:**446–451.

Scher, A. M., T. H. Weigert, and A. C. Young. 1953. Compact flowmeters for use in the unanesthetized animal, an electronic version of Chauveau's hemodrometer. *Science* **118:**82–84.

Spencer, M. P., and A. B. Denison. 1959. The square wave electromagnetic flowmeter: Theory of operation and design of magnet probes for clinical and experimental applications. *IRE Trans. Med. Electron.* **ME-6:**220–227.

Togawa, T., O. Okai, and M. Oshima. 1967. Observation of blood flow emf in externally applied strong magnetic field by surface electrodes. *Med. Biol. Eng.* **5:**169–170.

Tucker, M. J. 1952. A linear transducer for the electrical measurement of displacement. *Electron. Eng.* **24:**420–422.

Westerstein, A., G. Herrold, E. Abbott, and N. S. Assali. 1959. Gated sine wave electromagnetic flowmeter. *IRE Trans. Med. Electron.* **ME-6:**312–316.

Wetterer, E. 1937, 1938. Eine neue Methode zur Registrierung der Blutstromungsgeschwindegkeit am uneröffneter Gefass. *Z. Biol.* **98:**26–36, 1938, **99:**162.

Wetterer, E. 1943. Eine neue manometrische Sonde mit elektrischer Transmission. *Z. Biol.* **101:**333–350.

Wheeler, H. A. 1928. Simple inductance formulas for radio coils. *Proc. IRE* **16:**1398–1400.

Yanof, H. M. 1961. A trapezoidal-wave electromagnetic blood flowmeter. *J. Appl. Physiol.* **16:**566–570.

Yanof, H. M., A. L. Rosen, and W. C. Shoemaker. 1963. Design of an unplantable flowmeter transducer based on the Helmholtz coil. *J. Appl. Physiol.* **18:**227–230.

Young, F. B., H. Gerrand, and W. Jevous. 1920. Electrical disturbances due to tides and waves. *Philos. Mag.* (Ser. 6) **40:**149–159.

4

Capacitive Transducers

SIMPLE CAPACITORS

A capacitor or condenser consists of two conducting surfaces separated by an insulator (dielectric), which can be solid, liquid, gaseous, or a vacuum. The capacitance is measured in farads. The magnitude of the capacitance depends on the nature of the dielectric and varies directly with the area of the conducting surfaces and inversely with their separation. The capacitance can be altered by changing any of these three factors.

A typical parallel-plate capacitor has identical plates, each of area A cm^2, which are separated by a distance d cm; between them is placed a material of dielectric constant K. The capacitance is given by

$$C_{pF} = 0.0885 \frac{A}{d} K.$$

Because the dielectric constant of air is only very slightly higher than that of a vacuum, K can be given the value of unity for air capacitors. Thus a practical figure for rapid calculation of the capacitance of an air capacitor can be derived. A capacitor consisting of two plates 1 cm^2 in area separated by 1 mm has a capacitance of 0.885 pF, that is, slightly less than 1 pF. In nonmetric dimensions, a capacitor having plates 1 in.^{2} in area separated by 0.1 in. exhibits a capacitance of 2.17 pF, or slightly more than 2 pF. Although the equation for a parallel-plate capacitor indicates that the capacitance varies inversely with the distance between plates, this relationship holds only for distances that are small in comparison to the size of the plates. If the separation between the plates is large compared to their size, the capacitance–distance relationship deviates from that of a hyperbola.

CAPACITOR CONFIGURATIONS

In addition to the well-known parallel-plate capacitor, it is possible to construct variable capacitors having a variety of shapes. Foldvari and Lion (1964), pioneers in the use of capacitance for transduction, presented a compilation of useful configurations; Fig. 1 summarizes some of these.

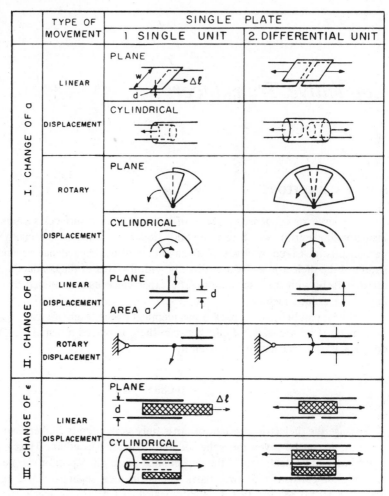

TYPE OF MOVEMENT		SINGLE PLATE	
		1 SINGLE UNIT	2. DIFFERENTIAL UNIT
I. CHANGE OF a	LINEAR DISPLACEMENT	PLANE	
		CYLINDRICAL	
	ROTARY DISPLACEMENT	PLANE	
		CYLINDRICAL	
II. CHANGE OF d	LINEAR DISPLACEMENT	PLANE AREA a	
	ROTARY DISPLACEMENT		
III. CHANGE OF ε	LINEAR DISPLACEMENT	PLANE	
		CYLINDRICAL	

Figure 1   Synopsis of capacitive displacement transducers. [From T. Foldvari and K. Lion, *Instrum. Control Syst.* **37**:77–85 (1964).]

CAPACITANCE-MEASURING CIRCUITS

Series Circuit

Alternating current is usually employed to obtain a signal that reflects the value of a capacitance. Depending on the application, the voltage proportional to the static value of the capacitance is often disregarded, and only the change is processed for ultimate reproduction. This method is illustrated in Fig. 2a. In this circuit the capacitance transducer is in series with a large resistance R. A small change in capacitance will produce a proportional change in the voltage across the capacitor and resistor.

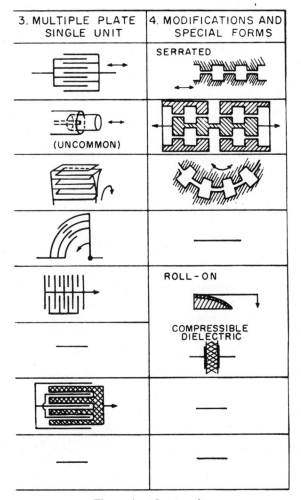

3. MULTIPLE PLATE SINGLE UNIT	4. MODIFICATIONS AND SPECIAL FORMS

Figure 1   (*Continued*)

Bridge Circuit

A more convenient method of employing capacitance involves placing the capacitance transducer in a bridge circuit as shown in Fig. 2*b*. Frequently it is possible to create a differential capacitance transducer, the two halves being placed in adjacent arms of a bridge. The event being detected is caused to increase the capacitance of one side of the bridge and to decrease that of the other side. When this method is employed, the output signal is twice that obtainable by varying one capacitive element. This technique is characterized by a high degree of temperature stability.

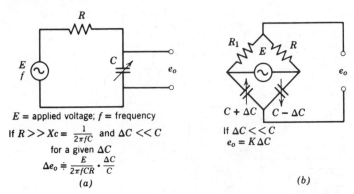

R

E
f

C

e_o

R_1 E R

e_o

$C + \Delta C$ $C - \Delta C$

E = applied voltage; f = frequency

If $R >> Xc = \dfrac{1}{2\pi fC}$ and $\Delta C << C$

for a given ΔC

$\Delta e_o \doteq \dfrac{E}{2\pi fCR} \cdot \dfrac{\Delta C}{C}$

(a)

If $\Delta C << C$
$e_o = K\Delta C$

(b)

Figure 2   Capacitive transducer circuits: (a) series circuit; (b) bridge circuit.

When capacitance transducers are employed in bridge circuits, either of two methods can be used to obtain direction sensitivity. Either the bridge is operated slightly off balance or a phase-sensitive detector is employed. With the first method the output of the bridge increases or decreases with a change in capacitance. The amount of initial imbalance chosen is dictated by the maximum expected change in C required to drive the bridge toward the balance point. With a phase-sensitive detector, direction sensitivity on either side of the balance is automatically obtained.

Resonant Circuit

Occasionally a single-element capacitive transducer is placed across a tuned circuit, which is detuned by the change in capacitance, thereby causing a current change in the associated circuitry. Sometimes the tuned circuit constitutes the frequency-determining component in an oscillator. A change in the capacitance of the transducer alters the frequency of the oscillator, giving rise to a frequency-modulated signal that is detected and displayed with the aid of appropriate circuitry.

Diode Twin-T Circuit

An ingenious method of employing the capacitance method has been described by Lion (1964). He pointed out that in a bridge circuit either the transducer or the oscillator must be operated above ground potential and that meeting this requirement frequently presents difficulties, surmountable only by the addition of special components and circuits. Instead of a bridge circuit he proposed the use of the diode twin-T circuit shown in Fig. 3. With this circuit configuration, one side of the oscillator, transducing capacitor, and output signal are all at the same potential, which can be ground.

In Lion's circuit, S is a radiofrequency oscillator producing sine or square waves of an amplitude E_i. During the positive half-cycle, diode D_1 conducts and charges C_1. During the next negative half-cycle, D_1 does not conduct, and C_1 discharges through R_1 and R_L and also through R_2 and D_2. Similarly, during the first positive

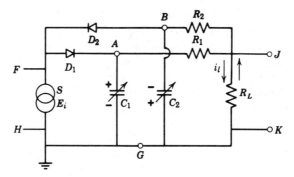

Figure 3 Diode twin-T circuit.

half-cycle, D_2 does not conduct; but during the second negative half-cycle, D_2 conducts and charges C_2. During the following half-cycle, C_2 discharges through R_2 and R_L and also through R_1 and D_1. If diodes D_1 and D_2 are identical, $C_1 = C_2$ and $R_1 = R_2$, the currents through R_1 and R_2 are equal in magnitude and opposite in sign, and when flowing through R_L, the output circuit, the net current is zero. Any variation in C_1 and C_2 causes current to flow through R_L, the load, which can be a resistor or a direct-reading microammeter. If display by a rapidly responding recorder is desired, the voltage across R_L can be amplified and displayed appropriately.

Lion (1964) and Foldvari and Lion (1964) gave the following expression, in which $R = R_1 = R_2$, for the current through R_L:

$$I = E_i \frac{R + 2R_L}{(R + R_L)^2} Rf(C_1 - C_2 - C_1 e^{-k_1} + C_2 e^{-k_2}),$$

where

$$k_1 = \frac{R + R_L}{2RfC_1(R + 2R_L)} \quad \text{and} \quad k_2 = \frac{R + R_L}{2RfC_2(R + 2R_L)}.$$

Maximum sensitivity of the circuit occurs when $1/k_1 = 1/k_2 = 0.57$. In commercially available transducers (Lion Research Corp., Cambridge, Massachusetts) consisting of a two-plate capacitor with a separation of 0.005 in., a sensitivity on the order of 1000 V/in. can be obtained.

The output impedance of the diode twin-T circuit is determined by the choice of R_1 and R_2 and is virtually independent of C_1 and C_2. By suitable choice of R_1 and R_2 an output impedance of 1–100 kΩ can be obtained. Optimum selection of these components will permit display of the capacitance change with a microammeter. If the output is to be displayed by means of a rapidly responding indicator, the rise time available is also dependent on the load resistance R_L and the oscillator frequency. With an R_L of 1000 Ω and an oscillator frequency of 1.3 MHz, for an instantaneous change in capacitance a rise time of 20 μsec is attainable.

Foldvari and Lion (1964) called attention to some of the highly desirable characteristics of their interesting circuit. Because the diodes operate at high level and in the linear portion of their characteristic, selection of matched diodes is not necessary. Another attractive feature is that changes in oscillator frequency do not adversely affect the sensitivity of the circuit; for example, a 10% change in frequency results in only a 1% alteration in sensitivity to capacitance change. Extremely desirable also is the remarkably high output. For example, with 46 V (rms sinusoidal) for E_i at a frequency of 1.3 MHz, a capacitance change from -7 to $+7$ pF produces an output of -5 to $+5$ V across a 1-MΩ load (R_L).

BIOMEDICAL APPLICATIONS

The capacitance method has been applied to the measurement of many physiological events, particularly the determination of blood pressure, since the late 1930s. This transducer was developed because higher fidelity and sensitivity were needed than were available from optical manometers, which had been perfected to a remarkably high degree by reducing mass, increasing stiffness, and recovering the lost sensitivity by increasing the distance to the photographic recording surface. The practical inconvenience of the optical methods was a major factor in stimulating the application of electrical transduction systems.

In applying the capacitance method to measure blood pressure, an elastic member exposed to blood pressure constitutes one plate of the capacitor; the other plate is nearby and fixed. For high sensitivity each investigator has placed the distensible plate as close as possible to the fixed plate. To obtain a rapid response time, the elastic member is made as small and as stiff as possible. This combination guarantees that only a small amount of fluid will be displaced when pressure is applied. The displacement is usually expressed in terms of cubic millimeters of fluid entering the transducer per 100 mmHg of applied pressure. In practical terms this figure describes the ability of the transducer to measure transient pressure changes applied to interconnecting catheters and needles. Transducers having low-volume displacement figures can be employed to record faithfully pressure transients with small-bore interconnecting tubing.

Schutz (1937) appears to have been one of the first to use the capacitance method to measure blood pressure. In his transducer the elastic member was a silvered glass membrane. The smallness and stiffness of the membrane he employed produced a natural frequency of 207 Hz. Following his lead, many other investigators constructed pressure transducers. Among these were Lilly (1942), Frommer (1943), Buchtal and Warburg (1943), and Hansen and Warburg (1947). In all these transducers the elastic members were small and stiff, providing a short response time and a small volume displacement. In all, the fixed and movable plates were in very close proximity. Ratios of area to separation varying from 10 to 10,000 have been employed.

One manufacturer (Hewlett-Packard) provides a pressure transducer in which the elastic member deflected by blood pressure is a quartz diaphragm coated with

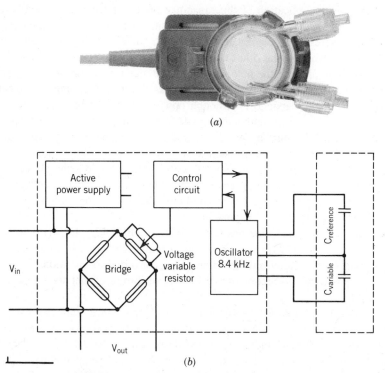

(a)

(b)

Figure 4 (*a*) The HP-1290 quartz diaphragm capacitive pressure transducer and (*b*) a block diagram of the circuit used with it. (Courtesy Hewlett-Packard Co., Waltham, Massachusetts.)

a conducting film that forms the moving electrode of the capacitor; Fig. 4*a* illustrates the device, and Fig. 4*b* is a block diagram of the circuit used with it. The application of pressure to the quartz diaphragm increases the capacitance, which is measured using an 8.4-kHz carrier. A reference capacitor in the transducer is used to provide temperature stability. The capacitance-change signal is caused to vary the resistance of one element in a resistive bridge circuit. The bridge is unbalanced by the application of pressure to the quartz diaphragm. Viewed from the output terminals, the device simulates a strain gauge bridge, the output impedance of which is 400 Ω.

The performance characteristics of the quartz capacitive pressure transducer are very good. The dynamic range is −30 to +300 mmHg, with a maximum range of −400 to +4000 mmHg. The output is 5 μV/mmHg per volt of excitation; typically 5–10 V (dc) is used to drive the transducer. The volume displacement is 0.2 mm^3/100 mmHg. The leakage current is low, being less than 5 μA for the application of 120 V, 60 Hz to a fluid-filled catheter connected to the disposable dome. The high-voltage breakdown is 16,000 V, to accommodate defibrillation voltages.

An interesting application of the capacitive method to measure blood pressure is due to Beyne and Gougerot (1939), who converted the height of mercury in a U-tube manometer to an electrical signal. One "plate" of the capacitor was the mercury itself, whereas the other consisted of tinfoil wrapped around the outside of the glass tube forming the manometer. As the mercury column rose, the capacitance between the mercury and the tinfoil increased, causing a change in the current flowing through the capacitor. Although application of the principle in no way improved the fidelity of the manometer, it permitted remote location of the pressure-indicating device. The fluid in such a manometer need not be mercury. Any solution of lower specific gravity can be used to produce a sensitive manometer or fluid-level transducer. Beyne and Gougerot (1939) used the same principle to convert small air-pressure changes in the respiratory system of a dog to an electrical signal by fitting the diaphragm of a Marey tambour with an electrode of tinfoil, which became the movable plate of a capacitor.

The condenser microphone has seen service in physiology for the detection of heart sounds. Asher (1932) recognized its potential and used it to detect human heart sounds, which, after amplification, were converted to variations in light intensity. A photographic record of the light beam produced phonocardiograms of high fidelity.

Luft (1943) and Liston (1950) employed a capacitance transducer to detect infrared radiation to create a gaseous carbon dioxide analyzer. Gaseous carbon dioxide absorbs infrared radiation at 15, 4.26, 2.77, and 2.69 μm. Therefore, radiant energy at any one or all of these wavelengths will be attenuated on passing through a gas sample containing CO_2. Measurement of the incident and emergent infrared energy will allow quantification of the concentration of CO_2 in the gas sample.

The manner in which the infrared-absorption principle is employed to measure the concentration of CO_2 in a sample of gas is shown in Fig. 5. A broad-band radiator emits infrared radiation, which was reflected from two front-surfaced mirrors. One of the two beams passed directly into a reference chamber (R). The other beam reached another chamber (S) after passing through a sampling chamber (C) that contains the gas to be analyzed for its CO_2 content. Very close to the diaphragm were two plate electrodes (P_1 and P_2), which, with the intervening diaphragm (d), constituted a differential capacitor. With no CO_2 in the sample cell C, the amounts of infrared radiation entering the measuring (S) and reference (R) chambers are the same. Since both chambers contain CO_2, which absorbs infrared energy, the temperature will rise equally, and therefore the pressure will rise equally in each chamber. Because the rise in pressure is the same in each chamber, the elastic diaphragm between them will not be deflected, and the capacitance measured between terminals 1 and 2 and between 2 and 3 will not be altered.

If a gas sample containing CO_2 is admitted to the sample cell C, the intensity of the emerging infrared energy will be less and the pressure rise in the measuring chamber S will be less than that in the reference chamber R. The elastic diaphragm will be deflected toward the measuring chamber S, thereby increasing the capacitance by an amount that is dependent on the concentration of CO_2 in the sample cell C.

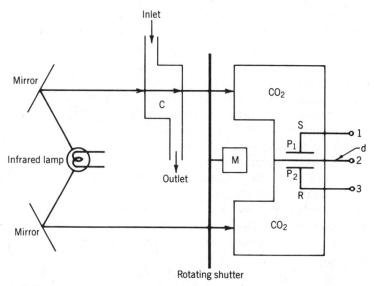

Figure 5 Principle employed in the Luft instrument to measure gaseous CO_2. 1, 2, and 3 constitute a differential capacitor; d is the diaphragm; M is the motor.

The infrared radiation that enters both chambers is interrupted by a shutter that is rotated by a motor. In this way, each chamber receives only a pulse of infrared energy, and there are only short-duration pulsatile changes in pressure in the chambers. With gas containing CO_2 in the sampling cell C, the pulses of pressure in the measuring chamber are of smaller magnitude than those in the reference chamber. Therefore there will be a pulsatile differential change in capacitance measured between terminals 1 and 2 and between 2 and 3.

A tiny hole was placed in the elastic diaphragm to equalize pressure over a long period. The leak through this tiny hole is so small that pressure does not become equalized between pulses of pressure. The pulsatile change in capacitance produces a voltage that is enlarged by a narrow-band amplifier. The amplified peak voltage is displayed on a meter calibrated in percent CO_2. An output is also provided for graphic recording.

In a typical infrared CO_2 analyzer, the gas to be analyzed for its CO_2 concentration is drawn into the sample chamber by a small aspirator pump. In some models the sample cell is larger and permits a continuous flow with low resistance, allowing the detector to be placed in series with the airway.

Because other gaseous compounds absorb infared energy and may be present in samples containing the CO_2 to be measured, the effect of these contaminating gases can be eliminated or reduced by "negative" filtering. This technique requires two optically similar gas-containing cells, one in each infrared beam ahead of the sample cell. If these filter cells are filled with a contaminating gas (or gases), equal amounts of infrared energy will be absorbed from each beam at the absorption wavelengths of the interfering gas. The remaining infrared energy is then passed on through the system as described previously. It is obvious that if negative filtering is used the absorption wavelengths of the interfering gas (or gases) must not completely overlap those of CO_2. The absorption of infrared energy is not a linear function of the amount of CO_2 in the sample, so linearizing networks are required in the amplifier to provide a linear percent CO_2 scale.

The response time of the infrared CO_2 analyzer is dependent on the speed with which the gas sample can be admitted to the sampling chamber and the response time of the detecting system in the analyzer. The latter is limited by the interruption rate of the rotating shutter. Response times (0–90%) on the order of 0.1 sec are attainable for the detecting system.

The CO_2 signal is calibrated in percent CO_2. Calibration is carried out using bottled gases of known concentrations of CO_2 in nitrogen or other diluent gases that will not absorb infrared energy.

When measuring respiratory gases, pCO_2 is the quantity desired, and it is necessary to convert percent CO_2 to pCO_2, and to include the correction for water vapor pressure at the temperature of measurement (see the section Respiratory Gases in Chap. 8).

Adams et al. (1960) described a miniature capacitance microphone that they used as a high-fidelity pulse pickup. This device consisted of a small chamber containing a fixed electrode. Covering the chamber (and a short distance from the fixed electrode) was a metallized mylar film, which constituted the other plate of the capacitor. In use the device was placed with the mylar film applied to the skin over a pulsating vessel. The film tracked the skin motion and thereby modulated the capacitance. By means of a suitable processing apparatus, a recordable electrical signal was developed.

Calibration of the capacitance pulse transducer applied to the radial artery was achieved first by occluding the artery at a point central to the transducer. This procedure established zero pressure. With the occlusion removed, the sensitivity was calibrated by requesting the subject to raise his arm 33.8 cm, which is equivalent to a change in pressure of 25 mmHg.

An interesting use of the capacitance-change principle for the measurement of stroke volume in a diaphragm-type blood pump was described by Normann et al. (1973a). In one application (see Fig. 6a) the blood within the pump on one side of the diaphragm was one "plate" of the capacitor (1); a metal foil in the air dome, into which positive and negative pressure was applied, constituted the other plate of the capacitor (2). The dielectric was therefore air and the plastic of the diaphragm. A capacitance change of slightly less than 1 pF was obtained for a pump stroke volume of 50 mL. The capacitance change varied the frequency of a 700-kHz oscillator, and the frequency change was processed to provide a signal that was linear with stroke volume. This system was used to monitor the amount of extracorporeal assistance provided to animals experiencing left-ventricular bypass.

Other configurations are possible with the capacitance method described by Normann. For example, in Fig. 6b the blood could constitute the dielectric in the diaphragm pump. When metal foil is wrapped around the conical plastic housing

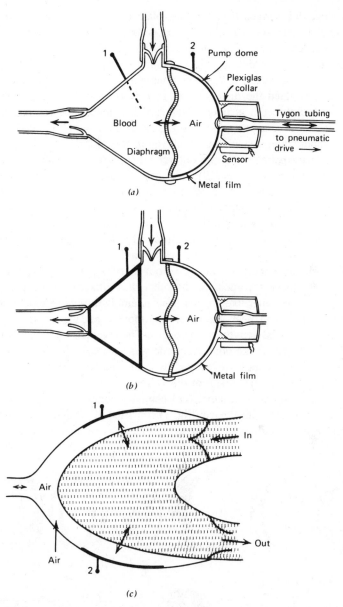

Figure 6 Three methods of using capacitance change to measure pump stroke volume. (*a*) Blood is one plate of the capacitor (1); metal film (2) in the air dome is the other. (*b*) Blood forms the changing dielectric between electrodes 1 and 2. (*c*) Blood in the sac (hatched area) forms the dielectric between the two electrodes (1 and 2). [Redrawn from N. A. Normann et al., *Cardiovasc. Res. Cent. Bull.* **12**:3–12 (1973).]

of the pump, this surface becomes one plate (1) of the capacitor, and the foil applied to the inner surface of the dome constitutes the other plate (2). In this way, no electrical contact with the blood is required.

Normann et al. (1973b) described another method of using the capacitance-change technique to measure stroke volume in a sac-type pump in which the blood in the sac constituted the dielectric, as in Fig. 6c. Two capacitor plates (1, 2) were applied to the conical plastic chamber that housed the sac and into which positive and negative air pressure was applied to fill and empty the sac. The same frequency modulation system was employed to record the stroke volume.

An ingenious application of the differential capacitance principle (Fig. 2b) was described by Boucek et al. (1959), who used it to construct a myograph for recording the contractions of the chick embryo heart at the 72-hr stage. At this time the heart is in a dynamic stage of development, changing from a tube to a four-chambered organ, which a little later produces an adult electrocardiogram. It is, however, incapable of exerting much force. To detect these feeble movements, Boucek and his colleagues placed the heart in a drop of plasma or saline solution. One end of a lightweight lever was made to rest on the part of the heart from which movement was to be recorded; to the other was affixed a metal plate centrally placed between two other fixed plates. The assembly thus constituted a differential capacitor. As the heart beat, the lever was moved, and its recorded motion described the mechanical activity of the organ. The lever also constituted one of the electrodes for the ECG; the other electrode was a wire dipping into the plasma or saline solution. Thus these investigators were able to record and correlate the embryo ECG with the movement of the various chambers of the heart.

An interesting differential capacitor pneumotachograph was described by Krobath and Reed (1964). This device (Fig. 7) consisted of a 0.1-mil aluminized mylar diaphragm with six radial slits, mounted in the center of the $\frac{5}{8}$-in.-diameter breath-

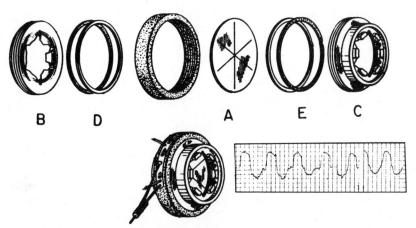

B   D   A   E   C

Figure 7 Exploded view (upper) and assembled view (lower left) of a differential capacitance pneumotachograph along with a typical record (lower right). [Redrawn from M. Krobath and C. Reed, *Am. J. Med. Electron.* **3**:105–109 (1964).]

ing tube. With inspiration and expiration, the six leaves would move in the direction of the air flow. On each side of the aluminized mylar leaves were concentric hexagonal-hole electrodes. The leaves of the mylar diaphragm and the two electrodes constituted a differential capacitor that formed two arms of a bridge circuit; the other arms were constituted by diodes. With 25 V at 200 kHz applied to the bridge, the output was 2 mV for a flow velocity of 1 mL/sec. The sine wave frequency response was 0–41 Hz, with 10 dB attenuation at 60 Hz. In the record shown in Fig. 7, during the expiratory phase of breathing the tiny cardiac-induced changes in airflow can be identified, demonstrating the short response time of the transducer.

The diode, twin-T (Lion) circuit was employed by Bourland (1974) to create a high-fidelity pneumotachograph, a device used to measure respiratory airflow. In this application, the respiratory air was caused to flow through an air resistor (Fleisch), which provides a pressure drop (ΔP) that is linear with airflow velocity. Figure 8a illustrates the air resistor and the capacitive differential pressure transducer connected to it. A cross section of the transducer, shown in Fig. 8b, dem-

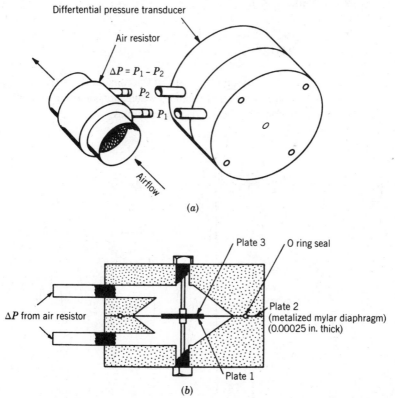

Figure 8 (a) Sketch of the Fleisch air resistor and the capacitive differential pressure transducer designed by Bourland (1974). (b) A cross section of the differential pressure transducer designed by Bourland (1974).

onstrates that the pressure-sensing diaphragm is an aluminum-coated sheet of mylar, 0.25 mil thick placed between two chambers communicating with the air resistor. A fixed plate is located on each side of the aluminized mylar membrane. Thus the plates and the aluminized mylar membrane constitute a differential capacitor, which is connected to the Lion circuit operating at 5 MHz.

The viscosity, stiffness, and low mass of the mylar membrane combine to provide an extremely short response time and critical damping. The frequency response extends from 0 to 1000 Hz, thereby providing high-fidelity recordings of airflow velocity. In fact, the sounds of respiration and vocalization can be heard easily by monitoring with a loudspeaker.

Figure 9 illustrates a typical airflow-velocity signal, revealing the biphasic inspiration–expiration signal. The small oscillations on the baseline are the cardiac-induced flow of air. The ECG has been included to make this point.

The small cardiac-induced airflow signal is called the pneumocardiogram (PNCG). On the right of Fig. 9 the recording sensitivity and chart speed have been increased to reveal the contour of the PNCG signal. The waves have letter designations, and the area under the HIJ component is proportional to cardiac stroke volume (Wessale et al., 1985).

BIOLOGICAL CAPACITORS

In those cases where living tissue forms part of the capacitor, the term biological capacitor is used. There are many circumstances when such an arrangement is very practical. The literature contains the following examples.

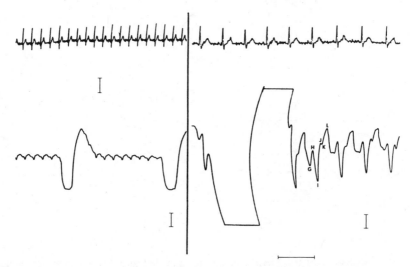

Figure 9   The ECG and pneumotachogram (left) at low sensitivity and (right) high sensitivity, showing the pneumocardiogram. (Courtesy of J. L. Wessale.)

Cremer (1907) inserted a beating frog heart between the plates of a condenser and recorded the capacitance change as the heart filled with blood and emptied of it. A similar system was described by Joseph (1944), who placed electrodes over the thoraxes of human subjects. Using a 90-V battery in series with a 2-MΩ resistor, he was able to detect pulsatile changes in capacitive current. A simultaneous record of the ECG showed that the capacitive changes were associated with cardiac activity, but calibration was not attempted.

In blood flow studies, Atzler and Lehman (1932) and Atzler (1935a, b) applied a capacitance-change method to human subjects by placing one electrode above the chest and the other below a glass plate that was mounted flush with the top of the examining table. The glass insulated the subject from the metal electrode. Using an ultrahigh-frequency current modulated by respiration and the systolic discharge from the heart, they detected the capacitance changes, calling their method "Dielektrographie." Whitehorn and Pearl (1949) carried out studies similar to those of Atzler and his associates. Their electrodes were 15 cm square and were placed before and behind the thorax. The pulsatile changes in capacitive reactance frequency modulated a 10.7-MHz oscillator. Calling these records "cardioelectrograms," they attempted calibration of the tracings and stated,

"Values for stroke volumes, cardiac output and cardiac indices, calculated from such records on the basis of preliminary calibration of the instrument by introduction of known volumes of saline between the plates, fall within the range of accepted normal values but conclusions as to the validity of this method are not yet possible."

Another application of the capacitance method was made by Fenning (1936–1937), who described an instrument he later called the "Oscillatocapacitograph." A rat was laid on one plate of the capacitor, and the other plate, 1 cm square, was placed 5 mm above the thorax of the animal. These plates were connected across the tuned circuit of a Hartley oscillator. Respiratory movements, which changed the capacitance by varying the area, separation, and distribution of the dielectric, altered the anode current of the oscillator tube. By monitoring this current, a good record of respiration in the rat was obtained. In the hands of Fenning and Bonnar (1936–1937), the same instrument was used to record maternal respiration, uterine contractions, and fetal respiration in the rat. Employing a slight modification of this technique, Tomberg (1963, 1964) detected human respiration by placing electrodes on the thorax without making ohmic contact with the chest wall. Frequencies between 50 and 300 MHz were employed.

Heart sounds have been detected in an ingenious application of the capacitance-change principle. For example, Yamakawa et al. (1954) placed a metal electrode near the tip of a closed catheter, which was then advanced into the hearts of dogs and human subjects. When the changes in capacitive reactance, measured between the catheter tip and the body of the subject, were recorded, heart sounds were clearly identified. So sensitive was the system that the sounds of vocalization were clearly recordable.

A similar investigation of heart sounds was carried out by Groom and Sihvonen

(1957a,b) and Groom et al. (1964), who constructed a monopolar electrode condenser microphone consisting of a chamber in contact with the thorax. Inside the chamber was the other electrode, mounted concentrically so that it did not contact the thoracic wall. Thus the heart sounds and all cardiac vibrations communicated to the thorax modulated the capacitance. The frequency response they attained extended from 0 to 50,000 Hz. In all probability cardiac vibrations had never been detected previously with such a wide bandwidth.

When the capacitive method is applied by placing electrodes in, on, or near living tissue, it is often difficult to know whether capacitance changes are the only ones measured. Usually the circuit contains both resistive and reactive components, and what is measured is in reality an impedance change. Only by using a detector for the capacitive (quadrature) current can one be assured that the signal obtained is capacitive in nature. The various physiological events that have been measured by impedance change are described in Chapter 11.

CHARACTERISTICS OF CAPACITIVE TRANSDUCERS

The extreme flexibility of capacitive transducers is perhaps their most attractive feature. In many applications they can be employed to detect dimension change without direct mechanical contact with the moving member. For this reason, capacitive transducers, which are often called proximity detectors, are free from loading, frictional, and hysteresis errors. With careful design of the capacitive element, extremely small or relatively large displacements can be measured. Another attractive feature of the capacitive transducer is the fact that the capacitance does not depend on the conductivity of its plates. Thus temperature errors from this source are extremely small, although not entirely absent, since the dimensions of the plates depend on temperature. The variation in the dielectric constant of air with temperature is small. Stability is achieved through the mechanical design of the capacitive transducer and the electrical circuitry connected to it. With efficient mechanical and electrical design, these sources of error can be reduced to insignificant levels.

Because the output impedance of a capacitive transducer is usually high, shielding is necessary, and a coaxial cable is frequently required to connect the transducer to the electronic equipment. In many applications the type of cable employed merits special consideration because its capacitance is in parallel with that of the transducing capacitor. Therefore a mechanically stable, low-capacitance coaxial cable is required. Often movement of the cable produces an undesirable capacitance change owing to a slight displacement of the outer shield relative to the inner conductor, which produces a signal indistinguishable from that made by the transducer. The use of special coaxial cables in which a layer of conducting powder has been applied to the dielectric directly below the shielding and in contact with it greatly attenuates this source of error. In many instances the problems presented by the high output impedance can be eliminated by locating some of the processing circuitry at the capacitive transducer. With this technique it is usually possible to incorporate an impedance transformer that provides a low output impedance, permitting location of the transducer at a distance from the processing equipment.

A most attractive feature of the capacitive-change principle is its low inherent noise, because the series-equivalent resistance is negligible. The use of two well-designed capacitors in a differential configuration provides excellent stability and low noise.

REFERENCES

Adams, R., B. S. Corell, and N. H. Wofesboro. 1960. Cuffless, noncannula, continuous recording of blood pressure. *Surgery* **47**:46–54.

Asher, A. G. 1932. Graphic registration of heart sounds by the argon glow tube. *Arch. Intern. Med.* **50**:913–920.

Atzler, E. 1935a. Dielektrographie. *Hand. Biol. Arbeitsmethoden* **5**:1073–1184.

Atzler, E. 1935b. Neues Verfahren zur Funktionsbeurteilung des Herzens. *Dtsch. Med. Wochenschr.* **59**:1347–1349.

Atzler, E., and G. Lehman. 1932. Über ein neues Verfahren zur Darstellung der Herztätigkeit. (Dielektrographie). *Arbeitsphysiologie* **5**:636–680.

Beyne, J., and L. Gougerot. 1939. Une méthode de transmission électrique et d'enregistrement à distance de la pression artérielle et du débit respiratorie. *C. R. Seances Soc. Biol.* **131**:700–774.

Boucek, R. J., W. P. Murphy, and G. H. Paff. 1959. Electrical and mechanical properties of chick embryo heart chambers. *Circ. Res.* **7**:787–793.

Bourland, J. D. 1974. The pneumocardiogram. Ph.D. Thesis, Baylor Medical College, Houston, TX.

Buchtal, F., and E. Warburg. 1943. A new method for direct electrical registration of intraarterial pressure in man with examples of its application. *Acta Physiol. Scand.* **5**:55–70.

Cremer, H. 1907. Über die Registrierung Mechanischer Vorgänge auf Menschen. *Med. Wochenschr.* **54**:1629.

Fenning, C. 1936–1937. A new method for recording physiologic activities. I. Recording respiration in small animals. *J. Lab. Clin. Med.* **22**:1279–1280.

Fenning, C., and E. B. Bonnar. 1936–1937. A new method of recording physiologic activities. II. The simultaneous recording of maternal respiration intrauterine fetal respiration and uterine contractions. *J. Lab. Clin. Med.* **22**:1280–84.

Foldvari, T., and K. Lion. 1964. Capacitive transducers. *Instrum. Control Syst.* **37**:77–85.

Frommer, J. C. 1943. Detecting small mechanical movements. *Electronics* **16**:104–105.

Groom, D., and Y. T. Sihvonen. 1957a. High sensitivity pickup for heart sounds and murmurs. *IRE Trans. Med. Electron.* **PGME-9**:35–40.

Groom, D., and Y. T. Sihvonen. 1957b. A high sensitivity pickup for cardiovascular sounds. *Am. Heart J.* **54**:592–601.

Groom, D., L. H. Medena, and Y. T. Sihvonen. 1964. The proximity transducer. *Am. J. Med. Electron.* **3**:261–265.

Hansen, A. T., and E. Warburg. 1947. An improved manometer for measuring intra-arterial and intra-cardiac pressures. *Am. Heart J.* **33**:709–710.

Joseph, N. R. 1944. Direct current dielectrograph for recording movements of the heart. *J. Clin. Invest.* **23**:25–28.

Krobath, H., and C. Reed. 1964. A new method for the continuous recording of the volume of inspiration and expiration under widely varying conditions. *Am. J. Med. Electron.* **3**:105–109.

Lilly, J. C. 1942. The electrical capacitance diaphragm manometer. *Rev. Sci. Instrum.* **13**:34–37.

Lion, K. 1964. Non-linear twin-T network for capacitance transducers. *Rev. Sci. Instrum.* **35**:353–356.

Liston, M. 1950. Performance of a double-beam infra-red recording spectrophotometer. *J. Opt. Soc. Am.* **140**:93–101.

Luft, K. F. 1943. Uber ein neue Methode der registrierung Gasonalyse mit Hilfe der absorption ultraroter Strahlen. *Z. Tech. Phys.* **24**:97–104.

Normann, N. A., M. E. DeBakey, G. P. Noon, and J. N. Ross. 1973a. Monitoring and closed-loop control of pneumatic blood pumps. *Cardiovasc. Res. Cent. Bull.* **12**:3–12.

Normann, N. A., G. P. Noon, and J. N. Ross. 1973b. Monitoring and automatic control of pneumatic blood pump. *Proc. Annu. Conf. Eng. Med. Biol.* **15**:334.

Schutz, E. 1937. Konstruktion einer manometrischen Sonde mit elektrischer Transmission. *Z. Biol.* **91**:515–521.

Tomberg, V. T. 1963. The high frequency spirometer. *Proc. Int. Congr. Med. Electron.*

Tomberg, V. T. 1964. Device and a new method of measuring pulmonary respiration. *Proc. Annu. Conf. Eng. Med. Biol.* **6**.

Wessale, J. L., J. D. Bourland, and C. F. Babbs et al. 1985. Correlation of the cardiogenic air flow in the respiratory airway. *Jpn. Heart J.* **26**(5):777–785.

Whitehorn, W. V., and E. R. Pearl. 1949. The use of change in capacity to record cardiac volume with human subject. *Science* **109**:262–263.

Yamakawa, K., Y., Shionoya, K. Kitamura, T. Nagai, T. Yamamoto, and S. Ohta. 1954. Intracardiac phonocardiography. *Am. Heart J.* **47**:424–431.

5

Photoelectric Transducers

INTRODUCTION

In the measurement of physiological events in living subjects, photoelectric transducers are employed in two ways. In the first method the photosensor functions as a detector of the changes in the intensity of light of a given wavelength, as in conventional colorimetry or spectrophotometry; in the second, it serves as a detector of changes in the intensity of light in which wavelength is relatively unimportant. There are numerous applications in both categories.

There are three basic types of photoelectric transducers: (1) the photoemissive (phototube), in which electrons are released from a metallic surface (usually alkali); (2) the photovoltaic, in which a potential difference is produced between two substances in contact; and (3) the photoconductive (photoresistor), in which a change in conductivity occurs. Although there is some overlap in applicability, each is recommended for certain tasks because of its particular spectral response, light sensitivity, output current, and voltage characteristics. The following sections describe the principles of operation, characteristics, and applications of each type.

PHOTOEMISSIVE TUBES

The photoemissive tube consists of an evacuated or gas-filled bulb with two electrodes. On one, the cathode, is a coating of a specially prepared material that releases electrons when illuminated. The other electrode, the anode, usually consists of a thin rod or loop of wire. For electron emission to occur, there are certain restrictions on the type of surface and the wavelength of the impinging light. Electron emission is possible only if the wavelength is shorter than a certain threshold value, which depends on the amount of energy required to release an electron from the cathode (work function). Thus there is a long-wave limit of sensitivity.

The materials most frequently employed for the emissive surface are cesium, antimony, silver, and bismuth in combination with trace amounts of other substances. Each type of surface exhibits its own spectral characteristics. Some surfaces are designed to be highly sensitive to narrow spectral regions; others are designed to have a fairly broad spectral sensitivity.

Photoemissive tubes come in a variety of configurations and sizes. In general, they, like other photodetectors, are described in terms of the direction of the light with respect to the location of the terminals connected to the internal electrodes. For example, if the terminals are on one end or on both ends of the device and the light enters at right angles, the device is designated a "side-on" photodetector. If the electrode terminals are on one end or on both ends and the light enters at one end, the term "end-on" photodetector is employed. Typical configurations for the photoemissive tube are illustrated in Fig. 1, which illustrates both side-on and end-on types.

With the photoemissive detector, a relatively high voltage (10–200 V) must be applied between the two electrodes. The electrons released by the light quanta are attracted to the anode. The electron flow constitutes a current that is linearly proportional to the intensity of the incident light. In the vacuum type the current produced is small and is not used to operate an indicator directly; it is usually led through a high resistance, and the voltage thus developed is applied to an amplifier having a high input impedance.

When higher currents are required, gas mixtures are often incorporated into the photoemissive detector. With this technique the primary electrons released by the incident light collide with gas molecules and produce secondary electrons and positive ions, thereby increasing the available current. To avoid the occurrence of a glow discharge, lower anode-to-cathode voltages must be employed. Although

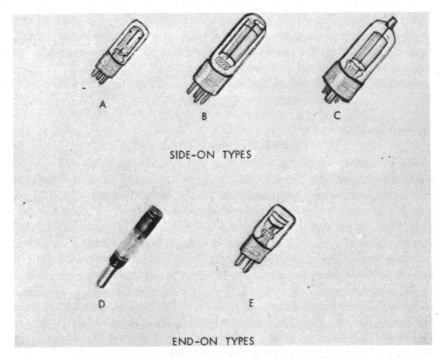

Figure 1   Photoemissive tubes: (*A, B, C*) side-on types; (*D, E*) end-on types. (Courtesy of Radio Corporation of America, Lancaster, Pennsylvania.)

the current intensity is increased about tenfold, the linear current–light relationship is compromised at higher intensities.

Both vacuum and gas-filled photoemissive photodetectors respond quickly to changes in light intensity. The response time of the former is approximately 10^{-9} sec, whereas that of the latter is much longer, approximately 10^{-3} sec. Both exhibit a small current flow with no light (dark current). Typical values are 10^{-8}–10^{-9} A for vacuum phototubes and 10^{-7}–10^{-8} A for gas-filled phototubes.

Although photoemissive surfaces respond to ultraviolet radiation, unless special materials that transmit ultraviolet energy are used in constructing the bulb the spectral sensitivity of photoemissive tubes seldom extends below 200 nm. The use of a special bulb will permit operation farther into the ultraviolet region. Figure 2 and Table 1 illustrate the transparency of the various materials used as windows in photodetectors.

It is obviously necessary to enclose the detecting material (or a radiator) that is transparent to ultraviolet or infrared radiation. In such cases, a window of radiation-transparent material is fused to the enclosure. It must be recognized that when a window material is fused to the enclosure, both must have the same thermal coefficient of expansion; otherwise the structure will fracture when the temperature change is large. Sometimes thermal coefficients cannot be matched exactly. In such circumstances, the use of one or more intervening materials with a similar coefficient of expansion distributes the thermal stress, creating a thermally stable structure.

Most photoemissive tubes are sensitive to visible light, and a few respond to infrared radiation down to 800 nm. The spectral sensitivity of a photoemissive surface is designated by the letter S and a number. This designation refers to a spectral curve recognized by all manufacturers. Data showing some of the spectral characteristics described by the various S numbers are presented in Fig. 3 and Table 2.

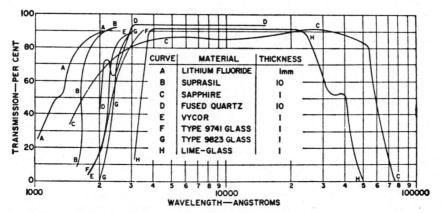

Figure 2 Transmission characteristics of various substances used in phototube windows. (From *RCA Phototubes and Photocells*, Radio Corporation of America, Lancaster, Pennsylvania, 1963. By permission.)

TABLE 1   Transmission Properties of Various Materials

	Useful Transmission (μm)		Crystal Structure	Melting Point (°C)	Solubility in H_2O at RT (g / 100 g H_2O)
	λ_{min}	λ_{max}			
LiF	0.105	7	Cubic—NaCl	848	0.27
MgF_2	0.11	7.5	Tetragonal—rutile	1255	0.01
CaF_2	0.125	9	Cubic	1418	0.16
BaF_2	0.14	15	Cubic—CaF_2	1320	0.001
SrF_2	0.12	10	Cubic—CaF_2	1190	0.01
Al_2O_3	0.14	6	Hexagonal	2050	0
SiO_2	0.15	5	Hexagonal	< 1470	0
NaCl	0.18	16	Cubic	801	36
KCl	0.19	20	Cubic—NaCl	776	35
KBr	0.20	25	Cubic—NaCl	730	54
KRS5	0.5	40	Cubic	414	0.05
CsBr	0.2	40	Simple cubic	636	124
CsI	0.2	50	Simple cubic	621	44
NaF	0.17	11	Cubic—NaCl	997	4.2
AgCl	0.4	25	Cubic	455	0
Si	1.1	20	Cubic—diamond	1420	0
Ge	1.7	20	Cubic—diamond	959	0
InSb	7.0	18	Cubic—zincblende	523	0
Pyrex	0.3	4	—	—	0

Source: D. L. Greenaway, and G. Harbeke, *Optical Properties and Band Structure of Semiconductors.* Pergamon Press, Oxford, 1968.

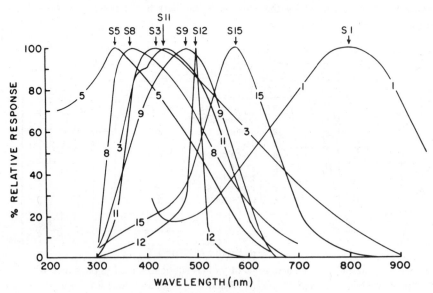

Figure 3   The S curves.

TABLE 2   Characteristics of the S Numbers

Designation	Photocathode	Window	Maximum Sensitivity	50% Point
S-1	AgO–Cs	Lime glass	800	620–950
S-3	AgO–Rb	Lime glass	420	350–640
S-4	Cs–Sb	Lime glass	400	320–540
S-5	Cs–Sb	"9741" glass	340	230–510
S-8	Cs–Bi	Lime glass	370	320–540
S-9	Cs–Sb (Semiopaque)	Lime glass	480	350–580
S-10	BiO–Ag–Cs (Semiopaque)	Lime glass	450	340–590
S-11	Cs–Sb (Semiopaque)	Lime glass	440	350–560
S-13	Cs–Sb (Semiopaque)	Fused silica	440	Narrow band
'S-13'	Cs–Sb (Semiopaque)	Sapphire	440	260–560
S-14	Ge	Lime glass	1500	700–1700
S-16	Cd–Se	Lime glass	750	—
S-17	Cs–Sb	Lime glass (refl. substrate)	490	310–580
S-19	Cd–Sb	Fused silica	330	190–460
S-20	Sb–K–NA–Cs (Semiopaque)	Lime glass	420	325–595
(S-20)	Sb–K–Na–Cs (Semiopaque)	Fused silica		3600–400
S-21	Cs–Sb (Semiopaque)	Special 9741 glass	440	260–560
	Cs–I	MgF₂		115–200
	Cs–Te	UV glass / Fused silica		185–320 / 160–320
	Sb–Cs	Borosilicate glass / UV glass		300–660 / 185–650
	Ga–As–Cs	Fused silica		160–910
	AgO–Cs	Borosilicate glass		300–1100
	Na–K–Sb–Cs	Borosilicate glass / UV glass		300–850 / 185–850

Source: RCA Phototubes and Photocells, RCA, Harrison, Pennsylvania, C. A. Harper, Handbook of Electronic Components, McGraw-Hill, New York, 1987; 1984 Hamamatsu catalog: Phototubes, Hamamatsu, Hamamatsu City, Japan.

PHOTOMULTIPLIER PHOTOTUBE

A photomultiplier is a high-sensitivity multianode photoemissive tube in which the primary electrons emitted from the photoemissive surface are caused to collide with successive anodes (dynodes), thereby giving rise to more electrons. Figure 4a is a schematic that illustrates the principle of operation; Fig. 4b shows the physical arrangement of dynodes in a typical photomultiplier.

A photon entering the window of the photomultiplier strikes the photoemissive surface (cathode) and liberates, say, one electron. This electron is accelerated to the first anode by a potential of about 100 V. On striking the first dynode, it liberates two secondary electrons, which in turn are attracted to the second dynode, which is at a potential 100 V higher (200 V above the cathode). Each electron striking the second dynode gives rise to two electrons, which are collected by the next dynode at a potential another 100 V higher. Thus, four electrons are liberated

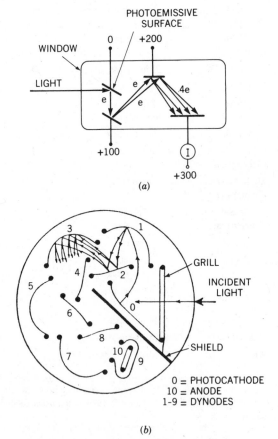

(a)

(b)

Figure 4   (a) Principle of electron multiplication used in a photomultiplier phototube; (b) arrangement of dynodes in a typical photomultiplier.

by the second dynode; this process can be continued by adding more dynodes. In the illustration, the current I_3 in the third dynode is four times the current flowing in the first dynode. This electron multiplication process can be continued by including more dynodes, each at a higher potential than its predecessor. Typically 10 or more dynodes are used, and current multiplications of 2^{10} or more can be achieved.

The spectral sensitivity depends on the type of photoemissive surface and the window on the envelope that houses the photomultiplier. Since the photomultiplier is a photoemissive tube, it has the same spectral characteristics. The spectral sensitivity is described by the S curves (Fig. 3 and Table 2).

Typically, the photomultiplier is exquisitely sensitive to visible light, with less sensitivity toward the infrared region. The sensitivity of the emissive surface to ultraviolet light is excellent, but the performance is limited by the type of window through which the light enters. For sensitivity to ultraviolet light, windows of materials such as sapphire or lithium fluoride are required along with the appropriate photoemissive material for the cathode.

As with other members of its family, the photomultiplier tube has a small dark current of about 10^{-7} A. The response time is extremely short, on the order of 10^{-8}–10^{-9} sec. Because of its very high sensitivity and short response time, the photomultiplier is an ideal detector for brief flashes of light of low intensity, such as those produced when radiation strikes the specially prepared crystals employed in scintillation counters.

SCINTILLATION COUNTER

A scintilla is a flash of light; a scintillation counter counts the number of light flashes. Such a device is used to monitor the decay of radioactive elements. Figure 5 illustrates the components of a typical instrument.

When an energetic particle, for example, an alpha particle or a photon, strikes certain crystals (and some materials dissolved in liquid), a faint flash of light is produced. The scintillation is detected by a photomultiplier phototube, which delivers a short pulse of current to the counting circuit that accumulates and displays the counts.

The light emitter, or scintillator, is specially prepared to be sensitive to ema-

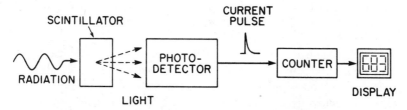

Figure 5   Principle employed in a typical scintillation counter.

nations from radioactive materials. Crystals of sodium iodide and zinc sulfate that have been activated by doping with thallium or silver are commonly used. Organic substances such as benzene, naphthalene, and anthracene are also used as scintillators. The spectral sensitivity of the photomultiplier is, of course, matched to the spectrum emitted by the scintillator.

PHOTOVOLTAIC AND JUNCTION DIODES

The photovoltaic (photogalvanic) cell is encountered frequently in biomedical studies. Unlike the photoemissive tube, which requires a relatively high voltage and produces a small current when illuminated, the photovoltaic cell develops a voltage that can drive a substantial current through a galvanometer or other low-impedance circuit.

One popular photovoltaic cell consists of a sandwich of a thin coating of selenium on an iron or steel backing. Above the selenium is a thin transparent film of metal. The film and selenium are insulated from each other, and the insulating region constitutes the barrier layer. When the barrier layer is illuminated, light quanta are absorbed, electrons are released, and a potential difference appears across the barrier. The transparent metal film becomes negative and the selenium positive. Completion of a circuit between the two electrodes causes a current to flow. The resistance between the electrodes decreases with illumination. This feature makes it possible to use photovoltaic cells in parallel; only those that are illuminated will supply current; those not illuminated do not load the others. In the solar power supplies used on board satellites, a diode is placed in series with a group of photodetectors to eliminate possible loading by partially illuminated or damaged photocells. This technique guarantees maximum current (Acker et al., 1960).

Other substances are used in voltaic cells. Cuprous oxide in contact with gold or platinum is sometimes employed in barrier-layer cells. Although these devices are available, they are not common because, compared to the selenium cell, they have low sensitivity to light. The spectral peak of the cuprous oxide cell is around 560 nm.

Selenium photocells cover the visible spectrum (300–700 nm) with a spectral sensitivity curve peaking around 550–570 nm. With an inexpensive filter it is easy to obtain a spectral curve closely resembling that of the human eye. For this reason these devices are used in illumination meters, exposure meters, and simple colorimeters, all of which operate without electronic amplification. The spectral sensitivity curves of many of the photovoltaic cells commercially available are plotted in Fig. 6.

The relationship between light intensity and the voltage developed by the photovoltaic sensor is not linear if the device is operated without a resistive load. At saturation a typical open-circuit voltage is approximately 200–600 mV. If a resistive load is placed across the device, the current flow becomes more linearly related to light intensity as the resistance is decreased. Hence it is necessary to employ a

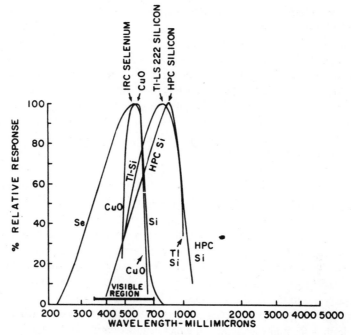

Figure 6 Spectral characteristics of photovoltaic cells, redrawn from data in manufacturers' bulletins. (TI = Texas Instruments; HPC = Hoffman Electronics Corp., IRC = International Rectifier Corp.)

low-resistance galvanometer or measuring circuit to indicate light intensity if a linear scale is to be obtained. When a galvanometer having an internal resistance of approximately 100 Ω is employed, a current of 0.5 mA can be obtained from many standard photovoltaic cells when they are adequately illuminated.

Because of the large capacitance of the barrier layer, the response time of a typical photovoltaic cell is seldom less than 5 msec, although a few miniature types exhibit response times of 0.1 msec. Perhaps the most undesirable feature of the photovoltaic cell in biomedical application is its sensitivity to temperature changes as the load resistance is varied. Many cells have an optimum value for the resistance that can be connected across the device to minimize the sensitivity change with temperature. This resistance value is not necessarily the one that yields the maximum power transfer or linearity of current with light intensity.

The absorption of light quanta by a semiconductor (P–N) junction results in the creation of hole–electron pairs and a voltage across the junction. Connection of an external load resistance produces a flow of current. Thus the junction photocell is a photovoltaic device that converts light (electromagnetic radiation) to electrical energy.

The most interesting photodiode is the solar battery that is used to convert sunlight into electrical power. It consists of a layer of boron diffused onto the surface of N-type silicon. When it is illuminated with bright sunlight, a voltage of about 0.5 V is developed. Connection of a load resistor across its terminals results in a current flow.

When a junction photocell is operated as a photovoltaic device, the current–voltage characteristic reveals that the device is nonlinear. Decreasing the value of the load resistor R_L increases the output current but decreases the voltage (see Fig. 7). The optimum value of load resistance is the value that corresponds to maximum power output (i.e., when the area of the rectangle $0-I_q-Q-V_q$ is maximum). The power available from a given unit is dependent on the area of the photojunction that is illuminated and the intensity of the illumination. The conversion efficiency is on the order of 5–10%.

The junction photocell can also be operated with forward or reverse bias applied to the P–N junction. Figure 8b illustrates the manner in which the current–voltage characteristic is altered when the cell is illuminated. To operate the device as a photoconductor, the P–N junction is reverse biased (i.e., P to negative, N to positive). The current–voltage characteristic of such a device is plotted upward, as in Fig. 8c. Thus, by placing a battery (E_{bb}) in series with a load resistor (R_L) and the junction photocell, an output voltage (ΔV) and current (ΔI) can be obtained for an increase in illumination from 0 to ϕ, as indicated by movement of the operating point up the load line (slope $1/R_L$) as in Fig. 8c.

There are many different types of junction photovoltaic cell, each designed to have a desired spectral sensitivity. In general, junction photocells tend to have their spectral peak sensitivity toward the red and infrared regions. For example, silicon cells exhibit their peak around 800 nm, whereas germanium units exhibit their maximum sensitivity around 1550 nm. Indium arsenide and indium antimonide exhibit response peaks at 3200 and 6800 nm, respectively. Frequently the latter

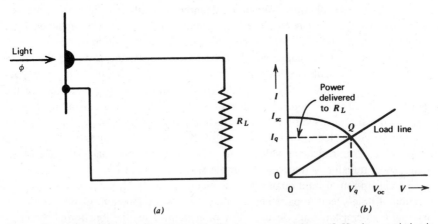

(a)   (b)

Figure 7   (a) The photojunction photocell; (b) the current–voltage (I–V) characteristics in response to illumination: I_{sc} is the short-circuit current; V_{oc} is the open-circuit voltage. The power delivered to the load resistor (R_L) for the illumination ϕ is equal to the area of the rectangle represented by the dashed line. The load line has a slope equal to $1/R_L$. I_q and V_q are the current and voltage of the circuit at the operating point Q, which is determined by the light intensity.

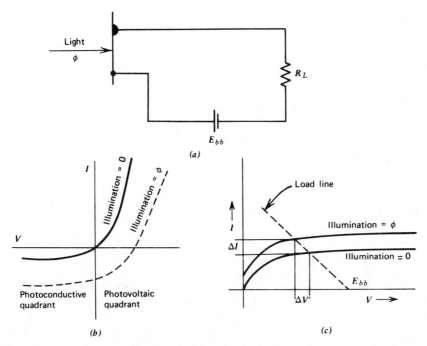

Figure 8 (*a*) Photojunction photocell; (*b*) its current–voltage characteristics in the dark and when illuminated. The graph in (*c*) illustrates operation of the device with a polarizing voltage E_{bb} to obtain an output voltage ΔV and current ΔI. (Redrawn from *Phototubes and Photocells*, Technical Manual PT60. Radio Corporation of America, Lancaster, Pennsylvania, 1963.)

types are cooled with liquid air to increase their sensitivity and reduce their thermal noise voltage.

The response time of junction photocells to light is short enough (microseconds to nanoseconds) to be used as light detectors in which there is rapid modulation of illumination. Because of their small size, high sensitivity, and short response time, junction photocells see a wide variety of uses as light detectors. One use, becoming increasingly important in the life sciences, is in optically coupled isolators. In these devices, a photojunction cell is used to detect the light produced by a light-emitting diode (LED) mounted a few millimeters away. Thus the desired signal modulates the light produced by the LED, and the light is detected by a junction photocell. In this way, a signal is coupled from one circuit to another without any electrical interconnection, thereby providing excellent electrical isolation.

PHOTOCONDUCTIVE CELLS

The photoconductive or photoresistive cell consists of a thin film of a material such as selenium, germanium, silicon, or a metal halide or sulfide. When exposed to certain types of radiant energy, it exhibits the photoconductive phenomenon, that is, a decrease in resistance. When light quanta are absorbed by the material, electrons are released into the conduction band, and if a voltage is applied to the film a current will flow. The resistance change with illumination is considerable. In most photoconductive cells the conductance is nearly linear with high intensity. Resistance therefore varies reciprocally with intensity. Most photoconductive cells will exhibit a drop in resistance from many megohms in the dark to a few hundreds of ohms when highly illuminated. Such devices are extremely sensitive photodetectors and are often employed as light-controlled switches.

The resistance R versus illumination intensity ϕ characteristic of a photoconductive cell is usually of the form $R = K/\phi^{\alpha}$, where K and α are constants depending on the type of photoconductor; Fig. 9 presents the data for a typical unit. This logarithmic relationship with illumination (i.e., $\log R = \log K - \alpha \log \phi$) is useful in many colorimetric applications. However, when it is desired to obtain a signal that is linearly related to light intensity, obvious difficulties arise. Nonetheless, over a limited range of illumination intensity, a reasonably linear current–light relationship can be obtained by connecting the photoresistor across a low-impedance voltage source (E) and measuring the current through the photoconductor with a current-measuring device having a resistance many times lower than the lowest resistance of the photoconductive cell with the maximum illumination to be employed. Since in many photoconductive cells α is not far from -1.0, the current I in the circuit is E/R, and if $R = K/\phi$, the current is equal to

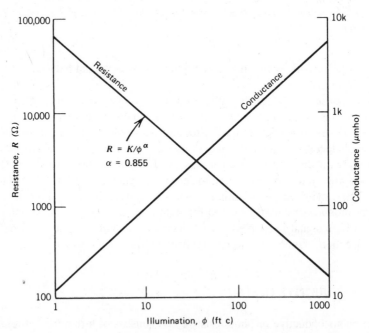

Figure 9   Resistance and conductance versus illumination for a typical photoconductive cell.

$E\phi/K$. If a low-resistance current-measuring device is not available, a low value of resistor can be employed, and the voltage across it can be measured using an amplifier.

Figure 10a illustrates two of the standard configurations of photoconductive cells. A wide range of diameters are available; some card-reading cells are as small

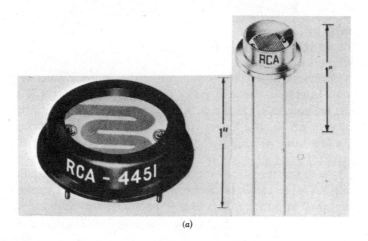

(a)

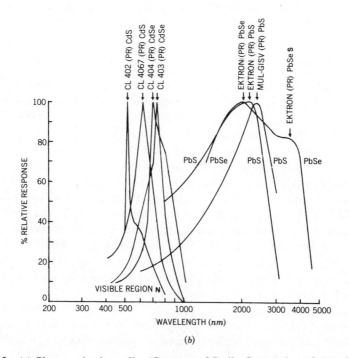

(b)

Figure 10 (a) Photoconductive cells. (Courtesy of Radio Corporation of America, Lancaster, Pennsylvania.) (b) Spectral characteristics of photoconductive cells: PR = photoresistive; CL = Clairex Corp.; EKTRON = Kodak Corp.; MUL = Mullard Corp.

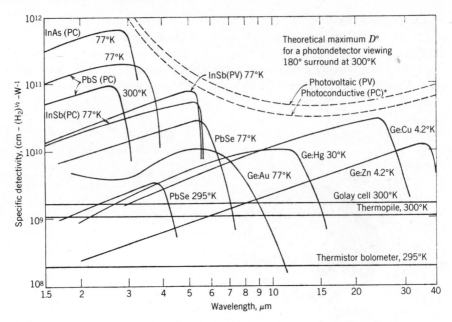

Figure 11 Spectral response of infrared detectors operated at the indicated temperatures. Chopper frequency is 1800 Hz, ferroelectric bolometer (100 Hz), thermocouple (10 Hz), and thermistor bolometer (10 Hz). (Redrawn from *Infrared Systems Imagery*, and R. D. Hudson, Wiley, New York, 1969.)

as 5 mm; others used in photoelectric relays are as large as 25 mm. Many manufacturers supply the same photosensitive material in side-on and end-on models.

Many of the photoconductive cells show good sensitivity to visible light; a few are sensitive to the ultraviolet and X-ray spectra. A large number, however, are exquisitely sensitive to the infrared region, a characteristic that prompted their development for spectroscopy and self-guiding infrared-seeking missiles. The sensitivity peaks of many units can be shifted by cooling; for example, Moss (1949) showed that the spectral peaks of lead sulfide, lead selenide, and lead telluride can be shifted farther into the infrared region by cooling to 20 K. The spectral characteristics of several of the photoconducting surfaces operated at room temperature are shown in Fig. 10b. Jacobs (1960) has listed the characteristics of many of the commercially available photoconductors when they are operated at reduced temperatures. Figure 11 illustrates the characteristics of many infrared-sensitive photoconductive cells operated at reduced temperatures.

The response and decay times vary widely with the type of material and are not independent of the illumination level. In general, the response time is shorter with a high light level. Typical response times for photoconductors operated at room temperatures vary between 0.1 and 30 msec.

THE PHOTOTRANSISTOR

With the photodiode, the current change for an illumination change is small, although the response time is very short. If some response time can be sacrificed, a considerable increase in current sensitivity can be obtained by using a phototransistor (see Fig. 12). In such a device, the area of the base–collector junction is large and the area of base–emitter junction is small. The incident radiation is caused to strike the base region, which is intentionally left unconnected. With this arrangement, the holes generated in the base region by the radiation cause the base potential to rise, forward biasing the base–emitter junction. Electrons then flow into the base from the emitter to neutralize the excess holes. Because of the close proximity of the collector junction, the probability of an electron combining with a hole is small, and most of the electrons are immediately drawn into the collector region, which is at a high positive potential. As a result, the total collector current is much larger than the photogenerated current; in fact, it is β times as large.

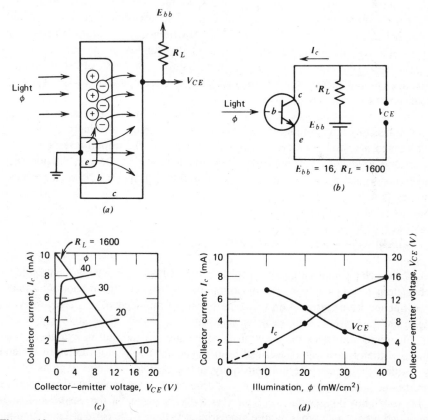

Figure 12 (a) Principle of operation of the phototransistor; (b) circuit employed with it; (c), operating characteristics in response to light flux ϕ.

Since the base is left unconnected, there are only three variables associated with operation of the phototransistor: collector-to-emitter voltage V_{CE}, collector current I_c, and illumination intensity ϕ. The operational characteristics of such a device can be predicted if one knows the collector characteristics; a typical example appears in Fig. 12c. The current–voltage characteristic resembles that of a conventional transistor, the parameter being illumination intensity ϕ rather than base current.

To employ the phototransistor as a light detector, it is merely necessary to connect it in series with a load resistor (R_L) and power supply (E_{bb}), as in Fig. 12b. By choosing a supply voltage and plotting the load line (slope $1/R_L$) on the collector characteristics, it is possible to predict the change in collector current and collector–emitter voltage in response to illumination (see Fig. 12c). The complete collector circuit response to light from 10 to 40 mW/cm^2 is plotted in Fig. 12d for a supply voltage of 16 V and a load resistance of 1600 Ω. Clearly the device is linear over a considerable range of illumination.

The phototransistor is a high-gain photodetector whose spectral peak sensitivity lies in the red and infrared regions of the spectrum. The high collector–base capacitance causes the device to have a longer response time than a photodiode. Nonetheless the response time is on the order of 5 μsec, which allows operation up to 100 kHz in many models. Because of the flatness of the current–voltage characteristic, the output impedance is high, being on the order of many kilohms. The temperature sensitivity of phototransistors is comparable to that of other semiconducting devices.

Despite their small size, high efficiency, and reasonably short response time, phototransistors have found little application in the biological sciences. They also see limited industrial application, primarily because of their inferior response time compared to that of a photodiode. It would appear that the combination of a photodiode with an appropriately designed amplifier provides a better light-detection system.

COMPARISON OF PHOTOELECTRIC TRANSDUCERS

With such an array of photodetectors, it is worthwhile reviewing the prominent characteristics of each type. The most important characteristics of photosensors are spectral sensitivity, response time, type of output provided (e.g., current or voltage), and linearity with illumination intensity.

Figure 13 illustrates the spectral characteristics of the human eye along with those of the photosensors described in this chapter. The photoemissive tubes tend to exhibit their peak spectral sensitivity in the visible and blue regions of the spectrum, possessing a rather short response time (microseconds). The response time is slightly longer but the light sensitivity is higher in the gas-filled photoemissive tubes; both types require a polarizing voltage. The current–light relationship is very nearly linear with illumination intensity, but there is a small residual dark current. Only a small output current is produced with illumination. However,

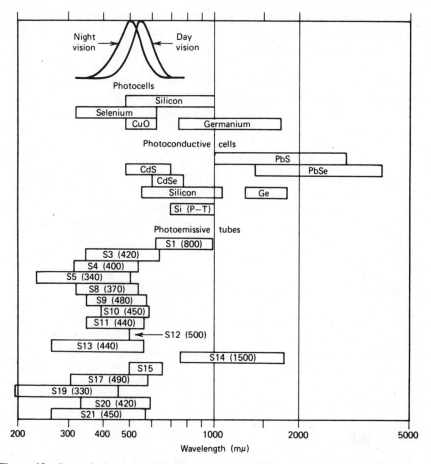

Figure 13   Spectral response of the human eye for night and day vision, along with the spectral sensitivities of photocells, photoconductors, and photoemissive tubes. The numbers in parentheses identify the spectral peaks for the *S* curves; P–T denotes a phototransistor.

when the small current is passed through a high resistance, a large output voltage is obtained. The fragility of the glass envelope restricts operation of the device to situations in which only small acceleration forces are encountered. Photomultiplier tubes are photoemissive tubes in which auxiliary electrodes (dynodes) are required to achieve electron multiplication.

Photovoltaic cells (photocells and photojunction cells) tend to have their peak spectral sensitivity in the visible and infrared regions. The response time depends on the type, the shortest response times being found in the photojunction cells. No polarizing voltage is needed, and current is delivered to the load resistor when the photovoltaic cell is illuminated. Photovoltaic cells are temperature sensitive and rugged and can be used as low-efficiency energy converters.

Photoconductive cells (photoresistors, biased junction photocells, and phototransistors) tend to be red- and infrared-sensitive. The response times depend on the type of device; the biased junction photocell exhibits the shortest response time, the phototransistor has a longer response time, and the photoresistor has the longest response time. All types require a polarizing voltage, and the resistance of the photoconductive cell varies almost inversely with illumination. The current–illumination relationship of the biased junction photocell and phototransistor is quite linear. All types are temperature-sensitive and rugged.

In choosing a photodetector for a particular colorimetric task, it is highly desirable to choose a device having a spectral peak at the wavelength of interest. If there is no photosensor with a spectral peak at the desired wavelength, a filter is chosen so that the combined spectral response of the photodetector and the transmission characteristics of the filter provide maximum spectral sensitivity at the desired wavelength. It is important to note that the use of filters decreases the efficiency of the photodetector; however, this price must frequently be paid to obtain the desired spectral purity.

COLORIMETRIC (SPECTROPHOTOMETRIC) APPLICATIONS

Apart from their use in spectrophotometers to analyze the composition of biological fluids (see Chapter 8), photoelectric detectors are used for the measurement of quantities in the living subject. Typical applications are the determination of cardiac output, the measurement of blood oxygen, and the measurement of bilirubin. Another application is thermography, in which the infrared radiation emitted from the body is used to identify skin temperature.

Cardiac Output

It is possible to measure the output of the heart (in liters per minute) by injecting a known amount of indicator into the venous system and measuring its passage in the arterial system with a calibrated detector (densitometer). The technique is known as the indicator-dilution method and is shown in Fig. 14. With a stable blood flow for the period of measurement, the prime requisites are that the indicator mix uniformly with the blood and that it not become lost from the circulation in the time between injection and measurement. A variety of indicators have been employed, the most popular being dyes (Table 3).

The dye-injection method was widely accepted after Hamilton et al. (1948) demonstrated that results obtained with it agreed with those obtained with the Fick technique. Since recording cuvette-densitometers for arterial blood became available, the method has been even more commonly employed. Although many dyes have been used, the three that became the most popular are Evans blue (T1824), indocyanine green (Cardio-green), and Coomassie Blue. These dyes are nontoxic and nonstimulating. Each has its own characteristics that recommend it for certain purposes. Table 3 summarizes the two most important characteristics of each dye: the wavelength of maximum absorption and the retention time in the vascular system.

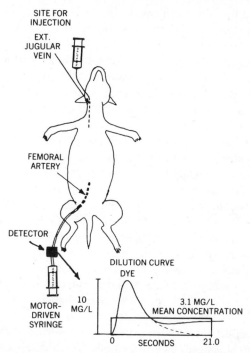

SITE FOR
INJECTION

EXT.
JUGULAR
VEIN

FEMORAL
ARTERY

DETECTOR

MOTOR-
DRIVEN
SYRINGE

10
MG/L

DILUTION CURVE
DYE

3.1 MG/L
MEAN CONCENTRATION

0   SECONDS   21.0

Figure 14 The dye-dilution method of measuring cardiac output. The dye is injected into the right heart and detected in arterial blood by withdrawal through a calibrated densitometer to obtain the dilution curve. In this example 2.5 mg of Evans Blue was injected. The mean height of the dilution curve was 3.1 mg/L, and the duration of the curve was 21 sec. Therefore, the cardiac output was $(60 \times 2.5)/(3.1 \times 21) = 2.30$ L/min.

A few comments will help to identify the relative advantages of each dye. Those that are retained in circulation for a long time yield the highest accuracy. Because of the long retention time, however, the circulation soon becomes loaded with the dye if repeated determinations are made. Although they may be harmless, such dyes often discolor the skin if large amounts are injected. Dyes that disappear

TABLE 3 Characteristics of Dyes

Name	Absorption Wavelength (nm)	50% Retention Time	Reference
Evans blue (T1824)	640	5 days	Connolly and Wood (1954)
Indocyanine green (Cardio-green)	800	10 min	Fox and Wood (1960); Wheeler et al. (1958)
Coomassie Blue[a]	585–600	15–20 min	Taylor and Shillingford (1959); Taylor and Thorp (1959)

[a]Sodium anazolene.

rapidly permit more frequent measurements, but because they leave the circulation, accuracy is compromised.

The wavelength for measurement of the dye concentration merits special consideration. Oxygenated blood transmits maximally around 640 nm; blood without oxygen (reduced blood) and fully oxygenated blood transmit equally well around 805 nm. Measurements with dyes that absorb around 640 nm are subject to errors with changes in oxygen saturation. Dyes with maximal transmission around 805 nm are immune to such errors.

The type of dilution curve following the injection of a dye appears in Fig. 14. Cardiac output is calculated by measuring the area under the first time–concentration curve as shown and dividing this quantity into the amount of indicator injected. Because recirculation usually obscures identification of the end of the first pass, the falling phase is extrapolated to the baseline, using the method developed by Kinsman et al. (1929), which employs a semilogarithmic plot of this portion of the curve and linear extrapolation to a negligible concentration (ca. 1% of maximum), thereby identifying the end of the first pass. The area under the first pass is then determined, and the mean concentration for that time is calculated. The mean concentration c for 1 min is calculated. Cardiac output is calculated by dividing ct into the amount of indicator injected. A sample calculation is included in the legend to Fig. 14.

When the optical density of flowing blood is recorded continuously, scattering and reflection from blood cells cause variations. The transmission therefore varies with the velocity of the bloodstream. For this reason it is often difficult to obtain a stable baseline in the recording. A method of overcoming some of these difficulties was reported by Sutterer (1960), who described a compensating densitometer for dye-dilution studies using indocyanine green. In this instrument he placed two photodetectors, one sensitive to a wavelength of 800 nm and the other sensitive to all wavelengths except 800 nm. By combining the outputs of the two photocells, he was able to compensate for changes in transmission due to blood flow.

If the dye is retained in the circulation, after several circulations a stable concentration called the end-tail is obtained. This is often used in calibrating the densitometer by withdrawing a sample of blood and analyzing it for dye concentration. This calibration technique is sometimes employed when ear oximeters are used to determine cardiac output. It is apparent that calibration by this technique is inaccurate if the dye is cleared rapidly. Because the end-tail calibration point is low on the concentration scale, high accuracy is difficult to achieve.

There is another use for the end-tail concentration: the calculation of blood volume. With total mixing of the dye and no loss from the cardiovascular system, blood volume is calculated by dividing the amount injected by the end-tail concentration. The figure obtained in this way assumes that the sample analyzed is representative of all the blood in the body.

Oximetry

The redness of blood indicates its oxygen content, and an oximeter is used to measure this property. More specifically, an oximeter measures oxygen saturation

(SaO_2), the amount of oxygen in the blood in relation to what it is capable of carrying. SaO_2 is therefore a relative quantity.

Oxygen is carried in the blood mainly by the iron pigment hemoglobin (Hb) in the red cells. Only a very small amount of oxygen is dissolved in the plasma. Oxygen saturation (in percent) is defined as

$$\% SaO_2 = \frac{HbO_2}{Hb + HbO_2} \times 100,$$

where HbO_2 is oxyhemoglobin (which is bright red) and Hb is hemoglobin (which is blue-grey).

The fundamental principle underlying operation of all oximeters is the difference in spectral transmission of hemoglobin and oxyhemoglobin; Fig. 15 presents this information. Since the ear helix (pinna) is a site frequently used to measure the transmission of light through blood, its spectral characteristics are included. Figure 15 shows that the transmission of light through a sample of oxygenated (100% saturated) blood, i.e., HbO_2, is a maximum around 640 nm. Figure 15 also shows that the transmission of light through oxygenated blood (HbO_2) and blood containing no oxygen (Hb) is equal at 805 nm which is called the isobestic point. Therefore, if two colorimetric channels are used to measure the oxygen content of the blood, the transmission of light at 640 nm depends on the amount of oxygen in the blood and the thickness of the blood–tissue path. The transmission at 805 nm is independent of the oxygen saturation but dependent on the thickness of the blood–tissue path. Therefore to measure oxygen saturation, at least two colorimetric channels are required, one providing information on total Hb and the other indicating the amount of HbO_2. Figure 16 illustrates the basic transmission oximeter.

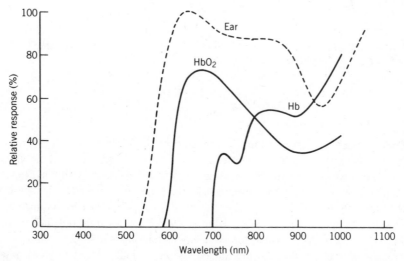

Figure 15 Spectral characteristics of Hb, HbO_2, and the ear. (Redrawn from Elam et al., 1949.)

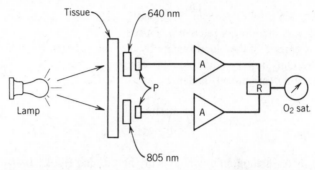

Figure 16   The essential components of a two-wavelength transmission oximeter. A lamp transilluminates a fold of tissue containing blood vessels. The transmitted light is detected by filtered red and infrared detectors (P). Amplifiers (A) enlarge the signals and logarithmic and ratio circuit. (R) processes them and drives a display device calibrated in percent saturation.

The fundamental spectral properties of blood are used in several ways to measure and/or record oxygen saturation. For example, with direct oximetry, blood is either placed in a sample cell (cuvette) or caused to flow through it. The blood is transilluminated, and the red and infrared transmissions are measured to indicate the saturation. Let T_r and T_{ir} be the transmission (emergent intensity divided by the incident intensity) for the red and infrared channels, respectively. According to the Beer–Lambert law, the optical density D identifies the concentration of a substance in solution. The optical density is equal to $\log(1/T)$, where T is the transmission. The percent oxygen saturation is

$$\% \mathrm{SaO_2} = \frac{D_r}{D_{ir}} \times 100,$$

where D_r and D_{ir} are the optical densities for the red and infrared channels, $D_r = \log(1/T_r)$, and $D_{ir} = \log(1/T_{ir})$; therefore

$$\% \mathrm{SaO_2} = \frac{\log(1/T_r)}{\log(1/T_{ir})} \times 100.$$

Oxygen saturation is proportional to the ratio of the logarithms of the reciprocal of the transmissions in the red and infrared bands (i.e., 640 and 805 nm). Studies of the optical density versus blood oxygen have been made by many investigators to demonstrate the importance of choosing the proper wavelengths for measuring $\mathrm{HbO_2}$ and Hb. Figure 17 illustrates the results of the studies by Kramer et al. (1951) and Shepherd et al. (1984). Kramer plotted the logarithm of the emergent intensity versus oxygen content for wavelengths ranging from 653 to 1056 nm and demonstrated that for 805 nm the transmission was independent of oxygen saturation. Similarly, Shepherd plotted the change in optical density versus the change

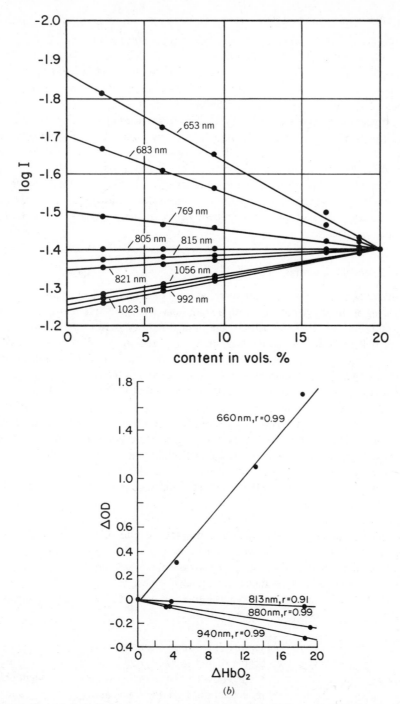

Figure 17 (*a*) Optical density versus oxygen content for various wavelengths. For whole blood, $d = 0.5$ mm, $\lambda = 653$–1056 nm, and oxygen capacity $= 20.0$ vol %. (Redrawn from Kramer et al., 1951) (*b*) Change in optical density versus change in oxygen content for various wavelengths. (Redrawn from Shepherd et al., 1984.)

in oxygen content for wavelengths extending from 600 to 940 nm, showing that at 813 nm the transmission is almost independent of oxygen saturation. Both studies demonstrate the importance of using the isobestic point (805 nm) for one of the measuring channels. They also demonstrate that the change in transmission with oxygen saturation is large in the 653–660-nm range.

The spectral measurement of oxygen saturation is accomplished by transmitting light through blood (transmission oximetry) or by measuring the light reflected from blood (reflectance oximetry). Transmission oximeters have been described for blood flowing in a cuvette and for blood flowing in a tissue bed that is capable of being transilluminated, such as the pinna or lobe of the ear, the lip, tongue, or nasal septum. Reflectance oximeters have been made for flowing blood as well as for the forehead, finger pad, and nailbed. Many of these types will now be described.

Whole Blood Oximetery

Cuvette oximeter. Oxygen saturation has been measured in flowing arterial blood by passing it through a cuvette with a light source on one side and filtered photodetectors on the other. Sometimes the optical density is recorded at two wavelengths (640 and 805 nm); at other times only red light (640 nm) is used. A continuous record of the optical density provides a record of the temporal changes in oxygen saturation. One of the earliest to describe a two-channel instrument was Kramer (1934, 1935), who used an unopened dog artery as the cuvette. Later others reported the use of cuvette oximeters.

One of the interesting facts demonstrated by continuous recordings of oxygen saturation in flowing blood is that with high-gain recording and a low respiratory rate, blood oxygen saturation reveals the intermittent nature of respiration; Fig. 18 presents an example. Such respiration-induced changes in oxygen saturation were discussed by Matthes (1934). If a truly representative sample of arterial blood is to be obtained in such a situation, it is clear that the sample should be withdrawn slowly during several breaths.

Despite its attractiveness and simplicity, the cuvette oximeter is rarely used today, probably because of the need to gain access to the bloodstream and to use an anticoagulant to inhibit clotting. However, there are instances when arterial blood is caused to flow in transparent plastic tubes, as when cardiopulmonary bypass is used. In such cases, oxygen saturation could be measured by transillumination of the blood-carrying plastic tubes.

Fiber-optic oximeter. The earliest fiber-optic oximeter was described by Enson et al. (1962). In this device beams of red (660 nm) and infrared (805 nm) light were transmitted 20 times per second down a fiber bundle in one lumen of a double-lumen catheter. The diffusely reflected light from the blood at the tip of the catheter was conducted to the external photodetector via a second fiber bundle in the other lumen of the catheter. The photodetecting apparatus consisted of a photomultiplier and an oscilloscope whose screen showed the red and infrared signals. The ratio

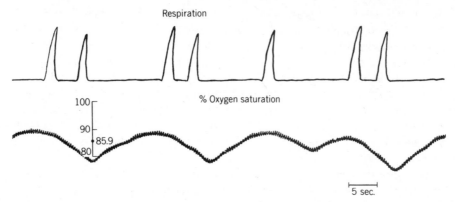

Figure 18 Rhythmic changes in oxygen saturation with respiration. The saturation changes were recorded with a cuvette oximeter calibrated at 85.9 and 100% O_2 saturation.

of these signals was found to vary linearly with oxygen saturation. The calibration graph presented showed a standard deviation of $\pm 1.9\%$ around the regression line.

A high-efficiency intravascular fiber-optic catheter oximeter was described by Johnson et al. (1971). Two light-emitting diodes (LEDs) alternately transmitted red (685 nm) and infrared (920 nm) light down fiber-optic bundles at a rate of 200 pulses per second. The light reflected from the blood was transmitted up a third fiber bundle and detected by two silicon photodiodes. It was found that the ratio of the two reflected signals very nearly cancelled reflectance variations due to blood flow and that this ratio was inversely related to oxygen saturation. The relationship between oxygen saturation (SaO_2) and the reflected red (I_r) and infrared (I_{ir}) signals was of the form $SaO_2 = A - B(I_{ir}/I_r)$, where A and B are constants determined experimentally. A very careful in vitro evaluation of the accuracy of this oximeter was presented by Woodroof and Koorajian (1973), who found that it exhibited its highest accuracy when the hematocrit was in the normal range (40%). The standard error in this range was about 2%; larger errors were encountered with hematocrit values below 25 and above 90%.

A fiber-optic oximeter was developed by Wirtzfield (1980) for detecting changes in oxygen saturation in right-ventricular venous blood. A decrease in oxygen saturation, which accompanies exercise, caused a pacemaker to increase its rate, thereby improving exercise tolerance for the patient.

Fiber-optic oximeters are excellent for monitoring changes in saturation when accurate calibration is not required. Several methods have been proposed to develop a calibration technique. Typically calibration is achieved by placing the catheter tip in two blood samples of known saturations (e.g., arterial and venous blood). With the passage of time, other techniques have been developed to standardize the sensitivity of the instrument with a fiber-optic catheter. One of the first methods employed placement of the catheter tip in a milk of magnesia solution, which provided a reflectance that could be related to a measured oxygen saturation. Ostrowski (1974) and Polanyi and Ostrowski (1977) mounted a tiny caged reflecting ball on the catheter tip a short distance from the optical fibers, thereby creating a tiny transmission-reflectance cell at the catheter tip. When the catheter tip was placed in sterile saline, the reflectance so obtained was used to standardize the measuring instrument. Another method of obtaining a known reflectance was developed by Polanyi and Ostrowski (1977). It consisted of applying a diffuse reflector (a length of white-pigmented poly(vinyl chloride) tubing, 20 diameters long), to the tip of the fiber-optic catheter. When the catheter was filled with saline, the reflectance value was used to standardize the instrument used with the fiber-optic catheter. Such calibrating procedures permit setting the instrument so that it can be operated with the particular fiber-optic catheter.

Fiber-optic catheter oximeters are now available commercially; some use two wavelengths, while others use more. The instrument provided by Oximetrix (Mountain View, California) employs three wavelengths. Figure 19 is a sketch of the catheter, which contains two fiber-optic bundles and an open lumen for pressure monitoring or withdrawal of blood samples. The fiber-optic bundles terminate in a connector (optical module) that couples to the photodetector assembly. The catheter also contains a thermistor for measuring cardiac output by the thermal dilution method. Calibration is achieved by inserting the tip into a small optical reference chamber supplied with each fiber-optic catheter; details are proprietary.

Fiber-optic catheters are very useful for monitoring changes in oxygen saturation. They are valuable in the diagnosis of left-to-right cardiac shunts. For example, the change in saturation as the catheter tip passes through the right atrium, ventricle, and pulmonary artery can identify the presence of a defect (hole) between the atria or the ventricles. When such a defect is present, arterial blood can flow through it and as the catheter tip is advanced it encounters abnormal increases in saturation.

Tissue-Bed Oximeter. Measuring the transmission of light through, or the reflected light from, a tissue bed allows the measurement of oxygen saturation in the

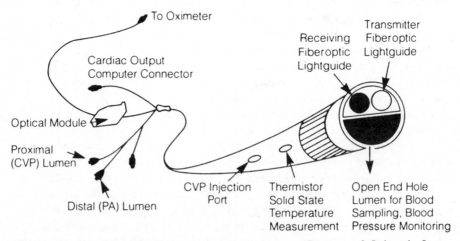

Figure 19 The Oximetrix fiber-optic catheter oximeter. (Courtesy of Oximetrix Inc., Mountain View, California.)

capillary bed. The former technique was introduced by Nicolai (1932), who ushered in oximetry by measuring the transmission of light through the palm of the hand. Matthes (1935) and Matthes and Gross (1939a, b) measured the transmission of red and infrared light through the human ear. Squire (1940) measured the redness of the blood in the web of the hand between the thumb and forefinger using two filtered phototubes; he also used a pressurizable, capsule to render the optical path bloodless for standardizing his instrument.

The first practical ear oximeter was developed by Millikan (1942). In it the photodetectors were mounted in a small fixture that fitted over the pinna of the ear. In an improved instrument described by Wood and Geraci (1949), the assembly was equipped with a pressure capsule that permitted rendering the optical path bloodless to make initial settings. Figure 20 shows a commercial version of the Wood-Geraci ear oximeter. In this device, which employs a small lamp and filtered CdS photoconductors, the blood is first expelled from the optical path by pressurizing the capsule to above systolic pressure. Then the instrument is adjusted to indicate 100% transmission. Releasing the pressure allows the blood to enter the optical path, and the red and infrared transmissions can be read to determine the saturation. Saunders et al. (1976) compared the oxygen saturation values obtained with the Waters oximeter with values obtained when samples of arterial blood were analyzed with the Van Slyke–Neill (chemical) method. Figure 21 illustrates the result.

A novel method of determining oxygen saturation of the blood in the fingertip was described by Yoshiya et al. (1980). With this technique, the absorption of red (650 nm) and infrared (805 nm) radiation are measured at the fingertip using a glass fiber-optic bundle, as shown in Figure 22a. The principle underlying the measurement is shown in Fig. 22b and is based on the fact that the pulsatile change

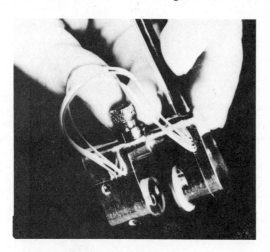
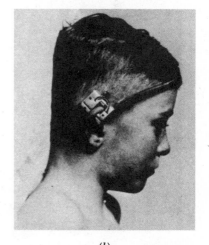

(a)   (b)

Figure 20   (a) The Wood–Geraci type of oximeter earpiece. The exciter lamp is enclosed in a housing and is covered by an inflatable transparent capsule. The red and infrared detectors are in the other housing. (b) The earpiece on the pinna. (Courtesy of the Waters Co., Rochester, Minnesota.)

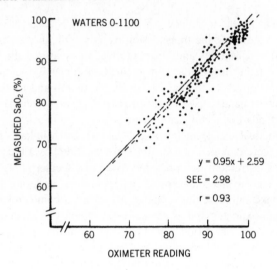

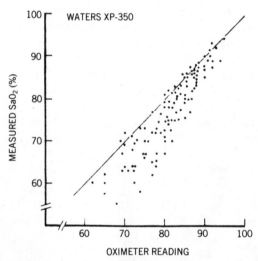

Figure 21 Relationship between oxygen saturation measured by the Van Slyke method and values obtained with two Waters oximeters. (Reproduced from Saunders et al., 1976.)

in absorbance A contains information on arterial saturation and the absorbances (V and T) by venous blood and tissues in the optical path are constant. An equation for arterial oxygen saturation (SaO_2) is derived that includes the ratio of the pulsatile (ac) and steady (dc) components at 650 and 805 nm:

$$SaO_2 = A - B(Y_{650}/Y_{805}),$$

where the Y values represent the logarithms of the transmission signal $(dc + ac)/dc$ at the two wavelengths.

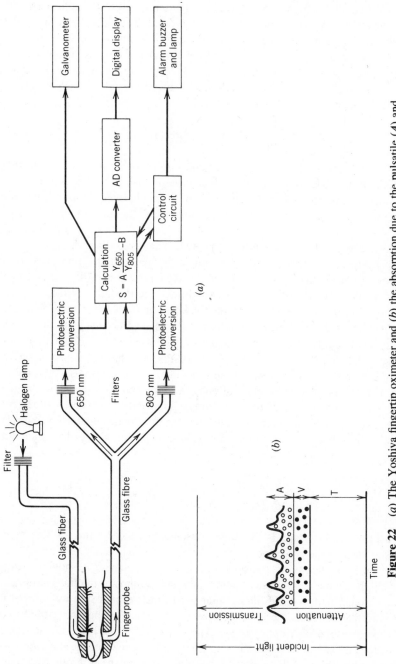

Figure 22 (*a*) The Yoshiya fingertip oximeter and (*b*) the absorption due to the pulsatile (*A*) and steady (*V*, *T*) components in the optical path. [Redrawn from I. Yoshiya et al., *Med. Biol. Eng. Comput.* **18**:27–31 (1980).]

Initial human studies with the Yoshiya (Minolta) oximeter by Sarnquist et al. (1980) revealed that the device overestimated arterial saturation; this fact was confirmed by Shimada and Yoshiya (1984), who found that light scattering by the intervening tissues caused the error. To accommodate this factor, the SaO_2 equation was altered to use the square of the ratio of the Y values. They then compared the fingertip oximeter values with those obtained from directly measured blood in three subjects in whom hypoxemia was produced by breathing low concentrations of oxygen in nitrogen. The result was

$$SaO_2(\text{oxim}) = 0.96 SaO_2(\text{direct}) + 3.97,$$

with a correlation coefficient of 0.98; the values given are in percent. The instrument was also modified to be inhibited when excessive peripheral vasoconstriction was encountered, being identified by the ratio of the ac/dc transmission. When this value fell below 0.5%, the instrument was automatically rendered inoperative.

Multiwavelength Transmission Oximeter. The preceding discussion has shown that oxygen saturation can be determined by measuring the transmission of light at two wavelengths. However, when the technique is applied to blood in a fold of skin, the intensity of the emergent light may be modified by factors other than hemoglobin, oxyhemoglobin, and the thickness of the blood sample. Skin and tissue pigments also absorb light, resulting in diminished accuracy and increased variability, particularly in the high-saturation range (e.g., 90–100%). To circumvent these problems, one manufacturer (Hewlett-Packard) has developed an eight-wavelength oximeter (Fig. 23), which was created by studying the spectral transmission of the ears of a wide range of subjects with both high and low oxygen saturations. Like the two-wavelength instrument, its operation depends on the Beer–Lambert law. The oxygen saturation is a function of the transmission T of light at the eight wavelengths. The manufacturer provides the following expression for saturation:

$$O_2(\text{sat}) = \frac{A_0 + A_1 \log T_1 + A_2 \log T_2 + \cdots + A_8 \log T_8}{B_0 + B_1 \log T_1 + B_2 \log T_2 + \cdots + B_8 \log T_8}.$$

In this expression the A and B terms are constants and the T terms are the transmissions at each of the wavelengths.

The manner of measuring transmission at each wavelength is shown in Fig. 23b. The light source is a tungsten iodide lamp that collimates the light beam and directs it through narrow-band filters, after which the beam is split by an optical fiber bundle that conducts the light to the ear. The emergent light is carried to a detector via a second fiber-optic bundle. The other half of the beam is conducted to a detector and serves as a reference intensity. In this manner the detector sees light that passes through the ear and light that does not pass through the ear. Therefore the photodetecting system identifies the difference in light transmitted through the ear, which contains information on Hb, HbO_2, thickness, and pig-

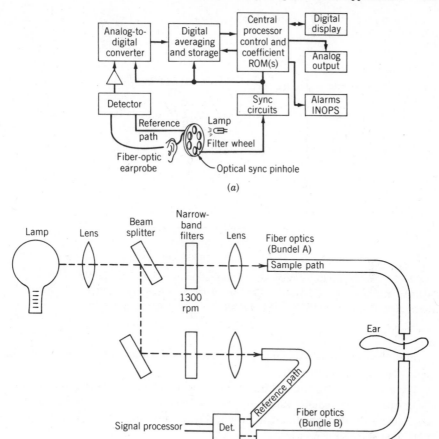

Figure 23   (*a*) Method of sequentially measuring the transmission of light through the ear at eight wavelengths in succession. (*b*) Principle employed in the multiwavelength fiber-optic ear oximeter. (Redrawn from Operating Guide for 47201A Oximeter, Hewlett-Packard, Waltham, Massachusetts.)

mentation, and light that is not affected by these absorbers. With this technique there is no need to make the ear bloodless.

The light transmission measurements are made sequentially at eight wavelengths in the region of 650–1050 nm; the particular wavelengths used were determined experimentally, and this information is proprietary. The wavelengths used were derived from a study that included black, Asian, American Indian, and Indian subjects of both sexes. Transmission measurements were made at various oxygen saturations.

Each of the eight filters is mounted at the periphery of a wheel that rotates at 1300 rpm. Thus the transmission is measured 21.67 times each second. An optical

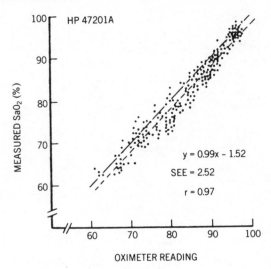

Figure 24 Relationship between oxygen saturation determined by the Van Slyke method and that obtained with the Hewlett-Packard oximeter. (Reproduced from Saunders et al., *Amer. Rev. Resp. Dis.* **113:**745–749 (1976).)

position detector on the rotating filter wheel reports which filter is in use to the logic circuitry of the oximeter.

The earpiece is standardized by placing a standardizing cavity in it; this permits the instrument to acquire values for the incident radiation at each of the eight wavelengths. The calibration can be checked at any time by inserting a special glass filter into the earpiece.

With all ear oximeters, the ear pinna is "arterialized" by rubbing it briskly to promote vasodilation before the earpiece is applied. The earpiece has a thermostatically controlled heater (41°C) that maintains the vasodilation.

The performance characteristics of the Hewlett-Packard multiwavelength oximeter were evaluated by Saunders et al. (1976). Figure 24 illustrates the results of plotting the intraarterial oxygen saturation against the oximeter value. The linear relationship and high correlation coefficient are impressive.

Reflectance Tissue-Bed Oximeter. After experimenting with the measurement of oxygen saturation in the blood sample using reflected red light, Zijlstra (1951) constructed a reflectance-type oximeter for human use. He employed a barrier-layer photocell in which was mounted axially a small lamp covered by a red filter transmitting light of 600–680 nm. A small box held the photocell and light bulb a short distance from the forehead of the subject. To obtain adequate stability in his first model, Zijlstra had to cool the photocell with a water chamber mounted behind it. In a second model, two photocells were used and a differential circuit was employed, which eliminated the need for a cooling chamber. In a later model, two spectral bands (red and green) were used, and a third photocell was added for compensation purposes. The output of the photocells was calibrated in terms of oxygen saturation by chemically analyzed blood samples. Zijlstra stated that if the oximeter was employed without calibration, the output of the photocells reflected only changes in saturation. He recommended use of the device for monitoring saturation during surgery.

Little attention was paid to Zijlstra's reflectance oximeter until recently when several manufacturers offered two-color models for sale. The main difference in the modern units is the use of light-emitting diodes to generate the red and infrared light and photoconductive cells or photodiodes as detectors.

Characteristics of Tissue-Bed Oximeters. Irrespective of whether the device is a transmission or reflectance oximeter, the relationship between the measured quantity and true arterial saturation depends on the state of the capillary bed. With all such instruments, it is recommended that the tissue bed be arterialized, which is accomplished by brisk rubbing (often with 70% isopropyl alcohol) or the application of heat, or both. Failure to arterialize will result in a measured oxygen saturation that is less than that in the major arteries. Vasoconstriction occurs with cold and with hypotension (mean blood pressure below 50 mmHg). In addition, the administration of vasoconstrictor drugs to raise blood pressure dramatically reduces capillary blood flow. Thus tissue-bed oximeters are difficult to use when there is vasoconstriction.

With all types of oximeters, it is essential to employ at least two spectral channels, one to respond to oxyhemoglobin (and the thickness of the blood path) and the other to respond to the hemoglobin (and the thickness of the blood path). This requirement dictates the use of wavelengths of 620–640 and 805 nm. The former is easily achieved; the latter is more difficult if light-emitting diodes (LEDs) are used as the light sources. At present there are no LEDs that emit at 805 nm; most are centered farther into the infrared region. The importance of the use of wavelengths other than 805 nm has been demonstrated by Kramer et al. (1951) and Shepherd et al. (1984); their results are shown in Fig. 17.

Operating Range of Oximeters. There are those who state that a good clinician does not need an oximeter to show that a subject is unsaturated, i.e., hypoxic. However, an extensive study carried out by Comroe and Botelho (1947) to illustrate the ability of clinicians to detect hypoxia showed that many experienced clinicians cannot detect hypoxia until the saturation has fallen to 80 or 85%. They demonstrated further that many other observers cannot recognize hypoxia by direct observation until the saturation has fallen to between 70 and 75%. Clinically, saturation is never permitted to fall below 50% for very long. Thus, the most valuable operating range can be arbitrarily set as 50 to 100% saturation. However, an oximeter has additional value in its ability to identify subtle changes in saturation that are undetectable by visual inspection.

Jaundice Meter

Jaundice is characterized by the yellow color imparted to the skin by an excess of bilirubin, the end product of the metabolism of heme, the iron pigment released from red blood cells. An excessive concentration of bilirubin indicates liver dysfunction, since the liver clears the circulation of bilirubin by secreting it in the bile. The jaundice meter is a reflectance colorimeter that quantifies the yellowness of the skin, which depends on the serum bilirubin concentration. Hannemann et al. (1978) demonstrated a method for determining bilirubin concentration from skin reflectance measurements, identifying the important spectral bands.

A two-channel jaundice meter (Minolta Camera Co., Osaka, Japan) that measures skin reflectance on the forehead is shown in Fig. 25. The light source is a 2 Joule xenon discharge tube that illuminates the skin surface through a fiber-optic bundle. The reflected light is split into two beams by a dichroic mirror. One beam passes through a 550-nm (green) filter, the other through a 460-nm (blue) filter, and the intensity of each beam is measured by a photodiode. The instrument is first standardized on a white reflector, and the difference in optical densities of the blue and green channels is displayed on a scale, the indication being related to serum bilirubin.

To use the jaundice meter, the fiber-optic surface (40 mm^2) is pressed against the forehead, and when a force of 200 g is reached the xenon discharge lamp flashes. This application of force blanches the skin and permits measurement of skin yellowness.

In a study of four neonates with serum bilirubin values ranging from 1.5 to 13.5 mg %, Yamanouchi et al. (1980) correlated the indication on the Minolta transcutaneous bilirubin meter with directly measured serum bilirubin determined by a spectrophotometer and chemical (alkali azobilirubin) analyzer. Figure 26 presents the results of both comparisons. A similar study conducted by Hannamenn et al. (1982) provided slightly different results in low-birth-weight and full-term infants.

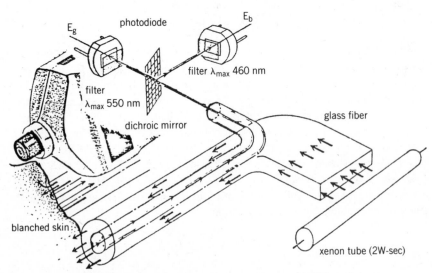

Figure 25   The Minolta bilirubin meter. [(Reproduced by permission from I. Yamanouchi et al., *Pediatrics* **65**(2):195–202. (1980).]

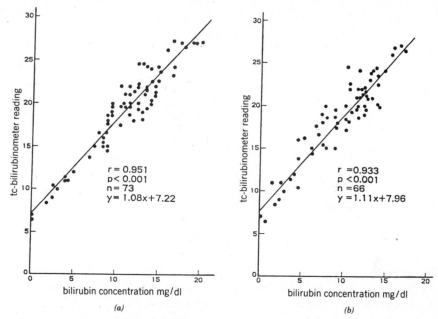

Figure 26 Correlation between transcutaneous (tc) bilirubinometry and serum total bilirubin concentration (*a*) measured with the American Optical spectrophotometer and (*b*) measured by the alkali azobilirubin method. [Redrawn with permission from I. Yamanouchi et al., *Pediatrics* **65**(2):195–202 (1980).]

These and other studies indicate that such an instrument is a useful screening tool and is perhaps of most value in following the results of therapy.

An important point should be recognized in jaundice assessment in neonates and other subjects. Whereas the serum bilirubin in a typical subject is about 1.1 mg %, when the subject is jaundiced it is 2–5 mg %. However, in neonates serum bilirubin concentration normally rises to about 10 mg % at day 3 and falls to about one-half this value by about day 8. This change reflects the development of liver function.

With a view to quantitatively establishing the accuracy of measuring bilirubin by transcutaneous reflectance, Hannemann et al. (1979) obtained reflectance spectra from 380 to 800 nm on 58 white and 45 black infants for three serum bilirubin concentration ranges (1 to 7, 7 to 13, and greater than 13 mg %). Their data are shown in Fig. 27 and indicate that there are differences between the results achieved with white and black infants. For this reason, they advocated the use of three wavelengths (420, 460, and 510 nm) for both white and black full-term infants.

The last word about jaundice meters has by no means been written. Such an instrument shares many of the problems of transcutaneous oximetry, which has evolved to eight channels of spectral data to improve accuracy in the presence of various skin pigmentations. Future jaundice meters need to be able to accommodate a wide range of skin pigments. How many and which spectral channels will be needed is for the future to establish.

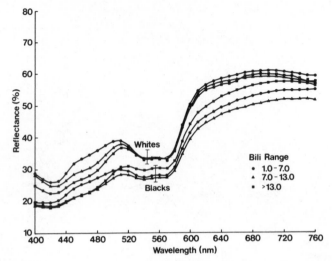

Figure 27   Representative reflectance spectra for ranges of bilirubin concentration (mg/100 mL serum) based on sample populations of 58 white and 45 black full-term infants. [From R. Hannemann et al., *Pediatr. Res.* **13**:1326–1329 (1979).]

THERMOGRAPHY

Principle

Photoconductive cells (photoresistors) are used to image the pattern of infrared radiation emitted by the human skin; the name given to this technique is thermography. The clinical uses of thermography will be presented following a description of the thermograph.

The temperature of the human skin is typically 32°C (89.6°F); the skin simulates a blackbody radiator. The wavelength of the radiation emitted by a blackbody is inversely proportional to its absolute temperature. From Wein's displacement law, the wavelength corresponding to 32°C (305 K) is

$$\lambda_{max} = \frac{2898}{305} = 9.50 \ \mu m.$$

Therefore the peak of radiant energy from the human body is in the infrared region. In order to use the radiated power as a measure of skin temperature, it is necessary to know the emissivity of skin.

The emissivity of the human skin has been investigated in vivo and in vitro. Hardy was one of the first to provide such data when he reported a value of 0.980 ± 0.01 in the wavelength range extending from 4 to 20 μm (Hardy and Muschenkeim, 1934; Hardy, 1939). He also stated that more than 70% of the radiated energy from human skin falls in this region. Mitchell et al. (1967) reported a value within 1% of unity for human skin; they also reviewed the reported data. Watmough and Oliver (1968) reported a value within 2% of unity for the 2–5.4-μm region and later a value that increased monotonically. From these data it can be concluded that the emissivity of human skin (black or white) is very nearly unity in the region around 9.5 μm, where the maximum amount of energy is radiated. Lloyd-Williams (1964) stated, "the human skin, whether white or black is, in a thermal sense, an almost perfect blackbody radiator and painting or blackening its surface cannot increase its radiation." Therefore, measurement of the radiant energy from human skin provides an indication of its temperature.

The Thermograph

At the heart of the thermograph is the detector for the infrared radiation emitted by the scene. To acquire data to form an image, the detector must be made to examine or scan the whole scene. Thus the two other important components are the scanning mirrors and focusing optics. Figure 28 identifies the essential parts of typical thermographs. Electronic circuitry is used to amplify the detected infrared signal and to control the scanning system so that a display can be synchronized to reproduce the thermal scene.

Detectors for infrared radiation consist of specially prepared compounds, which often include rare earth materials. Essentially such detectors are photoconductors, i.e., their resistance decreases with increasing incident radiation. The peak spectral sensitivity of each detector depends on the particular combination of materials employed. Many of the infrared detectors operate at very low temperatures in order to reduce their resistive noise and thereby attain an adequate signal-to-noise ratio. Liquid nitrogen, which boils at 77 K, is often used to cool the detector.

In addition to having an adequate sensitivity for the radiation to be measured, the infrared detector must have a short enough response time to indicate the temperature of a region of the scene before it moves to examine a region of different temperature. The importance of this fact will become more apparent when the scanning methods are described.

Scanning Methods

To form the thermographic image, the scene must be scanned by the infrared detector from left to right and from top to bottom. Many different techniques are used to accomplish this goal. Perhaps the easiest method of visualizing how this is accomplished is to refer to Fig. 28a, which illustrates the technique employed in the Texas Instruments Thermoscope. The infrared detector looks at the scene to be imaged through a front-surfaced converging mirror and a hexagonal front-surfaced mirror that rotates at 20 rev/sec. As this mirror rotates, it is tilted continuously so that the point of examination by the detector is moved across the scene with a slight angle. The rate of tilt of the mirror is such that the whole scene is examined with 125 lines in 4.5 sec. Then the tilt on the mirror is reversed, and it returns to its untilted position in 1.5 sec, and the scene is scanned again. In this way, the detector provides an output as it continuously examines the infrared energy emitted

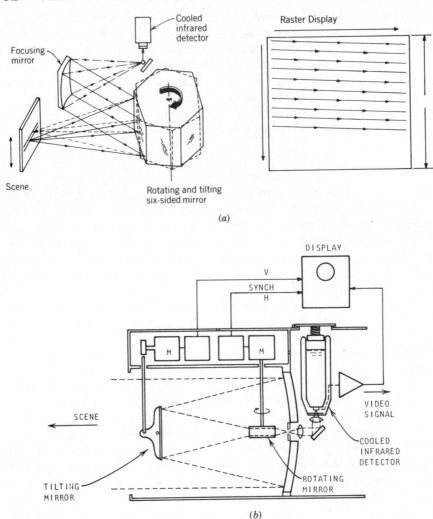

Figure 28 (*a*) Scanning method used in the Texas Instruments thermograph. The rotating and tilting mirrors cause the infrared detector to examine the scene from left to right and top to bottom. (*b*) The AGA thermograph. The rotating mirror causes the infrared detector to examine the scene from left to right, and the tilting mirror allows the detector to examine the scene from top to bottom. The motors M that drive the mirrors provide synchronizing (SYNCH) signals to the vertical (V) and horizontal (H) sweeps of the display oscilloscope.

by the object under investigation. The detector output is led to an amplifier, which in turn modulates the intensity of the beam of a cathode ray display tube.

In order to form the thermal image on the cathode ray tube, the excursion of the beam (sweep) must be synchronized with the rotating and tilting mirror. As it rotates, the mirror provides a signal that synchronizes the horizontal scan (time base). The vertical sweep of the cathode ray tube is synchronized with the tilting.

Thus, with no thermal image, a white raster, i.e., a series of slightly slanting parallel lines (120 in 4.5 sec), is seen on the cathode ray tube. When the infrared detector encounters a warm area in the scene, the intensity of the cathode ray display is reduced for the time taken to scan the warm region. Thus, a black-and-white image of the warmer and cooler regions appears on the face of the cathode ray tube.

The method of scanning in another thermograph (AGA Thermovision) is shown in Fig. 28*b*. A cooled InSb infrared detector scans the image horizontally via an eight-sided mirror rotating at 20 rev/sec, providing a line frequency of 1600 lines per second. Vertical scanning is accomplished by vibrating a front-surfaced mirror at 16 per second; thus the frame (picture) frequency is 16 per second. In summary, a 100-line picture is formed each $\frac{1}{16}$ sec. The motors driving the rotating and oscillating mirrors provide synchronizing signals for the cathode ray tube, which displays the thermal image.

With many thermographs, the display on the face of the cathode ray tube provides a temperature resolution of about 0.2°C. The display is usually photographed with a 70-mm film camera. Sometimes a Polaroid film or print is taken of the display. Some thermographs provide an isothermal-line feature to highlight all the regions above a selected temperature. With some instruments, the isothermal-line feature allows a chosen temperature range to be accented.

Temperature Calibration

To convert the black-and-white areas in the display to degrees of temperature, several different techniques are used. In one instrument (Texas Instruments), at the beginning and end of each scanning line the infrared detector sees internal temperature standards, thereby providing reference points in the display. However, a more accurate temperature calibration can be achieved by including reference black-bodies (at known temperatures) in the scene. A simple two-temperature blackbody is shown in Fig. 29. It consists of two copper blocks blackened with high-emissivity paint. Inside each block is a heater and a temperature detector. Each block is maintained at the desired constant temperature to within 0.01°C. The actual reference temperatures used are dictated by the temperature of the object to be studied. For skin examination, one at 28°C and one at 35°C is satisfactory.

Two-point calibration may not provide the desired accuracy, particularly if a film recording is made of a thermal image. The density of exposed photographic film is nonlinear with exposure. Therefore, accurate calibration of film requires multiple temperature reference points in the desired temperature range.

A more accurate temperature gray scale can be made by using an array of 10 blackbodies, each at a slightly different temperature—e.g., 29–38°C. The array of blackbody temperature references appears as varying shades of gray on the photographic film of the display. To relate points in the scene to temperature, areas of equal grayness are matched. Matching can be achieved by eye or by using a photographic densitometer to measure light transmission through the film at the desired point in the scene and then at points along the temperature gray scale. Of course, the photographic film can be digitized by using a scanning densitometer.

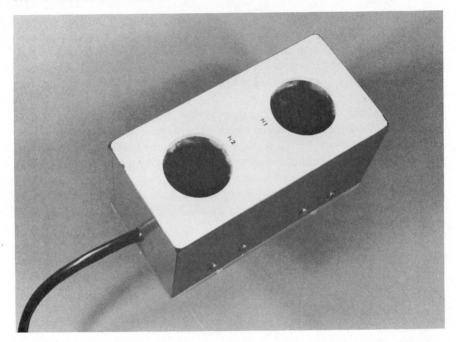

Figure 29   Reference blackbody temperature source consisting of two blocks of copper painted with flat black paint. Each block is maintained at a known and constant temperature. Inclusion of these blackbodies in the scene allows accurate temperature calibration of the scene. (Courtesy of J. A. Pearce.)

This provides a digital representation of the transmission at each point in the scene along with the temperature gray scale. Computer processing is then possible to write out isothermal line maps of the scene. However, the nonlinearity of the film makes direct digitization of the electrical signal from the infrared detector much more desirable.

By convention, the hotter areas in the scene are the darker areas in the display, although some thermographs can provide the opposite type of display also. The choice of black to represent increased temperature derives from the fact that the eye does not perceive equally well at the two ends of a gray scale. It has been shown that the minimum detectable change on the gray scale is smaller at the black end than at the white end. The case for the use of black to represent the hottest regions in the scene was championed by Wallace and Dodd (1969). In Fig. 30 both types of displays are presented. It is interesting to note that when black is used to represent the hotter areas (Fig. 30a) the cooler areas tend to fade into the background and help identify the boundaries of the object under study.

Physiological Basis for Thermography

The temperature of the skin is determined by the equilibrium between heat production and heat loss. As stated previously, exposed human skin in an envi-

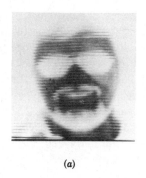 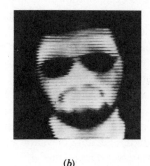

(a)   (b)

Figure 30   Thermograms of the face of a normal bearded subject wearing glasses. In (a) black is used to represent the hotter regions and in (b) the hottest regions are the whitest.

ronment of about 20°C (68°F) exhibits a temperature of about 32°C. Heat is lost to the environment by the evaporation of perspiration, conductive heat transfer to the air and supporting objects, convection, and radiation to all objects in the environment that are below skin temperature; those that are above skin temperature radiate heat to the body. For these reasons it is necessary to achieve an equilibrium with the environment before thermal imaging is carried out. With exposed skin, a period of about 10 min in a darkened room at a constant temperature and with little air movement is usually sufficient.

The source of skin heat is derived from the metabolic activity of the underlying tissues. Thus the local circulation and metabolism are the principal factors. It is useful to remember that venous blood, which drains metabolically active regions, is slightly hotter than arterial blood; therefore superficial veins will heat the skin more than superficial arteries. Tissues and organs with a high metabolic rate will be hotter than normal tissue, and their venous drainage will also be hotter than the venous drainage from normal tissue. Malignant tissue has a higher metabolic rate than normal tissue. These facts underlie the use of thermography to identify malignant tissue by its ability to elevate the overlying skin temperature. When the malignant tissue is deep, the skin temperature rise may be small. However, since clinical thermography has demonstrated an ability to detect both superficial and deep malignancies, it is necessary to find a reasonable explanation, which has been provided by Wallace and Cade (1975). From many studies in which cancer of the breast was identified by thermography, Wallace and Cade pointed out that the elevation in skin temperature resulting from a superficial tumor is due to conduction of heat from the tumor. The increased temperature due to deep-seated tumors reveals itself by an accentuated venous drainage pattern, which elevates skin temperature.

Clinical Applications

Normally the skin temperature has a fairly high degree of right-to-left symmetry after coming into equilibrium in a draft-free environment for about 10 min. It is only after this equilibration time that any subtle temperature differences of diagnostic significance are seen. The temperature difference due to an underlying pathophysiologic process may be on the order of $\pm 1°C$; therefore the thermograph should be able to resolve $\pm 0.1°C$. Very frequently the display device is set to cover a range of only about 5°C from the coolest to the hottest parts of the scene.

Any increased local blood supply or metabolism will raise skin temperature locally. Many diseases produce this effect; however, thermography has found its most frequent use in identifying cancer of the breast (Wallace and Dodd, 1969). Mammary malignancies may be small or large and superficial or deep. If superficial, the skin temperature elevation identifies the extent fairly well. If the tumor is deep, the elevated temperature of the venous drainage increases the skin temperature and provides the diagnostic information.

Figure 31 presents a thermogram of both normal female breasts, with the blacker

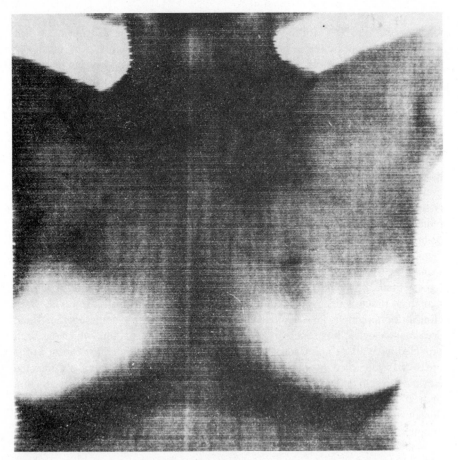

Figure 31 Thermogram of normal breasts showing a normal temperature distribution. The subject is seated with both hands on her head. (Reprinted with permission from J. D. Wallace, and C. M. Cade, *Clinical Thermography.* Copyright CRC Press, Boca Raton, Florida, 1975.)

areas being hotter. In this illustration, presented by Wallace and Cade (1975), the subject has both hands on her head. There is symmetry and normal temperature distribution. In another illustration from Wallace and Cade, Fig. 32 is a thermogram of a subject with a large carcinoma of the right breast. Another unilateral temperature elevation revealed by venous drainage is shown by the thermogram of the left breast illustrated in Fig. 33 from a subject with a small cancer.

Thermography has also been used to identify other pathophysiological processes. For example, decreased circulation due to vasospasm or blockage of an artery results in a reduction in the temperature of the region previously supplied by a blocked blood vessel. In the early days of vascular-repair surgery, thermography was used to identify the improvement in circulation resulting from vessel repair.

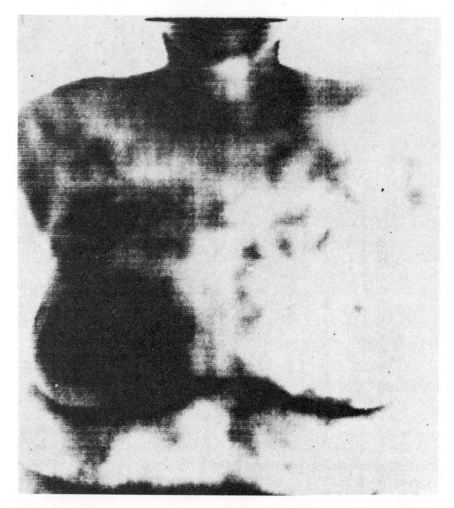

Figure 32 Thermogram of a subject with a large disseminated carcinoma of the right breast. (Reprinted with permission from J. D. Wallace and C. M. Cade, *Clinical Thermography*. Copyright CRC Press, Boca Raton, Florida, 1975.)

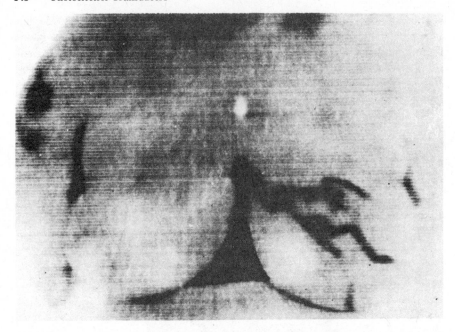

Figure 33   Thermogram of a subject with a small cancer of the left breast showing elevated temperature of the venous drainage type. (Reprinted with permission from J. D. Wallace and C. M. Cade, *Clinical Thermography*. Copyright CRC Press, Boca Raton, Florida, 1975.

Thermography has also been used to identify localized inflammation. For a time it appeared to offer promise in identifying arthritis. In their excellent monograph on clinical thermography, Wallace and Cade (1975) discuss a wide variety of uses for thermography, including some in veterinary medicine.

Thermography has been used to estimate the nonuniformity of current distribution under skin-surface electrodes carrying current. In these applications, the highest temperature rise identifies the region of highest current density. These applications are discussed in Chapter 13.

BODY TEMPERATURE

There has always been interest in the use of infrared emission to measure body temperature. An extensive investigation of the suitability of various body sites was undertaken by Barnes (1967). He used a calibrated thermistor bolometer that measured the infrared radiation emitted at various sites and compared the temperature obtained from each with body temperature measured with an oral thermometer. In 10 subjects he found that the only site that provided an accurate measure of body temperature was the ear canal. Figure 34 presents his results for the 10 subjects.

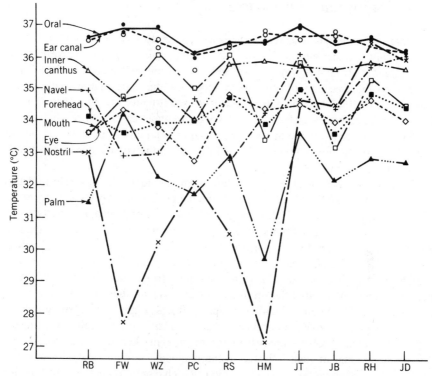

Figure 34 Temperature determined by infrared radiation at different sites on 10 subjects. The solid dark curve represents oral temperature measured directly. [Redrawn from R. B. Barnes, *J. Appl. Physiol.* **22**(6):1143–1146 (1967).]

In discussing the various sites for temperature measurement by infrared emission, Barnes stated that the ear canal is the ideal site because there is minimal air movement, the skin is dry (eliminating evaporative cooling), and there is minimal radiation loss to the environment. Ear wax, which is in thermal equilibrium, causes no difficulties. As a result of these findings by Barnes, tiny thermistors are being developed to measure the temperature in the ear canal.

Another colorimetric application of a photodetector is due to Baker (1961), who used the high-infrared-sensitivity characteristics of a lead selenide photoresistor to construct a rapidly responding carbon dioxide analyzer to record breath-by-breath changes in the concentration of this gas in expired air. The 4.26-μm absorption band of carbon dioxide was employed to detect the amount of this component in a gas sample passing between an infrared source and the photoconductive detector. The response time obtained was limited by the speed of admission of the gas sample and the frequency of the chopper amplifier. In practice, an overall response time of about 50 msec was obtained.

NONCOLORIMETRIC APPLICATIONS

There are numerous instances in which photodetectors have been used noncolorimetrically for the transduction of physiological events. One of the earliest was due to Rein et al. (1940), who constructed a blood pressure transducer by affixing a shade to the free end of a Bourdon tube. On one side of the shade was a photovoltaic cell, and on the other was a $\frac{1}{3}$-W exciter lamp. Pressure applied to the Bourdon tube moved the shade and exposed the photodetector to the light bulb, thereby producing a voltage that was recorded by a rapidly responding galvanometer. The response time reported was 12.5 msec, and the volume displacement was 13.5 mm^3/100 mmHg.

Gilson (1943) described the application of the photoelectric principle to detect the movement of the light beam of a Wiggers membrane manometer and the movement of a myograph lever. This method of transduction added sensitivity to an already high-quality photographic recording pressure transducer. His myograph was one of the first to produce an electrical signal from muscle pull. An ingenious method of using the photoelectric principle to develop a catheter-tip blood pressure transducer was described by Clark et al. (1965). In this device a tiny reflecting diaphragm was mounted at the tip of a catheter (0.11 in. diameter) that contained two concentrically mounted bundles of optical fibers. Light was transmitted down one bundle of 3-mil fibers and reflected back to a silicon photocell affixed to the end of the other. Pressure applied to the diaphragm changed the curvature and altered the amount of light reflected to the photocell. With a silvered mylar diaphragm of appropriate thickness (1–3 mils), the change in output was 200 μV for 0–50 mmHg change in pressure. The resonant frequency of the diaphragm was reported by these investigators to be 10 kHz, indicating that the device had an extremely high frequency response and was capable of recording the briefest of transients in the cardiovascular system.

Figure 35 summarizes several applications of the photoelectric principle described by Geddes et al. (1956, 1957, 1961). Figure 35a illustrates a blood pressure transducer that resembles Rein's except that a high-efficiency miniature photoemissive vacuum tube is employed instead of a photovoltaic cell. With a 15-psi Bourdon tube, a response time of 20 msec is easily attainable when the tube is filled with saline solution. A pneumograph (Fig. 35b) detects respiration by measuring changes in chest circumference. When the closed rubber bellows is wrapped around the chest, the pressure in it decreases with inspiration. The reduced pressure, sensed by the metal bellows, causes a shade to alter its position between a photoemissive tube and a light bulb. Figure 35c shows a photoelectric myograph. The stiff metal leaf with the hook carries the shade. When the muscle force is applied to the hook, the elastic leaf is deflected and the shade is made to move parallel to the face of the phototube by means of a parallelogram arrangement of springs. A series of metal leaves with different amounts of stiffness are employed to extend the range of the basic transducing element.

Photodetectors are ideally suited to detection of the arterial pulse. Usually the reflectance method introduced by Hertzman (1938) is employed in which the pho-

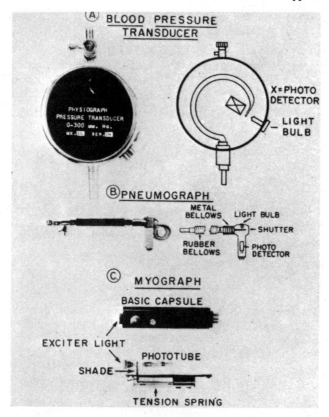

Figure 35 Photoelectric transducers: (*A*) blood pressure transducer; (*B*) pneumograph; (*C*) myograph.

todetector and light source are adjacent and are mounted in a small housing that is applied to the skin surface. The light is reflected and scattered from the underlying tissue bed, resulting in a pulsatile signal from the photodetector. Figure 36 illustrates the type of recording obtained with a reflectance photodetector, sometimes called a photoplethysmograph, applied to the fingerpad.

Although a small incandescent lamp or a light-emitting diode (LED) can be used to provide the light and a photoemissive, photodiode, or photoresistive cell can serve as the detector, several operating constraints favor certain choices. For example, to eliminate artifacts due to changes in ambient illumination, and to obtain immunity from changes in blood oxygen saturation, it is wise to choose an infrared light source and a detector operating at 805 nm. Consequently, an LED or a photoresistor or photodiode would be the preferred embodiment.

It is easy to obtain a pulse from a reflectance plethysmograph; however, the signal is derived from the capillary bed. For a time it was thought that blood flow could be determined from the photoplethysmogram; such a hope was not realized. Occlusion of the venous return immediately increases, rather than decreases, the

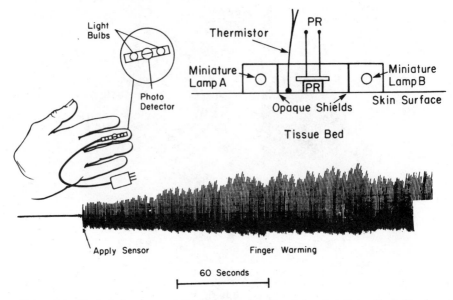

Figure 36 Photoplethysmograph (inset) and pulse record showing thermally induced vasodilation in the fingerpad resulting from tissue warming due to the small exciter lamp in the photoplethysmograph.

size of the pulsatile signal. Moreover, the signal amplitude depends on the degree of vasodilation of the small arterioles supplying the capillary bed. For example, vasoconstriction caused by the inhalation of cigarette smoke dramatically reduces the amplitude of the pulsatile signal. The vasoconstriction of cardiovascular shock is easily indicated by the photoplethysmogram, and such records have found use in monitoring anesthetized patients.

When employing photoelectric pickups, an important consideration is the amount of heat produced by the light source. Heat causes dilation of blood vessels, altering the state of the vascular bed under examination. Figure 36 illustrates this point. For this reason it is useful to include a temperature detector (thermistor) in the photoplethysmograph, as shown in Fig. 36. The skin temperature should never be allowed to exceed 42°C, to avoid tissue damage.

A photoelectric pulse pickup can be employed in systems that measure blood pressure and heart rate. Capacitance coupling with a relatively short time constant (0.3–1 sec for human subjects) can be used. If an artery central to a photoelectric pulse pickup is occluded by a pressurized cuff, the pulse disappears. As the pressure is reduced, the pulse appears when the pressure in the cuff is slightly below systolic. If the pressure is read at the first appearance of the pulse, the value obtained is very close to the systolic blood pressure in the artery under the cuff. As the pressure in the cuff is further decreased, the pulse increases in amplitude and reaches a stable level. There is no consistently identifiable transition point as the cuff pressure passes through mean or diastolic pressure.

An ingenious use of the photoelectric method to obtain a good approximation of systolic and diastolic pressures was described by Wood et al. (1950). With their method an oximeter earpiece with a pressure capsule was employed. A continuous record was made of the capsule pressure and the optical pulse. With a capsule pressure above systolic, the optical pulse record showed almost no oscillations. As the capsule pressure was reduced, the pulse appeared at a pressure near the systolic value. As the pressure was further reduced, the amplitude of the photoelectric pulse increased, passed through a maximum, and then stabilized at a reduced amplitude. When the pulses were maximal, the capsule pressure was taken as diastolic pressure. A simultaneous record of direct blood pressure in the radial artery revealed a good degree of correspondence for systolic and diastolic pressures. However, we now know that cuff pressure for maximal oscillations is mean arterial pressure.

Geddes et al. (1961) employed the photoelectric transduction principle to obtain an electrical signal related to the partial pressure of oxygen in a gas sample by the method represented in Fig. 37. In this illustration the detector is the Pauling paramagnetic oxygen analyzer (Pauling et al., 1946), which is now available commercially. By replacing the scale with a photodetector having a triangular aperture and replacing the light source with an illuminated slit, the position of the mirror-carrying sensor in the analyzer was converted to an electrical signal.

When fluids flow at low rates, it is advantageous to count drops. Although the size of a drop depends on many factors, in most situations 15–30 drops constitute 1 mL of aqueous fluid. With a given orifice, drop size is fairly constant. Drop counters in which the fluid strikes a pair of contacts have never been dependable.

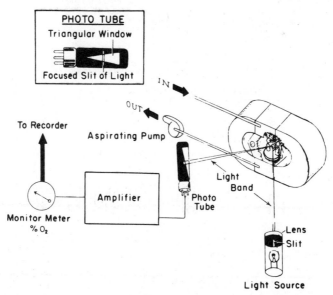

Figure 37 Photoelectric transducer applied to paramagnetic Beckman oxygen analyzer, model C (modified). [From L. A. Geddes et al., *IRE Trans. Bio-Med. Electron.* **BME-8**:38(1961). By permission.]

To eliminate direct contact with the drops of fluid, the photoelectric principle has been employed with considerable success. In some instances the drop interrupts the beam of light entering the photodetector; in others the drop reflects and scatters the light sensed by the photodetector. Among the investigators who have described such drop counters are Goetz (1948), Clementz and Ryberg (1949), Hilton and Lywood (1954), Lindgren and Unvas (1954), Peiss and McCoole (1958), and Geddes et al. (1969). The unit used by Geddes et al. (1969) is illustrated in Fig. 38 and consists of a miniature incandescent lamp and an infrared-sensitive photoresistor mounted in an assembly that is easily applied to any drip tube. The frame of the transducer consists of two 90 degree V-shaped plastic blocks. In the apex of one V is mounted the miniature lamp, and in the apex of the other is the photoresistor to which an infrared filter has been applied. Both the lamp and the

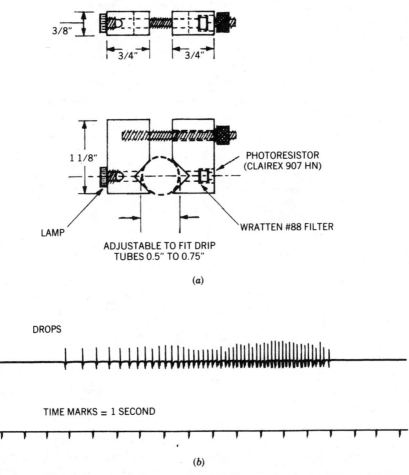

Figure 38 (*a*) Photoelectric drop counter employing infrared light. (*b*) Record of drops. [Redrawn from L. A. Geddes et al., *Med. Res. Eng.* **8**(4):27–29 (1969).]

photoresistor are mounted in small tunnels in the plastic blocks. The tunnels for the lamp and photoresistor collimate the optical path so that the falling drop alters the transmission, which is detected as a change in resistance by the photoresistor. The V shape of the blocks permits application of the transducer to drip tubes of different diameters.

The infrared filter (Wratten No. 88) in front of the photoresistor cuts out virtually all radiation shorter than 800 mm. The visible spectrum is largely excluded, which renders the transducer immune from ambient lighting interference, in particular from fluorescent lamps, which emit very little if any infrared energy. Although incandescent room lighting contains infrared energy, the collimated optical system and the sharp cutoff of the filter–photodetector assembly virtually eliminate detection of changes in room lighting caused by switching incandescent lamps on and off.

An ingenious photoplethysmograph-controlled servosystem for continuously measuring blood pressure noninvasively in humans was developed by Yamakoshi et al. (1980) and Yamakoshi and Kamiya (1983), who originally devised the method for application to the rat tail (Yamakoshi et al., 1979). The method relies on the principle of vascular unloading, the pressure in an occluding cuff continuously tracking the pressure to achieve this condition, which is the criterion for obtaining mean pressure with the oscillometric method (Geddes et al., 1983).

The system developed by Yamakoshi et al. is illustrated in Fig. 39a. A finger is placed in a sleeve surrounded by a fluid-filled annular compression chamber connected to an actuator that controls the counterpressure. A transducer on the piston of the actuator identifies its position to the feedback system. The sleeve surrounding the finger is translucent, and on one side is placed a light-emitting diode (LED); opposite it, and on the skin, is placed a photoelectric transducer (PT). The LED and PT constitute a direct-coupled photoelectric plethysmograph. The pressure in the fluid is recorded with a pressure transducer, and when the device is set for operation the recording reflects intraarterial pressure.

The method of setting the system involves finding the operating point in the open-loop condition; this is accomplished by increasing the counterpressure in the fluid while recording the pulsatile oscillations detected by the photoplethysmograph, as shown in Fig. 39b. The cuff pressure (and hence position of the actuator) for maximal oscillations is identified. The plethysmograph signal for this point identifies the condition for vascular unloading and provides the reference signal for the servosystem, which can now be activated to find this point. Figure 39c illustrates a typical pressure recording obtained from the fluid in the compression chamber and an intraarterial pressure recording; note the similarity. Yamakoshi et al. (1980) compared indirectly and directly recorded brachial artery blood pressure (I and D, respectively) from 50 to 125 mmHg in human subjects. The relationship obtained was $I = 0.97D - 9.76$ mmHg, with a correlation coefficient of 0.978.

The photoelectric servosystem described by Yamakoshi et al. measures and tracks digital arterial pressure, which is known to be below brachial artery pressure (Geddes, 1970), so the results obtained are not surprising. In fact, at 80 mmHg brachial artery pressure, the regression equation of Yamakoshi provides 68 mmHg, well within the known brachial-to-digital artery pressure difference.

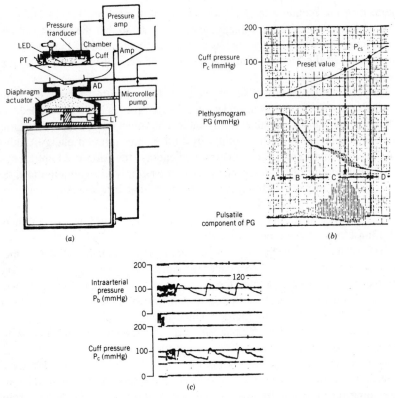

Figure 39   (*a*) The servocontrolled fluid-filled finger cuff for continuous indirect pressure. (*b*) Pulsatile oscillations detected by the plethysmograph as cuff pressure is increased. The system is preset at the value corresponding to the maximum of the pulsatile component. (*c*) Comparison of intraarterial pressure record obtained directly with record obtained indirectly from the fluid in the plethysmograph. (Redrawn from Yamakoshi et al., 1980.)

The dynamic response of the system is demonstrated by the similarity of the directly and indirectly recorded pressures shown in Fig. 39*c*. Further proof of the rapidity of response of the system can be seen by the presence of the dicrotic notch in the pressure recording obtained from the fluid in the plethysmograph. However, it is important to recognize that this servotracking method, while continuous, is still partially occlusive and reduces the perfusion of blood in the finger. Thus it cannot be applied for long periods of time without risk.

Another interesting use of the photoelectric principle is in the recording of the movements imparted to the body when the heart beats. Such a recording is called a ballistocardiogram, and from it may be derived body displacement, velocity, and acceleration. To record body movements directly rather than those of a table on which a subject was placed, Dock and Taubman (1949) developed a photoelectric transducer that was coupled to the shins or head of a supine subject. Body movements altered the position of a shade placed between a photodetector and a light source. For a time it was hoped that this signal could be calibrated directly in terms of the systolic discharge from the heart, but this has not been possible to date. In a given subject, however, ballistocardiograms do indicate changes in stroke volume.

A practical method for detecting rotary motion features a pair of polarizing filters. One filter is used to polarize the light from a source, and the other is placed between the source of polarized light and a photodetector. The amount of light reaching the photodetector depends on the relation between the planes of polarization of the filters. Rotation of either filter from the position of maximum or extinction will allow the frictionless detection of angular movement photoelectrically.

In using photoelectric transducers, suitable choice of the type of photodetector will produce an appreciable voltage or current for a small change in light level. Thus a high conversion efficiency is easy to obtain. Because the mask mounted on a moving member usually can be made small and lightweight, it adds little inertia to the system. Freedom from contact also eliminates frictional and hysteresis errors. With a proper choice of photodetector, the response time is determined by the mechanical characteristics of the moving element. Alternating and direct current can energize the light source. If alternating current is employed, the photodetector output contains a ripple signal with twice the frequency of the current used to excite the lamp.

There are disadvantages in using phototransducers. In most applications it is necessary to provide shielding to prevent stray light from entering the transducer; in nearly all, a constant-intensity light source is required. In addition, the light output of many lamps varies nearly as the square of the applied voltage; hence the lamp voltage must be well regulated. One way of reducing the need for regulation is to use two identical photodetectors in a differential configuration. In such a circuit arrangement one photodetector monitors the light intensity and the other senses the changes in light produced by the event being transduced. In practice, a signal derived from the difference in the outputs of the two photodetectors is immune to changes in light intensity over a considerable range.

REFERENCES

Acker, R. M., R. P. Lipkis, R. S. Miller, and P. C. Robinson. 1960. Solar cell power supplies for satellites. *Electronics* **33**:167–172.

Baker, L. E. 1961. A rapidly responding narrow-band infrared gaseous CO_2 analyzer for physiological studies. *IRE Trans. Bio-Med. Electron.* **BME-8**:16–24.

Barnes, R. B. 1967. Determination of body temperature by infra-red radiation. *J. Appl. Physiol.* **22**(6):1143–1146.

Clark, F. J., E. M. Schmidt, and R. F. De La Croix. 1965. Fiber optic blood pressure catheter with frequency response from DC into the audio range. *Proc. Natl. Electron. Conf.* **21**:213–216.

Clementz, B., and C. E. Ryberg. 1949. An ordinate recorder for measuring drop flow. *Acta Physiol. Scand.* **17**:339–344.

Comroe, J. H., and S. Y. Botelho. 1947. Unreliability of cyanosis in recognition of arterial anoxemia. *Am. J. Med. Sci.* **214:**1-6.

Connolly, D. C., and E. H. Wood. 1954. Simultaneous measurement of the appearance and disappearance of T1824 (Evans Blue) in blood and tissue after intravenous injection in man. *J. Appl. Physiol.* **7:**73-83.

Dock, W., and F. Taubman. 1949. Some techniques for recording the ballistocardiograph directly from the body. *Am. J. Med.* **7:**751-755.

Elam, J. O., J. F. Neville, W. Sleator, and W. N. Elam. 1949. Sources of error in oximetry. *Ann. Surg.* **130:**755-773.

Enson, Y., W. A. Briscoe, M. L. Polanyi, and A. Cournand. 1962. *In vivo* studies with an intravascular and intracardiac reflection oximeter. *J. Appl. Physiol.* **17:**552-558.

Fox, I. J., and E. H. Wood. 1960. Indocyanine green: Physical and physiologic properties. *Proc. Staff Meet. Mayo Clin.* **35:**732-744.

Geddes, L. A. 1970. *The Direct and Indirect Measurement of Blood Pressure.* Year Book Medical Publishers, Chicago, IL, 1970, 196 pp.

Geddes, L. A., H. E. Hoff, and W. A. Spencer. 1956. *IRE Natl. Cond. Rec.* **9:**29-37.

Geddes, L. A., H. E. Hoff, and W. A. Spencer. 1957. The Physiograph—An instrument in teaching physiology, *J. Med. Educ.* **32:**181-198.

Geddes, L. A., H. E. Hoff, and W. A. Spencer. 1961. The center for vital studies—A new laboratory for the study of bodily functions in man. *IRE Trans. Bio.-Med. Electron.* **BME-8:**33-45.

Geddes, L. A., A. G. Moore, J. Bourland, J. Vasku, and G. Cantrell. 1969. An efficient drop transducer. *Med. Res. Eng.* **8**(4):27-29.

Geddes, L. A., M. Voelz, C. Combs, and D. Reiner. 1983. Characterization of the oscillometric method for measuring indirect blood pressure. *Ann. Biomed. Eng.* **10**(6):271-280.

Gilson, W. E. 1943. Applications of electronics to physiology. *Electronics* **16:**86-89.

Goetz, R. H. 1948. A photoelectric drop recorder. *Lancet* **1:**830-831.

Goldie, E. A. G. 1942. A device for the continuous indication of oxygen saturation of circulating blood in man. *J. Sci. Instru.* **19:**23-25.

Greenaway, D. L., and G. Harbeke. 1968. *Optical Properties and Band Structure of Semiconductors.* Pergamon, Oxford.

Grodins, F. 1962. Basic concepts in the determination of vascular volumes by indicator dilution methods. *Circ. Res.* **10:**429-446.

Hamilton, W., R. L. Riley, A. M. Attyah, A. Cournand, D. M. Powell, A. Himmelstein, R. P. Noble, J. W. Remington, D. W. Richards, N. C. Wheeler, and A. C. Witham. 1948. Comparison of the Fick and dye injection methods of measuring the cardiac output in man. *Am. J. Physiol.* **153:**309-321.

Hannemann, R. E., D. P. DeWitt, and J. F. Weichel. 1978. Neonatal serum bilirubin from skin reflectance. *Pediatr. Res.* **12:**207-210.

Hannemann, R. E., D. P. DeWitt, E. J. Haley, R. L. Schreiver, and P. Bonderman. 1979. Determination of serum bilirubin by skin reflectance: Effect of pigmentation. *Pediatr. Res.* **13:**1326-1329.

Hannemann, R. E., R. Schreiver, D. P. DeWitt, S. A. Norris, and M. K. Glich. 1982. Evaluation of the Minolta bilirubin meter. *Pediatrics* **69:**107-109.

Hardy, J. D. 1939. The radiating power of human skin in the infrared. *Am. J. Physiol.* **127:**454-462.

Hardy, J. D., and C. Muschenkeim. 1934. The radiation from the human body. IV. The emission, reflection and transmission of infra-red radiation by the human skin. *J. Clin. Invest.* **13:**817-831.

Hertzman, A. 1938. The blood supply of various skin areas as estimated by the photoelectric plethysmograph. *Am. J. Physiol.* **124:**328-340.

Hilton, S. M., and D. W. Lywood. 1954. Photoelectric drop counter. *J. Physiol.* **123:**64.

Jacobs, S. F. 1960. Characteristics of infra-red detectors. *Electronics* **33:**72-73.

Johnson, C. C., R. D. Palm, D. C. Stewart and W. E. Martin, 1971. A solid-state fiberoptic oximeter. *J. Am. Assoc. Adv. Med. Instrum.* **5:**77–83.

Kinsman, J. M., J. W. Moore, and W. F. Hamilton. 1929. Studies on the circulation. *Am. J. Physiol.* **89:**322–330.

Kramer, K. 1934. Fortlaufende Registrierung der Sauerstoff sattigung. *Klin. Wochenschr.* **13:**379–381.

Kramer, K. 1935. Ein Verfahren zur fortlaufenden Messung des Sauerstoffgehaltes. *Z. Biol.* **96:**61–75.

Kramer, K., J. O. Elam, G. A. Saxton, and W. A. Elam. 1951. Influence of oxygen saturation, erythrocyte concentration and optical depth upon the red and near infrared light transmission in whole blood. *Am. J. Physiol.* **165:**229–246.

Lindgren, P., and B. Unvas. 1954. Photoelectric recording of the venous and arterial blood flow. *Acta Physiol. Scand.* **32:**259–263.

Lloyd-Williams, K. 1964. Pictorial heat scanning. *Phys. Med. J. Biol.* **9:**433.

Matthes, K. 1934. Uber der Einfluss der Atmung auf die Sauerstoffsattigung des arterienblutes. *Naunyn-Schmiedebergs Arch. Exp. Pathol. Pharmakol.* **176:**683–698.

Matthes, K. 1935. Untersuchungen uber die Sauerstoffsattigung des menschlichen arterien Blutes. *Naunyn-Schmiedebergs Arch. Exp. Pathol. Pharmakol.* **179:**698–707.

Matthes, K., and F. Gross. 1939a. Untersuchungen uber de absorption von ratem und ultrarotem licht durch kohlenoxydegesattigtes sauerstoffgesattigtes und reduziertes. *Blut Arch. Exp. Pathol. Pharmakol.* **191:**369–380, 381–390, 391–406.

Matthes, K., and F. Gross. 1939b. Uber den nachweis von Methamoglobin und cyanethamoblobin in stromeden. *Blut Arch. Exp. Pathol. Pharmakol.* **191:**706–714.

Millikan, C. A. 1942. The oximeter, an instrument for measuring continuously the oxygen saturation of arterial blood in man. *Rev. Sci. Instrum.* **13:**434–444.

Mitchell, D., C. H. Wyndham, T. Hodgson, and P. R. N. Nabarro. 1967. Measurement of the total normal emissivity of skin without the need for measuring skin temperature. *Phys. Med. J. Biol.* **12:**359–366.

Moss, T. S. 1949. The temperature variation of the long wave limit of infra-red conductivity in lead sulphide and similar substances. *Proc. Phys. Soc. London, Ser. B* **62:**741–748.

Nicolai, L. 1932. Uber Sichtbarmachtung, Verlauf und chemische kinetik der Oxyhamoglobin-reducktion in lebenden Gewebe, besonders in der menschlichten Haut. *Pfluegers Arch. Gesamte Physiol.* **229:**372–384.

Ostrowski, D. S. 1974. U.S. Patent 3,807,390, April.

Pauling, L., R. E. Wood, and J. H. Strudivant. 1946. An instrument for determining the partial pressure of oxygen in a gas. *Science* **103:**338.

Peiss, C., and R. D. McCoole. 1958. Simple optically recording flowmeter for drop or integrated flow measurement. *J. Appl. Physiol.* **12:**137–139.

Polanyi, M. L., and D. S. Ostrowski. 1977. Reflection standard for fiber optic probe. U.S. Patent 4,050,450, September 27.

Radio Corporation of America. 1963.

RCA Phototubes-Photocells, Bull. 1G1018. RCA, Electron Tube Div., Harrison, PA.

Rein, H., A. A. Hampel, and W. A. Heinemann. 1940. Photoelectric Transmissionmanometer zur Blutdruckschreibung. *Pfluegers Arch. Gesamte Physiol.* **243:**329–335.

Sarnquist, F. H., C. Todd, and C. Whitcher. 1980. Accuracy of a new non-invasive oxygen saturation monitor. *Anesthesiology* **53:**S163.

Saunders, N. A., A. E. P. Fowles, and A. S. Rebuck. 1976. Ear oximetry: Accuracy and practicability in the assessment of artercal oxygenation. *Am. Rev. Respir. Dis.* **113:**745–749.

Shepherd, A. P., J. W. Kiel, and G. L. Riddel. 1984. Evaluation of light-emitting diodes for whole blood oximetry. *IEEE Trans. Biomed. Eng.* **BMF-31**(11):723–728.

Shimada, Y., and I. Yoshiya. 1984. Effects of multiple scattering and peripheral circulation on arterial oxygen saturation measured with a pulse-type oximeter. *Med. Biol. Eng. Comput.* **22:**476–478.

Squire, J. R. 1940. Instrument for measuring quantity of blood and its degree of oxygenation in web of hand. *Clin. Sci.* **4**:331–337.

Sutterer, W. F. 1960. A compensated densitometer for indocyanine green. *Physiologist* **3**:159.

Taylor, S. H., and J. P. Shillingford. 1959. Clinical applications of Coomassie blue. *Br. Heart J.* **21**:497–504.

Taylor, S. H., and J. M. Thorp. 1959. Properties and biological behavior of Coomassie blue. *Br. Heart J.* **21**:492–496.

Wallace, J. D., and C. M. Cade. 1975. *Clinical Thermography. CRC Press*, Cleveland, OH, 1975.

Wallace, J. D., and G. D. Dodd. 1969. Thermography in the diagnosis of breast cancer. *Radiology* **91**:679–695.

Watmough, D. J. and R. Oliver. 1968. Emissivity of human skin in the waveband between 2 μ and 6 μ. *Nature* **219**:622–624.

Wheeler, H. O., W. I. Cranston, and J. I. Meltzer. 1958. Hepatic uptake and biliary excretion of indocyanine green in the dog. *Proc. Soc. Exp. Biol. Med.* **99**:11–14.

Wirtzfield, A. 1980. Cardiac pacemaker. U.S. Patent 4,202,339.

Wood, E. H., and J. E. Geraci. 1949. Photoelectric determination of arterial oxygen saturation in man. *J. Lab. Clin. Med.* **34**:387–401.

Wood, E. H., J. R. B. Knutson, and B. E. Taylor. 1950. Measurement of blood content and blood pressure in the human ear. *Proc. Staff Meet. Mayo Clin.* **25**:398–405.

Woodroof, E. A., and S. Koorajian. 1973. *In vitro* evaluation of an *in-vivo* fiberoptic oximeter. *Med. Instrum.* 7:287–292.

Yamakoshi, K., and A. Kamiya. 1983. Noninvasive automatic monitoring of instantaneous arterial blood pressure using the vascular unloading technique. *Med. Biol. Eng. Comput.* **21**:557–565.

Yamakoshi, K., H. Shimazu, and T. Togawa. 1979. Indirect measurement of instantaneous blood pressure in the rat. *Am. J. Physiol.* **6**(5):H632–H637.

Yamakoshi, K., H. Shimazu, and T. Togawa. 1980. Measurement of instantaneous arterial blood pressure in the human finger by the vascular unloading technique. *IEEE Trans. Biomed. Eng.* **BME-27**(3):150–155.

Yamanouchi, I., Y. Yamauchi, and I. Igarashi. 1980. Transcutaneous bilirubinometry. *Pediatrics* **65**(2):195–202.

Yoshiya, I., Y. Shimada, and K. Tanaka. 1980. Spectrophotometric monitoring of arterial oxygen saturation in fingertip. *Med. Biol. Eng. Comput.* **18**:27–31.

Zijlstra, W. G. 1951. *Fundamentals and Applications of Clinical Oximetry*. Van Gorcum, The Netherlands.

6

Piezoelectric Devices

PIEZOELECTRIC DEVICES

The piezoelectric (piezo = pressure) effect, discovered in 1880 by Pierre and Jacques Curie, is the property of some natural crystalline substances to develop electrical potential along certain crystallographic axes in response to the movement of charge as a result of mechanical deformation. Figure 1 diagrams the method of designating crystallographic axes in some of the more familiar crystals. A necessary condition for the presence of the effect is the absence of a center of symmetry of charge distribution. Of the 32 crystal classes, 21 lack this symmetry, and crystals in all but one of these classes can exhibit the piezoelectric phenomenon. Although about 1000 crystalline substances have been observed to have the property, quantitative data are available for only about 100. The magnitude of the effect is of practical value in about 10 substances.

In addition to the naturally occurring crystals, certain ceramics, notably barium titanate, can be induced to acquire the piezoelectric property. With the application of a high voltage to electrodes in contact with the material, there is a reorientation of the crystalline structure that persists after removal of the polarizing voltage. The induction process is carried out at an elevated temperature. This technique, in addition to producing a material with a high piezoelectric constant, removes the geometrical constraints of crystallographic axes and makes it possible to cast piezoelectric crystals having any desired form.

To observe the piezoelectric effect, electrodes must be placed on specific faces of the crystal and the deforming force applied in the appropriate direction (Fig. 2). The voltage appearing between the electrodes is linearly related to the deformation. In practice, piezoelements are slabs removed from the parent crystal by cutting along appropriate crystallographic axes. The magnitude of the piezoelectric effect is dependent on the axis of the cut. The unit employed to designate the magnitude of the effect is the picocoulomb per square meter per newton per square meter $[(pC/m^2)/(N/m^2)]$. Table 1 lists the constants for some of the more common piezoelectric materials.

The slabs cut from the parent crystal can be mounted to permit the development of a piezoelectric voltage in response to bending, twisting, or shearing forces. Frequently the slabs are assembled in pairs or in stacks. One configuration, the bimorph (Clevite Corp., Bedford, Ohio), is particularly useful because it permits

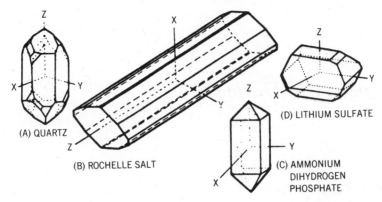

Figure 1 Crystals and axes. (Clevite Corp., Bedford, Ohio. By permission.)

a greater range of motion than is attainable with a single plate. Some of the typical mounting arrangements are illustrated in Fig. 2.

Except for quartz, naturally occurring piezoelectric crystals are less used nowadays, mainly because their performance deteriorates in the presence of high humidity. Ceramic piezoelements are much less hygroscopic and are readily available in a variety of shapes, including rods, cylinders, and disks.

A piezoelectric crystal need be distorted only a tiny amount to obtain a potential in the fractional volt range. For this reason it may be called an efficient isometric transducer. The stiffness of piezocrystals is high, and the permissible deformations are small. Donaldson (1958) stated that the deformation of crystals used in phonograph pickups is 10 μm per gram of force and that crystals used in accelerometers are distorted only 1 μm per kilogram of force.

A close electrical analog to the piezoelectric crystal is a capacitor that is charged by the application of mechanical force. Figure 3 illustrates the simplest equivalent circuit. Typical phonograph crystals develop signals in the fractional volt range. With very large crystals and high forces, it is possible to develop many hundreds of volts.

Piezoelectric materials lose their piezoelectric property when they are heated. The temperature at which this occurs is called the Curie point. Most piezoelectric materials have an upper and a lower temperature limit for retention of the property. The safe operating range is usually much smaller than these two temperature extremes indicate. The upper temperature limits for many piezoelectric crystals are shown in Table 1. With an increase in temperature, a slight deterioration of the piezoelectric effect occurs in the piezoelectric ceramics. Although the effect is small, it is nonetheless present and must be considered if techniques requiring high accuracy are employed. Some natural crystals are deliquescent, and therefore their performance is adversely affected by high humidity.

Piezoelectric crystals, being high-impedance devices, can deliver only very small currents. Connecting a resistive load across them markedly reduces the output voltage and the time constant. A more serious drawback is that, because of leakage

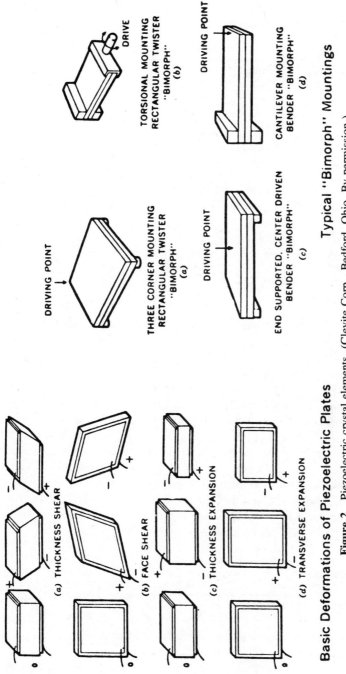

DRIVE

TORSIONAL MOUNTING
RECTANGULAR TWISTER
"BIMORPH"
(b)

DRIVING POINT

CANTILEVER MOUNTING
BENDER "BIMORPH"
(d)

DRIVING POINT

THREE CORNER MOUNTING
RECTANGULAR TWISTER
"BIMORPH"
(a)

DRIVING POINT

END SUPPORTED, CENTER DRIVEN
BENDER "BIMORPH"
(c)

Typical "Bimorph" Mountings

Basic Deformations of Piezoelectric Plates

(a) THICKNESS SHEAR

(b) FACE SHEAR

(c) THICKNESS EXPANSION

(d) TRANSVERSE EXPANSION

Figure 2   Piezoelectric crystal elements. (Clevite Corp., Bedford, Ohio. By permission.)

TABLE 1   Characteristics of Piezoelectric Materials

Piezoelectric Material	Piezoelectric Constant $[(pC/m^2)/(N/m^2)]$	Maximum Humidity Range (%)	Dielectric Constant[a]	Temperature (°C)
Rochelle salt (30°C)	$d14 + 500$		350	−18 to +24
	$d25 - 54$	40–70	9.2	45
	$d36 + 12$		9.5	45
Quartz	$d11 + 2.3$		4.5	550
	$d14 - 0.7$		4.5	550
Ammonium dihydrogen	$d14 - 1.5$	0–94	56	120–125
phosphate (ADP)	$d36 + 48$		15.5	120–125
Barium titanate	$d31 - 34$		170	125
(crystal)	$d33 + 86$		170	125
	$d15 + 392$		2900	125
Barium titanate (ceramic)	$d31 - 7.8$		1700	
	$d33 + 190$		1700	70–100
	$d15 + 260$		1450	

[a]Relative to air.

Source: Encyclopedia Britannica, Chicago, London, Toronto, Geneva, 1963.

resistance, the voltage cannot be maintained when a sustained force is applied. Therefore piezoelectric crystals are only suited to the measurement of changing mechanical forces. They can develop a voltage for changes in mechanical deformation having a frequency of a few hertz to many megahertz. The upper limit is determined by the thickness of the moving system. Because of the high stiffness and low mass of such crystals, they see extensive service in devices to convert force to an electrical signal and in devices to generate mechanical displacement by the application of a voltage. Both modalities are used in many ultrasonic measuring and imaging systems. In the former, the relatively large voltages produced make piezoelements ideal devices to convert physiological events to electrical signals. Because piezoelements can be used to generate continuous-wave or pulsed ultrasound (i.e., above 20 kHz), they are ideally suited to insonate living tissue. Low energies are used for imaging, while higher energies are used for heat therapy. High-energy focused ultrasound can be used to destroy selected regions of tissue.

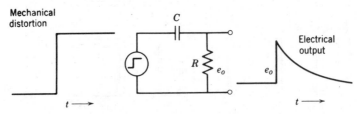

Figure 3 Piezoelectric crystal equivalent circuit. The decrease in output during the sustained deformation is due to internal leakage.

Piezoelectric Detectors

The piezoelectric transducer is particularly well suited to the detection of the pressure pulse and low-energy acoustic phenomena such as heart and Korotkoff sounds. Just after the piezoelectric crystal appeared in industry, Gomez and Langevin (1937) recognized its value for pulse-wave recording in the human subject and discussed this application extensively. Miller and White (1941) employed a crystal microphone air-coupled to a chamber placed on the skin to measure arterial and venous pulses. The small pulsations seen in blood pressure cuffs were recorded with good fidelity by Rappaport and Luisada (1944) and Lax et al. (1956). Both teams rebuilt crystal microphones to operate as differential pressure transducers in which the mean cuff pressure was applied to one side of the diaphragm and the total pressure (mean plus oscillations) to the other. Malcolm (1946) described a piezoelectric crystal in a holder of unique design that served as a general-purpose transducer for ballistocardiography, heart sounds, pulse-wave recording, drop counting, muscle pull, and respiration.

In many respects the piezoelectric element is ideal for heart-sound transduction; almost as soon as the crystal microphone was available commercially, it was called into service for this purpose. Sachs et al. (1935) and Bjerring et al. (1935) used the crystal microphone and described an amplifying device for heart sounds. This instrument, one of the first of its kind to become available commercially, was described in more detail by Lockhart a few years later (1938). Narat (1936) eliminated the air coupling from the surface of the body to the microphone diaphragm by developing a contact crystal microphone for the transduction of all vibrations produced by the heart; however, this technique did not attract much attention. Nearly all subsequent workers have used the air-coupling method, probably to attenuate the large amount of low-frequency vibrational energy generated by the beating heart. Boone (1939) employed a crystal microphone with a cathode ray oscilloscope to guarantee maximum fidelity in reproduction of all the cardiac vibrations. Mannheimer (1941) used the high-efficiency and high-fidelity qualities of the crystal microphone in an attempt to calibrate phonocardiography by separating the sounds into four frequency bands. Rappaport and Sprague (1941, 1942) also selected the crystal microphone for their extensive studies on the nature of heart sounds and the frequency response of stethoscopes. The high-efficiency feature of the crystal microphone showed itself again in the transduction of fetal heart sounds. Wood and Gunn (1953) recorded, counted, and monitored these feeble sounds with the aid of an amplifying system with variable frequency tuning.

Wallace et al. (1957) and Lewis et al. (1957) constructed miniature phonocatheters by mounting hollow tubular barium titanate crystals on the ends of catheters to detect the intracardiac sounds during heart catheterization studies. Geddes et al. (1974) developed a catheter-tip unit containing a piezoelectric bimorph crystal transducer for monitoring breath and respiratory sounds in the esophagus. This device permits audible presentation of these sounds to an audience with very little interference from acoustic feedback. Figure 4 is a record of the electrocardiogram (ECG), aortic blood pressure, and the esophageal phonocardiogram (PCG) in a dog with arterial fibrillation. The PCG shows splitting of the first (S_1S_1') and second

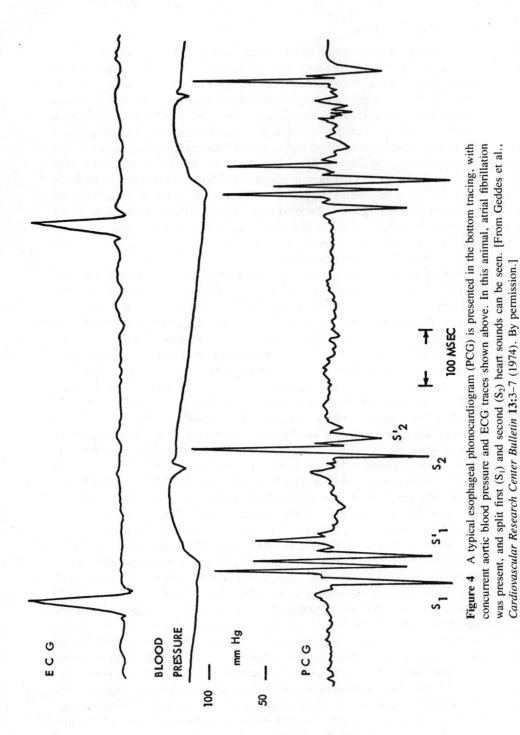

Figure 4 A typical esophageal phonocardiogram (PCG) is presented in the bottom tracing, with concurrent aortic blood pressure and ECG traces shown above. In this animal, atrial fibrillation was present, and split first (S₁) and second (S₂) heart sounds can be seen. [From Geddes et al., *Cardiovascular Research Center Bulletin* **13**:3–7 (1974). By permission.]

(S_2, S_2') heart sounds. By placing the catheter-tip piezoelement at different sites in the esophagus, any of the four heart sounds can be enhanced. The addition of a pair of electrodes (Geddes, 1984) permits acquisition of the ECG and respiration by impedance change as well as the impedance cardiogram. Such a catheter transducer has been used by the authors in the dog laboratory for over 15 years.

Among the feeblest of auscultatory phenomena are the Korotkoff sounds, and the high-efficiency feature of the piezoelectric crystal has been put to use in their detection. Omberg (1936) used a crystal microphone to control the cycling of a pump connected to a blood pressure cuff. As the cuff pressure decayed, the systolic sounds detected by the microphone restarted the pump; when they disappeared, the pump stopped, thereby maintaining the cuff pressure very nearly equal to systolic blood pressure. Gilson et al. (1941; Gilson, 1942) recorded human blood pressure indirectly by presenting two-channel records of cuff pressure and Korotkoff sounds detected by a crystal microphone. These sounds, as they appeared in a smaller cuff located below the blood pressure cuff on the subject's arm, were detected by Rappaport and Luisada (1944). Like Omberg, Gilford and Broida (1954) used a crystal microphone as the primary detector in their fully automatic recording machine, which plotted and indicated both systolic and diastolic human blood pressures. Detection of the Korotkoff sounds by crystal elements and their superposition on the occluding cuff pressure were described by Currens et al. (1957) and Geddes et al. (1959).

Figure 5 shows a piezoelement from a phonograph cartridge mounted in the lower third of a blood pressure cuff (Geddes et al., 1959) to detect the Korotkoff sounds in the measurement of blood pressure. In a subsequent report, Geddes and Moore (1968) mounted the piezoelectric crystal within the bladder in the same position. This technique maintains the crystal close to the source of the Korotkoff sounds and provides good coupling with the tissues. In addition, the cuff acts as an acoustic shield and reduces detection of environmental noise.

Virtually all of the automatic blood-pressure-measuring instruments that use the Korotkoff (auscultatory) sound method employ a piezoelectric element. For convenience, the element is placed in a pocket in the lower third of the cuff so that it faces the skin.

Accelerometers. According to Newton's law, force F is equal to mass m multiplied by acceleration a, i.e., $F = ma$. Conversely, acceleration $a = F/m$. Therefore by measuring the force exerted on a mass, it is possible to determine acceleration. Force is easily measured using a piezoelectric element. This technique is employed by one manufacturer (PCB Piezotronic, Inc., Depew, New York) in the manner shown in Fig. 6a. Two quartz crystals are mounted below a spring-loaded mass. Acceleration in the direction of the arrow causes the mass to be forced against the crystals. The voltage developed is enlarged by an amplifier within the housing. The output is specified in terms of millivolts per unit (m/sec^2) of acceleration.

It should be recalled that acceleration is a change in velocity. No output is produced by an accelerometer unless it is subjected to a changing velocity, i.e., an acceleration.

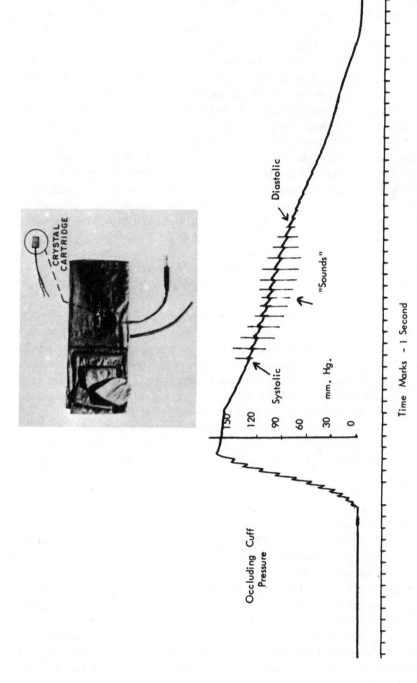

Figure 5   Korotkoff sound detector.

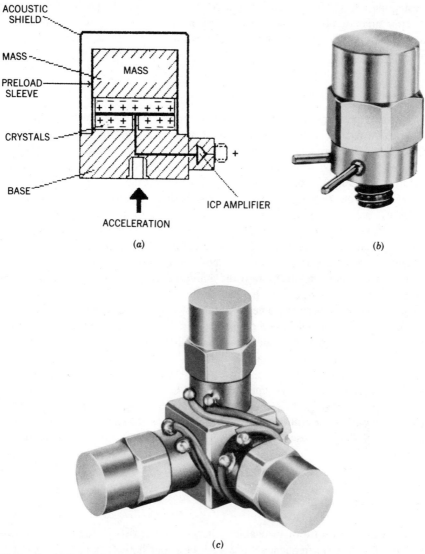

ACOUSTIC
SHIELD

MASS

PRELOAD
SLEEVE

MASS

+ + + + + +
+ + + + + +

CRYSTALS

BASE

ICP AMPLIFIER

+

ACCELERATION

(a)

(b)

(c)

Figure 6 (a) Principle employed in the piezoelectric accelerometer. (b) single-axis and (c) triaxial accelerometers. (Courtesy of PCB Piezotronics, Inc., Depew, New York.)

Figure 6b illustrates a single-axis miniature accelerometer, and Fig. 6c shows three such units assembled to detect acceleration in three directions. The accelerometers shown are small, being just over $\frac{1}{4}$ in. in diameter and mounted by a 5–40 threaded shaft. With 18–24 V of excitation (for the built-in amplifier), a typical output is 10 mV/(m/sec^2), with a frequency response extending from 1 to 10,000 Hz.

Miniature accelerometers, such as those shown in Fig. 6, are very practical for sensing motion. Often they are used to detect the activity of animals in cages that are appropriately mounted. Accelerometers are also useful in sensing body motion in exercising animals and humans. Sometimes cardiac vibrations, the arterial pulse, and tremor are sensed with accelerometers.

Piezoelectric Reproducers

As stated previously, when a voltage is applied to a piezoelectric element, a deformation results. This feature permits the use of piezoelements in a variety of devices such as earphones, loudspeakers, and ultrasonic instruments. This mechanical deformation property was used by Offner in the mid-1940s to create a rapidly responding graphic recorder, which he called the "crystograph." In this device two large, thin square crystals were clamped at three corners; the fourth corner of each crystal was free to move in response to the applied voltage. The crystals were driven in phase opposition, and the free corners were coupled to a pulley system that drove a direct-inking recording stylus. A frequency response extending from less than 1 Hz to well above 60 Hz was achieved.

Another ingenious application of the ability of the piezoelectric crystal to produce movement was described by Pascoe (1955). He faced the problem of advancing a microelectrode into a nerve cell that was enveloped in a tough membrane. By mounting the microelectrode on a piezoelectric crystal and applying a pulse of voltage, the electrode was suddenly advanced 20 μm, and the tip of the electrode penetrated the cell without damage.

The ultrasonic ranging and imaging devices to be described use both properties of piezoelectric crystals, their ability to distort rapidly in response to the application to a voltage and their ability to develop a voltage in response to a short-duration deformation. Prior to describing these devices it is useful to review the properties of ultrasound.

PROPERTIES OF ULTRASOUND

Ultrasound is a form of mechanical energy that consists of high-frequency vibrations. Because the frequency lies above the upper limit of human audition (20 kHz), it cannot be detected by the human ear; however, some birds and animals can perceive low-frequency ultrasound. Low-intensity ultrasound passes through living tissue without altering tissue function. Higher energy ultrasound can produce heating and cavitation, both of which can alter cell function. Cavitation, which occurs at high power density, is the process by which a high local pressure gradient causes the development of gas bubbles.

Ultrasound cannot travel through a vacuum. Being mechanical in nature, ultrasound does not ionize the medium—as X rays and gamma rays do. Another difference relates to the way ultrasound is generated—by electrically inducing a deformation in a solid. The particles of the solid are made to oscillate with the frequency of the applied ultrasonic energy. Energy is transferred from one particle to its neighbor; there is no net translation of the individual particles.

As a beam of ultrasonic energy traverses a medium, the medium's constituent particles oscillate. The distance between the points of maximum (or minimum) amplitude is known as the wavelength λ. The frequency f of the ultrasound is expressed in hertz (Hz), or number of cycles per second. The period T is the time required to complete one cycle and is the reciprocal of frequency.

$$T = 1/f$$

The wavelength λ and the frequency f are related to the propagation velocity c by

$$c = f\lambda.$$

Velocity

In an isotropic medium, the propagation velocity c is dependent on the medium and its temperature. Table 2 presents velocity data for various media. The velocity of propagation is determined by the delay between the movement of adjacent particles. This delay depends on the elasticity E and the density ρ of the medium. In fact,

$$c = \sqrt{E/\rho}.$$

Note that for a given density the velocity will be higher in harder tissues such as bone.

TABLE 2 Ultrasonic Properties of Some Common Materials, Including Biological Tissues

	Propagation Velocity (m/s)	Characteristic Impedance (10^6 kg/m^2 s)	Attenuation Coefficient at 1 MHz (dB/cm)	Frequency Dependence of Attenuation Coefficient
Air	330	0.0004	10	f^2
Aluminium	6400	17	0.02	f
Bone	2700–4100	3.75–7.38	3–10	f–$f^{1.5}$
Castor oil	1500	1.4	1	f^2
Lung	650–1160	0.26–0.46	40	$f^{0.6}$
Muscle	1545–1630	1.65–1.74	1.5–2.5	f
Perspex	2680	3.2	2	f
Soft tissues (except muscle)	1460–1615	1.35–1.68	0.3–1.5	f
Water	1480	1.52	0.002	f^2

Data obtained from P. N. T. Wells, *Ultrasonics in Clinical Diagnosis*, Churchill Livingstone, Edinburgh, 1977.

Since the velocity is medium-dependent, the wavelength will depend on the medium as well as on the frequency. For example, in water the propagation velocity is 1480 m/sec. Therefore, the wavelength for 1-MHz ultrasound is 1.48 mm.

Attenuation

On passing through a uniform medium, ultrasound intensity decreases along the transmission path; this loss of amplitude is called attenuation. Attenuation can result from three processes: beam divergence, absorption, and scattering. On entering a medium, the beam may broaden or diverge, in which case the energy becomes spread out over a larger area as the beam progresses through the medium, and the energy per unit area decreases.

The amount of absorption depends on the type of medium. Absorption identifies the difficulty with which the particles of the medium transfer energy. Viscosity and frictional factors consume energy, which is lost as heat. Absorption is frequency-dependent. Figure 7 illustrates the absorption characteristic for a variety of media over an extended frequency range. Although attenuation varies almost as the square

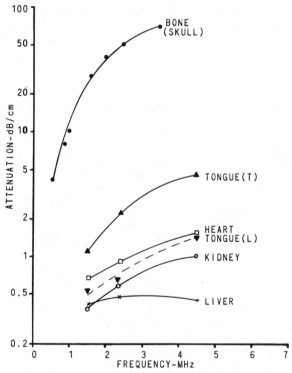

Figure 7 Attenuation versus frequency for various tissue specimens; T and L refer to transverse and longitudinal. (Human skull data from Hueter, 1952; all other data from Hueter, 1976.)

of frequency in air and liquids, in soft tissues it is approximately linear with frequency over a limited range, above which it is less frequency-dependent.

Scattering also causes attenuation of ultrasound. For example, an ultrasonic beam may be scattered by small inhomogeneities in the medium; the beam will be diffused, and less energy will flow through a given cross-sectional area along the path.

The attenuation coefficient is the measure used to describe the ability of a uniform substance to attenuate ultrasound. For convenience, the decibel per centimeter (dB/cm) is the most frequently used unit. A simple example will serve to illustrate absorption. Consider a 1-cm thick specimen ($L = 1$) in which the acoustic power emerging is one-half of that entering. The attenuation coefficient α is defined as 10 times the logarithm (to the base 10) of the ratio of emergent power P_e to incident power P_i, all divided by the distance L traversed by the ultrasound:

$$\alpha = \frac{10 \log \left(P_e/P_i \right)}{L} \text{ dB/cm.}$$

In the example selected, $L = 1$ and $P_e/P_i = 1/2$, the attenuation coefficient is

$$\alpha = 10 \log \left(1/2 \right) = -3.01 \text{ dB/cm.}$$

The negative sign indicates that attenuation has taken place. Usually the incident and emergent powers are not known. However, the incident amplitude A_i and emergent amplitude A_e are known or easily measured. Because power is proportional to the square of the amplitude, the attenuation coefficient α is given by

$$\alpha = \frac{20 \log \left(A_e/A_i \right)}{L} \text{ dB/cm.}$$

The significance of the attenuation of ultrasound in a medium should not be underestimated. To demonstrate this point, Fig. 8a illustrates an incident beam traveling through a uniform medium 3 cm thick with an attenuation coefficient of 3.01 dB/cm. After passing through 1 cm, the power is one-half and the amplitude is $1/\sqrt{2}$ of the incident value. Similarly, as the beam traverses the full 3 cm, the emergent power is one-eighth and the emergent amplitude $1/2.82$ of the incident value.

Interactions at Boundaries

When a beam of ultrasound traveling in one medium encounters a second medium, several phenomena occur. For example, in Fig. 8b the ultrasonic beam enters the medium with normal incidence, i.e., at right angles to the direction of travel. In this case, part of the energy is reflected by the interface, and the remainder continues on without beam deviation. The reflected energy is called the echo and

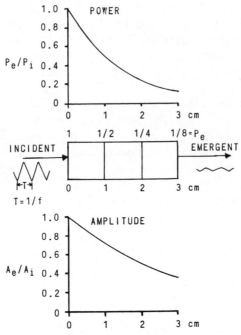

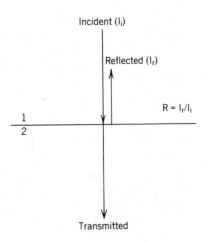

Figure 8a The attenuation of ultrasound on passing through a specimen 3 cm thick. P is the acoustic power and A is the acoustic amplitude; i and e refer to the incident and emergent values, respectively.

depends on the characteristic impedances of the two media. Characteristic (specific) impedance is defined as the ratio of the instantaneous acoustic pressure to the velocity of the particles. Table 2 includes a listing of typical values. Numerically, the characteristic impedance Z is equal to the product of the velocity c and the density ρ, i.e.,

Figure 8b Reflection at an interface when the incident beam strikes a reflecting surface at 90 degrees.

$$Z = c\rho.$$

For normal incidence, the reflectance coefficient R is defined as

$$R = \left(\frac{Z_1 - Z_2}{Z_1 + Z_2}\right)^2.$$

In this expression, Z_1 and Z_2 are the characteristic impedances of the two media. Note that if $Z_1 = Z_2$ (i.e., $c_1\rho_1 = c_2\rho_2$), the reflectance coefficient is zero, and no reflection takes place. Conversely, if a beam of ultrasound traveling in water ($Z = 1.52 \times 10^6$) impinges normally on the surface that is in contact with air ($Z = 0.0004 \times 10^6$), the reflection coefficient is 0.999; therefore 99.9% of the incident energy is reflected, and only 0.1% enters the air. The larger the difference in characteristic impedance, the larger the reflection coefficient. A reflection coefficient of 1.0 means that all incident energy is reflected.

The difference in characteristic impedance has important implications in the use of ultrasound. For example, structures that lie behind air-filled organs (e.g., lung), do not return measurable echoes. Likewise, a tissue mass (e.g., tumor) with a characteristic impedance that is similar to that of surrounding tissue will return a very small amplitude echo.

If the incident beam of ultrasound does not strike the interface between two media at right angles, several interesting events occur. As shown in Fig. 9, the angle between the incident beam and a perpendicular to the interface ($c_1\rho_1/c_2\rho_2$) is known as the angle of incidence θ_i. The reflected beam will travel with an angle θ_r with respect to the normal. For a plane interface, $\theta_r = \theta_i$.

The ultrasonic beam that enters and is transmitted by the second medium will be diverted (refracted) from its original path and travel at an angle θ_t with respect to a perpendicular erected to the interface. The angle θ_t will not equal θ_i; the

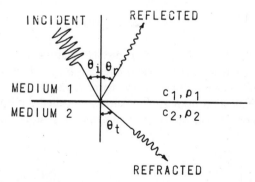

Figure 9 An incident beam in medium 1 strikes the interface with medium 2, producing a reflected beam and a refracted beam. θ_i and θ_r are the angles of incidence and reflection (which are equal), and θ_t is the angle of the refracted beam, which is transmitted by the second medium. All angles are measured with respect to a line normal to the interface.

difference will depend on the ratio of the velocities of ultrasound in the two media. The following relationship (Snell's law) defines the angles in terms of the velocities:

$$\frac{\sin \theta_i}{\sin \theta_t} = \frac{c_1}{c_2}$$

where θ_i and θ_t refer to the incident and transmitted angles, respectively, and c_1 and c_2 are the velocities of ultrasound in media 1 and 2, respectively.

An interesting situation can develop when the angle of incidence θ_i is increased as shown in Fig. 10. Note that there will be a critical angle of incidence for which the refracted ray will have an angle of 90 degrees (ray 5). In such a situation, which is called total internal reflection, the refracted beam travels within the interfacial plane and is not transmitted into medium 2. In essence there is no refracted beam. The conditions necessary for this situation can be derived by putting $\theta_t =$ 90 degrees, the sine of which is 1.0; then

$$\sin \theta_{ic} = \frac{c_1}{c_2}$$

where θ_{ic} is the critical angle of incidence and c_1, c_2 are the velocities of sound in the two media.

The concept of a critical angle is important when there is a hard tissue–soft tissue boundary. For example, in echoencephalography, where the ultrasound crosses a bone–soft tissue boundary, if the angle of incidence is greater than the critical angle the ultrasound will not enter the brain. If the velocities of ultrasound in soft tissue and bone are 1500 and 4000 m/sec, respectively, the critical angle of incidence θ_{ic} is given by

$$\sin \theta_{ic} = \frac{1500}{4000} = 0.375$$

$$\theta_{ic} = 22 \text{ degrees}.$$

Up to this point, the discussion of reflectance has dealt with a narrow beam and a smooth interface. Reflection at a smooth interface is called specular (mirrorlike). However, ultrasonic beams are not always narrow, and reflecting surfaces are not always smooth. Reflection from a rough surface is called diffuse, and the combination of a beam of finite cross section impinging on a surface that is not smooth

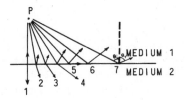

Figure 10 The critical angle of incidence is illustrated by ray 5 emanating from a point source P. Rays 1–4 enter medium 2, but rays 5–7 experience total internal reflection.

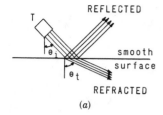

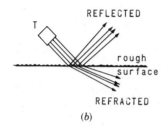

Figure 11 Reflections and refraction of a parallel-ray beam from a transducer T. (*a*) When the beam encounters a smooth surface rays in the reflected and refracted beams remain parallel. (*b*) The beam encounters a rough surface; note the divergence among the rays in the reflected and refracted beams.

results in considerable scattering of the reflected beam. Figure 11*a* shows idealized reflection and refraction for a beam of parallel rays striking a smooth surface, and Fig. 11*b* shows the effect of a rough surface on the reflected and refracted beams.

Doppler Frequency Shift

The Doppler frequency shift is familiar to anyone who has listened to the approach and passage of a high-speed vehicle moving with a constant velocity and emitting a constant-frequency sound. When the vehicle is approaching, the frequency of the sound it emits is perceived to become higher and higher. After it passes, the sound frequency is perceived to be lower and lower despite the fact that it actually remains the same. This frequency shift was described by Doppler (1803–1853), an Austrian physicist.

An explanation of the frequency shift is obvious. When the source (or observer) is approaching, more cycles per second arrive at the point of observation; the converse is true when the source (or observer) recedes. For these four situations, the perceived frequency f' is given by the following equations.

Observer moving toward source:

$$f' = f\left(\frac{c + v}{c}\right).$$

Observer moving away from source:

$$f' = f\left(\frac{c - v}{c}\right).$$

Source moving toward observer:

$$f' = f\left(\frac{c}{c - v}\right).$$

Source moving away from observer:

$$f' = f\left(\frac{c}{c + v}\right).$$

In these expressions, f is the frequency of the source, v is the velocity of the source relative to the observer, and c is the velocity of sound in the medium.

In the biomedical applications of ultrasound, the source is fixed and the target moves. The most frequent use for Doppler ultrasound is for the measurement of blood flow velocity. In this case the moving target consists of the blood cells that reflect the ultrasound.

GENERATION OF ULTRASOUND

For the production of ultrasound, ceramics such as lead zirconate titanate and barium titanate are most popular because of their strong piezoelectric effect. Such materials, called ferroelectrics, have the piezoelectric property induced during fabrication. This polarization procedure is carried out at elevated temperature. On cooling, the piezoelectric property is retained. Such materials can be cut into a variety of shapes without significant loss of piezoelectricity.

In most applications, the piezoelement is required to produce a narrow beam of ultrasound. To do this, a small disk of piezoelectric material is used. There are some interesting facts that must be remembered when coupling the element to the specimen. The interface with the specimen constitutes a reflecting surface, and energy is reflected back into the piezoelement. In order to obtain constructive interference (i.e., reinforcement), the thickness of the transducer is made one-half wavelength for the frequency used. The velocity of ultrasound in lead zirconate titanate is 4000 m/sec. At a frequency of 1 MHz, $\lambda/2 = 2$ mm.

Reflections from structures behind the piezoelement are eliminated by the use of an air backing or an acoustically absorbing material. Often the transducer is matched to the specimen by a layer of material of intermediate characteristic impedance, having a thickness of one-quarter wavelength ($\lambda/4$) at the frequency of operation; Fig. 12 illustrates this arrangement.

The ultrasonic field in front of the transducer merits attention because its character depends on the radius of the transducer, the frequency, and the medium. Figure 12 illustrates the principal components of the field in front of a transducer of diameter $2r$ and thickness $\lambda/2$.

The ultrasound beam enters the medium, and two regions are defined. If the piezoelement is circular, the beam of ultrasound is cylindrical near the transducer.

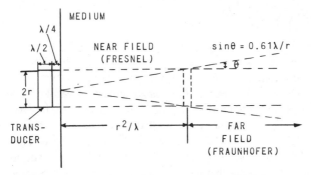

Figure 12 Transducer ($\lambda/2$ in thickness) coupled to a medium by a quarter-wavelength ($\lambda/4$) material of intermediate characteristic impedance. The idealized near (Fresnel) and far (Fraunhofer) fields are identified.

Farther from the transducer, the beam diverges; the region between this point and the element is called its near field or Fresnel zone. The region beyond is called the far field or Fraunhofer zone. In practice, of course, the demarcation between these two regions is not sharp; one merges into the other in a transition zone.

In the near field, ultrasound radiated from different parts of the element travels as spherical waves that interfere constructively and destructively. Thus, there are regions of maxima and minima along and across the beam. The length of the near field depends on the radius r of the transducer and the wavelength λ of sound in the medium in front of the element. The length L of the near field is given by

$$L = r^2/\lambda.$$

In the far field, the ultrasound diverges and appears to be coming from a point source located at the center of the transducer. The angle of divergence θ also depends on the radius r of the transducer and the wavelength λ of sound in the medium. The angle of divergence θ is shown in Fig. 12 and is given by

$$\sin \theta = 0.61\lambda/r.$$

Thus, the radius of the transducer and the wavelength of the ultrasound in the medium determine the nature of the field in front of the transducer. The length of the near field increases with increasing transducer diameter and with increasing frequency of the ultrasound. The beam divergence in the far field decreases with increasing transducer diameter and with increasing frequency.

To illustrate typical dimensions, the first echocardiographic studies were conducted at 2.5 MHz using a piezoelement 12 mm in diameter. The transition between the near and far fields was 6 cm, and the angle of divergence was about 3.5 degrees.

It should be noted that the discussion has centered on the behavior of a plane piezoelement. Control of the ultrasonic beam can be achieved by focusing with lenses or curved reflectors. In addition, elements can be made with curved surfaces. These options have not been used very extensively.

PULSE-ECHO TECHNIQUES

Pulse-echo techniques are used widely to identify structures within the body. The underlying principle entails delivery of a short burst of ultrasound into the subject and detection of the echoes returned from structures with differing acoustic impedances. Usually the transmitting piezoelement is employed to receive the echoes after the pulse of ultrasound is delivered. Occasionally a second piezoelement is used to detect the echoes. Recall that the reflection coefficient is the square of the ratio of the difference of the acoustic impedances of two adjacent media to their sum. Obviously, then, the greater the difference in acoustic impedance, the larger the echo. Also recall that the absorption coefficient increases with frequency for typical tissues. Therefore, it is necessary to use a low frequency if a deep target is to be located. Moreover, resolution is also frequency dependent: The lower the frequency, the less the resolution. In many pulse-echo systems the echo amplifier gain is increased logarithmically with time after delivery of the burst of ultrasound. This technique permits enhancement of the weaker echoes from deep-lying tissues. In designing ultrasonic systems, all of these tradeoffs must be considered carefully.

Pulse-Echo Display Modes

Basically, there are two types of pulse-echo display, the A-scan and B-scan (B for brightness) methods. Originally, the A-scan method plotted amplitude against time, and the B-scan method plotted range against azimuth (bearing on the ground with respect to a reference point).

A-Scan Method. In ultrasonics, the A-scan method plots amplitude of echo against distance, which is proportional to time, since the velocity of ultrasound in the medium is known. This technique was developed by Firestone (1945) to detect echo-producing flaws in metal. Soon thereafter, French et al. (1950, 1951) developed a 15-MHz pulse-echo system to examine tumor-containing human brains removed post mortem. They noted that the echoes produced by tumors (confirmed histologically) were larger than those returned by normal tissue. Reid and Wild (1952) used a 15-MHz pulse-echo system to examine human breast tumors. They found that the echo amplitudes from cancer were larger than those from normal tissue. There soon arose a growing desire to obtain cross-sectional images or tomograms of internal organs.

The A-scan method shows the distance (range) to the echo-producing target. Figure 13a shows that the ultrasonic transducer was pulsed at the beginning of the sweep (X or time axis) and the amplitudes of the echoes (1, 2) reflected by the interfaces are applied to the vertical (Y) axis of the cathode ray tube (CRT). Thus, the distance along the X or time axis of the CRT identifies the range or distance to reflecting interfaces 1 and 2.

As shown in Fig. 13a, the ultrasonic echoes consist of several cycles of ultrasound, i.e., positive and negative amplitude deflections. In most applications, the onset of the echo complex and its envelope contain the useful information. For

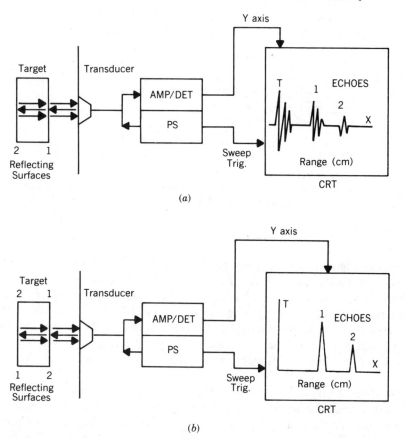

Figure 13 (*a*) A-scan display (echo amplitude versus range). T is the transmitter pulse; 1 and 2 are the target echoes; and PS is the power supply that drives the transducer. (*b*) The same signals as in (*a*) have been demodulated and smoothed for this A-scan display.

these reasons, the ultrasonic echo is demodulated and smoothed so that the negative and positive amplitudes of the echo are displayed in the same direction on the range axis as illustrated in Fig. 13*b*.

With normal incidence, the amplitude of an echo depends on its distance from the transducer, the attenuation coefficient of the medium, the reflectance coefficient of the target interface, and any scattering or divergence that occurs along the path. More distant targets return echoes that are usually smaller in amplitude.

Note that the time *t* of a returning echo represents twice the distance *d* from the transducer to the target. Therefore, $2d = ct$, where *c* is the velocity of ultrasound in the medium and *t* is the time of the returning echo. Since *c* is known, the distance *d* to the reflector is

$$d = ct/2.$$

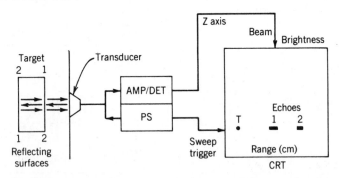

Figure 14 B-scan display (range displayed by brightness modulation). T is the transmitter pulse; 1 and 2 are the target echoes, and PS is the power supply that drives the transducer.

B-Scan Method. The B-scan method employs brightening of the CRT beam to identify the target. For example, if instead of using the echo signal to produce a vertical deflection on the CRT, as shown in Fig. 13*b*, it is used to brighten the CRT beam, a B-mode display is produced as shown in Fig. 14. With this type of presentation, a linear sweep is applied to the X axis of the CRT. The beam brightness is adjusted so that it becomes visible only when an echo is present. Thus, the positions of the bright spots represent the ranges to the targets.

M-Mode Method. A popular variant of the B-scan method is called the M-mode display (M: for motion). The easiest way to visualize this presentation is to consider that the target in Fig. 15 moves rhythmically. Thus, the distance between the two bright-spot echoes 1 and 2 and the transmitter pulse T will vary rhythmically. To obtain a record of these movements, it is customary to place a lens in front of the CRT and focus the image on a moving photographic paper behind a narrow slit (∼0.5 mm) as shown in Fig. 15. Thus, the spots move back and forth at right angles to the movement of the photographic paper. When developed, the excursions of the spots, representing the target motion, are clearly seen as curved lines; this is the M-mode display.

In some instruments, the motion of the bright spots on the CRT face is brought to the moving photographic surface by using a short bundle of optical fibers arranged in a line. The photographic surface contacts the line of optical fibers, which is at right angles to the motion of the photographic surface. Self-developing paper is used, and the image is available within a few minutes.

The M-mode display can also be created on the face of a CRT. For example, starting from the position shown in Fig. 15, rotate the CRT by 90 degrees clockwise. Now movement of the target will cause the spots to move up and down along a vertical line. If this line is caused to move slowly across the face of the CRT, by applying a slowly rising potential to the horizontal axis of the CRT, the M-mode display is created as shown in Fig. 16. A long-persistence phosphor CRT is used so that the image can be retained for several seconds.

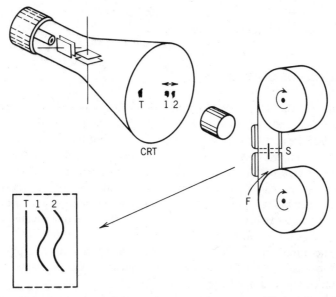

Figure 15 The M-mode display employing a camera to record the motion of the target echoes 1, 2.

Resolution

With pulse-echo techniques, there is a limit in distinguishing two closely spaced structures. This limit is about one wavelength for the ultrasound in the medium. Since the velocity of ultrasound in soft tissue is typically 1500 m/sec, the resolution δ in millimeters can be expressed as a function of the frequency f,

$$\delta = \frac{1.5}{f},$$

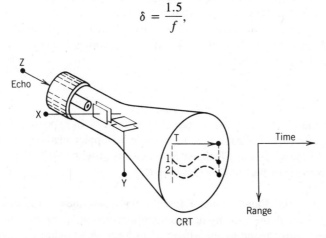

Figure 16 The M-mode display. The range is indicated along a vertical line, and movement of the echo-producing target (1, 2) is displayed by applying a linearly rising potential to the horizontal axis of the CRT.

where δ is in millimeters and f is in megahertz. For example, at 15 MHz the theoretical resolution is about 0.1 mm.

APPLICATIONS OF ULTRASOUND

Moderate-intensity ($0.5-5$ W/cm^2), low-frequency ($1-3$ MHz) ultrasound has been used to treat inflammatory diseases. It has been found useful for muscle and joint pain (DeForest, 1955). In this application it is not known whether the therapeutic effect is related only to the temperature rise produced by the ultrasound or is due to alteration of biochemical reactions or membrane permeability. High-intensity ultrasound can destroy cells, both thermally and by cavitation, which ruptures cell membranes. Focused high-intensity ultrasound (e.g., 1 MHz at 50–1500 W/cm^2) has been used to produce very small (fraction of a square millimeter) or larger thermal lesions in the human brain (Fry and Fry, 1960).

Diagnostic ultrasound employs low energy to detect a variety of physiological events and to image internal organs. Figure 17 presents data on energy levels and exposure times reported by Ulrich (1974).

Techniques to determine blood flow velocity and the location, size, and movement of internal organs use a beam of ultrasound that is reflected from the target. The frequency of the returning echo, or the echo return time, contains the desired information. Scanning methods, which cause the beam of ultrasound to traverse the tissue, permit cross-sectional imaging (tomography).

The use of ultrasonic energy to obtain diagnostic information enjoys several advantages over other techniques. For example, it is very easy to use and does not stress the subject. It can be applied noninvasively and, at the energy level used presently, is nonhazardous. This is particularly valuable with imaging techniques and permits repeated and prolonged examinations. There are no known cumulative effects as there are with X-ray examination. This feature makes ultrasonics very useful in obstetrics, gynecology, and pediatrics. Finally, when used for imaging, ultrasound can permit visualization of soft tissues, which do not reveal themselves very well with X-ray techniques.

Blood Flowmeters

Ultrasound is used to measure blood flow velocity in exposed vessels as well as transcutaneously. Both the time-of-flight and Doppler methods have been employed. The transcutaneous Doppler flowmeter is in wide use clinically; the principles of both types will now be described.

Direct Arterial Flowmeters. Kalmus (1954) described a 100-kHz ultrasonic flowmeter in which the velocity of water was detected by measuring the phase shift between an upstream and a downstream transducer. A switching system operating at 10 Hz permitted interchange of the transmitting and receiving transducers; this method was used extensively in later instruments. The technique was soon applied to the measurement of blood flow by Herrick and Anderson (1959). The pulsed

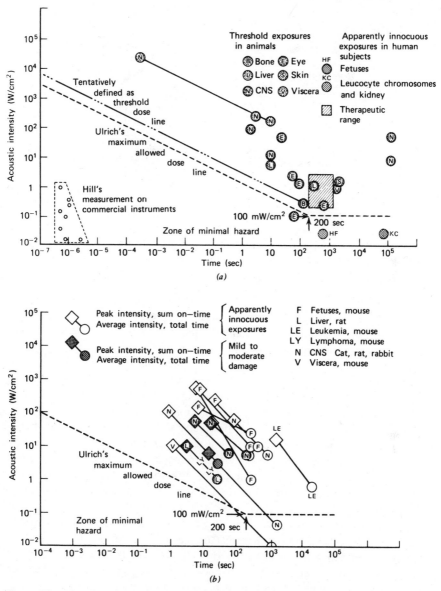

Figure 17 The effects of ultrasound on living tissues, illustrating the safe and hazardous exposure times for 0.5–6 MHz ultrasound. [Redrawn from W. D. Ulrich, *IEEE Trans. Biomed. Eng.* **21**:48–51 (1974).]

(transit-time) ultrasonic flowmeter (Fig. 18*a*) was developed by Franklin et al. (1959). In this device, 3-MHz ultrasound was applied to a barium titanate piezo-electric crystal mounted in a 1.3-cm Lucite sleeve. The ultrasound pulse consisted of 8 cycles of the 3-MHz ultrasound; a similar piezoelectric transducer located downstream detected the arrival of the ultrasound, as shown in Fig. 18*a*. Electronic

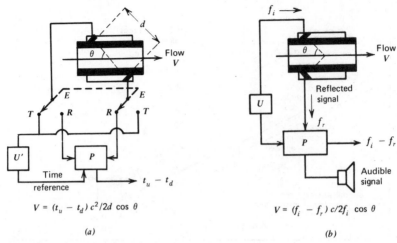

$$V = (t_u - t_d)\, c^2/2d\, \cos\theta$$

(a)

$$V = (f_i - f_r)\, c/2f_i\, \cos\theta$$

(b)

Figure 18   (a) Transit-time (time-of-flight) flowmeter; (b) Doppler frequency-shift flow-meter.

switching (E–E) permitted the downstream receiver to become the transmitter (T) and the upstream transmitter to become the receiver (R). The switching rate for measurement of upstream and downstream times was 800/sec. A time difference on the order of nanoseconds was obtained with the transducer assembly applied to the dog aorta. An overall flow-velocity frequency response extending from 0 to beyond 15 Hz was obtained, which allowed high-fidelity recording of the contour of the velocity-flow wave at rest and during exercise.

The Doppler frequency-shift blood flowmeter was developed by Franklin et al. (1961) after preliminary experience with a pulse transit-time flowmeter (Franklin et al., 1959). Figure 18b illustrates a typical arrangement for measuring blood flow velocity using continuous-wave ultrasound. A perivascular sleeve contains two piezoelectric elements: one transmits the incident ultrasonic energy of frequency f_i into the flowing blood. The blood cells reflect a part of the beam to a second receiving piezoelement. With the flow direction shown, the received frequency f_r of the reflected echo is lower than that of the incident ultrasound because the reflector (blood cells) is moving away from the source. It should be noted that because the blood cells have different velocities, the frequency range of the back-scattered ultrasound will be broad and dependent on the velocity profile. The idealized velocity V for a profile that is uniform across the vessel (plug flow) is:

$$V = (f_i - f_r)c/(2f_i \cos\theta)$$

where f_i and f_r are the frequencies of the incident and received ultrasound, respectively, c is the velocity of ultrasound in blood, and θ is the angle of incidence of the ultrasound. The difference-frequency $(f_i - f_r)$ signal is processed to provide an output that can be recorded graphically. With the ultrasonic frequencies used

(~ 5 MHz) and typical blood flow velocities encountered, the difference frequency lies in the audible range, thereby allowing presentation of the flow signal by a loudspeaker. In a typical case, a flow velocity of 0–100 cm/sec, the frequency shift extends from about 0 to 5000 Hz.

Transcutaneous Flowmeters. With a suitable fluid or gel coupling between two adjacent piezoelements and the skin, ultrasound can be transmitted into a superficial artery (or vein) and the backscattered flow signal can be detected from the skin surface. Figure 19a illustrates a typical arrangement for the piezoelements. Several types of transcutaneous (sometimes called percutaneous) flowmeters are available commercially and are ideal for examining both arterial and venous flows.

The transcutaneous blood flowmeter was developed by Baker (1964). A typical instrument contains two piezoelements; one is for transmitting, and one is for receiving the continuous-wave ultrasound as shown in Fig. 19a. Because the vessel is subcutaneous, the two piezoelements must be placed in line and have different angles with respect to the axis of the vessel. Both transducers are coupled to the skin with a gel to provide a suitable low-loss path for the ultrasound. The coupling agent also constitutes an "acoustic hinge," which allows the operator to adjust the transducer so that the ultrasound beam can intercept the blood flow in the vessel.

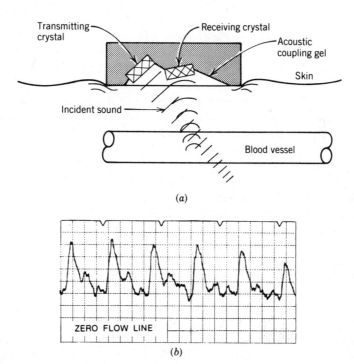

(a)

(b)

Figure 19   (a) Principle employed in the transcutaneous Doppler frequency-shift flowmeter; and (b) a typical record obtained from a digital artery. (Courtesy Parks Medical, Portland, Oregon.)

It should be noted that the echo contains information on blood flow and a component due to vessel-wall movement. Fortunately, the latter has a lower frequency spectrum and can be filtered out electronically without serious compromise to the operation of the flowmeter. Figure 19*b* illustrates a typical record from the digital artery of the index finger.

With the transcutaneous ultrasonic blood flowmeter, it is easy to differentiate arterial from venous flow, even when an artery and vein are in close proximity. Arterial flow is characterized by a tone with an increasing and decreasing frequency in synchrony with the cardiac cycle. Venous flow is characterized by a low-pitched rumbling sound with little change in frequency. With practice, it is possible to use the transcutaneous flowmeter to estimate the flow in superficial vessels and to compare the flow in homologous vessels.

The transcutaneous blood flowmeter has been used to detect the fetal heartbeat as early as 10 weeks and consistently at 12 weeks after the first day of the last menstrual period. Johnson et al. (1965) described the use of a continuous-wave 5-MHz instrument for this purpose. The transducer was hand-held over the lower abdomen, and the position and orientation were varied until a definite fetal pulse was heard. Fetal blood flow could be easily distinguished from maternal blood flow. At present, there are several versions of this instrument available commercially.

Characteristics of Doppler Flowmeters. Certain important facts must be borne in mind when Doppler-type flowmeters are used. Of paramount importance is the fact that they indicate velocity, not volumetric flow. Calibration in terms of volumetric flow requires a knowledge of the velocity profile, the vessel diameter, and the angle of incidence. According to Roberts (1973), mean flow is accurately reproduced by the frequency shift when the flow profile is uniform over the diameter of the vessel. When the profile is parabolic, Roberts stated that the indicated flow is expected to be 16% above true flow. A few of the commercially available flowmeters indicate the direction of flow, toward or away from the transducer; many do not. Nonetheless, an excellent indication of the presence of flow and a decrease or increase can be obtained. Because the reflector is constituted by blood cells, it is obvious that Doppler frequency-shift flowmeters cannot be used with solutions that do not have reflecting particles. Care must be exercised to attain good acoustic coupling between the transducers and the flowing blood; however, direct contact with the blood is not required.

Baker (1970) combined the pulse-echo and Doppler shift techniques in a single instrument that provided a velocity profile of blood flow across the diameter of an unopened artery. Figure 20 is an isometric projection sketch of the flow profile.

Air bubbles are excellent reflectors of ultrasound, which can be used to detect their presence. Using the Doppler frequency-shift method, Martin and Colley (1983) employed a cylindrical (6.5 × 6.5 mm) piezoelement placed in the esophagus to detect air bubbles (air emboli) in the vascular systems of dogs. The cylindrical shape of the piezoelement provided a 360-degree ultrasonic (4-MHz) field that

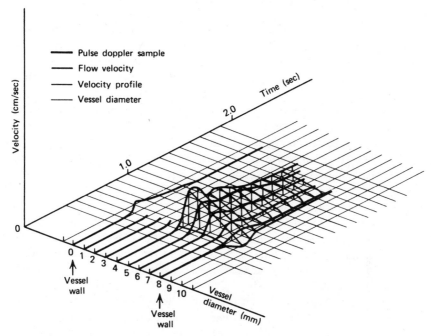

Figure 20 Blood flow velocity profile across the diameter of a blood vessel determined with a pulsed ultrasonic Doppler blood flowmeter. [From D. W. Baker, *IEEE Trans. Sonics Ultrason.* **SU-17**:170–185 (1970). By permission.]

was pulsed at 1–2 kHz. The device functioned as a blood velocity flowmeter, the output of which was monitored aurally and, after processing, on a graphic recorder. They found that intravascular injections of air as small as 0.05–2 mL were detectable. This sensitivity is greater than that obtainable with a precordial flowmeter. They also showed that at the power level used (7 mW/cm^2) there was no damage to the esophagus, which firmly embraced the transducer.

Pulse-Echo Applications

Echoencephalography. Echoencephalography employs the pulse-echo A-mode display to identify the location of midline structures of the brain. The technique was developed by Leksell (1955–1956), who applied 0.5-MHz ultrasound to a transmitting piezoelement on the scalp; a second receiving element was placed alongside. This study provided the first clinically useful echoencephalograms from patients with intracranial space-occupying lesions.

The echoencephalogram provides quantitative, noninvasive information on the location of the midline structures of the brain. Displacement of these structures indicates the presence of an expanded lesion in one hemisphere. A brain tumor or hemorrhage displaces the midline toward the opposite side; brain atrophy displaces the midline toward the same side. With generalized brain swelling, there may not be a midline displacement, but the midline echo pattern is altered. In hydrocephalic children the echograms provide a means of monitoring head and ventricular size. The echoencephalogram is of decisive value in head injury and often dictates whether surgery should be performed. A midline displacement of 2 mm in children and 4 mm in adults is considered pathological (Lithander, 1961).

Several techniques are employed with the various instruments. However, the underlying objective is the same—the accurate location of midline structures. To attain this goal, a pulse-echo transducer is placed on the scalp, usually above the ear, and coupled to the skin with a gel or oil. The ultrasonic beam (1 to 2 MHz), which travels normal to the face of the transducer, is considerably attenuated ($\sim$ 30–40 dB) by the skull. Careful alignment is necessary, because the only echoes that can be obtained are small in amplitude; the largest arise from the surfaces of structures that are perpendicular to the beam. It is noteworthy that the skull and its convoluted contents are by no means normal to the beam. Nonetheless, reflection occurs for certain midline structures such as the third ventricle–pellucidum complex (White, 1977). These midline structures return the strongest signal, which is called the M echo.

To determine whether the M echo arises from the midline, the head is examined first with the transducer on one side and an echo pattern is obtained. Then the transducer is placed on the other side of the head, and another echo pattern is obtained. Sometimes two transducers are used simultaneously, one on the left and the other on the right. Usually both patterns are photographed. Figure 21*A* illustrates schematically an echogram from a normal midline, and Fig. 21*B* illustrates schematically an echogram from a displaced midline. The difference in distance from the transmitter pulse T to the M echoes, measured along the horizontal axis, is equal to twice the midline displacement.

Figure 22 illustrates typical echoencephalograms presented by Wells (1970).

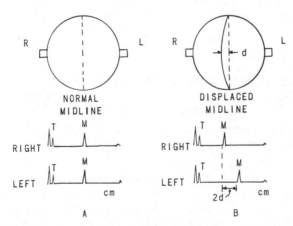

Figure 21   Principle underlying M-mode echoencephalography. (*A*) Echoes from a normal midline; (*B*) midline displacement.

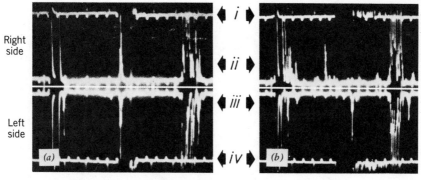

Distance from transducer (cm)

Figure 22 (a) Typical normal echoencephalogram; (b) echogram from a patient with displacement of the midline. [From P. N. T. Wells, *Biomed. Eng.* **6**:378–385 (1970). By permission.]

Figure 22a is an echogram from a normal subject. The top and bottom recordings identify 1-cm range markers, and the midline is identified ultrasonically. The two middle A-scan recordings were obtained from the right and left sides of the head of a normal subject. In both cases, the sweep travels from the left to the right of the display. To aid in identification, the left-side recording is inverted. In this normal subject, both midline echoes are in the center of the recording. Figure 22b presents an echogram from a subject with a deviation of the midline due to a left-sided intracranial hemorrhage, which deviated the midline toward the right. Note that both M echoes are displaced from the center of the recording and indicate a midline deviation to the right.

The accuracy of midline identification has been investigated; Lithander (1961) reported a standard error of 0.4 mm, using 2- and 4-MHz ultrasound. The clinical accuracy of echoencephalography has been studied by White (1977), who reported on a series of 484 patients in which only 8% provided unsatisfactory echoes. False negatives were obtained in only 17%. The percentage of false positives is difficult to identify from his data, but it appears to be about 2% of all the patients studied.

Although conventional echoencephalographs display the M echo on an oscilloscope, automatic devices that do not display the echoes are available commercially. In such instruments, sophisticated logic circuitry examines the echoes obtained and provides a digital display of midline displacement.

Ophthalmology. Pulse-echo ultrasound is used to measure the dimensions of the various structures of the eye. Figure 23a is a sketch showing the cross section of a human eye, which is almost spherical and about 1 in. in diameter. With this dimension as a guide, it can be seen that the various structures are small, calling attention to the need for using high-frequency ultrasound to resolve the structures.

The eye has a hard white scleral coat that is transparent in the anterior (corneal) region. The sclera is about 1 mm thick, and the cornea is about 0.5 mm thick at the center. Behind the cornea is the anterior chamber, which is about 3 mm deep

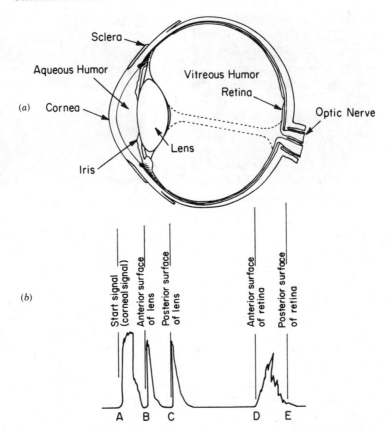

Figure 23 (*a*) The eye; (*b*) echograms from the anterior surface of the cornea. [Redrawn from G. A. Leary, *Ultrasonics* **6**:84–87 (1967).]

at its center and contains the aqueous humor and iris. This dimension decreases when the eye focuses on nearby objects. Behind the iris is the crystalline lens, which changes curvature to focus the image on the retina. The crystalline lens is about 3.6 mm thick. Behind the lens is a large chamber filled with a gel, the vitreous humor. The distance from the lens to the retina at the posterior of the eye is about 16.8 mm. The retina consists of photoreceptors (rods and cones) and nerves that are nourished by blood vessels in the adjacent choroid.

Ultrasound (6–20 MHz) A-scan presentations provide clear echoes from the anterior surface of the cornea, the anterior and posterior surfaces of the lens, and the anterior surface of the retina. The axial length of the anterior chamber, lens, and distance to the retina can be measured (Fig. 23*b*). This is a valuable asset because there is a normal development rate to this dimension in children. Retinal detachment, the presence of a tumor behind the retina, and the presence of foreign bodies can be identified. Because ultrasound passes through optically opaque structures, examination of eyes with cataracts and intraocular hemorrhage is possible.

The transducer may be placed directly on the cornea after application of a topical anesthetic. A coupling solution or natural tears will allow easy passage of the ultrasound into the eye. Sometimes the transducer is coupled to the cornea by a column of fluid about 3 cm long. With this technique, the echo from the anterior corneal surface can be clearly distinguished from the transmitter pulse. Water-filled goggles have been used for corneal imaging. The length of the fluid column is important because the first echo from the cornea is reflected back by the transducer and appears a second time and could interfere with intraocular echoes. It has been found that a fluid column about 30 mm deep eliminates the problem and allows acquisition of anterior corneal surface echoes.

There is no doubt that satisfactory results are obtained only when the operator has an intimate knowledge of the anatomy of the eye and when he or she can interact with the display, i.e., adjust the transducer to optimize the echo pattern.

M-Mode Echocardiography. The movements of a variety of cardiac structures can be recorded from the chest wall using the M-mode pulse-echo technique. Originally, echocardiography was the name applied to this technique when it was used to visualize movements of the mitral valve. However, it was soon realized that the M mode could be altered to create images that provide even more useful cardiac information. Therefore, echocardiography has come to mean the use of ultrasound to visualize the heart, its valves, and its vessels.

Edler (1955, 1961, 1967; Edler et al., 1961) developed the M-mode technique to track the motion of the anterior leaflet of the mitral valve. When this valve, which is the gateway to the left ventricle, becomes diseased, its orifice narrows (stenosis) and its cusps do not open enough to allow adequate ventricular filling. Often the cusps do not come together, and regurgitation occurs. Thus, the noninvasive M-mode technique, which promised assessment of the operation of this important valve, became of intense interest to cardiologists, who soon learned the art of aiming the beam of ultrasound to intercept the mitral valve.

Because of the multiple moving targets in the heart, Edler and Hertz included the electrocardiogram as an aid to identify the echoes of the valve-leaflet motion. In this way, the echoes could be located temporally in the cardiac cycle, and the transducer could be adjusted to optimize visualization of the mitral valve motion.

The method of acquiring an echocardiogram of the mitral valve is shown in Fig. 24a. The transducer T is placed on the left chest over the third intercostal space about 1 to 3 cm from the sternum. Occasionally the fourth or fifth intercostal space is used. A suitable coupling gel is applied, and the transducer axis is varied until the beam intercepts the mitral valve leaflet and the maximum amplitude record is obtained. With careful adjustment, echoes can be obtained from both anterior and posterior mitral valve leaflets.

Figure 24a also illustrates the ECG and an echogram from a normal mitral valve. The line E–F identifies opening of the mitral valve during the early passive-filling phase of ventricular relaxation. Figure 24b illustrates an echogram from a subject with stenosis of the mitral valve. Note that the slope of the line E–F is much less, indicating an inability of the valve to open rapidly.

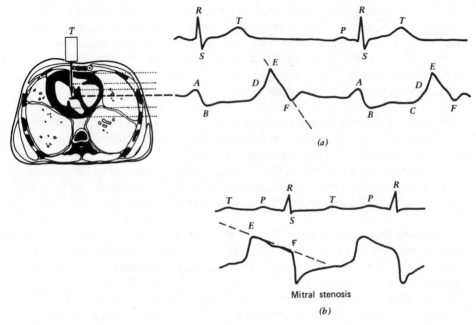

Figure 24 (*a*) Recording an M-mode echocardiogram from the normal anterior mitral valve leaflet. Diagram at left shows transducer T placed over left chest. (*b*) Recording from a diseased mitral valve. Note the difference in rate of motion (E–F).

Because echograms are calibrated in amplitude (range of motion) and time, it is possible to obtain quantitative data on the distance moved (mm) and the rate of movement (mm/sec). It has been found that a reduced rate of movement correlates with a decreased area for the mitral valve (Segal et al., 1966). Data have been tabulated for the normal rates and amplitude of movement (Wells, 1977).

M-mode echocardiography is also used to track aortic valve motion and to identify aortic valve stenosis and regurgitation. The tricuspid and pulmonary valves are difficult (and often impossible) to track ultrasonically. Portions of the atrial and ventricular walls and septa can be targeted and their thicknesses measured. Data have been tabulated for many of these dimensions (Wells, 1977).

Pericardial effusion is readily detected with M-mode echoes. It has been demonstrated that with the intracardiac injection of saline solution (so that microbubbles or a thermal gradient are produced), intraventricular shunts and valvular regurgitation can be identified. Prosthetic mitral and aortic valves produce characteristic echoes. M-mode echocardiography is particularly useful in congenital heart disease. In fact, echocardiographic examination of the heart in children provides better echoes than in adults because the small thorax is much more transparent to ultrasound.

Gordon and Kerber (1977) and Kerber et al. (1975, 1979; Kerber and Marcus,

1976) reviewed the echocardiographic literature on reduced movement of the ventricular wall seen in patients with coronary heart disease. Kerber et al. (1975) had shown that M-mode echoes could be used to identify ventricular dyskinesias in patients with coronary occlusion, and later (Kerber et al., 1979) were able to demonstrate the changes in ventricular wall thickness in normal and underperfused ventricular walls.

Present experience indicates that in about 20% of adults, satisfactory precordial echoes are unobtainable. This failure rate can be due to obesity (especially in women with large breasts), large muscular chests, emphysema (which causes the heart to be surrounded by large, air-filled lungs), and deformity of the chest cage. A rapid heart rate provides echoes of poor quality that are difficult to interpret.

Perhaps the major limitation to precordial examination with ultrasound is the limited number of ultrasonic windows for cardiac examination. The left parasternal site, where the heart is least obscured by the lungs, provides the most diagnostic ultrasonic information. Frazin (1978) circumvented this difficulty by passing a catheter-borne transducer down the esophagus and obtained M-mode echoes from structures that cannot be examined from the chest surface. However, the development of two-dimensional, real-time imaging diminished the popularity of M-mode echocardiography. Nonetheless it is well to remember that it provides an amplitude-versus-time record of the motion of cardiac structures that is not easily obtained with two-dimensional imaging.

The feasibility of obtaining stroke volume using a precordial ultrasonic transducer was investigated by Feigenbaum et al. (1967). In this study it was found that the amplitude of motion of the mitral ring (MRE_a), recorded by M-mode ultrasound as shown in Fig. 25a, when multiplied by the left ventricular diameter LVD, measured as shown in Fig. 25b, provided a quantity that was linearly proportional to stroke volume, as shown in Fig. 25c. In this study of 16 patients, average stroke volume was measured by the Fick method. The correlation coefficient was 0.973.

The use of ultrasound to determine stroke volume noninvasively was again investigated by Matsumoto et al. (1980). To obtain the best ultrasonic echoes, the ventricular dimensions were measured with an esophageal transducer operating at 5 MHz. In a series of 21 patients, the relationship between ultrasonically measured cardiac output (CO) and that measured with Cardio-green dye was CO = 0.85CO(dye) + 1.01 with a correlation coefficient of 0.72.

Over the years, investigators have developed many equations for calculating stroke volume from ventricular dimensions. Kronik et al. (1979) investigated the validity of eight of these expressions. They found that of the eight formulas for computing stroke volume (SV) using M-mode echocardiography to measure internal ventricular diameters D, the Teichholz expression provided the best correlation ($r = 0.68$–0.74) with stroke volume measured by thermodilution. The expression is

$$SV = V_d - V_s,$$

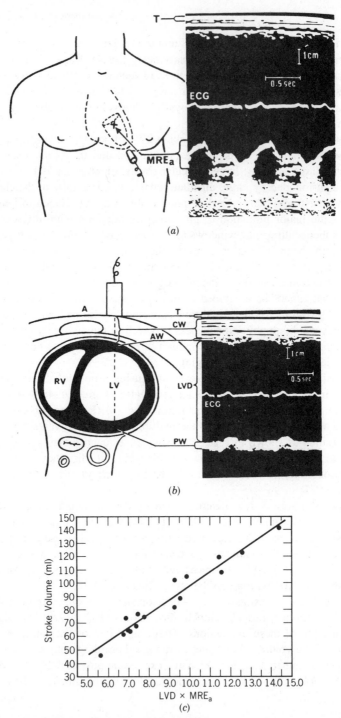

Figure 25 (*a*) Method of recording the amplitude of the mitral valve echo (MRE$_a$); (*b*) the left ventricular diameter (LVD); (*c*) correlation of the product LVD × MRE$_a$ with stroke volume. [Redrawn from H. Feigenbaum et al., *Circulation* **35**:1092–1099 (1967).]

where V_d and V_s are the diastolic and systolic volumes, respectively, calculated from the diastolic and systolic diameters D by substituting first one D (diastolic) and then the other (systolic) into the empirical expression

$$V = 7D^3/(2.4 + D).$$

The accuracy obtainable with ventricular dimensions used to measure stroke volume is limited because of the geometric assumptions needed to enter the dimension changes into an equation to yield stroke volume. Even before ultrasound was used for this purpose, X-ray images were employed, and similar limitations were recognized, particularly in diseased hearts.

Using the M-mode signal to record the aortic diameter noninvasively, and with the Doppler flow probe placed over the suprasternal notch (to obtain aortic flow velocity), Darsee et al. (1980) were able to determine cardiac output noninvasively. By multiplying the integral of aortic flow velocity by the average aortic cross-sectional area, cardiac output was calculated. In a group of 15 patients, these cardiac output values were compared with those obtained by the thermodilution method. An excellent correlation was obtained between ultrasonically and directly measured cardiac outputs, except in the case of one patient who was anemic. Because it is the red cells that produce the Doppler signal, the signals were poor in the anemic patient. The excellent correlation in the other patients is to be expected because left-ventricular output is the quantity that is being measured.

The system described by Darsee et al. is being embodied into an instrument for clinical use. The applicability of the combined M-mode and Doppler flowmeter system to a wide variety of patients is yet to be established. Initial results indicate that good signals can be obtained on about 80% of patients.

Verlangieri et al. (1984), using monkeys, combined B-mode imaging at 20 frames/sec and the Doppler frequency-shift technique to determine the blood flow in the common and internal carotid artery and the carotid sinus. Vessel diameters were measured with 10-MHz B-mode ultrasound; the blood flow velocity was measured with 3.5-MHz ultrasound. Imaging was possible to a depth of 3.8 cm. These authors pointed out that the technique could be applied to humans and were solving the problems for such application.

Intravascular Applications. Many studies have been reported in which a piezoelement was placed in the vascular system to obtain echoes from adjacent structures. Omoto (1967) called attention to the improvement in detail obtainable when the ultrasonic transducer assembly is located within the vascular system. To prove his point, he developed a miniature ultrasonic transducer mounted in a long catheter with a lateral window to allow passage of the ultrasound. The catheter was advanced into the vena cava to image the cardiac structures in front of it, using the brightness modulation presentation. Figure 26 gives the principle employed. Rotation of the transducer allowed imaging in different directions. To obtain a spatial display, the angular position of the transducer was coupled to the Y axis of an oscilloscope in which the X axis identified the head–foot position of the transducer. An X–Y plotter, in which the pen could be lifted electronically, was also

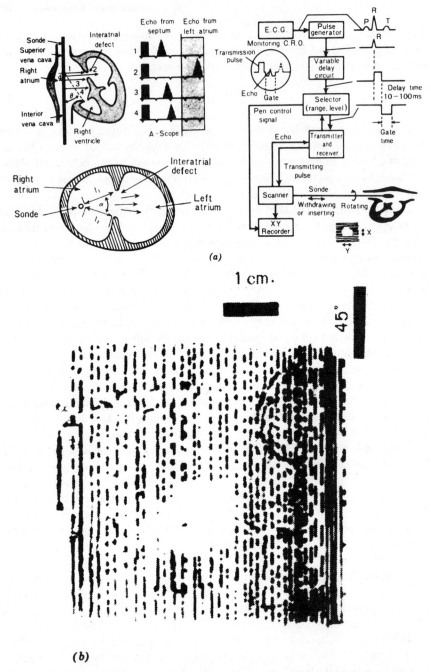

Figure 26 (a) Ultrasonic imaging of the interatrial septum using a transducer mounted on the side of a venous catheter that can be rotated to image the structures at a fixed head–foot level and placed at different head–foot levels to produce an ultrasonic tomogram of the heart and its chambers. (b) Ultrasonic tomogram of the interatrial septum in which there is a hole measuring 25 × 15 mm. [From R. Omoto, *Jpn. Heart J.* **8:**569–581 (1967). By permission.]

used as a display device. Thus by choosing a point in the vena cava and rotating the transducer through ± 90 degrees, images of the structures at the level of the transducer were obtained. Then the catheter-borne transducer assembly was moved to a new position and rotated again ± 90 degrees, thereby imaging at a new level. The procedure was repeated until the region of interest was completely examined.

The method developed by Omoto (1967) was used to identify the presence of a hole in the interatrial septum. Figure 26b presents an ultrasonic tomogram displayed with an X–Y plotter, revealing a hole measuring 25×15 mm. At the time of surgery, the size of the hole was found to be 27×16 mm.

Eggelton et al. (1969) devised a catheter-borne transducer with four 10-MHz ultrasonic piezoelements spaced 10 degrees apart. The four piezoelements were pulsed and sampled serially. They placed the catheter transducer in the left ventricle of a dog, and by acquiring dynamic echo information throughout the cardiac cycle with catheter positions from 0 to 90 degrees they were able to plot the contour of the ventricular shapes throughout the cardiac cycle.

Hughes et al. (1979a, b) reported the use of a 10-MHz ultrasonic triaxial M-mode catheter-borne transducer to measure aortic diameter and wall thickness throughout the cardiac cycle. With aortic pressure, diameter, and thickness, the essential components are available for the calculation of Young's modulus (Posey and Geddes, 1973). The triaxial (10-MHz) catheter transducer provided three pairs of inner- and outer-wall echoes (Fig. 27a), from which diameter and wall thickness could be computed on a beat-by-beat basis. Blood pressure was recorded from the same site; Fig. 27b illustrates a typical record. From this investigation (Hughes et al., 1979b), it was shown that the modulus of elasticity E of the aorta was pressure-dependent according to $E = E_0 e^{\alpha P}$, where E_0 is the zero-pressure modulus (E and E_0 in dynes per square centimeter), α is a constant that depends on the site in a particular aorta, and P is pressure in millimeters of mercury. Typical values for α for the canine aorta are 0.016 to 0.017. Typical values for E_0 are 667 to 687 mmHg.

Despite the remarkable achievements with intravascular imaging, the technique has not survived, probably because the information provided can be obtained more easily in other ways.

Two-Dimensional Imaging

The ability of a beam of pulsed ultrasound to provide echoes from targets along its path led directly to ultrasonic imaging. Some techniques provide cross-sectional views in which target motion is not important; other techniques provide multiple tomograms in rapid sequence in which motion is displayed. The terminology used to describe these images is by no means standardized.

To create a two-dimensional image, the ultrasonic beam must be made to traverse (scan) the subject, and the position of the beam must be reported to the display CRT. Thus, there are two possible scan methods, rectilinear and angular (sometimes called polar or sector). In the former case, the transducer is moved across the subject along a line and the CRT beam moves horizontally with the transducer. As the transducer moves, the echoes brighten the beam, thereby pro-

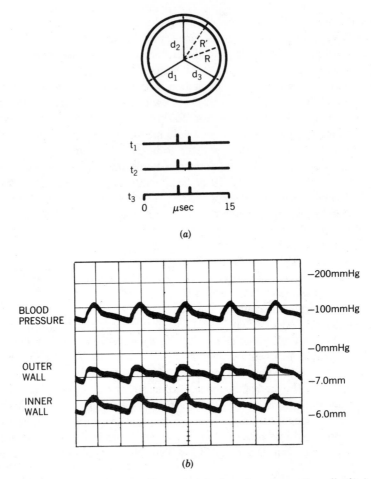

(a)

(b)

Figure 27 (a) Method of obtaining three pairs of echoes from the aortic wall. (b) A record of aortic pressure and inner and outer aortic wall diameters throughout the cardiac cycle. [From D. J. Hughes *et al.*, *Med. Biol. Eng. Comput.* **23**(3): 197–202 (1985). By permission.]

ducing an ultrasonic tomogram. This type of scan is sometimes called a compound B-scan when several transducers are used. In some applications the transducer is caused to follow the surface of the body; contact scanning is the name usually applied to this technique. A complex linkage is used, and the spatial position of the transducer is continually reported to the display device.

A very popular ultrasonic imaging technique employs a piezoelement that is oscillated through an angle of about 40 degrees to provide a sector scan. To eliminate the need for mechanically oscillating the piezoelement, a linear array of tiny piezoelements is excited so that the resultant ultrasonic beam scans the subject; such a scanner is called a phased array.

Although virtually all of the two-dimensional imaging techniques employ the pulse-echo method, it is possible to use absorption to obtain a two-dimensional image. Such a method was described by Jacobs et al. (1962; Jacobs, 1965). At the heart of the instrument was the Sokoloff image-converter tube, which provided images that were displayed on a conventional television monitor.

The Sokoloff tube consists of a quartz faceplate that receives the ultrasonic energy that has passed through the object to be imaged. The acoustic energy pattern on the faceplate is dependent on the spatial absorption characteristics of the object. The image pattern produces an oscillating potential pattern because of the piezoelectric property of quartz. The quartz plate is scanned by a high-velocity electron beam. The secondary electrons emanating from the quartz faceplate are modulated by the potential distribution pattern. The collected secondary electrons enter an electron multiplier within the tube and produce a substantial output current. The standard NTSC television scanning system was used by Jacobs, and with this first biomedical application of the Sokoloff tube, real-time black-and-white absorption images were produced. In a later application, the signal from the Sokoloff tube was processed to obtain color imagery to represent the ultrasonic absorption pattern.

Unfortunately, Jacobs' development of the Sokoloff tube produced absorption images that, although bright and clear, were difficult to obtain practically, owing to the complexities in coupling the ultrasonic generator and Sokoloff tube to the subject. A second difficulty with the device was the limited image size (~ 4 in.) due to the diameter of the quartz plate. The elegant real-time television compatibility could not surmount this difficulty, and it was never adapted clinically for imaging.

Tomography. The simplest method of acquiring cross-sectional images using ultrasound is shown in Fig. 28. The specimen to be imaged is immersed in a fluid with the transducer located below the surface of the liquid and above the subject. A series of echoes are obtained, which appear as bright spots along the sweep when the B-scan display is employed. In this particular case, it is convenient to apply the sweep to the Y axis of the oscilloscope. With ultrasonic tomography, the position of the X axis of the cathode ray tube indicates the position of the transducer assembly; thus as the transducer scans the subject, the bright-spot echoes represent the distances to the underlying reflecting tissues and organs, and their positions along the horizontal axis indicate their locations. Therefore a single scan across a subject will display a cross-section view of all the reflecting structures intercepted by the scanning ultrasonic beam.

One of the earliest, two-dimensional pulse-echo ultrasonic scanners was described by Baum and Greenwood (1958), who used 15 MHz to obtain echoes from the eyes of human subjects. The transducer was coupled to the eye via a column of water, and the transducer was moved slowly to obtain a tomogram of the eye. Olofsson (1963) constructed a different type of scanner, which consisted of two piezoelectric elements and two curved acoustic reflectors. One element was used to produce bursts of 1-MHz ultrasound and the other to receive the echoes from the object under examination. Olofsson used this transducer assembly, which measured approximately 15 $\times$ 5 cm, to image an isolated calf heart suspended in a water tank. The transducer assembly was moved to and fro in the tank to scan the

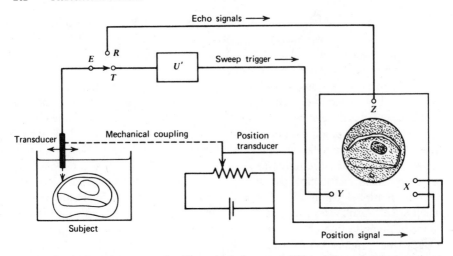

Figure 28 Ultrasonic tomography. The pulsed ultrasound (U′) is delivered to the transducer assembly and at the same time triggers the sweep, which is applied to the Y axis of the oscilloscope. The echoes returned from the reflecting surfaces in the subject are applied to the Z axis of the cathode ray tube to brighten the beam when an electronic switch (E) allows the transducer to act as a receiver nanoseconds after the initial pulse of ultrasound is delivered. Repetitive ultrasonic pulsing and electronic switching are carried out while the transducer is moved to examine a cross section of the subject. The horizontal position of the transducer is displayed on the X axis of the oscilloscope.

heart. The resulting tomogram compared very well with a picture of the heart cut in cross section along the imaging plane.

Perhaps the most outstanding slow-speed mechanical scanner was developed by Ebina et al. (1967). This instrument permitted linear scanning of the subject and allowed rotation of the transducer as well. The instrument employed 2.25-MHz ultrasound, and the heart was imaged through a water bag coupled to the chest with olive oil. An ingenious ECG triggering system was developed to allow imaging at any chosen instant in the cardiac cycle. The ultrasonic tomograms required several seconds to complete, and those presented by Ebina et al. were remarkably clear. Some clinical use was made of this equipment, which is shown in Fig. 29.

Acquiring cross-sectional images using the water-immersion and water-bag methods is inconvenient for clinical studies, despite the diagnostic value of the images. A solution to this problem was reported by Donald (1964, 1966), who created a hand-held transducer that could be moved over the abdominal surface while the transducer position was being continuously reported to the display device. Figure 30 illustrates the general principle employed in this instrument. The ultrasound (usually 2.5 MHz) is coupled to the abdomen with a liberal coating of oil. The transducer is moved over the abdomen, usually in a head-to-foot direction at first, while the operator views the display. Then oblique or transverse scans are made as dictated by the imagery. The goal is to obtain an ultrasonic tomogram of

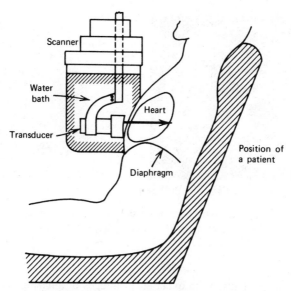

Figure 29 Ultrasonic tomography in the human. [From T. Ebina et al., *Jpn. Heart J.* **8**:331–353 (1967). By permission.]

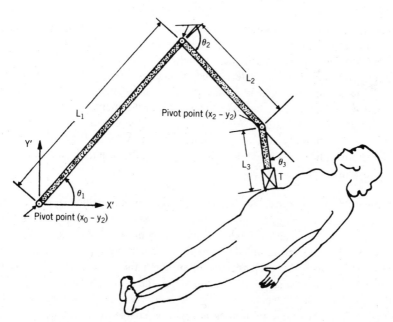

Figure 30 The contact scanner in which the transducer T is moved over the abdominal wall to obtain tomograms of the pregnant uterus. The position and angle of the transducer are identified by the transducer at the joints in the scanning arm.

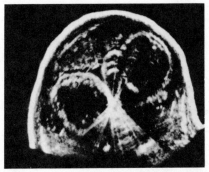 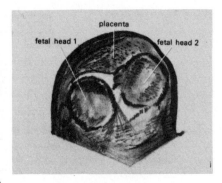

TWIN PREGNANCY (35 TH WEEK)

Figure 31   (Left) Ultrasonic tomogram of the uterus containing twins in the 35th week of pregnancy. (Right) Sketch identifying the features in the tomogram. (Courtesy Aloka Co. Tokyo 181, Japan.)

the uterus and its contents. With experience, images of amazing clarity and detail can be obtained. Figure 31 illustrates a twin pregnancy in utero.

The amount of information that can be obtained during pregnancy is remarkable. Donald (1977) summarized the major indications for using ultrasound in early, middle, and late pregnancy and following labor (puerperium). According to Donald, a gestational sac can be detected and its volume estimated after the fifth week of pregnancy. The size, position, and number of fetuses are easily determined. At present there is enough crown-to-rump data to be able to specify normal or abnormal development. Moreover, if measurements are made regularly within the first 10 weeks, the fetal maturity date can be estimated to within 1 week. Information on the position of the fetus is a valuable aid for amniocentesis (withdrawal of amniotic fluid for genetic studies). Anatomic developmental defects of the head and spine are easily identified. Also detectable are hydatiform mole, ovarian cyst, blighted ovum, fibromyoma, and placenta praevia. Viewing beyond the opaque, gas-filled bowel has been made possible by causing the urinary bladder to be filled, which displaces the intestine.

Linear Array Imaging.   An interesting all-electronic method of constructing a two-dimensional image of a subject employs a linear array of transducers that are excited sequentially. The CRT beam is moved by an increment each time the next transducer is pulsed and sampled. (Sometimes several are pulsed simultaneously.) The echoes returned by each transducer brighten the CRT beam. The resulting tomogram consists of a series of lines on which the echo information is displayed. If the individual transducers are not small and closely spaced, the distance between the lines will be large and the tomogram will be coarse in appearance.

A 10-element array for imaging the eye in cross section was described by Buschmann (1965). The 10 piezoelements were mounted in a curved holder having the same radius of curvature as the eyeball. The 10 elements were pulsed and sampled in sequence, one cycle being completed in 30 msec. The curved pattern improved the lateral resolution of the B-mode display of the interior of the eye.

A 20-element linear array was used by Bom et al. (1971) and Kloster et al. (1973) to image the human heart in cross section. King (1973) employed a similar 24-element array for the same purpose. The technique of exciting multiple elements was used to increase the echo amplitude. Although there are several developments under way to increase the number of elements and to improve the lateral resolution, the appearance of the phased array is making these developments less attractive.

Dynamic Imaging. Dynamic reflective imaging developed slowly from the slow-scan mechanical systems. One of the earliest was described by Asberg (1967), who modified Olofsson's (1963) instrument. This two-transducer, two-mirror system, operating at 1 MHz, acquired images of the human heart at 7 frames/sec. To accomplish this feat, Asberg mounted a water tank on the subject's chest and moved the position of the transducer rapidly with a motor. Asberg pointed out that this image rate (7/sec) was too slow to capture the movements of the heart. He used motion-picture film to record the images, which showed that the slow frame rate produced an objectionable flicker in the picture.

An interesting rotating ultrasonic transducer for real-time imaging from the body surface was described by Patzold et al. (1970). In this device, two ultrasonic elements were mounted on a rotating shaft at the focus of a large cylindrical parabolic mirror. Rotation of the transducers scanned the field transversely 16 times per second. With a pulse repetition rate of 2000 pulses/sec, each picture was constituted by 140 lines. The size (width) of the mirror was not given, nor was the frequency of the ultrasound. The device was designed for imaging the pregnant uterus. An interesting feature of the design is rectilinear scanning of the subject with a beam of almost uniform width.

Sector Scanners. Sector scanners present a two-dimensional image by oscillating the ultrasonic beam back and forth through an angle to scan the object. A simple real-time sector scanner was described by Griffith and Henry (1974). A 12-mm-diameter transducer, with a 6-degree beam width, was mounted on a servo-controlled dc motor with a shaft that swept through a 30-degree angle 15 times per second. The angular position of the transducer was reported to the display equipment by a rotary variable differential transformer. Thus, the position of the (radial) sweep on the CRT moved with the transducer angle. The ultrasonic frequency emitted by the transducer was 2.5 MHz, and the repetition rate was 2000/sec. Thus, the object was scanned 30 times each second, and each picture was made up of 66 radial lines.

At the same time as Griffith and Henry were developing their sector scanner, Eggelton and Johnston (1974) created an elegantly simple sector scanner by mounting the transducer of an M-mode echocardiograph on the end of the oscillating shaft of an electric toothbrush. Straightforward modification of the electronics of the M-mode instrument allowed real-time sector tomograms to be presented on the display cathode ray tube. This technique was responsible for the immediate avail-

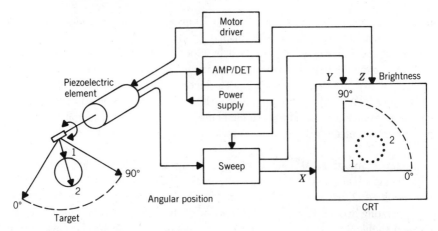

Figure 32 Sector scanner. The target is scanned by a beam of ultrasound derived from a piezoelectric element that is made to oscillate through an angle. The echoes from the target are amplified, detected, and caused to modulate the brightness of a cathode ray tube (CRT). The angular position of the piezoelectric element is reported to the CRT circuitry so that the display on the CRT is constituted by a series of radial lines that are brightness-modulated by the target.

ability of sector scanners. With such an instrument, a 30–90-degree sector tomo- gram is produced on the face of a cathode ray tube; Fig. 32 illustrates the principle underlying the mechanical sector scanner in which an ultrasonic transducer is os- cillated to scan the subject. A B-mode display presents the sector tomogram.

The first real-time sector scanners were developed by Griffith and Henry (1974) and Eggelton and Johnston (1974), although a variety of slower scanners had been described earlier. However, with these early instruments, it was difficult to couple the ultrasonic energy to the subject. Water immersion or the use of water chambers was necessary, making patient examination impractical. The advent of the oscil- lating transducer, coupled to the subject via a mound of gel, made real-time sector scanning a practical clinical procedure.

The scanner developed by Eggelton and Johnston (1974) employed a 12.5-mm piezoelement with a 10-cm focus and delivered pulses of 2.5-MHz ultrasound with a repetition frequency of 4500/sec. The frame rate was variable from 0 to 60 frames/sec; usually a rate of 40 frames/sec was used, which provided a 125-line picture for the 30° sector.

Sector scanners with characteristics like those just described are available com- mercially and are used clinically for real-time two-dimensional imaging of the heart, its valves, and outflow tracts. In some cases the ultrasonic imagery is re- corded on videotape, thereby allowing replay and closer examination.

To date the sector scanner has been used almost exclusively for imaging the heart. In the study by Griffith and Henry, (1974), the mitral and aortic valves were imaged as they opened and closed (Fig. 33). It was also possible to image the aorta, pulmonary artery, and ventricles in cross section. Because of its ability to

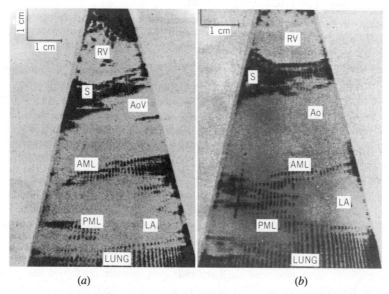

(a)   (b)

Figure 33   Sector scans of human hearts obtained with the transducer on the anterior chest wall. (a) A normal heart in diastole with open mitral and closed aortic valve. (b) A systolic frame from the same subject with open aortic and closed mitral valve. (Ao = aorta, AoV = aortic valve, LA = left atrium, AML = anterior mitral valve leaflet, PML = posterior mitral valve leaflet, PM = papillary muscle, RV = right ventricle, S = ventricular septum. [From J. M. Griffith and W. L. Henry, *Circulation* **49**:1147–1151 (1974). By permission of the American Heart Association, Inc.]

image the ventricular outflow tracks, these authors pointed out the value of sector scanning in the study of cardiac anomalies.

Weyman et al. (1976) and Dillon et al. (1977) used the sector scanner to measure the diameter of the left main coronary artery in patients with coronary artery disease and to image interatrial septal defects. In the former study, confirmation of the image was achieved by contrast injection while imaging. In the latter study, dye injected into the right atrium confirmed the presence of the septal defect and verified the accuracy of the ultrasonic images.

The images obtained with the sector scanner are limited by the available ultrasonic windows—those regions on the surface of the thorax where ultrasound can gain access to internal structures. As stated previously, bone attenuates and the air-filled lungs reflect ultrasound dramatically; hence distant structures are virtually invisible to ultrasound. Viewing sites must be chosen with these facts in mind. At present, the popular transducer locations are the apical, subxiphoid, suprasternal notch, and parasternal.

Intraesophageal Imaging.   Because of the limited number of ultrasonic windows on the chest, not all parts of the heart can be visualized ultrasonically with a conventional sector scanner. To overcome this limitation, Eggelton and Weidner (1973), Fearnot et al. (1978; Fearnot, 1980), and Hisanaga et al. (1978) developed intraesophageal scanners. Use of this site eliminates the restrictions on viewing imposed by the air-filled lungs and rib cage.

Eggelton's scanner consisted of multiple piezoelements at the tip of a flexible rotating shaft. The elements were pulsed and sampled in succession to provide a horizontal-plane tomogram of the thoracic contents. The scanner described by Fearnot consisted of four piezoelectric elements mounted at the end of a shaft rotating at 450 rev/min within a concentric tube that had a window and was filled with mineral oil. The piezoelements were connected to a slip-ring commutator, and each element was pulsed and sampled for 90 degrees of rotation of the shaft. Thirty 166-line sector-scan horizontal-plane images were produced each second using 5-MHz ultrasound. The scanning format permitted recording the sector scans on standard videotape.

The esophageal scanner developed by Hisanaga et al. (1978) consisted of an oil-filled catheter in which a piezoelement was caused to move up and down with an excursion of 7 cm, 4–10 times per second. The ultrasound frequency used was 2.25 MHz, and the pulse repetition frequency was 6 KHz. Thus, 8–20 vertical-plane pictures were produced each second; each picture contained 300 or more lines. In the following year, Hisanaga et al. (1978) described a sector scanner similar to that reported by Fearnot, with which they obtained horizontal-plane echograms of the ventricles.

With both esophageal cardiac imagers, the authors described pictures of good clarity. Hisanaga et al. reported that both atrioventricular valves, the aorta, and bifurcation of the pulmonary artery were observed in human subjects. Only a few subjects gagged while swallowing the catheter, which was 13–15 mm in diameter. There is no doubt that there will be continued development of esophageal scanners.

Phased-Array Imaging. The phased-array imaging technique employs a linear arrangement of piezoelements that are serially excited and sampled in a special sequence to enable synthesis of tomograms of much higher lateral resolution than are obtainable when the pulse-echo technique is applied to each element sequentially. Although there are many ways of exciting the piezoelements, it should be noted that the phased-array scheme permits acquiring sector- and rectangular-scan images without mechanical movement of the transducer. In essence, with the phased-array technique, the beam of ultrasound is steered electronically by exciting the piezoelements in a special way.

The first phased-array imaging system was described by Somer (1968, 1969), who employed a 20-element array. The elements were spaced 0.5 mm ($\lambda/2$) apart, and the entire array measured 11 × 11 mm. The elements were pulsed and sampled to produce a 90-degree sector scan of 32 lines, repeated 30 times/sec. A unique feature allowed increasing the image to 128 lines by reducing the frame rate to 8 frames/sec. Another feature allowed acquiring A-scan information along any two of the 32 radial directions. The device was used for imaging the pregnant uterus.

An improved phased-array sector scanner with dynamic focusing was described by von Ramm and Thurstone (1976). In this device, 16 piezoelements were excited

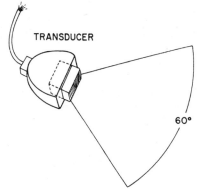

TRANSDUCER

60°

Figure 34 A phased-array transducer consisting of 24 elements. [Redrawn from J. A. Kisslo et al., *Yale J. Biol. Med.* **50**:355–365 (1977).]

and sampled to provide a 60-degree sector scan of 256 lines. A digital computer was used to control the pulsing and sampling of the piezoelements. The use of an improved model was reported by Kisslo et al. (1977). The transducer, shown in Fig. 34, consisted of twenty-four 2.25-MHz piezoelements. The array measured 24 by 14 mm and provided a 60-degree, 256-line picture at 20 frames/sec, or a 90-degree, 160-line picture at 30 frames/sec. The depth range was 18 cm, and the resolution was measured with a wire target in water. The range resolution was 1.5 mm, and the azimuthal resolution was 1.5 degrees in the visual field (3.5–18 cm).

Kisslo et al. (1977) reported that in clinical trials the transducer was placed on the chest over the sternal border, at the level of the second or fifth rib, these sites being the ultrasonic windows for cross-sectional imaging of the heart. They reported that in over 2 years experience the system was used to identify valvular heart disease, endocarditis, pericardial effusion, and congenital heart defects.

A different type of phased array was described by Selbie et al. (1980). The 2-MHz transducer consisted of 31 piezoelements occupying 10 by 120 mm. The method of exciting and sampling the elements produced a 93-line rectangular image repeated at the (British) television frame rate. The device, known as the Aberdeen Phased Array, has not been used clinically.

The options for imaging with a linear array of piezoelements are many. Pulsing and sampling of the elements can provide an almost real-time tomogram. Because the processing techniques employ digitized signals, a considerable variety of processing algorithms can be applied. Tape storage of the images in digital form is simple and convenient. Although great flexibility is possible with the phased array, it is subject to the same limitation as other ultrasonic imaging systems in assessing cardiac function—the limited number of sites on the thorax suitable for image acquisition.

REFERENCES

Asberg, A. 1967. Ultrasonic cinematography of the living heart. *Ultrasonics* **6**:113–117.

Baker, D. W. 1964. A sonic transcutaneous blood flowmeter. *Proc. Annu. Conf. Med. Biol. Eng.* **6**:76.

Baker, D. W. 1970. Pulsed ultrasonic Doppler blood-flow sensing. *IEEE Trans. Sonics Ultrason.* **SU-17**:170–185.

Baum, G., and I. Greenwood. 1958. The application of ultrasonic locating techniques to ophthalmology. *Arch. Ophthalmol.* **60**:263–279.

Bjerring, W. L., H. C. Boone, and M. L. Lockhart. 1935. Use of electrostethophone for recording heart sounds. *JAMA* **104**:628–637.

Bom, N., C. T. Lancee, J. Hornkoop, and P. G. Hugenhold. 1971. Ultrasonic viewer for cross-sectional analyses of moving cardiac structures. *Biomed. Eng.* **6**:500–503.

Boone, B. R. 1939. An amplifier for recording heart sounds through use of the cathode ray tube. *J. Lab. Clin. Med.* **25**:188–193.

Buschmann, W. 1965. New equipment and transducers for ophthalmic diagnosis. *Ultrasonics* **3**:18–21.

Currens, J. H., G. L. Bramwell, and S. Aronow. 1957. An automatic blood pressure recording machine. *N. Engl. J. Med.* **17**:780–784.

Darsee, J. R., P. F. Walter, and D. D. Nutter. 1980. Transcutaneous Doppler method of measuring cardiac output. *Am. J. Cardiol.* **15**:613–618.

DeForest, R. E. 1955. Ultrasonic energy for therapeutic purposes. *JAMA* **157**:1407–1408.

Dillon, J. C., A. E. Weyman, H. Feigenbaum, R. C. Eggelton, and K. Johnston, 1977. Cross-sectional echocardiographic examination of the inter-atrial septum. *Circulation* **55**(1):115–120.

Donald, I. 1964. Ultrasonography in two dimensions. *Med. Biol. Illus.* **14**(4):216–224.

Donald, I. 1966. Sonar examination of the abdomen, *Ultrasonics* (July):119–124.

Donald, I. 1977. Ultrasonic investigation in obstetrics and gynaecology. In *Ultrasonics in Clinical Diagnosis*, 2nd ed. P. N. T. Wells (ed.). Churchill-Livingstone, Edinburgh and London, 195 pp.

Donaldson, P. E. K. 1958. *Electronic Apparatus for Biological Research*. Butterworth, London.

Ebina, T., S. Oka, M. Tanaka, S. Kosaka, Y. Terasawa, K. Unno, Y. Kikuchi, and R. Uchida. 1967. The ultrasono-tomography for heart and great vessels in human subjects by means of the ultransonic reflection technique. *Jpn. Heart J.* **8**:331–353.

Edler, I. 1955. The diagnostic use of ultrasound in heart disease. *Acta Med. Scand.* **152**(Supp.):304–308.

Edler, I. 1956. Ultrasound-cardiogram in mitral valvular disease. *Acta Chir. Scand.* **111**:230–232.

Edler, I. 1961. Ultrasoundcardiography. In *Studies on the Cardiopulmonary Function in Sarcoidosis*, Supp. 370, Parts 1 and 2. N. Svanbarg (ed.). Bjurstrom Co., Stocholm.

Edler, I. 1967. Ultrasound cardiography. *Ultrasonics* **6**:72–79.

Edler, I., A. Gustafson, T. Karlefors, and B. Christensson. 1961. Ultrasound cardiography. *Acta Med. Scand., Suppl.* **370**:68–82.

Eggelton, R. C., and K. W. Johnston. 1974. Real time B-mode mechanical scanning system. *Proc. Soc. Photo-Opt. Instrum. Eng.* **47**:96–100.

Eggelton, R. C., and A. W. Weidner. 1973. Ultrasonic catheter with rotating transducers. U.S. Patent 3,779,234, December 18.

Eggelton, R. C., C. Townsend, G. Kosoff, et al. 1969. Computed ultrasonic visualizations of dynamic ventricular configuration. *Proc. 8th Int. Conf. Eng. Med. Biol., 1969.*

Fearnot, N. E. 1980. Dynamic imaging of the dog heart from the esophagus using ultrasound. Ph.D. thesis, Purdue University, West Lafayette, IN.

Fearnot, N. E., J. D. Bourland, L. A. Geddes, and R. E. Eggelton. 1978. An esophageal echocardiographic scanner. *Proc. 13th AAMI Conf.* p. 90.

Feigenbaum, H., A. Zaky, and W. Nasser. 1967. Use of ultrasound to measure left ventricular stroke volume. *Circulation* **35**:1093–1099.

Firestone, F. A. 1945. The supersonic reflectoscope, an instrument for inspecting the interior of solid parts by means of sound waves. *J. Acoust. Soc. Am.* **17**(3):287–299.

Franklin, D. L., D. W. Baker, R. M. Ellis, and R. F. Rushmer. 1959. A pulsed ultrasonic flowmeter. *IRE Trans. Med. Electron.* **ME-6:**204–206.

Franklin, D. L., W. Schlegel, and R. F. Rushmer. 1961. Blood flow measurement by Doppler frequency shift. *Science* **134:**564–565.

Frazin, L. I. 1978. The development of esophageal echocardiography. *Appl. Radiol.* **7**(2):108–113.

French, L. A., J. J. Wild, and D. Neal. 1950. Detection of cerebral tumors by ultrasonic pulses. *Cancer* **3:**705–708.

French, L. A., J. J. Wild, and D. Neal. 1951. The experimental applications of ultrasound to the localization of brain tumors. *J. Neurosurg.* **8:**198–203.

Fry, W. J., and F. J. Fry. 1960. Fundamental neurological research and human neurosurgery using intense ultrasound. *IEEE Trans. Med. Electron.* (7):166–181.

Geddes, L. A. 1984. Intraesophageal monitoring of the ECG and respiration in anesthetized animals. *Med. Biol. Eng. Comput.* **22:**90–91.

Geddes, L. A., and A. G. Moore. 1968. The efficient detection of Korotkoff sounds. *Med. Biol. Eng.* **6:**603–609.

Geddes, L. A., W. A. Spencer, and H. E. Hoff. 1959. Graphic recording of the Korotkoff sounds. *Am. Heart J.* **57:**361–370.

Geddes, L. A., J. Bourland, and E. Arriaga. 1974. Recording esophageal heart sounds with a catheter-tip microphone. *Cardiovasc. Res. Cent. Bull.* **13:**3–7.

Gilford, S. R., and H. P. Broida. 1954. Physiological monitoring equipment for anesthesia and other uses. *Natl. Bur. Stand. (U.S.), Annu. Rep.* **3301** (Project 1204-20-5512).

Gilson, W. E. 1942. Automatic blood pressure recorder. *Electronics* **15:**54–56.

Gilson, W. E., H. Goldberg, and H. Slocum. 1941. Automatic device for periodically determining and recording both systolic and diastolic blood pressure in man. *Science* **94:**194.

Gomez, D. M., and A. Langevin. 1937. *La piézographe directe et instantanée.* Hermann, Paris.

Gordon, M. J., and R. E. Kerber. 1977. Interventricular septal motion in patients with proximal and distal left anterior descending coronary artery lesions. *Circulation* **55:**338–341.

Griffith, J. M., and W. L. Henry. 1974. A sector scanner for real-time two-dimensional echocardiography. *Circulation* **49:**1147–1151.

Herrick, J. F., and J. A. Anderson. 1959. An ultrasonic flowmeter. *IRE Trans. Med. Electron.* **ME-6:**195–197.

Hisanaga, K., and A. Hisanaga. 1979. A transesophageal real-time sector scanner with an oil-filled cell. *Amer. Inst. for Ultrasound in Med., 1979* Paper 1116.

Hisanaga, K., A. Hisanaga, and Y. Ichie. 1978. A new transesophageal real-time linear scanner and initial clinical results. *Proc. A.I.U.M. Meet., 1978.*

Hueter, T. F. 1952. Ultrasonic measurements in human skull bone and their dependency upon frequency. *Naturwissenschaften* **39**(1):21–22.

Hueter, T. F. 1976. Measurement of ultrasonic absorption in animal tissues and its dependence on frequency. In *Ultrasonic Biophysics.* F. Dunn and W. D. O'Brien (eds.). Dowden, Hutchinson & Ross, Stroudsburg, PA, 410 pp.

Hughes, D. J., L. A. Geddes, J. D. Bourland, and C. F. Babbs. 1979a. Dynamic imaging of the aorta with 10-MHz ultrasound. In *Acoustical Imaging.* A. R. Metherell (ed.). Plenum, New York.

Hughes, D. J., C. F. Babbs, L. A. Geddes, and J. D. Bourland. 1979b. Measurement of Young's modulus of elasticity of the canine aorta with ultrasound. *Ultrason. Imaging* **1:**356–367.

Jacobs, J. E. 1965. Applications of ultrasound image converters in biology. *Biomechanics and Related Engineering Topics.* Pergamon, Oxford, Chap 5.

Jacobs, J. E., D. W. Cugell, J. R. Wennemark, and W. J. Collis. 1962. Cinesonography in applied biological problems. *Dig. 15th Annu. Conf. Eng. Med. Biol.* Paper No. 8, p. 28.

212   Piezoelectric Devices

Johnson, W. L., H. F. Stegall, J. N. Lein, and R. F. Rushmer. 1965. Detection of fetal life in early pregnancy with an ultrasonic Doppler flowmeter. *Obstet. Gynecol.* **26**:305–307.

Kalmus, H. P. 1954. An electric flowmeter. *Rev. Sci. Instrum.* **25**:201–206.

Kerber, R. E., and M. E. Marcus. 1976. Evaluation of regional myocardial function in ischemic heart disease. *Prog. Cardiovasc. Dis.* **20**(6):441–450.

Kerber, R. E., M. L. Marcus, J. Ehrhardt, R. Wilson, and F. M. Aboud. 1975. Correlation between echocardiographically demonstrated segmental dyskinesis and regional myocardial perfusion. *Circulation* **52**:1097–1104.

Kerber, R. E., J. B. Martins, and M. L. Marcus. 1979. Effect of acute ischemia, nitroglycerin and nitroprusside on regional myocardial thickening, stress and pressure. *Circulation* **60**(1):121–129.

King, D. L. 1973. Real-time cross-sectional ultrasonic imaging of the heart using a linear array multi-element transducer. *J. Clin. Ultrasound* **1**(3):196–200.

Kisslo, J. A., O. T. Von Ramm, and F. L. Thurstone. 1977. Clinical results of real-time ultrasonic scanning of the heart using a phased array system. *Yale J. Biol. Med.* **50**:355–365.

Kloster, F. E., J. Roelandt, F. J. Ten-Cate, N. Bom, and P. G. Hugenholtz. 1973. Multi-scan echocardiography. *Circulation* **48**:1075–1084.

Kronik, G., J. Slany, and H. Mosslacher. 1979. Comparative value of eight M-mode echocardiographic formulae for determining left ventricular stroke volume. *Circulation* **60**:1308–1316.

Lax, H., A. W. Feinberg, and B. M. Cohen. 1956. Studies of the arterial pulse wave. *J. Chronic Dis.* **3**:618–631.

Leary, S. A. 1967. Basic techniques for applying ultrasonics to ophthalmic measurement and diagnosis. *Ultrasonics* **6**:84–87.

Leksell, L. 1955–1956. Echo-encephalography. *Acta Chir. Scand.* **110**:301–315.

Lewis, D. H., G. W. Dietz, J. D. Wallace, and J. R. Brown. 1957. Intracardiac phonocardiography in man. *Circulation* **16**:764–775.

Lithander, B. 1961. Clinical and experimental studies in echoencephalography. *Acta Psychiatr. Neurol. Scand.* **36**:1–53.

Lockhart, M. L. 1938. The stethograph. *Am. Heart J.* **10**:72–78.

Malcolm, J. L. 1946. A piezoelectric unit for general purpose physiological recording. *J. Sci. Instrum.* **23**:146–148.

Mannheimer, E. 1941. Calibrated phonocardiography. *Am. Heart J.* **21**:151–162.

Martin, R. W., and P. S. Colley. 1983. Evaluation of transesophageal Doppler detection of air embolism. *Anesthesiology* **58**(2):117–123.

Matsumoto, M., Y. Oka, J. Strom et al. 1980. Application of transesophageal echocardiography to continuous intraoperative monitoring of left ventricular performance. *Am. J. Cardiol.* **46**:95–105.

Miller, A., and P. D. White. 1941. Crystal microphone for pulse wave recording. *Am. Heart J.* **21**:504–510.

Narat, J. K. 1936. New electronic stethoscope and stethograph. Preliminary report. *Ill. Med. J.* **70**:131–134.

Olofsson, S. 1963. An ultrasonic optical mirror system. *Acustica* **18**:361–367.

Omberg, A. C. 1936. Apparatus for recording systolic blood pressure. *Rev. Sci. Instrum.* **7**:33–34.

Omoto, R. 1967. Intracardiac scanning of the heart with the aid of ultrasonic intravascular probe. *Jpn. Heart J.* **8**:569–581.

Pascoe, J. E. 1955. A technique for introduction of intracellular electrodes. *J. Physiol.* **128**:26P–27P.

Patzold, J., W. Krause, H. Kresse, and R. Soldner. 1970. Present state of an ultrasonic cross-section procedure with rapid image rate. *IEEE Trans. Biomed. Eng.* **BME-17**:263–265.

Posey, J. A., Jr., and L. A. Geddes. 1973. Measurement of the modulus of elasticity of the arterial wall. *Cardiovasc. Res. Cent. Bull.* **111**(4):83–103.

Rappaport, M. B., and A. Luisada. 1944. Indirect sphygmomanometry. *J. Lab. Clin. Med.* **29:**638–665.

Rappaport, M. B., and H. B. Sprague. 1941. Physiologic and physical laws that govern auscultation and their application. *Am. Heart J.* **21:**257–318.

Rappaport, M. B., and H. B. Sprague. 1942. Graphic registration of normal heart sounds. *Am. Heart J.* **23:**591–623.

Reid, J. M., and J. O. Wild. 1952. Ultrasonic ranging for cancer diagnosis. *Electronics* (July):136–138.

Roberts, V. C. 1973. The measurement of flow in intact blood vessels. *CRC Crit. Rev. Bioeng.* **1:**419–447.

Sachs, H. A., H. Marquis, and B. Blumenthal. 1935. A modification of the Wiggers-Dean system measuring heart sounds using audio amplification. *Am. Heart J.* **10:**965–8.

Segal, B., W. Lekoff, and B. Kingsley. 1966. Echocardiography. *JAMA* **195:**99–104.

Selbie, R. D., J. M. S. Hutchison, and J. R. Mallard. 1980. The Aberdeen phased array. *Med. Biol. Eng. Comput.* **18**(3):335–343.

Somer, J. C. 1968. *Ultrasonics* **6**(3):153.

Somer, J. C. 1969. Electronic sector scanning with ultrasonic beams. *Proc. 1st World Conf. Ultrasound Diagn. Med., 1969.*

Ulrich, W. D. 1974. Ultrasound dosage for non-therapeutic use in human beings—Extrapolation from a literature survey. *IEEE Trans. Biomed. Eng.* **BME-21:**48–51.

Verlangieri, A. J., M. J. Bush, and J. C. Kapeghian. 1984. Duplex ultrasound analysis of the carotid arteries in macaca fasciculares. *J. Cardiovasc. Ultrasonogr.* **1**(4):293–302.

von Ramm, O. T., and T. L. Thurstone. 1976. Cardiac imaging using a phased array ultrasound system. *Circulation* **53:**258–262.

Wallace, J. D., J. R. Brown, D. H. Lewis, and G. W. Dietz. 1957. Phonocatheters: Their design and application. Part 1. *IRE Trans. Med. Electron.* **PGME-9:**25–30.

War Department Technical Manual 1944. *Radar System Fundamentals*, TM-11-467. U.S. Govt. Printing Office, Washington, DC.

Wells, P. N. T. 1970. The present status of medical ultrasonic diagnostics. *Biomed. Eng.* **5:**376–385.

Wells, P. N. T. (ed.). 1977. *Ultrasonics in Clinical Diagnosis*. Churchill-Livingstone, Edinburgh and London, 195 pp.

Weyman, A. E., H. Feigenbaum, J. C. Dillon, K. W. Johnston, and R. G. Eggelton. 1976. Noninvasive visualization of the left main coronary artery by cross-sectional echocardiography. *Circulation* **54**(2):169–174.

White, O.N. 1977. Ultrasonic investigation of the brain. In *Ultrasonics in Clinical Diagnosis*. P. N. T. Wells (ed.). Churchill-Livingstone, Edinburgh and London, 195 pp.

Wood, M. C., and A. C. Gunn. 1953. The amplification and recording of foetal heart sounds. *Electron. Eng.* **25:**90–93.

7

Thermoelectric Devices

THERMOELECTRICITY

When two dissimilar metals are joined, a temperature-dependent potential, called the contact potential, develops. First demonstrated in 1821 by Seebeck, this phenomenon has been used extensively for the measurement of temperature for more than a century. The contact potential is related to the differences in the work functions of the two metals. Although a single junction of two metals can be employed to develop the potential, such a simple arrangement is often impractical; the usual configuration for utilization of the thermoelectric effect is illustrated in Fig. 1a. The two metals (1, 2) constitute the thermocouple, and the potential developed is dependent on the temperature difference between the two bimetal junctions J_{1-2} and J_{2-1}. In practice, it is customary to keep one junction at a reference temperature, employing the other to measure the unknown temperature. Usually the reference point chosen is 0 or 100°C, although ambient temperature is sometimes employed.

Because the measuring junction often must be located some distance from the reference junction and the indicating instrument, it is usually impractical to choose the same metal for both the interconnecting cable conductors and the thermojunctions. For this reason conducting wires of a different material are introduced into the circuit. Under these conditions the thermodetector takes the form shown in Fig. 1b. Thus there are really three important thermal junctions: J_{1-2}, J_{1-3}, and J_{2-3}. The temperature $T_{J_{1-2}}$ can be measured only if the temperatures of the two remaining junctions are kept constant. Usually the connecting wires are made of materials chosen so that the thermal voltages between junctions J_{1-3} and J_{2-3} are small. Thus minor variations in the temperature at J_{1-3} and J_{2-3} will contribute only insignificant error voltages, and the voltage presented to the indicator is largely a function of $T_{J_{1-2}}$.

The ability of a particular thermojunction to develop a voltage is specified by its thermoelectric power, an old term now of dubious merit. The voltages developed by couples of various metals are usually small. Certain special alloys that produce a nearly linear voltage with temperature have been developed. It is customary to specify the thermoelectric sensitivity S of a material with respect to platinum, which can be obtained with high purity; moreover, platinum has a high melting point. Table 1 lists the thermoelectric sensitivities in microvolts per degree Celsius for

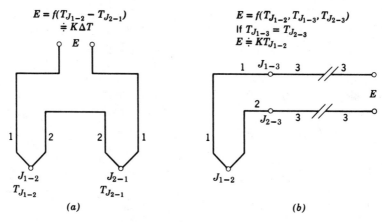

$$E = f(T_{J_{1-2}} - T_{J_{2-1}})$$
$$\doteq K\Delta T$$

$$E = f(T_{J_{1-2}}, T_{J_{1-3}}, T_{J_{2-3}})$$
If $T_{J_{1-3}} = T_{J_{2-3}}$
$$E \doteq KT_{J_{1-2}}$$

(a)

(b)

Figure 1   Thermojunctions.

many popular substances. To determine the thermoelectric sensitivity of a couple consisting of any two substances listed in Table 1, it is only necessary to subtract their thermoelectric sensitivities. For example, a couple of selenium and bismuth would provide $900 - (-72) = 972 \; \mu V/°C$. A couple of nichrome and iron would provide $6.5 \; \mu V/°C$. However, it should be emphasized that the voltage–temperature relationship is not linear over a wide temperature range.

For accurate measurement of temperature with a thermocouple, the voltage must be measured with a potentiometer. If current passes through the junctions, one is warmed and the other is cooled. This phenomenon is known as the Peltier effect, and although its magnitude is small it must be considered in terms of both changing the resistance of the circuit and adding heat to or abstracting heat from what is being measured.

TABLE 1   Thermoelectric Sensitivity $S = dE/dt$ of Thermoelement Made of Materials Listed against Platinum[a]

Material	$S \; (\mu V/°C)$	Material	$S \; (\mu V/°C)$
Bismuth	−72	Silver	6.5
Constantan	−35	Copper	6.5
Nickel	−15	Gold	6.5
Potassium	−9	Tungsten	7.5
Sodium	−2	Cadmium	7.5
Platinum	0	Iron	18.5
Mercury	0.6	Nichrome	25
Carbon	3	Antimony	47
Aluminum	3.5	Germanium	300
Lead	4	Silicon	400
Tantalum	4.5	Tellurium	500
Rhodium	6	Selenium	900

[a]Reference junction kept at a temperature of 0°C.

Source: K. S. Lion, *Instrumentation in Scientific Research.* McGraw-Hill, New York, 1959.

The potential difference depends on the species of the metals, not on the size of the conductors that constitute the junction. If the thermoelectric voltage is used to deliver current, the total circuit resistance must be kept low.

Although the thermocouple has been somewhat overshadowed by the thermistor as a temperature sensor, new techniques of fabrication indicate that it may see wider application in biomedicine. For example, Reed and Kampwirth (1964), Reed (1966), and Cain and Welch (1974) described thermocouples of micron dimensions (Fig. 2) that could easily be inserted into single living cells to measure the temperature of the cytoplasm.

The response time for miniature thermocouples (25 μm) was given by Gelb et al. (1964) as 116 msec for 95% response. Thermocouples made from 40-gauge wire (High Temperature Instruments Corp., Philadelphia, Pennsylvania) are advertised as having a time constant of 0.1 sec, and the time constant of its ultraminiature couples is given as 0.05 sec. Another supplier (Omega Engineering Inc., Springdale, Connecticut) has advertised fine-wire (0.002–0.005 in.) iron–constantan thermocouples having time constants in the range of 0.002–1 sec.)

Certain precautions must be observed in the construction of thermocouples. The material from which the junctions are made must be homogeneous, and considerable attention is needed in the fusing of the elements to form the active junction. Bulletin 15A-RP 1.4 of the Leeds and Northrup Co. covers the important details of construction and describes gas, electric arc, and resistance welding of the thermojunctions.

An ingenious laboratory method of arc-welding thermocouple junctions electrically, described by Riley (1949), employs a metal cup in which is placed a small quantity of mercury, which is then covered with mineral or motor oil to a depth

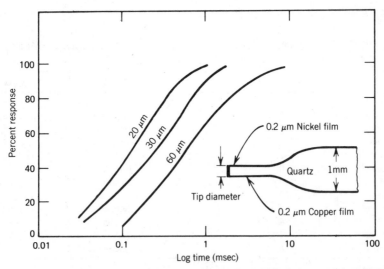

Figure 2 Copper–nickel thermojunctions and their response times. (Courtesy of A. J. Welch, University of Texas, Austin, 1974.)

of 2–3 cm. The metal cup and the mercury within it constitute one electrode connected to a 115-V power source. The ends of the thermocouple wires are cleaned and are then twisted tightly together for a distance of several millimeters. The distal end, which is to become the thermojunction, is then cut, leaving only a little more than a single turn of the twisted wires. The other ends of the wires are then joined and connected by way of a variable resistor to the other side of the power source. The resistor that Riley used consisted of a 400-W heating element to fabricate a 0.3-mm thermocouple. Welding is accomplished by lowering the twisted ends of the thermocouple wires into the oil to make contact with the surface of the mercury and then withdrawing them. As contact is broken, the high-temperature arc formed between the wires and the pool of mercury fuses the ends to form the thermojunction. Iron–constantan, platinum, platinum–rhodium, chromel–alumel, and copper–constantan wires have been welded by using this easily mastered technique. Riley reported that the magnitude of the resistor is dictated by the diameter of the wires chosen for the thermocouple. In his experience wires ranging from 0.1 to 4 mm have been successfully welded.

New fabrication techniques are available for the construction of microthermocouples and thermopiles (which consist of an array of thermocouples in series). Guilbeau and Mayall (1981) described a 1-μm thermojunction made by vapor deposition of tellurium on a glass-insulated fine platinum wire. The couple provided an output of 300 μV/°C. The resistance was several hundred megohms, and the response time was less than 50 msec.

Integrated-circuit technology was used by Lahiji (1981) to fabricate a thermopile of 60 bismuth–antimony junctions on a 2 $\times$ 2 $\times$ 1 mm chip. The output was 176 μV/°C, and the response time was 15 msec.

Towe et al. (1985) employed thin-film technology to create a thermopile of 150 bismuth–antimony thermojunctions on a 1.8-mm-square substrate. One series of junctions were coated with a glucose-oxidizing enzyme, and the heat of oxidation was measured by the coated junctions, providing a voltage proportional to glucose concentration.

BIOMEDICAL APPLICATIONS

In biomedical studies thermocouples find a variety of uses as detectors of temperature that reflect circulation in the regions measured. Scott (1930) described the use of four couples in series (a thermopile) for measuring skin temperature. Hardy (1934) measured radiant heat from the body with such a device. Miniature thermocouples for determining the temperatures of deep tissues and blood have been constructed and placed in hypodermic needles by Clark (1922), Bazzett and McGlone (1927), Sheard (1931), and Foster (1936). Bazzett and McGlone have reminded investigators that thermocouples were used to measure the temperature in human muscle as long ago as 1835. In all probability the thermocouple was the first electrical transducer in physiology. In the hands of Hill (1932), the thermocouple showed that the temperature rise in nerve cells during the passage of an impulse was 7×10^{-8} °C.

Rein (1928) described his blood flow transducer, the thermostromuhr, which employed a pair of small thermocouples and a heating element to measure blood flow. The apparatus consisted of a tube with the heating element located in the axial stream; the thermocouples were mounted proximal and distal to the heating element. Blood flowing past the heating element was warmed. The upstream couple detected the temperature of the blood before heating, and the downstream unit monitored the temperature of the warmed blood. The temperature difference was thus dependent on blood flow. By improving Rein's instrument, Baldes et al. (1933) were able to measure very tiny blood flows. Their contribution consisted of warming the blood with dielectric heating instead of using a heating element in the bloodstream.

For a considerable time the thermostromuhr was a standard blood flow transducer. Burton (1938) analyzed the theoretical considerations underlying the functioning of the device. Applications, advantages, and limitations were set forth by Gregg (1948) and Linzell (1953).

Thermocouples were used by Gibbs (1934) and by Grayson et al. (1952) to measure tissue perfusion using the thermal clearance method (see Chap. 2). With this technique heat is deposited in the tissue, and after cessation of heating the rate of decrease in temperature (due to bloodflow) describes the blood perfusion. Gibbs used the method to measure brain perfusion; Grayson et al. used it to measure kidney perfusion (in millimeters per minute per gram of tissue).

Although thermocouples can be used to measure the temperature change indicative of blood flow, the thermistor is more popular, largely because of the larger signal obtainable. Nonetheless if it is desired to measure very small temperature changes, the thermocouple is superior.

NUCLEAR POWER SUPPLIES

In the early days of cardiac pacemaking (before introduction of the lithium cell by Greatbatch et al. in 1971), battery life was short, and considerable research was devoted to the development of nuclear power supplies. Two types were ultimately perfected: the thermonuclear and the betavoltaic. The former employed plutonium-238 (^{238}Pu) and a series of thermocouples to convert heat to electrical energy, and the betavoltaic converter employed promethium-147 (^{147}Pm) and a series of P-N junctions to produce the electrical energy. Although nuclear energy supplies are no longer used in pacemakers, they were successful. The energy available from the thermonuclear unit is substantial and the unit is long-lived, and, although no longer needed for pacemakers, it is a candidate for energizing implanted power-hungry devices such as the implanted artificial heart.

Plutonium-238 emits alpha particles as it decays. The alpha particles strike the inner wall of the container as shown in Fig. 3. Absorption of the alpha particles by the wall raises its temperature to about 110°C. Applied to the wall are a series of thermojunctions, the other ends of which are in contact with the case of the implant which is maintained very nearly at body temperature. Thus, the two thermojunctions are at different temperatures and produce a voltage. To obtain a sub-

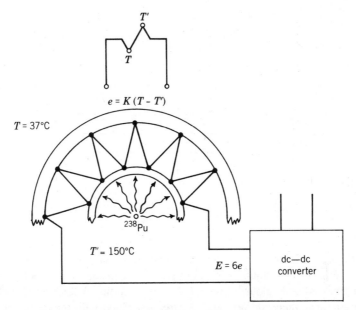

$$T'$$

$$e = K(T - T')$$

$$T = 37°C$$

$$^{238}Pu$$

$$T' = 150°C$$

$$E = 6e$$

dc—dc
converter

Figure 3   Alpha particles emitted by a plutonium (^{238}Pu) energy source strike its container and raise its temperature. The outer container is at body temperature; the temperature difference between the two containers is detected by a series of thermojunctions. The voltage produced thereby is used to drive a dc–dc converter to obtain a higher voltage.

stantial voltage, a series configuration of about 30 bismuth-tellurium thermojunctions is used.

In summary, the energy-exchange process starts with the ejection of alpha particles from the ^{238}Pu, which produce heat when they collide with the container wall, giving rise to a temperature difference that is then converted to a voltage by the series-connected thermocouples.

Although there is more than adequate current developed by the thermocouples, the output is only about 1 V. In order to raise the voltage, a dc-to-dc converter is used. This device is merely an oscillator that is driven by the low-voltage thermocouples. A transformer is used to step up the alternating voltage to the desired level, and it is then rectified and filtered to obtain a constant voltage of the desired magnitude (e.g., 10–20 V).

The amount of plutonium required is small; for cardiac pacing the amount needed is $\frac{1}{4}$ g in the oxide form. The half-life of ^{238}Pu is 86.4 yr, so the life expectancy of such an energy source exceeds a typical lifetime. Of course, for higher power requirements, more plutonium would be required.

PELTIER EFFECT

In 1831 Peltier discovered that if direct current is applied to a thermocouple circuit, one junction is cooled and the other is warmed. Thus was born the heat

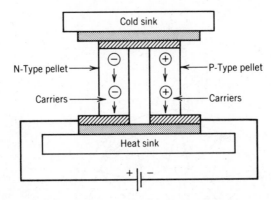

Figure 4   Thermoelectric cooler. (Courtesy of Marlow Industries, Dallas, Texas.)

pump. Figure 4 illustrates a modern embodiment of the principle. In a practical device, a series of thermojunctions are used. To obtain substantial cooling the heat must be removed continuously from the heated junctions. Although the conversion efficiency is low, there are no moving parts associated with the device, which is employed in small refrigerators. Smaller thermoelectric coolers are used to pump heat from solid-state devices deep within an electronic device. They are also used to cool photoconductive cells to shift the spectral sensitivity and improve the signal-to-noise ratio. Peltier converters are available in a variety of sizes, ranging from about 0.5 to 50 W of cooling.

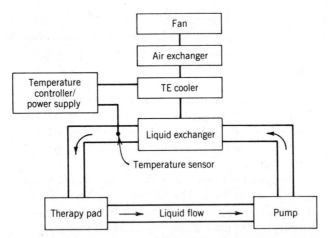

Figure 5   Thermoelectric (TE) cooler consisting of a series of P–N junctions arranged in series. The cold sides are coupled to the liquid heat exchanger, which circulates the chilled water through the pad. The heat is removed from the warmed thermojunctions by an air-cooled heat exchanger. (Redrawn from E. J. Burke and R. J. Buist, *Adv. Bioeng.* pp. 80–83. Copyright American Society of Mechanical Engineers.)

Biomedical Applications

Peltier devices are beginning to be used in biomedical research as heat pumps. Yamazaki (1965) and Hayward et al. (1965) reviewed many of the applications in which the Peltier effect has been used to cool tissues and fluids. An interesting thermoelectric cooler designed to create a cold pack (pad) was described by Burke and Buist (1982). The pad was cooled to 42°F (7.2°C) by circulating water cooled by a series of Peltier junctions. Figure 5 illustrates the method by which the thermoelectric (TE) cooler was coupled to the heat exchanger. Direct current was applied to a series string of Peltier (P–N) junctions. The cold side of each was in contact with the heat exchanger that circulated the cold water through the pad. The hot sides of the Peltier units were cooled by a heat exchanger, which was cooled by a fan blowing ambient air through it.

It should be obvious that the pad could be heated by merely reversing the current flow through the P–N junctions. This is an attractive feature if it is desired to reheat the site after cooling.

REFERENCES

Baldes, E. J., J. F. Herrick, and H. E. Essex. 1933. Modification in thermostromuhr method of measuring flow of blood. *Proc. Soc. Exp. Biol. Med.* **30:**1109–1111.

Bazzett, H. C., and B. McGlone. 1927. Temperature gradients in tissues in man. *Am. J. Physiol.* **82:**415–451.

Burke, E. J., and R. J. Buist. 1982. A thermoelectric cooling/heating system for a hospital therapy pad. *Adv. Bioeng.* pp. 80–83.

Burton, A. C. 1938. Theory and design of the thermostromuhr. *J. Appl. Phys.* **9:**127–131.

Cain, C., and A. J. Welch. 1974. Thin-film temperature sensors for biological measurement. *IEEE Trans. Biomed. Eng.* **BME-21**(5):421–423.

Clark, H. 1922. The measurement of intravenous temperatures. *J. Exp. Med.* **35:**385–389.

Foster, P. C. 1936. Thermocouples for the medical laboratory. *J. Lab. Clin. Med.* **22:**68–81.

Gelb, G. H., B. D. Marcus, and D. Dropkin. 1964. Manufacture of fine wire thermocouple probes. *Rev. Sci. Instrum.* **35:**80–81.

Gibbs, F. A. 1934. Thermoelectric blood flow recorder in the form of a needle. *Proc. Soc. Exp. Biol. Med.* **31:**141–146.

Grayson, T. 1952. Internal calorimeter in the determination of thermal conductivity and blood flow. *J. Physiol.* **118:**54–72.

Greatbatch, W., J. Lee, W. Mathias, M. Eldridge, J. R. Moser, and A. Schneider. 1971. The solid-state lithium battery. *IEEE Trans. Biomed. Eng.* **BME-18:**316–324.

Gregg, D. E. 1948. *Thermostromuhr: Methods in Medical Research*, Vol. 1. Yearbook Publishers, Chicago, IL.

Guilbeau, E., and B. I. Mayall. 1981. Microthermocouple for soft tissue temperature determination. *IEEE Trans. Biomed. Eng.* **BME-28**(3):301–305.

Hardy, J. D. 1934. The radiation of heat from the human body. *J. Clin Invest.* **13:**593–620.

Hayward, J. N., L. H. Ott, D. G. Stuart, and F. C. Cheshire. 1965. Peltier biothermodes. *Am. J. Med. Electron.* **4:**11–19.

Hill, A. V. 1932. A closer analysis of the heat production of nerve. *Proc. R. Soc. London, Ser. B* **III:**106–164.

Lahiji, G. R. 1981. *A Monolith Thermopile Detector Fabricated Using Integrated-Circuit Technology*, Tech. Rep. No. 150. Electron Physics Lab., University of Michigan, Ann Arbor, 107 pp.

Leeds and Northrup Co. Bulletin 15A-RP 1.4. Instrument Society of America, Pittsburgh, PA.

Linzell, J. L. 1953. Internal calorimetry in the measurement of blood flow with heated thermocouples. *J. Physiol.* **121**:390–402.

Reed, R. P. 1966. Thin-film sensors of micron size and application in biothermology. Ph.D. dissertation, University of Texas, Austin.

Reed, R. P., and R. T. Kampwirth. 1964. Thermocouples of micron size by vapor deposition. *Direction* **10**:8.

Rein, H. 1928. Die Thermo-Stromuhr. *Z. Biol.* **87**:394–418.

Riley, J. A. 1949. A simple method for welding thermocouples. *Science* **109**:281.

Scott, W. J. M. 1930. An improved electrodermal instrument of measuring the surface temperature. *JAMA* **94**:1987–1988.

Sheard, C. 1931. The electromotive thermometer, an instrument for measuring intramural, intravenous, superficial and cavity temperatures. *Am. J. Clin. Pathol.* **1**:209–226.

Towe, B. C., E. Guilbeau, T. Mathis, H. Muehlbauer, J. McCall, and J. Coburn. 1985. A glucose sensor using a thin film thermopile. *Proc. Annu. Conf. Eng. Med. Biol.* **27**:93.

Yamazaki, Z. 1965. Medical application of thermoelectric cooling. *JEE, Jpn. Electron. Eng.* **2**:32–35.

8

Chemical Transducers

INTRODUCTION

Chemical transducers play an important role in medicine and physiology in the assessment of metabolism. In general, there are two types: (1) those that measure chemical composition of the blood, tissue, and organ fluids and (2) those that measure the composition of the respiratory gases. The most commonly encountered transducers are those used for measuring the blood gases (in solution). Such transducers measure the partial pressure of oxygen (pO_2) and carbon dioxide (pCO_2) and the concentration of hydrogen ions (pH). Complementing these transducers are those for the respiratory gases O_2, CO_2, and N_2. The latter is a diluent the measurement of which permits determining the only lung volume not measurable with a spirometer—the residual volume (RV), which is the quantity of air remaining in the lungs after a maximal expiration.

Although some chemical transducers employ a color change to identify a chemical species (for example, the oximeter), many are electrochemical cells in which the quantity to be measured causes a change in cell potential or a change in current flow through the cell. All such cells contain electrodes, sometimes of unusual design. Often one electrode constitutes the sensor, and the other (reference) electrode plays no active part. It is well to recall that such reference electrodes have a potential with respect to their environmental solutions. Electrodes are dealt with in Chapter 9.

BLOOD GASES

Perhaps the most frequently used chemical transducers are those for measurement of blood gases. Before describing them, it is important to understand the meaning of the term blood gases.

The term blood gases refers to the partial pressures of oxygen and carbon dioxide and the hydrogen ion concentration. The three quantities are measured with two quite different types of electrochemical sensors. In the pO_2 electrode it is current flow that is proportional to pO_2, whereas in the pH and pCO_2 electrodes it is the potential that identifies these two quantities. All three blood gas transducers will be described. However, it is useful to first review the concepts of partial pressure (Dalton's law) and dissolved gas (Henry's law).

TABLE 1 Composition of Air

Oxygen (O_2)	20.9%
Nitrogen (N_2)	79.0%
Carbon dioxide (CO_2)	0.03%
Residual gases	0.07%
Total	100%

DALTON'S LAW

Dalton's law of partial pressures states that the pressure exerted by a mixture of gases is equal to the sum of the pressures that each gas would exert if it alone occupied the whole volume. For example, if a sample of atmospheric air is analyzed, the result is shown in Table 1.

If the barometric pressure were 760 mmHg, then the partial pressures of these three gases would be

pO_2	$760 \times 20.9/100 =$	158.84 mmHg
pN_2	$760 \times 79.0/100 =$	600.40 mmHg
pCO_2	$760 \times 0.03/100 =$	0.228 mmHg
p(Residuals)	$760 \times 0.07/100 =$	0.532 mmHg
	Total $=$	760.0 mmHg

Thus the pressure of a gas sample is equal to the sum of the partial pressures of its components. In general, the partial pressure of a gas G, i.e., p_G, is

$$p_G = \frac{N_G}{V} RT.$$

where p_G = partial pressure of the gas,
    N_G = number of moles of gas in volume V,
    T = absolute temperature, and
    R = the gas constant.

HENRY'S LAW

Henry's law states that when a gas is exposed to a liquid, the volume V that goes into a simple physical solution depends directly on the partial pressure and the solubility of the gas in the solution. In this situation, there is no chemical combination between the gas and the solvent in which it dissolves.

The solubility of a gas is described in terms of the solubility constant a, which is determined experimentally and is usually expressed as the number of milliliters of a gas dissolved in 1 mL of solvent when the partial pressure of the gas is 760 mmHg (1 atm). The solubility constants for oxygen, nitrogen, and carbon dioxide at 0 and 37°C for water are shown in Table 2.

TABLE 2 Solubility of Gases

Gas	Solubility Constant a (mL/mL H_2O at 760 mmHg)	
	0°C	37°C
Oxygen	0.0489	0.0239
Nitrogen	0.0235	0.0123
Carbon dioxide	1.713	0.567

Source: *Handbook of Chemistry and Physics*, 44th ed., Chemical Rubber Publishing Co., Cleveland, Ohio, 1963.

Note that for all gases the solubility decreases with an increase in temperature. With the data in Table 2 it is possible to calculate the amount of each gas that will be dissolved in water for any partial pressure at the temperature for which the solubility constant is known. For example, it is of interest to know how much oxygen, nitrogen, and carbon dioxide will dissolve in water at 37°C when the gases are present in air at 760 mmHg. The following sample calculation, based on the previous example in which air was analyzed, provides this information:

$$pO_2 = 158.84 \text{ mmHg}, \quad pN_2 = 600.49 \text{ mmHg}, \quad pCO_2 = 0.228 \text{ mmHg};$$

$$\text{Volume of } O_2 \text{ dissolved} = \frac{158.84}{760} \times 0.0239 = 0.005 \text{ mL/mL } H_2O$$

$$\text{Volume of } N_2 \text{ dissolved} = \frac{600.40}{760} \times 0.0123 = 0.0097 \text{ mL/mL } H_2O$$

$$\text{Volume of } CO_2 \text{ dissolved} = \frac{0.228}{760} \times 0.567 = 0.00017 \text{ mL/mL } H_2O$$

The values so obtained are in milliliters of each gas per milliliter of water at 37°C. In biological studies it is customary to express the volume of dissolved gas in terms of the volume in 100 mL of solution. This unit is designated volume percent (vol %). Therefore, when the values obtained are multiplied by 100, the following values are obtained:

$$V_{O_2} = 0.5 \text{ vol \%}$$

$$V_{N_2} = 0.97 \text{ vol \%}$$

$$V_{CO_2} = 0.017 \text{ vol \%}$$

This rather lengthy example illustrates that the partial pressure of a gas in contact with a liquid is an indicator of the volume of gas dissolved in solution. To determine the actual volume dissolved it is necessary to know the solubility constant. However, in many physiological situations there is a loose chemical combination of the gas with a component of the solvent (e.g., blood) and different conditions obtain.

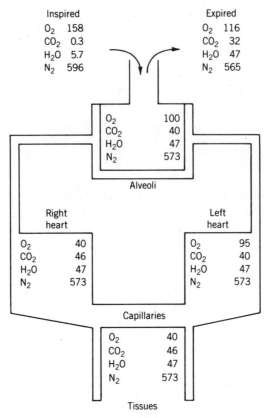

Figure 1   The partial pressures (mmHg) of the respiratory gases in the alveoli and in arterial and venous blood and the tissues. (Redrawn from J. Comroe, *The Lung*. Chicago Year Book Publishers, Chicago, Illinois, 1974.)

Nonetheless even in these situations the partial pressure of the gas is an indicator of the volume contained in solution at equilibrium.

Figure 1 illustrates the partial pressures of respiratory gases in the lungs and in arterial, capillary, and venous blood. These quantities are important measures of metabolic activity.

THE pO_2 OF BLOOD

The pO_2 electrode measures the partial pressure of oxygen in solution. The volume of oxygen in simple solution depends on the solubility coefficient for oxygen. When measuring the partial pressure of oxygen in blood, a different situation obtains because the red cells contain hemoglobin (Hb), an iron pigment that combines loosely with oxygen to become oxyhemoglobin (HbO_2). The volume of oxygen in blood is also proportional to the partial pressure, but in a special way.

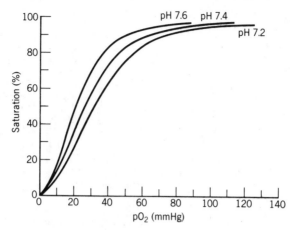

Figure 2   The oxygen–hemoglobin dissociation curves for pH 7.2, 7.4, and 7.6.

One gram of hemoglobin combines with 1.34 mL of oxygen. Typically, 100 mL of blood contains 15 g of hemoglobin. Therefore, 100 mL of blood is capable of carrying $15 \times 1.34 = 20.1$ mL oxygen. (In other words, the normal oxygen content of the blood is 20.1 vol %.) Typically, the 15 g of hemoglobin is contained in blood when the hematocrit (percentage of red cells) is 40%. The amount of oxygen carried by the red cells is expressed as percent saturation. Thus for a 40% hematocrit, 100% saturation would correspond to 20.1 mL O_2/100 mL blood. Of course, there is a little oxygen dissolved in the plasma, and the total oxygen in 100 mL of blood is slightly more than 20.1 vol % at saturation.

The percent saturation of blood depends on the partial pressure of oxygen to which it is exposed and the hydrogen ion concentration (pH). This relationship is embodied in the oxygen dissociation curve shown in Fig. 2.

REFERENCE ELECTRODES

In electrochemical methods for measuring blood chemistry one electrode serves as the sensing element, and the other constitutes a reference electrode. The two most common reference electrodes are the calomel half-cell and the silver–silver chloride electrode. The former is more complex and is used in electrochemistry; the latter is much simpler and easier to prepare (see Chap. 9) and is used extensively in physiological measurements. Both will now be described.

Calomel Electrode

The calomel electrode (Fig. 3) is one of the most stable of the practical reference electrodes. The potential is developed across a junction of pure mercury and potassium chloride solution, which is saturated with calomel (mercurous chloride). The potential of the calomel electrode is dependent on the concentration of the

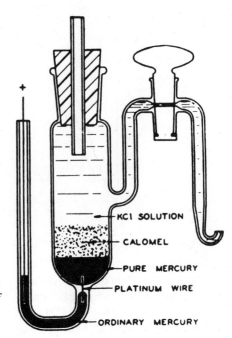

Figure 3 The calomel electrode. (From Wellard et al., *Instrumental Methods of Analysis*, Van Nostrand, Princeton, New Jersey, 1951.)

KCI SOLUTION

CALOMEL

PURE MERCURY

PLATINUM WIRE

ORDINARY MERCURY

potassium chloride solution. Use of a calomel electrode (or calomel half-cell as it is often called) to measure the potential of other half-cells which may likewise possess a fluid boundary, may give rise to a potential between the two liquid junctions. Such liquid-to-liquid junction potentials are minimized by the use of a "salt bridge," which usually consists of a saturated solution of potassium chloride held in an agar gel in a glass tube and serves as a conductor to connect the two liquids. Potassium chloride is especially useful for this purpose because the potassium and chloride ions possess approximately the same mobilities and hence minimize the formation of concentration gradients and resulting electrical potentials. If potassium chloride cannot be used because the presence of certain ions (such as silver) in one or both solutions may produce undesirable chemical reactions, ammonium nitrate may be substituted.

Apart from the practicality of the calomel cell, its chief advantage lies in the stability of its potential over long periods. Because it is a chemical cell, temperature influences the mobility of the ions, and therefore a small temperature correction is necessary. The EMFs of typical calomel cells are listed in Table 3.

Silver–Silver Chloride Electrode

In many electrochemical cells, the silver–silver chloride (Ag–AgCl) electrode is used as the reference electrode. The construction and properties of this electrode are described in Chapter 9. It is useful to recognize that when it is used in an electrochemical cell the Ag–AgCl electrode is a chloride ion electrode. In other

TABLE 3 The EMFs of Reference Cells

Mercury–Calomel Cell	EMF[a] (V)	Correction (V/°C)
$Hg\|HgCl_2\|0.01\ M$ KCl	+0.388	+0.00094
$Hg\|HgCl_2\|0.1\ M$ KCl	+0.333	+0.00079
$Hg\|HgCl_2\|1.0\ M$ KCl	+0.280	+0.00059 avg.
$Hg\|HgCl_2\|3.5\ M$ KCl	+0.247	+0.00047

[a]Referred to standard hydrogen electrode at 25°C.

Source: C. A. Hampel (ed.), *Encyclopedia of Electrochemistry*, Reinhold Publishing Corp., New York, 1964.

words, the potential E of an Ag–AgCl electrode is dependent on the activity A of the chloride ions in its vicinity. At 37°C the potential in volts is

$$E = 0.2251 - 0.06153 \log A.$$

The activity A is proportional to the Cl^- concentration.

The outstanding characteristics of an Ag–AgCl electrode are its simplicity and electrochemical stability in a constant environment. It is for this reason that it is used as an electrode for recording bioelectrical events and as a reference electrode in electrochemical cells.

THE pO₂ ELECTRODE

The pO₂ electrode indicates the partial pressure of oxygen in a liquid (or gas) by the current that flows through the oxygen cathode, the electrolyte, and the reference anode to which a constant polarizing voltage (0.6–0.8 V) has been applied. For practical reasons, the oxygen cathode and its reference electrode cannot be placed directly in a blood sample to measure its pO₂. An excellent discussion of the principles and technique was presented by Davies (1962) who prefers to call this electrode an oxygen cathode. This terminology serves to avoid possible confusion with the oxygen electrode as understood in physical chemistry, which operates under equilibrium conditions and possesses a standard potential of +1.229 V relative to the hydrogen electrode.

A method for applying the oxygen electrode to measure the partial pressure of dissolved oxygen is diagramed in Fig. 4. The oxygen electrode itself is a piece of platinum wire embedded in an insulating glass holder with the end of the wire exposed to the solution under measurement. According to Davies (1962), the principle of operation of the electrode is as follows:

1. When the platinum electrode is made slightly negative (about −0.2 V) with respect to the reference electrode, oxygen reaching the surface of the platinum is reduced electrolytically (i.e., the O_2 accepts electrons). The reaction at the cathode is, however, not fully understood.

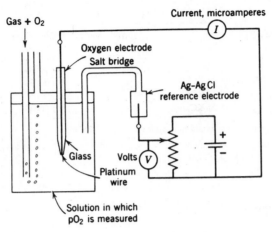

Figure 4   The pO_2 electrode.

2. When the platinum is made more negative (0.6–0.8 V) the velocity of the electrolytic reduction is limited by the maximum rate at which O_2 can diffuse to the electrode surface and is not affected greatly by the magnitude of the potential difference. In this voltage range it is found that the current flowing is proportional to the oxygen concentration in the body of the solution (Fig. 5).

The shape of the electrode current–potential relationship is shown in Fig. 5a. The electrode is operated in the "plateau" region over which the current shows very little dependence on the applied voltage. If the potential is held constant (at −0.7 V, for example), the current is a linear function of the partial pressure of dissolved oxygen, which is expressed as percent O_2 in Fig. 5b.

Although most of the commercially available pO_2 electrodes exhibit a response time of 30–60 sec, it is possible to construct electrodes with a very short response time. Figure 6 gives the response time of an open-type oxygen electrode to a sudden change in pO_2 as reported by Davies (1962). The 0–90% response time of the recording system, including the capacitance of the oxygen electrode and wiring, was determined to be about 25 μsec. The rise time of this particular electrode is seen to be approximately 0.3 msec (300 μsec), which is certainly adequate to continuously monitor locally varying changes in tissue oxygen content.

The oxygen electrode is not free of practical difficulties. The problem known as electrode aging presents itself as a slow reduction in current over time (minutes or hours), even though the oxygen tension of the test medium is maintained at a constant level. Aging requires frequent recalibration of the electrode. The exact cause of aging is not known, but the phenomenon is associated with material attaching itself to the electrode surface. Two measures are often used to combat this problem. First, the electrode is covered with a protective film such as polyethylene, which has the undesirable effect of shielding the electrode from the dis-

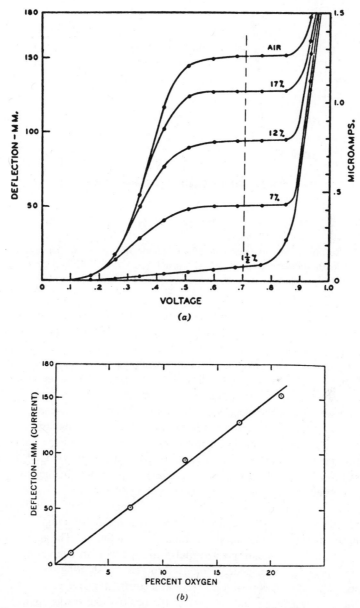

Figure 5 (a) Current–voltage characteristics of the pO₂ electrode. (b) Response of pO₂ electrode versus percent oxygen; values obtained from (a) for polarization voltage of 0.7 V. [From R. A. Olson, et al., *J. Gen. Physiol.* **32**:687–703 (1949). By permission.]

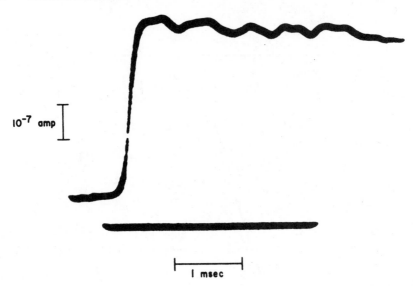

10^{-7} amp

⊢——⊣
I msec

Figure 6   Response time of open-type pO_2 electrode. [From P. W. Davies, in *Physical Techniques in Biological Research*. W. L. Nastuk (ed.), Vol. IV. Academic Press, New York, 1962. By permission.

solved O_2, consequently increasing the response time (0–90%) to as much as 2.5 min. The second procedure employed to minimize aging is to reverse the flow of current frequently to lower or reverse the accumulation of surface contaminants.

Another problem encountered with the oxygen electrode is created by the presence of the electrode itself. The O_2 diffusion field is maximal in the vicinity of the electrode, causing the concentration of O_2 there to be different from what would exist in the absence of the electrode. This source of error is reduced by constantly rotating or vibrating the electrode or by giving it a special geometrical shape.

Olson et al. (1949) reported an investigation that explored the application of alternating potential techniques to overcome the difficulties attending the use of open, static platinum electrodes. This method employed switching the potential pattern imposed on an electrolytic cell consisting of a platinum electrode of 20-gauge wire about 3 mm long versus a 0.1 M calomel half-cell, both immersed in a 0.1 M KCl solution. Dual cells were used as a means of comparing electrode performance in oxygen- and nitrogen-saturated KCl solutions. The applied potential pattern consisted of a square positive pulse followed by an interval during which the applied potential was suddenly reduced to zero by shorting the cell through a resistance. The short was then removed and a square negative pulse applied, after which the short was again induced before the positive pulse was applied to begin the next cycle. Observations were made over the range of 30 cycles/sec down to 6–12 cycles/min. Because of the time required for stabilization of the oxygen plateau, the maximum rate at which the potential could be switched and stable values of current output obtained was between 5 and 10 cycles/min.

The Clark (1956) type of oxygen electrode (Fig. 7) has been employed widely

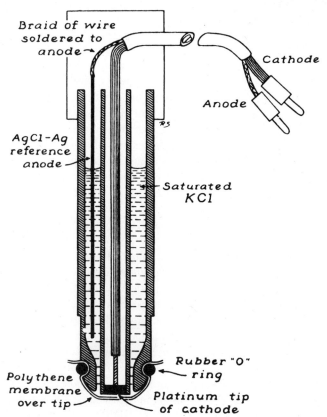

Figure 7 The Clark-type pO_2 electrode. [From B. J. Sproule et al., *J. Appl. Physiol.* **11**:365–370 (1957). By permission.]

by many biological investigators. It is of single-unit construction with a self-contained Ag–AgCl reference electrode. The entire device is isolated from the solution under measurement by a polyethylene membrane. This feature allows the electrode to be used for measuring oxygen tension in solutions of poor electrical conductivity or in the gas phase. The stability of response of the Clark electrode depends on the diffusion distance between the platinum surface and the membrane. Care must be exercised to ensure that the membrane is kept taut to maintain the diffusion distance constant.

In physiology the pO_2 electrode has been applied extensively to monitor the partial pressure of oxygen in biological fluids. Among the first to exploit the method were Davies and Brink (1942a, b), who described the construction of a bare platinum electrode paired with a calomel cell polarized with 0.6 V. Using this system they successfully recorded the oxygen tension changes in the arterioles of a cat's brain and in skeletal muscle during contraction. Their papers, which discuss the theory and electrode reactions, as well as many of the practical details of the method, are recommended reading for those wishing to enter the field. Kreuzer et al. (1958) compared the fidelity of the pO_2 electrode method with that of standard chemical procedures.

Two interesting and useful in vitro pO_2 electrodes were described by Tobias and Holmes (1947). One was built into a hypodermic syringe barrel, and on withdrawal of a blood sample from a vessel into the syringe, the oxygen tension was instantly read on a calibrated galvanometer; the other was built into a hypodermic needle, which Tobias used to measure pO_2 in the eyelid, lip, and vagina.

Detailed descriptions of use of the pO_2 electrode to measure the oxygen tension in the brain of a cat were presented by Davies and Brink (1942a, b). Davies et al. (1943–1944) presented multichannel recordings of the EEG and local oxygen tension changes in experimental animals during convulsions. Using an ingenious occlusion method, Davies et al. (1948) recorded the rate of oxygen consumption on the surface of the cortex of cats before and after electrical stimulation of the brain. Clark (1956) developed a unique electrode assembly for monitoring oxygen tension in heart–lung machines. Clark and Misrahy (1957) and Clark et al. (1958) also achieved the remarkable feat of chronically implanting pO_2 electrodes in the brains of cats, and they recorded the local oxygen tension over periods of months to years.

The rate of oxygen consumption at synaptic endings of sympathetic ganglia was measured by Bronk et al. (1946), using the occlusion technique. They found that 90 sec elapsed before the oxygen tension dropped to near-zero levels. Posternak et al. (1947), recording in the same region, found that the oxygen consumption was doubled when the ganglia were electrically stimulated at a rate of 15 pulses/sec.

In frog and crab nerve fibers, pO_2 microelectrodes were used by Bronk et al. (1947) and Carlson et al. (1948) to record the oxygen consumption during stimulation. They found that oxygen consumption outlasted heat production by as much as 30 sec.

Regional oxygen tensions have been measured on a variety of other tissues. Davies (1946), who recorded the consumption of oxygen in frog skeletal muscle during and following a single twitch, noted a fall in the oxygen tension during the first half-second and a return to the control level in 2 sec. Oxygen tension measurements have also been recorded by Cater et al. (1957b, c) in the intact lactating mammary gland and in tumors.

For the measurement of pO_2 in solution, the oxygen electrode offers several advantages; among them are (1) the current obtained is linearly related to the concentration of oxygen; (2) the electrode can be made small enough to measure concentrations in highly localized areas; (3) when used in vitro, only a small sample of fluid is required; and (4) the measurement requires only seconds as compared to minutes for chemical determination. Electrode configurations have been developed with a response time short enough for continuous recording of transient changes.

Probably the greatest difficulty in the use of the pO_2 electrode is the size of the electrical signal produced. Although provision of a known stable polarizing voltage offers no difficulties, measurement of the current representing the partial pressure of oxygen presents special problems. The current measured by Tobias (1949) was 0.650 μA for 500 mmHg oxygen tension. The total range of the indicator used by Davies and Brink (1942a, b) was 0.05 μA for an oxygen tension of 180 mmHg.

The recorder sensitivity employed by Kreuzer et al. (1958) was 0.96 μA, and that described by Clark et al. (1958) produced a full-scale deflection for 0.98 μA. The signal detected by Cater et al. (1957a, b, c) was 0.01 μA.

The partial pressure of oxygen can be measured transcutaneously with the pO_2 electrode. A description of this device and the transcutaneous pCO_2 electrode appear elsewhere in this chapter.

MEMBRANE ELECTRODES

A potential is developed if an interface is created by imposing a semipermeable barrier (membrane) between two liquid phases so that the membrane allows transfer of a particular ion. After equilibrium has been established, the potential created is proportional to the logarithm of the ratio of the concentrations of the ion to which the membrane is selectively permeable. For a membrane that is ideally selective, the potential developed is given by the Nernst equation:

$$E = -\frac{RT}{nF} \ln \frac{C_1}{C_2} = -2.303 \frac{RT}{nF} \log \frac{C_1}{C_2},$$

where n = valence of the ion,
   R = gas constant (8.315×10^7 J/(mol·K),
   T = absolute temperature (K),
   F = number of coulombs transferred (96,500 C, i.e., 1 faraday, is required to convert 1 equivalent of an element to 1 equivalent of ions), and
C_1 and C_2 = concentration of the selected ion on the two sides of the membrane.

This form of the Nernst equation is based on ideal thermodynamic considerations and is valid only for very dilute solutions. It has been found to be in error as the ionic concentrations are increased. This departure from ideal thermodynamic behavior is expressed in terms of the ionic activity, which is related to the ionic concentration in accordance with the expression

$$a = C \times \nu,$$

where a = the activity of a specific ion,
   C = the concentration of the ion, and
   ν = the activity coefficient.

The Nernst equation is usually written in terms of ion activity as follows:

$$E = -\frac{RT}{nF} \ln \frac{a_1}{a_2} = -2.303 \frac{RT}{nF} \log \frac{a_1}{a_2}.$$

The activity of an ion species is a measure of the effective concentration rather than the actual concentration. For very dilute solutions ν approaches unity, and the ideal situation in which the potential developed is proportional to the logarithm of the ratio of concentrations more nearly holds. Activity coefficients must be known if the ion concentration is to be determined in terms of the electrical potential developed. The Debye–Hückel equations have been found to yield accurate values for the activity coefficients of dilute solutions, such as those encountered in living systems. For a discussion of the application of the Debye–Hückel theory of electrolytes to biological systems, a textbook such as that of Bull (1964) is recommended.

The availability of a membrane that exhibits selective permeability for a particular ion provides a means of creating a transducer for that species of ion. Of course, a reference electrode must be used with ion-sensitive electrodes. The following will describe many of the popular types of ion-specific electrodes.

The pH Electrode

Because it is impractical to use the standard hydrogen electrode to determine pH, the glass electrode is ordinarily employed. A typical glass electrode is illustrated in Fig. 8. According to Bull (1943), the glass electrode was discovered by Cremer and was developed by Haber and Klemensiewicz. It consists of a thin glass membrane that permits the passage of only hydrogen ions (in the form of hydronium H_3O^+). The usual configuration consists of a spherical bulb 0.25 in. in diameter.

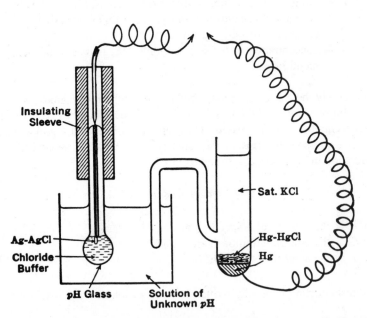

Figure 8   The glass electrode used with the calomel half-cell to measure pH. (From H. B. Bull, *Physical Biochemistry*. Wiley, New York, 1943. By permission.)

On the inside of the pH-responsive glass bulb is placed a buffer solution, usually of pH 1, in which is immersed an Ag–AgCl electrode. The other side of the glass bulb is exposed to the solution of unknown pH. The connection to the potential-measuring circuit and the solution being tested is completed through a potassium chloride salt bridge and a calomel reference electrode.

The mechanism underlying the operation of the glass electrode is far from simple, and several theories have been proposed to explain the origin of the pH-dependent potential. According to Eisenman (1967), opinion regarding the origin of the glass electrode potential was for many years divided into two schools of thought. One view held that the potential was exclusively a phase-boundary potential produced at the membrane–solution interface. The other view attributed it to a diffusion potential arising within the membrane. These views have been reconciled, and Eisenman states, "It now seems virtually certain that the glass electrode is nothing more or less than a perfect cation-exchange membrane, whose electrode potential represents a sum of contributions from both diffusion and phase-boundary processes." The total glass electrode potential is therefore expressed as the sum of the two boundary potentials produced at the membrane–solution interface and the diffusion potential arising within the glass. The interested reader is referred to Eisenman (1967) for detailed theoretical and practical information pertaining to glass electrodes.

The potential developed across the glass membrane is about 60 mV per unit of pH at 30°C. Operation at a different temperature requires the application of a small correction.

The glass electrode made the determination of pH in the laboratory a simple and routine procedure. Bull (1943) listed the following advantages of the glass electrode as compiled by Dole et al. (1941):

1. The glass electrode is independent of oxidation–reduction potentials.
2. It is not necessary to pass a gas through the solution or to add any material to it.
3. It is possible to use very small quantities of solution.
4. The electrode can be used in colored or turbid solutions.
5. The electrode gives accurate values in unbuffered solutions.
6. Equilibrium is reached rapidly.

The glass electrode does, however, possess some limitations. The range of pH over which accurate response is obtained may be restricted unless special glasses are used. For example, some error often exists in both highly acidic solutions (near pH = 0) and alkaline solutions (above pH = 9). Figure 9 shows the error in pH for both acid and alkaline solutions for electrodes constructed from the classic Corning 015 glass; the amount of error encountered because of sodium and potassium ion concentration can be seen. Errors in pH measurement in the range above pH = 9 are known as "salt" or "alkaline" errors. It is now possible to purchase pH electrodes constructed from special glass for use over the range pH = 0–14 with only a slight correction required above pH = 13.

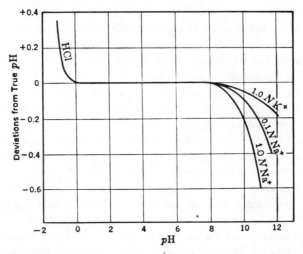

Figure 9   Glass electrode error as a function of solution pH. (From M. Dole, *Theoretical and Experimental Electrochemistry*. McGraw-Hill, New York, 1935. By permission.)

Because the pH is determined in terms of the potential developed by the pH electrode, the magnitude of the potential must be accurately measured. Since the potential is developed by the diffusion of relatively few ions across a glass surface, which in itself is a good insulator, the pH electrode has the characteristics of a potential source with a very high internal impedance. Typical values are in excess of 200 MΩ. To prevent the device used to measure this potential from drawing current from the electrode, it must possess an input impedance much higher than that of the pH electrode. This requirement is met by use of a potentiometer or a voltage-measuring instrument that employs an electrometer tube or a field-effect transistor in the input stage.

While in vitro measurements of pH abound in the life sciences, the continuous recording of pH changes in vivo has been carried out less frequently, although the number of investigations has increased with the improvement of pH-monitoring equipment. The stability and sensitivity requirements of pH-measuring devices for in vivo work can be appreciated by recalling that the range of hydrogen ion concentration compatible with normal cellular function is about one pH unit; therefore, in recording pH continuously in vivo the recording system is never presented with a signal greater than 60 mV. When measuring mammalian arterial blood, the normal pH range is about 7.36–7.44, and the signal obtainable is only 5 mV. Accordingly, this amplitude must be adequately displayed by the recording stylus or indicator. If smaller changes within the normal range are to be registered, the recording system must possess a sensitivity and stability in the microvolt range.

One of the earliest to measure pH in vivo electrically was McClendon (1915), who passed a platinum gaseous hydrogen–calomel electrode assembly into the stomachs and duodenums of adults and infants to make readings of the pH. Continuous recording of pH was introduced by Gesell and Hertzman (1926). Using a cuvette equipped with an MnO_2 electrode paired with a calomel cell affixed to a continuous aspirating device, they recorded pH changes of arterial and venous blood under a variety of circumstances to investigate the effect of pH on the respiratory center. Voegtlin et al. (1930) introduced the glass electrode for continuously measuring blood pH, using electrodes mounted in a flow-through cuvette. They referred to graphic recording and proved that such an electrode system is insensitive to changes in blood flow. A similar electrode system described by Fruhling and Winterstein (1934) was used to make recordings of the pH of carotid artery blood of dogs. Dubuisson (1937a, b) recorded a pH change of a few tenths of a pH unit within a second after the beginning of contraction of skeletal muscle. Continuous records of pH changes on the surface of the cortices of monkeys were made by Dusser de Barenne et al. (1937). They employed a glass electrode paired with a silver–silver chloride electrode filled with physiological saline to avoid the injurious action of the potassium ion in the calomel electrode.

The technique of prolonged recording of pH in the blood of experimental animals was investigated thoroughly by Nims and co-workers. In a series of papers (Nims, 1937; Nims and Marshall, 1937) they discussed the construction of electrodes suitable for recording pH in flowing blood and described experiments in which continuous records of pH changes were made for periods up to 8 hr. Elegant records of rhythmic changes of approximately 0.1 pH unit in the anesthetized dog were presented. Marshall and Nims (1937) recorded the blood pH response to a variety of injected substances, and Nims et al. (1938) showed that by careful adjustment of the respirator the pH could be maintained at a chosen level in the curarized dog.

Band and Semple (1967) developed a rapidly responding, indwelling arterial glass electrode for the continuous measurement of blood pH. The pH-sensitive cell consisted of a glass electrode and an Ag–AgCl reference electrode, both lying in the lumen of an intraarterial needle. The outside diameter of the pH-sensitive glass portion of the electrode measured 0.5–0.8 mm, the wall thickness 0.0025–0.005 mm, and the length 1.5–2.0 cm. The 90% response to a change in pH of blood flowing past the electrode at 2 mL/min was 0.5 sec. The two samples of blood used to measure the response time had been equilibrated previously with 4 and 6% CO_2. In a test performed by driving buffers past the electrode in situ at high flow rates (10 mL/min), 90% of the response occurred in about 40 msec.

For the most part, the glass electrode is an excellent device for monitoring pH and changes in pH. Some limitations and precautions, however, should be mentioned in connection with its use. The glass electrode exhibits a loss of sensitivity and decreased speed of response after a period of service (i.e., a couple of months). This deterioration may be accelerated, becoming more severe when the electrode is employed in solutions containing proteins. The electrode may be restored repeatedly by etching the glass surface to remove the inactive outer layer. According to Brems (1962), the sensitivity of the glass electrode increases by 0.34%/°C with rising temperature, and the electrical resistance of the glass increases with falling temperature, accordingly increasing the required input impedance of the recording device. Because the active portion of the electrode consists of a thin glass bulb, obvious precautions are required to prevent breakage.

Mattock and Band (1967) called attention to the limitations of glass electrodes for both pH and cation determinations. In regard to accuracy of measurement, these investigators state:

"It is probably true to say that the accuracy of most pH measurements in terms of interpretative values is relatively poor, and insufficient work has been done to establish how accurate are most of the measurements of cations by electrochemical methods. A good reproducibility or even a good discrimination does not imply good accuracy, since this, if related (as is usual) to an individual ion activity, depends mainly on the validity of the extrathermodynamic assumptions which have to be made in the interpretation of the Nernst equation."

These investigators give the following example showing the degree of difference that can arise between accuracy and discrimination:

"In blood pH measurements it is probably fair to say that a discrimination between samples to within ± 0.004 pH unit ($\equiv \pm 1\%$) is possible, but that accuracy in terms of translation to hydrogen ion activity cannot be any better than ± 0.02 pH unit ($\equiv 4.5\%$). This implies that an operational pH scale for blood can be defined quite closely, without involving interpretation of the pH numbers to beyond a 'notional' activity, but that an absolute activity determination from these numbers can only be uncertain."

The pCO_2 Electrode

The partial pressure of carbon dioxide is measured with a modified pH electrode. The modification developed by Stow and Randall (1954) and Stow et al. (1957) and later refined by Severinghaus and Bradley (1958) consists of covering the pH-sensitive glass membrane with a rubber membrane that is permeable to carbon dioxide. Between this covering membrane and the glass electrode is placed a weak aqueous bicarbonate solution. When this electrode assembly is introduced into a solution in which the pCO_2 is to be measured, the CO_2 diffuses through the permeable covering and the following reaction takes place:

$$CO_2 + H_2O \rightarrow H_2CO_3 \rightarrow H^+ + HCO_3^-$$

The pH electrode measures the concentration of hydrogen ions (H^+) that are formed. As in the case of pH measurement, a reference electrode is required to measure the pCO_2-dependent voltage. The principal components of the pCO_2 electrode are shown in Fig. 10, where the glass and reference electrodes are shown enclosed in a small chamber containing the HCO_3^- solution. The reference electrode is usually a chlorided silver wire.

Severinghaus and Bradley (1958) showed both analytically and experimentally that the sensitivity of the Stow electrode could be doubled by including bicarbonate ion in the aqueous medium between the rubber membrane and the glass electrode. These investigators also found that wet Teflon backed with a layer of cellophane

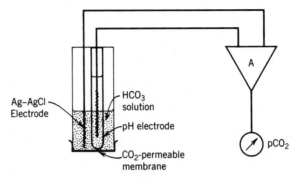

Figure 10 The pCO_2 electrode, consisting of a glass pH-sensitive electrode and an Ag–AgCl reference electrode in a dilute bicarbonate (HCO_3^-) solution. A thin CO_2-permeable membrane (e.g., Teflon) covers the end of the electrode. CO_2 diffusing through the membrane alters the pH of the bicarbonate solution, which is detected by the pH electrode. A high-input impedance amplifier (A) drives an indicator calibrated in pCO_2.

0.002 in. thick was a superior membrane. The optimum aqueous solution consisted of 0.01 M $NaHCO_3$ and 0.1 M NaCl in which the cellophane had been soaked for several hours. In addition to these modifications of Stow's electrode, Severinghaus and Bradley added NaCl to the solution surrounding the reference electrode, thus increasing the conductivity of this solution and stabilizing the reference electrode. The resulting modified pCO_2 electrode was twice as sensitive and drifted much less than before. The response time was such that equilibrium was reached in about 2 min after a fourfold rise in CO_2 and in about 4 min after a fourfold fall in CO_2.

Further improvements in stability and response time, achieved by utilization of a flat-plane-membrane glass electrode for tissue measurements, were reported by Hertz and Siesjö (1959). The increase in overall stability was also due to the use of a calomel cell (made an integral part of the electrode) instead of the Ag–AgCl reference cell. The response time was reduced to 25–30 sec for 90% response by employing a more dilute $NaHCO_3$ solution (0.0001 N). The use of this dilute solution, however, reduced the sensitivity slightly and introduced an initial rapid drift toward alkalinity, followed later by a slower drift. The use of a 0.001 N solution of $NaHCO_3$ appeared to provide a good compromise between drift and response time, although more dilute solutions (even distilled water) were required when rapid response time was the primary consideration. The response times for the electrode at 36°C in saline, equilibrated with different gas mixtures of known CO_2 concentrations, are shown in Fig. 11. Because of its unique construction, this electrode could not be used in the horizontal or inverted position.

Severinghaus (1962) reported improvement in both response time and linearity of the Severinghaus–Bradley electrode in the low pCO_2 range by replacing the cellophane spacer used to hold the water film on the surface of the glass electrode with very thin nylon mesh from a stocking. Glass wool fibers or powdered glass wool were also found to constitute good separators. By using a membrane of $\frac{3}{8}$-mil

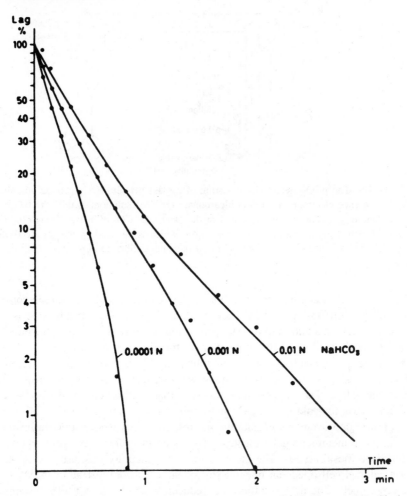

Figure 11   The response time of the pCO_2 electrode. [From C. H. Hertz and B. Siesjo, *Acta Physiol. Scand.* **47:**115–123 (1959). By permission.]

Teflon and glass wool for the separator, electrodes with 95% response in 20 sec were constructed. It was discovered that glass wool catalyzed the reaction of CO_2 with water. The response time was found to be almost entirely due to the diffusion rate, which was governed by the membrane thickness and temperature. According to Severinghaus, the response time was reduced further by the addition of hemolyzed blood to the electrolyte. The blood provides carbonic anhydrase activity for 1 or 2 days.

In an effort to reduce the response time further, Reyes and Neville (1967) used 0.5-mil polyethylene as a pCO_2 electrode membrane. No separator or spacing material was placed between the glass surface and the membrane. A commercial preparation of carbonic anhydrase was added to the electrolyte. The response time of this electrode was 6 sec for 90% of a step change from 2 to 5% CO_2.

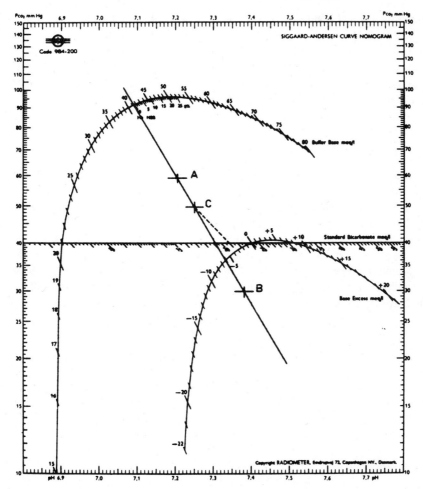

Figure 12 Acid–base nomogram according to Siggaard-Andersen and Engel. (From Radiometer Bulletin 21917E, Copenhagen. By permission.)

In commercially available equipment that uses the Astrup method (Radiometer Co., Copenhagen, Denmark), for the determination of blood pCO_2, the electrode employed for measuring pH directly also serves to determine pCO_2. The procedure makes use of a nomogram (shown in Fig. 12), the ordinate of which is pCO_2 in millimeters of mercury plotted on a log scale, and the abscissa is pH plotted on a linear scale. Briefly, the method employed is as follows. First, the pH of a small sample of heparinized blood (drawn from a capillary bed such as the lobe of the ear) is measured directly. This is the actual pH value, and it determines a vertical line passing through this point on the pH axis. Next, two other small samples taken at the same time as the first are equilibrated under temperature control with two different standard gas mixtures of known pCO_2—at 60 and 30 mmHg, for example. The pH of the equilibrated blood samples is then measured directly with the pH electrode. These two values are then plotted on the nomogram (points A and B, respectively), and a straight line is drawn between them. The intersection of line A–B with the vertical line through the actual pH value (point C) is projected to the pCO_2 axis, from which the actual pCO_2 is read. This construction also permits reading values of standard bicarbonate, base excess, and buffer base (all in milliequivalents per liter). The basis of this method was reported by Siggaard-Andersen and Engel (1960) and Siggaard-Andersen (1962).

BLOOD GAS ANALYSIS

The essential tool for monitoring the metabolic status of a patient is the blood gas analyzer. From a small blood sample, values for pO_2, pH, and pCO_2 are indicated. Because temperature is critically important, the transducer assembly in the blood gas analyzer is thermostatically controlled, usually at 37°C. For this reason the device is left on at all times. Every effort is taken to make the triple transducer assembly as small as possible so that only a very small volume of blood is required for analysis. The pO_2 and pCO_2 values are displayed as partial pressure (in millimeters of mercury). Hydrogen-ion concentration is displayed as pH, defined as

$$pH = -\log \frac{1}{[H^+]}$$

where $[H^+]$ is the concentration of hydrogen ions. For normal cellular function the pH can vary over only a relatively small amount around 7.40. The factors that determine pH are embodied in what is called the acid–base balance, a short review of which will now be presented.

ACID–BASE BALANCE

Cells consume oxygen and nutrients and produce carbon dioxide and metabolic acids. There are biochemical mechanisms to prevent buildup of these end products of metabolism. The carbon dioxide is excreted mainly by the respiratory system, and the metabolic acids are handled by the kidneys. By these two mechanisms, blood pH is regulated to within the rather narrow limits of 7.35–7.45.

Under normal circumstances the concentration of hydrogen ions ($[H^+]$) in arterial blood at 37°C is 40 nmol/L (40×10^{-9} mol). Therefore

$$pH = \log \frac{1}{[H^+]} = \log \frac{1}{40 \times 10^{-9}} = 7.3979 = 7.40.$$

If the hydrogen ion concentration increases, the pH falls, indicating acidosis. If the hydrogen ion concentration decreases, the pH rises, indicating alkalosis. Thus the acid–base status is indicated by the pH. The factors that underlie the acid or base balance will be discussed presently.

In addition to renal and respiratory control of pH, the blood contains buffers that minimize a change in pH despite the addition of hydrogen or hydroxyl ions. The mechanism of this action is via the formation of new compounds that are weakly ionized. The buffer value of a substance is the quantity of hydrogen (or hydroxyl) ions that can be added or removed from a solution with a change of one pH unit. In general, a buffer consists of a weak acid with a highly ionized salt of the same acid. In the blood there are three principal buffering agents: hemoglobin (Hb^-), bicarbonate (HCO_3^-), and phosphate ($H_2PO_4^-$). Of the three blood buffers, Hb^- and HCO_3^- dominate. How the acid–base balance is maintained will be described in the following paragraphs.

The Henderson–Hasselbalch Equation

The factors that underlie establishment of the pH are embodied in the Henderson–Hasselbalch (H-H) equation, which derives from the law of mass action. The H-H equation is

$$pH = pK + \log \frac{[HCO_3^-]}{[H_2CO_3]},$$

where pK is the buffering capability of the blood, typically 6.1, $[HCO_3^-]$ is the bicarbonate concentration, and $[H_2CO_3]$ is the carbonic acid concentration.

The H-H equation can be converted into a much more useful form by recognizing that the carbonic acid in the blood derives from the dissolved CO_2, which is identified by the pCO_2. It is easy to measure the pCO_2, which reflects the H_2CO_3. The solubility of CO_2 in water at 37°C is 1.32×10^{-3} g/L per millimeter of mercury of partial pressure, which is equal to 0.03 meq/L per mmHg partial pressure. Accordingly this value can be substituted for $[H_2CO_3]$ in the previous expression to give

$$pH = pK + \log \frac{[HCO_3^-]}{0.03 \ pCO_2}.$$

For the bicarbonate buffer system, the overall pK is about 6.1; the normal concentration of HCO_3^- is 24 meq/L, and arterial blood pCO_2 is 40 mmHg. Therefore, in a normal subject the arterial pH is expected to be

$$pH = 6.1 + \log \frac{24}{0.03 \times 40} = 6.1 + 1.3 = 7.40.$$

This expression, which is a modification of the H-H equation, can be used to illustrate how pH is expected to vary. In this connection, it is important to know that the blood HCO_3^- level is slowly regulated by the kidneys and the CO_2 level is regulated rapidly by respiration. Therefore the previous equation can be represented symbolically as:

$$pH = pK + \log \frac{kidney}{lung}.$$

From this it can be seen that both kidney and respiratory function regulate the pH. In addition, for a normal blood pH of 7.40, the ratio $[HCO_3^-]/(0.03\ pCO_2)$ equals 20. It therefore follows that the values of bicarbonate concentration and pCO_2 can depart significantly from their normal values, and as long as the ratio is 20 the pH will be normal. It should not be concluded that any values for HCO_3^- concentration and pCO_2 can be entered into the equation, although it is true that the values of these two quantities can depart from their normal values and pH can be normal if their ratio is maintained, i.e., $[HCO_3^-]/(0.03\ pCO_2) = 20$. For pH limits of 7.35 and 7.45, the corresponding ratios are 17.8 and 22.4.

The manner in which HCO_3^- concentration and pCO_2 vary in respiratory and metabolic acidosis is shown in Table 4. Although there are two types of metabolic imbalance (respiratory and metabolic) and two pH states (acidosis and alkalosis), the four conditions are not encountered with equal frequency. Respiratory acidosis and alkalosis and metabolic acidosis are not encountered with equal frequency. Respiratory acidosis and alkalosis and metabolic acidosis are the most commonly encountered, the latter with low cardiac output and the former with pulmonary dysfunction. Thus it can be seen that the blood gas values for pH and pCO_2, along with the pO_2, provide valuable information in guiding the therapy for metabolically deranged patients.

TRANSCUTANEOUS pO_2 TRANSDUCERS

The transducer designed especially for measuring the partial pressure of oxygen from the skin surface operates on the same principle as the conventional pO_2 electrode, although a heating element must be added to allow measurement of blood pO_2 from the skin surface. The pO_2 measured in this way is often designated $tcpO_2$ (transcutaneous pO_2).

TABLE 4 Summary of Acidosis and Alkalosis

	Respiratory	
Acidosis (CO$_2$ Excess)	Item	Alkalosis (CO$_2$ Deficit)
Low	pH	High
Always high	pCO$_2$	Always low
Usually high	[HCO$_3^-$]	Usually low
	Metabolic	
Acidosis (Acid Excess or Base Deficit)	Item	Alkalosis (Acid Deficit or Base Excess)
Low	pH	High
Usually low	pCO$_2$	Normal or high
Always low	[HCO$_3^-$]	Usually high

Figure 13a illustrates one of the popular tcpO$_2$ electrodes that was described by Huch et al. (1973, 1974, 1976) and Huch and Huch (1976). The transducer consists of a small plastic housing 18 mm in diameter and 9 mm high. An annular silver electrode constitutes the anode, and the cathode consists of three platinum wires, each 15 μm in diameter. The current in each cathode is measured, and when they are equal, equilibrium has been reached (Huch et al., 1973). A Teflon membrane about 12 μm thick encloses the electrolyte, which is in contact with the anode and cathodes. Surrounding the anode is a heating element that raises the temperature of the transducer and skin surface to about 42°C. Often, a second thin membrane, moistened with a drop of KCl solution, separates the face of the transducer (Teflon membrane) from the skin. Sometimes the skin is initially moistened with a drop of water to facilitate the diffusion of O$_2$. With the conventional polarizing voltage (~ 0.8 V), the current is linearly proportional to the partial pressure of oxygen on the skin surface.

For the transcutaneous pO$_2$ transducer to measure arterial pO$_2$, it is placed on the skin as shown in Fig. 13b. It is necessary, however, to "arterialize" the underlying capillary bed; this is accomplished by the heater. When the capillary bed is fully dilated, which requires about 10 min, the partial pressure of oxygen on the skin surface is usually close to that in the capillary bed. Failure to achieve this condition results in a falsely low pO$_2$ reading. Figure 14 illustrates the relationship between tcpO$_2$ and arterial pO$_2$ under typical conditions.

Calibration of the tcpO$_2$ transducer is accomplished by exposing the membrane of the transducer to humidified 100% nitrogen; this provides a zero pO$_2$ reading. Then the transducer is exposed to a humidified sample of oxygen of known concentration (known partial pressure). Often ambient air is used, which provides a pO$_2$ of about 20% of the barometric pressure.

According to Huch et al. (1974), there are two potential sources of error in tcpO$_2$ measurement: (1) The increased skin temperature tends to raise the skin pO$_2$, and (2) local oxygen consumption by the tissues tends to reduce the skin pO$_2$ below arterial pO$_2$. It is believed that, in practice, the net effect of these two errors is small. Despite some controversy about the meaning of the tcpO$_2$, it is well established that the output of the tcpO$_2$ transducer tracks arterial pO$_2$ very well, and therefore the tcpO$_2$ transducer is ideal for monitoring changes in pO$_2$.

It should be clear that the reading provided by the heated tcpO$_2$ transducer is highly dependent on the perfusion (blood flow per gram) in the subjacent tissue. In subjects with a normal cardiac index (cardiac output per square meter of body surface area), the heated tcpO$_2$ transducer will provide pO$_2$ values that are quite close to the arterial pO$_2$. However, when the subjacent tissue is poorly perfused, e.g., when the cardiac index drops to less than two-thirds normal, the tcpO$_2$ reading is substantially less than the arterial pO$_2$. In fact, the difference between the two is an index of the inadequacy of tissue perfusion. A low tcpO$_2$ is therefore a signal to investigate the cause and can be considered an alerting sign of impending shock.

Transcutaneous monitoring of pO$_2$ is especially valuable in premature infants and in subjects who have an impaired ability of the lungs to transport oxygen. In the case of the newborn, oxygen toxicity constitutes an important hazard. For

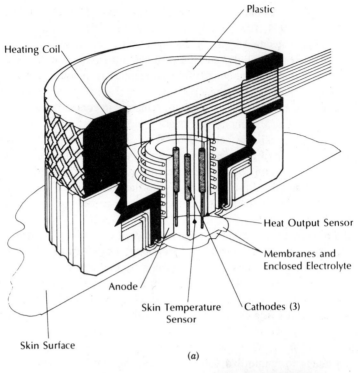

(a)

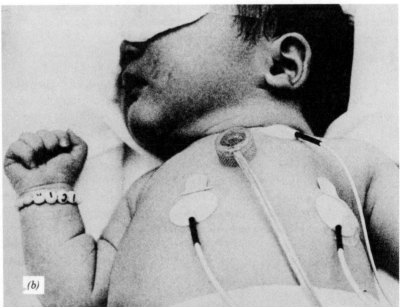

Figure 13   (a) The transcutaneous pO_2 electrode and (b) its application to an infant. (From Huch et al., 1976.)

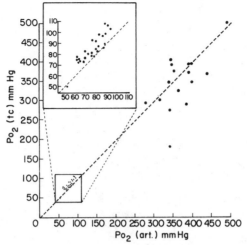

Figure 14 The relationship between transcutaneous (tc) pO_2 and arterial (art.) pO_2. [Redrawn from R. Huch et al. *Arch. Dis. Child.* **49**:213–218 (1974).]

example, in the premature infant, the lungs have not matured and hypoxia is usually present. However, exposing the subject to a high concentration of oxygen (more than 40%) in an incubator to alleviate the hypoxia can cause changes in the retina (retrolental fibroplasia) that can lead to blindness. Thus the oxygen therapy must be carefully managed to control the pO_2 to a level that is just adequate to avoid hypoxia.

TRANSCUTANEOUS pCO₂ TRANSDUCERS

The pCO_2 electrode has been miniaturized for transcutaneous measurement of blood pCO_2. Figure 15 illustrates a cutaway view of one popular type, which consists of a miniature glass electrode, a reference electrode, an electrolyte, and a CO_2-permeable membrane (Teflon). A thermostatically controlled heating coil maintains the device at a constant temperature. As in the conventional pCO_2 electrode, CO_2 gas passes through the Teflon membrane and changes the pH of the electrolyte, which is measured by the glass electrode. The voltage of the glass electrode with respect to the reference electrode is logarithmically proportional to the pCO_2. Because the glass electrode has a very high impedance ($\sim 10^9$ Ω), a miniature high-input impedance amplifier is mounted on the electrode assembly. The output of the amplifier is conducted to the recording apparatus by way of a shielded cable. The output is the Nernst value (55–63 mV/pH) and is temperature-dependent; this is one reason thermostatic control is employed; the other is to provide vasodilation.

Calibration of the pCO_2 electrode requires exposure to two known values of pCO_2. Typically 5 and 10% CO_2 gas mixtures are used. Ambient air is not sufficiently free of CO_2 to allow its use for a zero pCO_2 calibration.

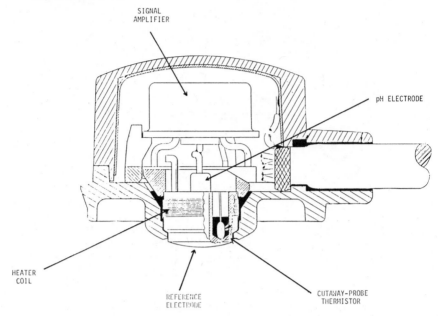

Figure 15   The transcutaneous pCO_2 electrode. (Courtesy Air Shields, a Healthdyne Co. Hatboro, Pennsylvania.)

Fiber-Optic Chemical Transducers

The fiber-optic oximeter (see Chap. 5) was the first of a long line of evolutionary fiber-optic transducers for chemical substances. Many of the transmission, reflectance, and fluorescent techniques used in analytical chemistry lend themselves to embodiment in fiber-optic catheters (Seitz, 1984). In general, one fiber (or bundle) carries incident radiation; a second brings the colorimetric information to a photodetector for measurement. Optical filters are used to filter the incident radiation or the returned radiation to accept only the spectrum that identifies the desired chemical substance. Often, two wavelengths are used, one providing the desired information and the other a reference signal. Figure 16 illustrates the general principle of a fiber-optic transducer in which the key to detecting the desired substance is a sensing material that changes its optical properties in response to the concentration of the substance to be measured. The sensing material is contained in a measuring chamber at the tip of the catheter. The walls of this chamber are made from a membrane that is permeable to the substance to be measured. Use of this technique allows measurement in blood and other tissue fluids.

Hydrogen Ion Concentration (pH)

Lubbers and Opitz (1975, 1976) reported that the fluorescent spectrum of beta-methyl umbelliferon depends on pH. Figure 17 illustrates this relationship. By

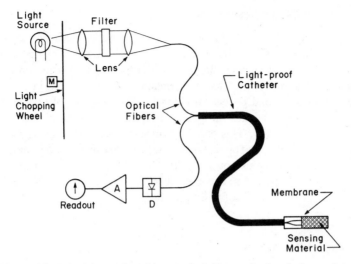

Figure 16 Principle employed in a typical fiber-optic chemical transducer.

measuring the emitted radiation at 330 and 357 nm, a signal proportional to pH can be obtained. Note that at 330 nm (the isobestic point), the emitted radiation is independent of pH and the emission at this wavelength provides a reference signal.

Peterson et al. (1980) reported the use of phenol red to construct a fiber-optic catheter transducer for pH. The phenol red was immobilized on acrylamide spheres placed in the measuring chamber; the membrane covering it was dialysis tubing. One optical fiber illuminated the spheres, and another detected the scattered and reflected light, which was measured with a photodetector, the readout being proportional to pH.

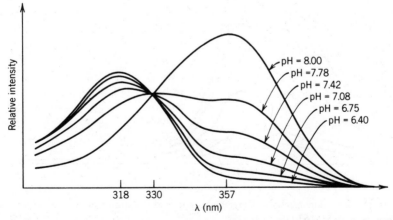

Figure 17 Emission spectrum of beta-methyl umbelliferon. [Redrawn from J. S. Schultz, *Med. Instrum.* **19**(4):158–163 (1985).]

Carbon Dioxide Partial Pressure (pCO$_2$)

The availability of a fiber-optic system for pH measurement provided the opportunity to create a pCO$_2$ transducer. Vurek et al. (1983) reported the use of phenol red in a CO$_2$-permeable chamber of Silastic mounted at the tip of a fiber-optic catheter. The measuring chamber contained the phenol red in a solution of potassium bicarbonate and potassium chloride. The principle of operation relates to the fact that pCO$_2$ changes the pH of the phenol red solution, which in turn changes its optical density. This change is measured colorimetrically by the scattered and reflected light. The optical properties were measured at 570 nm; a second wavelength, produced by use of a Wratten No. 70 filter, provided the reference signal. Vurek et al. reported an excellent correlation between directly and optically measured pCO$_2$ over a range of 0–80 mmHg.

Oxygen Partial Pressure (pO$_2$)

Lubbers and Opitz (1976) reported that pO$_2$ could be detected using pyrene butyric acid, the emission spectrum of which depends on pO$_2$. Figure 18 illustrates this relationship. The intensity of emission at 342 nm is proportional to pO$_2$.

Peterson et al. (1980) developed a fiber-optic pO$_2$ catheter transducer based on the fluorescence of pyrene butyric acid, which was immobilized on beads placed in the measuring chamber covered with a thin oxygen-permeable silicone rubber membrane. By measuring the emission at two wavelengths (342 and 330 nm), a signal was derived that was proportional to pO$_2$ from 0 to 500 mmHg.

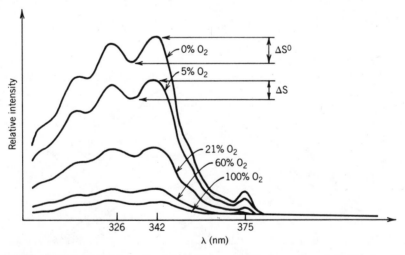

Figure 18 Emission spectrum of pyrene butyric acid. [Redrawn from J. S. Schultz, *Med. Instrum.* **19**(4):158–163 (1985).]

Characteristics of Fiber-Optic Transducers

The selectivity and sensitivity of fiber-optic transducers for chemical substances depends on the nature of the sensing material. Those created to date appear to have adequate selectivity. However, the signal tends to be small because of the nature of the sensing material and the constraints imposed by fiber optics. The response times of typical sensors is quite long, because time is required for the sensing material to come into chemical equilibrium with the solution being measured. Most types are designed for use in blood and produce an on-line signal.

A highly attractive feature of fiber-optic transducers is that their use does not produce an electrically conducting path from the measuring equipment to the patient. This is particularly desirable when transducers are used in operating rooms where electrosurgical equipment is employed. In addition, when electrochemical cells are used, electrode instability and contamination are often a problem; these are obviated by fiber-optic transducers.

ION-SPECIFIC ELECTRODES

Introduction

The familiar pH-sensitive glass electrode is the prototype of ion-selective electrodes. The pH sensitivity resides in the thin glass membrane, the potential across which is described by the Nernst equation (see under Membrane Electrodes earlier in this chapter). At 25°C, the change in potential is 59.2 mV per decade change in H^+. It is now possible to create membranes that are specific for cation and anion species. The term membrane is used in its broadest sense to identify a thin specimen of material that provides the selectivity. The ion selection can occur at the surface or within the membrane.

Before describing the membranes, the basic principles should be understood. Figure 19 illustrates a prototype ion-selective electrode consisting of an ion-specific membrane mounted at the end of an insulating tube containing a solution (S_i), in which an internal reference electrode is immersed. The ion-selective electrode is immersed in an outside solution (S_o) containing ion species $X_o^{\pm}$, which is to be measured. Into this solution is immersed the external reference electrode. The voltage E_{12} appearing across terminals 1 and 2 consists of three parts: (1) the half-cell potential (E_{1-S_i}) of the internal reference electrode in contact with the internal solution (S_i), (2) the Nernst potential (E_m) developed across the membrane, and (3) the half-cell potential (E_{2-S_o}) of the external reference electrode in contact with the outside solution (S_o) in which the concentration of the ion species $X^{\pm}$ is to be measured. That is,

$$E_{12} = E_{1-S_i} + E_m + E_{2-S_o}.$$

Obviously, it is the Nernst potential

$$E_m = \frac{RT}{nF} \ln \frac{X_i^{\pm}}{X_o^{\pm}}$$

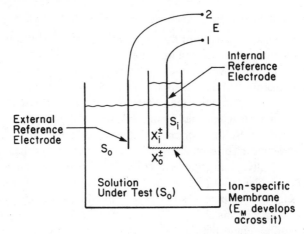

Figure 19 Prototype ion-specific membrane electrode for measuring the activity of the $X^{\pm}$ ion. Potential E_{1-2} appearing between electrode terminals 1 and 2 is the sum of the half-cell potentials of the internal and external reference electrodes plus the potential E_m developed across the ion-specific membrane.

that contains the information on the concentration of $X_o^{\pm}$. From the foregoing, it is obvious that the half-cell potentials of the internal and external reference electrodes must be constant for the measured voltage E_{1-2} to represent the concentration of $X_o^{\pm}$. The half-cell potential of the internal reference electrode is constant because changes in $X_o^{\pm}$ do not affect it. However, it is essential that the half-cell potential of the external reference electrode not be affected by changes in concentration of the ionic species ($X_o^{\pm}$) being measured. If, for example, the ion-selective membrane were designed for chloride ions, the reference electrode could not be of silver–silver chloride, because such an electrode is a chloride ion electrode (see Chap. 9). Therefore, in addition to an ion-specific membrane, the half-cell potential of the external reference electrode must not change with changes in the concentration of the ion that is to be measured. Perhaps the most important fact to remember is that ion-specific membranes have a very high impedance. Therefore, measurement of the potentials that they develop requires the use of a potential-measuring instrument with a very high input impedance, that is, an electrometer.

Ion-Selective Membranes

Ion-selective membranes take many forms. Often the active agent is contained in a chemically inert binder, which gives the membrane its mechanical properties. Membranes containing active substances have been made of paraffin, collodion, poly(vinyl chloride) (PVC), polyethylene (PE), and silicone rubber (Silastic). Membranes can also be of solid materials, such as specially treated (doped) glass or halide films. Doped and undoped crystals have been used. Those in which a binder is used are called inhomogeneous, the others being designated homogeneous. Irrespective of the type, it is the property of the active material that provides ion specificity.

It is obviously highly desirable that a membrane be specific for a single ionic species. However, there is usually some response to other ionic species; this phenomenon is known as interference. It appears that the degree of interference is often dependent on pH. In many cases, the interference is small, although this is not always true, and ion-selective membrane electrodes should be used only when interfering ions are present in low concentrations. Alternatively, if the interfering ions do not change in concentration, an ion-selective electrode can still be used if it is carefully calibrated.

A bewildering array of active materials are used to create ion-specific membranes. Covington (1979) presented an excellent review of these materials; Table 5 is based on his review. Note that both cation- and anion-selective electrodes have been fabricated.

Sodium Ion Electrode

Calling attention to the fundamental observation of von Lengyel and Blum (1934) that the addition of oxides of aluminum or boron to the melt used in making a glass pH electrode resulted in an electrode selectively sensitive to sodium ion, Eisenman et al. (1957) set themselves the task of developing a practical electrode for this purpose. They constructed glass electrodes from various mixtures of oxides of sodium, aluminum, and silicon, and produced one having 250 times more sensitivity to sodium than to potassium. They stated that the ultimate limits of specificity were unknown and that for biological work the electrode produced a sodium ion voltage with less than 0.2% error in the presence of potassium concentrations up to 30 mM at any pH greater than 5.6. They quote a voltage output of 160 μV for a 1-meq/L change in sodium at 150 meq/L. In addition, the electrode was insensitive to calcium, magnesium, ammonium, and lithium ions. Although the authors did not give data relating to the rapidity of response, they called attention to the fact that the drift was less than 1.3% per hour. Because of the resemblance of their electrode to the glass pH electrode, it may be inferred that the response time is similar. Moreover, they stated that their sodium-sensitive transducer could be used with any pH meter and was not poisoned by constituents of serum, cerebrospinal fluid, or brain homogenate when electrodes were soaked in these solutions for many hours.

Calcium Ion Electrode

Ross (1967) reported the development of a simple electrode capable of measuring calcium ion activity in the presence of many common interfering ions. The electrode utilizes a liquid ion-exchange membrane containing the calcium salt of a

TABLE 5   Ion-Selective Membranes and Ions They Identify

Ion	Construction^a
K^+	Glass/bulb; valinomycin/L(diphenyl ether) or PVC or SR; potassium tetrakis(*p*-chlorophenyl)borate/L
NH_4^+	Glass/bulb; monactin-nonactin/L(diphenyl ether)
Ca^{2+}	Calcium di-*n*-decylphosphate/L(di(*n*-octylphenyl)phosphonate) or PVC; thenoyltrifluoracetone/PVC; CaF_2-LaF_3/disk, calcium(di-*n*-octylphenyl)phosphate/G(di(*n*-octylphenyl)phosphonate), SSL
Ca^{2+}/Mg^{2+}	Calcium di-*n*-decylphosphate/L(decanol)
Ba^{2+}	Nonylphenoxypolyethyleneoxyethanol/L
Cu^{2+}	Ag_2S + CuS/disk or SR; $Cu_1{}'$ $_{79}S$/disk; CuS/G; chalcogenide glass/disk; $(R-S-CH_2COO)_2Cu/L$
Fe^{3+}	Chalcogenide glass/disk
Ag^+	Glass/bulb; Ag_2S/disk
Zn^{2+}	ZnSe + Ag_2S/disk
Mn^{2+}	MnSe + Ag_2S/disk
Cd^{2+}	CdS + Ag_2S/disk
Ni^{2+}	NiSe + Ag_2S/disk
Pb^{2+}	PbS + Ag_2S/disk or SR; $(R-S-CH_2COO)_2Pb/L$
F^-	LaF_3/single crystal or SR
Cl^-	AgCl + Ag_2S/disk; AgCl/SR; AgCl + Ag_2S/G; Hg_2Cl_2 + HgS/disk; dimethyldistearylammonium chloride/L
Br^-	AgBr + Ag_2S/disk; AgBr/SR; AgBr + Ag_2S/G
I^-	AgI + Ag_2S/disk; AgI/SR; $I_2/G(CCl_4)$
S_2^-	Ag_2S/disk; Ag_2S/SR; Ag_2S/G
ClO_4^-	Fe(II)tris(substituted 1,10-phenanthroline)perchlorate/L; tetra-*n*-heptylammonium perchlorate/L
NO_3^-	Ni(II)tris(substituted 1,10-phenanthroline)nitrate/L or PVC; tridodecylhexadecylammonium nitrate/L or PVC
BF_4^-	Ni(II)tris(substituted 1,10-phenanthroline)fluoroborate/L
SCN^-	AgSCN + Ag_2S/disk; AgI/SR
SO_4^{2-}	$PbSO_4$ + PbS + Ag_2S + Cu_2S/disk
CO_3^{2-}	Tri(*n*-octyl)methylammonium chloride/L(trifluoroacetyl-*p*-butylbenzene)

^{a}L, liquid ion-exchange form; G, graphite Selectrode; SR, silicone rubber heterogeneous membrane; PVC, poly(vinyl chloride) membrane; SSL, specially synthesized ligand.

Source: A. K. Covington (ed.), *Ion-Selective Electrode Technology*. CRC Press, Boca Raton, Florida, 1979.

disubstituted phosphoric acid and is able to measure free calcium ion activity in the presence of a thousandfold excess of sodium or potassium ions.

Sulfide Ion Electrode

An electrode to measure sulfide ion activity is available commercially, and the following information has been supplied by the manufacturer (Orion Research, Inc., Cambridge, Massachusetts). This electrode is constructed of unbreakable plastic; because it is a solid-state device, it requires no renewal. No interference is encountered from a wide variety of other anions. The electrode will detect any level of sulfide for which stable standard solutions can be prepared. Its ultimate sensitivity is below 10^{-17} M, and it will follow sulfide activity over the pH range 1–12.

Fluoride Ion Electrode

The development of an electrode for measurement of fluoride ion activity was reported by Frant and Ross (1966). The principle of construction of the electrode is similar to that of a conventional glass pH electrode, except that the membrane material is a disk-shaped section of a single-crystal rare-earth fluoride, such as LaF_3, NdF_3, or PrF_3. The disk-shaped section (1 cm in diameter, 1–2 mm thick) is cemented to the end of a rigid poly(vinyl chloride) tube filled with a solution containing both fluoride and chloride ions (typically 0.1 M NaF and 0.1 M KCl), and electrical contact is made by inserting an Ag–AgCl electrode into the solution. Electrical connection to the test sample is through a standard saturated calomel cell. Measurements were reproducible to within less than 1 mV.

Because the membrane is permeable only to fluoride ions, the potential developed is given by the Nernst equation. The only significant interference comes from the hydroxide ion, as would be expected on the basis of similarities in charge and ionic radii. The electrode response as a function of pH and fluoride concentration is given in Fig. 20.

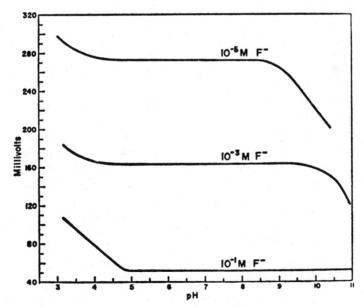

Figure 20 Sensitivity characteristics of the fluoride ion electrode. [From M. S. Frant and J. W. Ross, *Science* **154:**1533–1554 (1966). Copyright 1966 by the American Association for the Advancement of Science. By permission.]

TABLE 6   Concentrations of Plasma Ions

Ion Species	Concentration (mEq/L)
Na^+	135–145
K^+	3.5–5
Ca^{2+}	4.5–5.5
Cl^-	100–106

IONIC CONTENT OF BLOOD

In a healthy subject, the concentrations of the many ions in the blood are maintained within a narrow range. Table 6 presents a summary of these values in plasma. In disease states that cause metabolic imbalances, the concentrations of the ions will depart from their normal values. For this reason, it is desirable to have a simple, rapid, and easy way to measure the concentrations of plasma ions. The solution to this problem has been made possible by the availability of ion-specific electrodes. There are now many commercially available instruments for this purpose, the most familiar being the blood gas analyzer, which provides values for pO_2, pH, and pCO_2. However, it does not provide information on the other important ions, such as Na^+, K^+, and Cl^-. Accordingly, analogous instruments, containing ion-specific electrodes, have been developed to meet this need. One of these, the Chem-Pro (SenTech Medical Corporation, Arden Hills, Minnesota), embodies some unusually attractive features. For example, four ion-selective electrodes are mounted in a conduit leading to a sample chamber on a disposable plastic board like those used for printed circuits. In the conduit are four ion-sensing [K^+, Na^+, Cl^-, and H^+ (i.e., pH)] electrodes and a reference electrode. The four active electrodes are of carbon covered with proprietary ion-selective membranes. The reference electrode is Ag–AgCl, which communicates with the blood sample by way of a gel bridge (analogous to a salt bridge).

Figure 21 illustrates the Chem-Pro disposable transducer card with the cylindrical chamber that accepts the blood sample and the four active and reference electrodes. The blood sample (125 μL) is placed in the cylindrical sample chamber, which is then rotated one quarter turn. This act allows a calibrating solution to flow over the ion-selective electrodes in the conduit. In 30 sec the calibration is complete, and the sample cell is given a half turn, which allows the blood sample to access the ion-selective electrodes. The voltages that they develop are proportional to the activities of the ions for which they are selective. A digital readout displays the concentrations of each ion species (Na^+, K^+, Cl^-, and H^+). After measurement, the card can be retained for file purposes, since it provides space for the patient's name or identification number and date.

Continuous Monitoring of Blood Chemistry

The availability of ion-selective electrodes provided the opportunity to obtain analog recordings of blood chemistry. Friedman et al. (1958, 1959), using a flow-

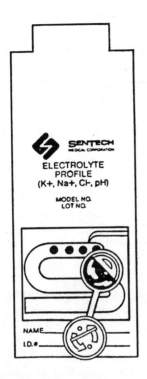 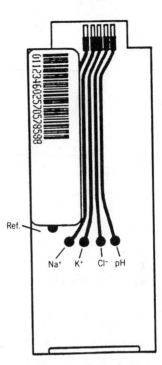

Figure 21 Disposable transducer assembly for measurement of K^+, Na^+, Cl^-, and H^+ concentrations. Blood to be analyzed is placed in the cylindrical chamber, which communicates with the ion-selective transducer. (Courtesy of SenTech, Arden Hills, Minnesota.)

through cuvette-type electrode, continuously recorded the concentration of sodium in the femoral arteries of dogs. They noted that the electrode was flow-sensitive in certain flow ranges but not in others. Their striking records, made with a direct recorder, illustrate changes of a few milliequivalents per liter in sodium concentration produced by a variety of pressor and depressor drugs.

Gotoh et al. (1966), in a study of cerebral blood flow and metabolism, reported the simultaneous use of several chemical transducers to monitor venous and arterial blood in more than 80 human subjects. Arterial and venous blood were passed through similar transparent acrylic cuvettes, which were maintained at body temperature. Transducers mounted in the cuvettes monitored the values of pO_2, pCO_2, pH, and Na^+ and K^+ concentrations in the circulating heparinized blood. Other physiological data, such as the EEG, ECG, blood pressure, temperature, expired pCO_2, and oxygen saturation, were also recorded. The primary advantage of this system lies in permitting the simultaneous detection of small changes in blood chemistry as rapidly as possible. Gotoh pointed out, however, that the response times are not the same for all the chemical transducers, and therefore the method is not suitable for studies in which time sequences within a second or two are important. The problems encountered with blood clotting were discussed, but the use of an adequate amount of heparin appears to have eliminated these difficulties.

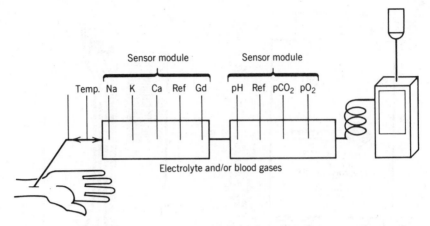

Figure 22 Multiple chemical sensors mounted in flow-through cuvettes for continuous recording. (Courtesy Ionetics, Inc., Costa Mesa, California.)

The concept described by Gotoh et al. (1966) is now being embodied in commercially available instruments. Figure 22 illustrates a multiple sensor in a flow-through cell in which sensors for temperature; Na^+, K^+, Ca^{2+}, and Gd^+ concentrations; pH; CO_2; and O_2 are mounted. Similar flow-through cuvettes are available for measurement of pO_2 and pCO_2 (Ionetics Inc., Costa Mesa, California).

McKinley et al. (1980) used a catheter-tip, ion-sensitive FET to record K^+ activity in the venous blood of dogs following the infusion of a KCl–glucose–insulin solution. They also recorded K^+ in a dog made hypokalemic and in hemorrhaged dogs. The venous activity of Ca^{2+} in dogs was recorded by McKinley et al. (1981). Both studies are described in the forthcoming section on FET chemosensors.

Niebauer et al. (1986) recorded the activity of K^+ in the blood from dog coronary arteries after the delivery of a pulse of defibrillating current. When cells are depolarized, K^+ exits and can be detected as shown in Fig. 23. In this study a blood-perfused beating dog heart was in an isoresistive and isotonic volume conductor that contained the defibrillating electrodes. The K^+ sensor was placed in the venous-drainage line as shown. The analog recording of Fig. 24 illustrates the transient increase in K^+ following a single defibrillating shock. It was found that the K^+ release was proportional to shock strength.

Undoubtedly more analog recordings will be made of the concentrations of blood constituents, by either flow-through or catheter-tip chemosensors. However, when interpreting such recordings, the response times and selectivities of such chemosensors should be borne in mind. In addition, many of the ion-selective electrodes are flow-sensitive, and care must be exercised in calibration.

FIELD-EFFECT TRANSISTOR CHEMOSENSORS

The very high impedance of the gate of a field-effect transistor (FET) makes it an ideal device for measuring the potential developed by an ion-selective mem-

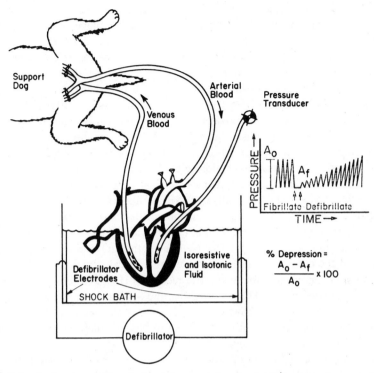

Figure 23 Perfused, working isolated heart used to study K^+ release in venous blood following a defibrillator shock applied to electrodes at the ends of the chamber in which the heart is suspended. [Redrawn from M. Niebauer et al., *Med. Instrum.* **20**(3):135–137 (1986).]

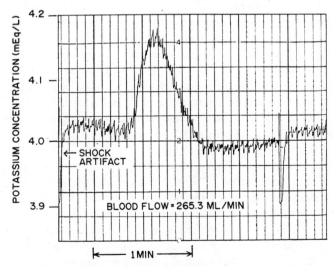

Figure 24 A record of the K^+ concentration increase in the coronary venous blood following a 0.6 A/cm², 5-msec rectangular wave defibrillator shock. [Redrawn from M. Niebauer et al., *Med. Instrum.* **20**(3):135–137 (1986).]

brane. This potential is described by the Nernst equation (see earlier in this chapter). Thus, the drain current, which is a function of the gate voltage, is proportional to the activity of the ion species for which the membrane was designed.

Two techniques have been used with the FET: (1) The ion-selective electrode is mounted very close to the gate terminal, and (2) the ion-selective membrane is deposited directly on the gate of the FET. In both cases, the voltage, which is measured with respect to a reference electrode, is on the order of 60 mV per decade change in concentration for monovalent ions; for others this value is divided by the valence. As stated previously, such electrodes measure the chemical activity, which is proportional to concentration. It is important to remember that it is the type of membrane that provides the ion selectivity, not the FET.

The first ion-sensitive field-effect transistor was described by Bergveld (1970, 1972). In this device, which he called an ISFET, the 2000-Å thick layer of SiO_2 on the gate constituted the ion-selective membrane that was exposed to the solution under test. He found that the FET drain current varied linearly with the concentration of Na^+ in a solution of pH 4.0. He likened the SiO_2 membrane to the glass membrane of the conventional pH electrode and advocated making ISFETs a few square micrometers in area for bioelectric recording (Bergveld et al., 1976). In a previous paper (Bergveld, 1972), showed that the SiO_2 layer on the gate of a FET is sensitive to Na^+ and H^+; however the device was also sensitive to K^+, Ca^{2+}, and Mg^+, to a lesser degree. It is interesting to observe that in all of Bergveld's studies, no reference electrode was employed.

Matsuo and Wise (1974) developed a pH-sensitive electrode using a metal oxide semiconductor FET (MOSFET) in which the gate was first covered with a layer of SiO_2, 1000 Å thick, upon which was placed a layer of SiN_4, also 1000 Å thick; the latter was employed to improve the long-term stability. A saturated KCl–calomel electrode was used as the reference. The drain current decreased linearly with pH, and the electrode exhibited a sensitivity predicted by the Nernst equation. The response time was short, in the range of pH 5–8; in higher H^+ concentration (pH < 4), the response time was longer. The sensitivity to Na^+ and K^+ was very small. The authors also reported using the transducer for biopotential recording in a constant-pH solution.

A potassium-ion-sensitive FET was described by Moss et al. (1975). A layer of SiO_2 was first deposited on the gate of a FET; then a layer of SiN_4 was added, on top of which was placed the K^+-selective membrane, the recipe for which is given in the paper. The sensitivity to K^+ was as predicted by the Nernst equation, the drain current being proportional to the logarithm of the K^+ activity. The sensitivity to Na^+ was tested and found to be small. A long-term test showed that the maximum stability was reached at 79 hr, with excellent stability to 313 hr and only a small drift thereafter. They attributed the drift to instability of the polymer membrane interface where the ion selection occurs.

Moss et al. (1978) developed ion-sensitive FETs for H^+ and Ca^{2+}. Two versions of the pH electrode were studied; one consisted of bare SiO_2 on the gate, and the other employed SiO_2/SiN_4. The sensitivity for pH was that predicted by the Nernst equation. The bare SiO_2 surface exhibited a shorter lifetime than that of the SiO_2–

SiN_4 surface, which becomes hydrated to form a gel, which results in development of sensitivity to Na^+ and K^+. With the passage of time, the gel dissolves, leaving bare silicon. It is for this reason that the SiO_2–SiN_4 surface is preferred for sensing pH.

The Ca^{2+} and K^+ FET electrodes described by Moss et al. (1978) employed poly(vinyl chloride) to hold the ion-selective material. Dodecyl phosphonate was used for Ca^{2+}, and valinomycin or crown ethers for K^+. The Ca^{2+} electrode exhibited little sensitivity to K^+ or Na^+. The sensitivity of the K^+-sensitive FET to Na^+ was small, being 1–2×10^{-3}, with a response time of about 1 min.

Cheung et al. (1978) showed how an ISFET could be mounted at the tip of a catheter. Figure 25 illustrates this embodiment in which the reference electrode (Ag–AgCl) and the gate region are shown. The ion-selective membrane would be on the gate.

Cheung et al. (1978) analyzed the suitability of three gate coverings of silicon: oxide (SiO_2), nitride (SiO_2/SiN_4), and oxynitride (40% silicon, 40% oxygen, and 20% nitrogen) as ion-selective membranes. Table 7 presents their results, which identify selectivity and response time. From Table 7 it is seen that the nitride-gate FET is the best candidate for a pH electrode, being least sensitive to Ca^{2+}, K^+, and Na^+.

McKinley et al. (1980) employed a catheter-tip ISFET to record the concentration of K^+ in femoral venous blood of the dog in response to an infusion of KCl

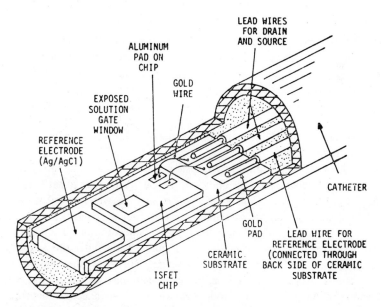

Figure 25 Catheter-tip, ion-sensitive field-effect transducer (ISFET). The ion-selective membrane is placed over the window, and the Ag–AgCl reference electrode is adjacent to it. [From P. W. Cheung et al., in *Theory, Design and Applications of Solid-State Chemical Sensors*. P. W. Cheung et al. (eds.). CRC Press, Boca Raton, Florida, 1978.]

TABLE 7 Summary of Chemical Response of Various ISFET Sensors

	Nitride	Oxynitride	Oxide
pH range tested	3–9	3–9	3–9
pH sensitivity (mV/decade)	45–58	25–40	15–30
Chemical response time (95%)	<1 sec	<1 sec	<2 sec
Ion (K^+, Na^+, Ca^{2+}) concentration	0.01–1.0 M	0.01–1.0 M	0.01–1.0 M
Selectivity coefficient ($\times 10^6$)(pH 6–8) $K_{H^+, M^{2+}}$			
K^+	0.1–5	50–1000	10–150
Na^+	0.1–4	3–100	1–15
Ca^{2+}	0.01–4	0.4–10	0.1–6
$K_{H^+, M^{2+}}$ comparison at pH 6–8	Approximately the same	$K^+ > Na^+ > Ca^{2+}$	$K^+ > Na^+ > Ca^{2+}$
Drift	+2 mV/4 days	±2 mV/8 days	±60 mV/4 days
Continuous operational lifetime	>60 days	>60 days	>60 days
Overall temperature sensitivity of total system	1 mV/°C	1 mV/°C	1 mV/°C

Source: P. W. Cheung and D. G. Fleming (eds.), *Theory, Design and Biomedical Applications of Solid-State Chemical Sensors.* CRC Press, Boca Raton, Florida, 1978, 296 pp.

into a jugular vein. Figure 26 illustrates the recording that they obtained. The data points on the record represent the K^+ values obtained by analyzing the K^+ concentration in blood withdrawn from the sampling point at the catheter tip.

McKinley et al. (1981) used a catheter-tip polymeric ISFET to record the Ca^{2+} activity in the vena cava of heparinized dogs. The sensor was first calibrated in solutions of known Ca^{2+} activity. They found that the sensitivity was 23–27 mV per decade change in Ca^{2+} activity; this is close to the Nernst value of 30 (recall that calcium is divalent).

The venous Ca^{2+} was reduced by infusion of sodium citrate; Fig. 27 illustrates this response. To demonstrate the ability of the Ca^{2+} electrode to serve as a sensor to control Ca^{2+}, they contrived a feedback system in which the Ca^{2+} was first reduced by continuous citrate infusion. The Ca^{2+} sensor control system directed the infusion of $CaCl_2$ to raise the venous Ca^{2+} concentration. The converse experiment was also performed successfully. Figure 28 illustrates this sequence.

In conclusion, ISFETs offer many advantages. However, they are not without their limitations. Although all are based on measurement of the Nernst potential, like the well-known pH glass electrode, they are not as advanced as this commonly used electrode. Among the advantages of the ISFET are the opportunity for continuous monitoring of the ion species for which it is designed. Response times depend on the design and range from less than 1 sec to several minutes, the time required to reach chemical equilibrium. ISFETs can be made very small and

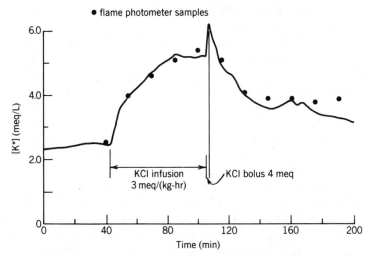

Figure 26 Venous potassium activity monitored continuously during venous KCl solution infusion in a dog with a precalibrated ISFET probe compared with arterial serum samples analyzed for K^+ concentration using an emission flame photometer. [Redrawn from B. A. McKinley et al., *Med. Instrum.* **14**(2):93–97 (1980).]

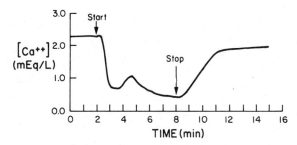

Figure 27 Calcium ion activity of venous blood in response to a sodium citrate dose of 96 mg/kg given to a dog. [Redrawn from B. A. McKinley et al., *CRC Crit. Care Med.* **9**(4):334–339 (1981).

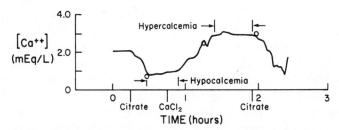

Figure 28 Calcium ion activity of venous blood, reduced first by sodium citrate infusion and restored automatically by feedback control, which directed the infusion of $CaCl_2$. [Redrawn from B. A. McKinley et al., *CRC Crit. Care Med.* **9**(4):334–339 (1981).]

capable of being mounted on a catheter tip or of being placed in a tiny cell, requiring only microliters of fluid to make the measurement. The dynamic range is very large, although this feature is not of great importance when used with biological fluids, the composition of which is controlled to rather narrow limits. ISFETs can be used in colored, turbid, or opaque solutions, a situation that is impossible when colorimetric analytical techniques are used. The output impedance of the ISFET is low, permitting the use of long leads to connect the device to the measuring instrument. Because integrated-circuit fabrication techniques are used, mass production is easy, and the unit cost can be low, offering the opportunity to create disposable devices. Finally, it is often possible to use the ISFET as one of the pair of electrodes to measure a bioelectric event.

ISFETs have their limitations and must be used in appropriate situations. Perhaps the most serious limitation is the selectivity. Although a unit can be designed to sense a specific ion, it may be sensitive to other ions; this phenomenon is known as interference. Ideally, an ISFET should be ion-specific; however, this limitation is overcome by using it in solutions in which the interfering ions are absent or are present only in low concentrations. ISFETs are temperature-sensitive, as predicted by the Nernst equation. Precautions must be taken to operate them isothermally or correct for this factor. The precision is quite good, typically 0.5%. It must be recognized that a reference electrode is needed, and its design must be such that it is not selectively ion-sensitive. Often a salt bridge is used with a reference electrode to eliminate this problem. The half-cell potential of the reference electrode also forms part of the bias voltage for the FET. The membrane employed in an ISFET can become coated with proteins or poisoned by the constituents of some solutions. Therefore, suitable precautions must be taken to protect it.

GLUCOSE ELECTRODES

Glucose is the essential metabolic input for many cells. The quantitative measurement of blood glucose is therefore very important and typically involves withdrawing a blood sample, separating the plasma from the cells, adding a reagent to the plasma, and processing the resultant solution to permit the colorimetric measurement of a new compound that identifies the concentration of glucose. This procedure is time-consuming and has stimulated research to create glucose sensors that provide an electrical signal proportional to glucose concentration. A comprehensive review of the attributes of 10 methods for measuring glucose concentration was presented by Passey et al. (1977), with the 1974 standard in view. Ongoing research is directed toward the creation of an implantable glucose sensor to permit the closed-loop control of an implantable insulin delivery system to maintain a constant blood glucose level in diabetic patients.

When glucose is metabolized, oxygen is consumed and gluconic acid and hydrogen peroxide are produced. In the presence of the enzyme glucose oxidase, the reaction proceeds rapidly, the enzyme not being consumed because it is merely a biological catalyst. The exothermic reaction is as follows:

$$C_6H_{12}O_6 + O_2 \rightarrow H_2O_2 + \text{gluconic acid}$$

It is obvious that the glucose concentration can be measured by determining the oxygen consumed, the heat liberated, and the H_2O_2 or gluconic acid produced. Alternatively, the glucose can be consumed in a fuel cell, the current from which would identify the concentration of glucose. Of the five possibilities, all but the measurement of gluconic acid are used in the creation of glucose electrodes. Prior to their description, it is useful to understand how the metabolism of glucose is altered in diabetes.

Diabetes

In normal subjects the blood glucose level depends on previous food intake. In a normal fasting subject, the glucose level is 60–90 mg/100 mL of blood (60–90 mg %). The upper limit for normal subjects is about 125; values higher than this are strongly indicative of diabetes mellitus (sugar or sweet diabetes), the pancreatic beta-cell disease of insulin deficiency. Insulin causes the glucose to enter the body's cells, where it is metabolized. In diabetes mellitus, the blood glucose level is high and can be on the order of 400–2000 mg %. When the blood level exceeds about 160 mg %, glucose can be detected in the urine, which is produced in large quantities (diuresis).

Glucose Tolerance Test

The diagnosis of diabetes mellitus involves measurement of the blood glucose after fasting and with glucose loading. The procedure is called the glucose tolerance test, which involves taking blood samples for analysis over a period of about 6 hr. In a normal, fasting subject, the glucose level is typically 60–90 mg %. Following the ingestion of 100 g of glucose, the blood level rises to 120–150 mg % in about 1 hr, returning to the control level in about 2 hr, as shown in Fig. 29. In the diabetic, the fasting glucose level is much higher, and it takes much longer for the blood glucose level to return to the fasting value.

Enzyme Electrode

Clark (1962) described the basic design for an enzyme electrode, the enzyme being placed between two membranes; this design was adopted in many later electrodes. Kadish and Hall (1965) paved the way for the creation of a glucose electrode by measuring blood glucose indirectly, using a dialysis membrane to allow passage of blood glucose into the dialysate. Using glucose oxidase in the dialysate, they measured the pO_2 decrease with a pO_2 electrode.

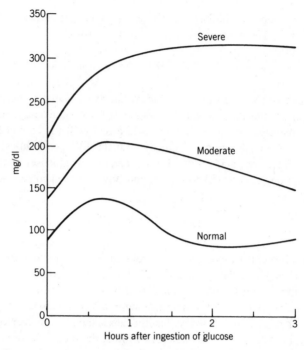

Figure 29   The glucose tolerance test, being the blood glucose level in response to the oral ingestion of 100 g of glucose. Typical blood glucose levels are shown for normal subjects and for patients with severe and moderate diabetes.

Updike and Hicks (1967) developed an interesting glucose oxidase pO_2 electrode for measuring glucose concentration. The device consisted of a platinum cathode and a silver anode covered by a membrane on which was a gel containing glucose oxidase. The decrease in pO_2 indicated the glucose concentration. To eliminate any error due to changing pO_2 in the blood, they used two identical electrodes in a differential circuit; the glucose oxidase activity on one electrode was reduced to zero by heat. Thus one electrode sensed pO_2, and the other sensed pO_2 and its reduction due to the oxidation of glucose.

Clark and Sachs (1968) contributed important improvements leading to a practical glucose sensor. The electrode consisted of a standard Clark pO_2 electrode coated with the enzyme glucose oxidase (EC 1.1.3.4) and covered with a cellophane membrane that is permeable to glucose and prevents the oxidase from being poisoned by substances in the fluid being measured. The decrease in pO_2 was a measure of the glucose concentration. Figure 30a illustrates this electrode design. Bessman and Schultz (1972) modified a Clark pO_2 electrode to sense glucose by the decrease in pO_2. The modification consisted of replacing the membrane with one of Teflon coated with a gold–platinum black film, which replaced the glucose oxidase as the catalyst. Although the electrode functioned adequately, the metal

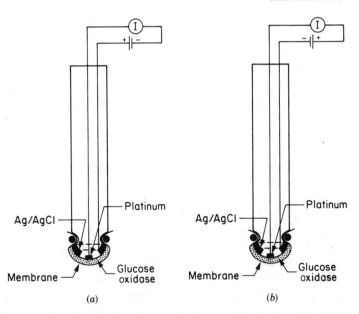

Figure 30 Enzyme electrodes for glucose. (*a*) The oxygen cathode, a Clark pO₂ electrode coated with immobilized glucose oxidase covered by a glucose- and oxygen-permeable membrane. (*b*) The peroxide electrode. In both cases the current *I* is proportional to the glucose concentration. [Redrawn from L. C. Clark, in *Theory, Design and Biomedical Applications of Solid-State Chemical Sensors.* P. W. Cheung and D. G. Fleming (eds.). CRC Press, Boca Raton, Florida, 1978, 296 pp.]

catalyst was easily poisoned by blood constituents. To solve this problem, they proposed periodic electrolytic cleaning of the catalyst by the use of dc pulses.

Bessman and Schultz (1973) devised a differential fuel cell glucose oxidase sensor suitable for implantation that measured 20 mm in diameter and 3 mm in height. The sensor consisted of a poly(vinyl chloride) membrane that carried two sensing areas; one was a plain matrix, and the other a matrix containing the glucose oxidase. Behind each were a silver cathode and a lead anode, in an acid-buffered solution. The ratio of the currents from the two pO₂ electrodes was found to be exponential with glucose concentration. The response time was about $2\frac{1}{2}$ min. It was found that the differential cell reduced artifacts due to mechanical motion.

Clark (1978, 1979) pointed out that hydrogen peroxide, which is produced when glucose is oxidized, is a labile product that is decomposed rapidly by many substances. When a cellophane membrane is used to separate the glucose oxidase from the fluid containing the glucose to be measured, the peroxide is available for measurement with a cell containing a platinum anode and an Ag–AgCl reference electrode (Fig. 30*b*). With a polarizing voltage of about 0.7 V, the current is proportional to the glucose in the sample being measured. Note that by making the platinum the anode, the cell is made to be specific for hydrogen peroxide; however, such a cell has some sensitivity to ascorbic acid. Clark (1970) described the differential technique to overcome this difficulty.

Silver (1976) developed two types of glucose oxidase microelectrode for the intracellular measurement of glucose. In one type the glucose oxidase was deposited on the bare area (3 μm $\times$ 3 μm) of a metal microelectrode. The other employed a conventional glass micropipet (tip diameter 0.1 μm), which was first covered with platinum over which glass insulation was applied, leaving the distal portion bare. The exposed platinum was covered with a resin that held the glucose oxidase. The platinum was polarized positively using a 0.6-V source connected to an Ag–AgCl reference electrode. Both electrodes were operated in the peroxide mode and were used to measure intracellular glucose in nerve cells, which was found to be remarkably constant except in spreading depression.

A small-diameter (175 μm) needle glucose sensor for subcutaneous use was described by Gardner and Silver (1979). The electrode consisted of a platinum anode polarized 0.7 V positive with respect to an Ag–AgCl electrode. The bare tip was covered with glucose oxidase and then covered by a cellulose acetate membrane. The response time for this peroxide–glucose electrode was about 20 sec; it was used for subcutaneous and intravenous measurement of glucose concentration.

As stated previously, there is an obvious need for a long-lived implantable sensor for closed-loop control of the delivery of insulin. Much research has been devoted to this subject, but the sensor problems are formidable. Nonetheless, steady progress is being made toward this goal. Clark and Duggan (1982) described an implantable glucose sensor consisting of a platinum ball at the end of a 28-gauge platinum wire. The wire was insulated up to the ball, which was coated with immobilized glucose oxidase and covered with a cellophane membrane. The platinum electrode was polarized positively, and an Ag–AgCl electrode was used as the reference. The current was proportional to the hydrogen peroxide resulting from the oxidation of glucose. The performance of the electrode was evaluated in buffered solutions containing known concentrations of glucose, as well as in freshly drawn whole blood. In the former, the behavior was excellent, but in whole blood the performance was not entirely satisfactory. Nonetheless, the performance was adequate to record glucose in jugular vein blood of a dog for a short time.

The longer-term performance of the platinum-ball glucose oxidase–peroxide electrode was investigated further by Clark and Noyes (1984). Because of previous difficulties with whole blood, Clark elected to measure blood glucose in the tissue fluid in the peritoneal cavity of the rat, a site in which he found the glucose level tracked blood glucose. The electrode (Fig. 31a) was implanted in the rat and paired with an Ag–AgCl reference electrode; the wires from both electrodes could be reached easily for measurement. The glucose-sensing characteristic of each electrode was measured before implantation and after removal. Figure 31b illustrates a typical electrode after 70 days. Although a fibrous tissue capsule covered the membrane, there was little change in performance (Fig. 31c, d). Such results are very promising, but the maximum lifetime has not been determined.

A glucose oxidase–peroxide needle electrode was described by Shichiri et al.

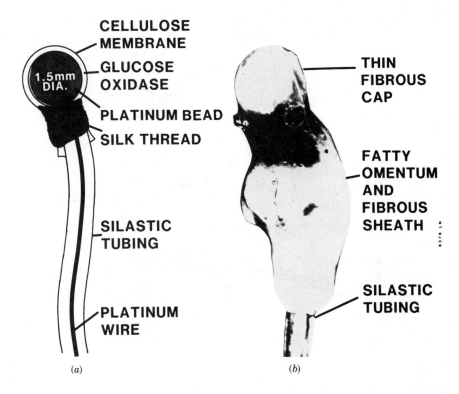

CELLULOSE MEMBRANE

1.5mm DIA.

GLUCOSE OXIDASE

PLATINUM BEAD

SILK THREAD

SILASTIC TUBING

PLATINUM WIRE

(a)

THIN FIBROUS CAP

FATTY OMENTUM AND FIBROUS SHEATH

SILASTIC TUBING

(b)

Figure 31 The platinum-anode, hydrogen peroxide electrode for sensing glucose in peritoneal fluid; (a) before implantation and (b) after 70 days of implantation. (c, d) Current-voltage curves (polarograms) of a similar electrode (S) before implantation and (d) after 99 days of implantation. The curves are for 100-mg % increments of glucose concentration. (Courtesy of L. C. Clark, Jr., 1985.)

(1985) that measured less than 1 mm in diameter. The device was inserted subcutaneously to monitor glucose concentrations in humans over prolonged periods using telemetry. Figure 32 presents a 36-hr record from a pancreatectomized patient. The points along the recording represent the glucose concentrations obtained from blood samples drawn at the various times. Actrapid, an insulin compound, was given at the times indicated to decrease the blood glucose. This sensor was used for the closed-loop control of insulin delivery in patients.

Chang et al. (1973) described a fuel cell glucose sensor consisting of two platinum electrodes, disk-shaped to have a large surface area. Between them was an ion-exchange membrane, and on the other side of the cathode was an oxygen-permeable membrane. On the other side of the fuel anode was a semipermeable membrane that separated it from a third pulsing (rejuvenating) electrode; this electrode and the oxygen-permeable membrane were exposed to tissue fluids. The short-circuit current was linearly proportional to glucose concentration. Implantable units measuring 2 cm in diameter and 0.3 cm thick were implanted in the abdominal

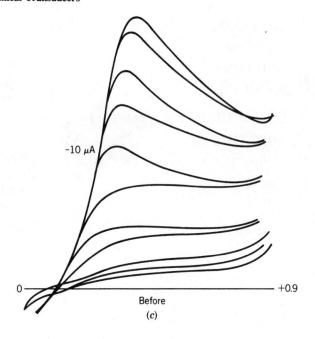

−10 μA

0 ──────────────────────── +0.9
Before
(c)

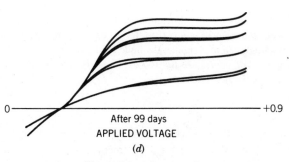

0 ──────────────────────── +0.9
After 99 days
APPLIED VOLTAGE
(d)

Figure 31   (*Continued*)

skin of monkeys and rabbits. The current produced by the fuel cell tracked blood glucose levels quite well. Due to oxidation of the platinum anode, the sensitivity to glucose concentration decreased with time. The anode was rejuvenated by passing a train of short-duration pulses between it and the pulsing electrode. Although this procedure is easily carried out, the need to do so has diminished the popularity of the fuel cell glucose sensor.

The tiny temperature rise produced when glucose is oxidized was used by Towe and Gilbeau (1985) to create a potentially implantable glucose sensor. Along the center of a 1.6-mm square glass substrate they mounted one row of bismuth–

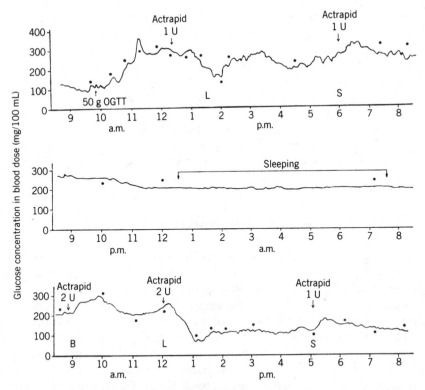

Figure 32 Glucose concentration monitored by telemetry for 36 hr using a subcutaneous peroxide needle electrode in the forearm. The data points along the analog record represent blood glucose levels determined from blood samples. [Redrawn from M. Shichiri et al., in *Implantable Sensors for Closed-Loop Prosthetic Systems*. W. Ko (ed.). Futura Publ. Co., Mt. Kisco, New York, 1985.]

antimony thermojunctions. Along the outer edges were two more rows; in all, 150 junctions were created. On the center row was placed glucose oxidase. Thus when glucose oxidase catalyzed the oxidation of glucose, a temperature rise on the order of 0.001 °C occurred, the temperature difference being indicated by the difference in voltage between the central and outer rows of thermojunctions. The overall sensitivity of the glucose sensor was about 1 μV/mmol glucose. Although the signal is small, the technique represents a new way to sense glucose.

Closed-Loop Glucose Control

Although long-term closed-loop control of blood glucose by insulin delivered by a totally implanted sensor–drug-delivery system has not been achieved, steady progress is being made. Closed-loop control of blood glucose with the glucose sensor outside the body has been achieved and is used clinically. It appears that Kadish (1964) was the first to apply closed-loop control of blood glucose to human patients. Blood was drawn into an automated analyzer for glucose concentration measurement. If the glucose level exceeded 150 mg %, insulin was infused. If the glucose concentration was below 50 mg %, glucagon (a substance that increases blood sugar) was infused. The post-meal increase in glucose was automatically reduced by injection of insulin. Since this report by Kadish, there have been an enormous number of papers on the automatic control of blood glucose, the improvements depending largely on the availability of improved glucose sensors. Among those who have contributed importantly to this field are Albisser et al. (1974a, b, 1977), Pfeiffer et al. (1974), Kraegen et al. (1978), Santiago et al. (1978), and Broekhuyse et al. (1981). These papers discussed glucose measurement techniques and algorithms for the control of insulin delivery.

COLORIMETERS AND SPECTROPHOTOMETERS

Colorimeters and spectrophotometers are instruments that measure the transmission of light through solutions that are colored by dissolved substances. The basic principle underlying the operation of both is the Beer–Lambert law, which relates the transmission of light to the length of the absorbing path and the concentration of the material that imparts color to the solution. In the colorimeter, the wavelength of the light (i.e., the color) used to measure the transmission is provided by a filter placed in front of a light source. In the spectrophotometer, the colored light is provided by a prism or diffraction grating; the light produced in this manner is confined to a relatively narrow spectral band. Figure 33a illustrates the essential components of the colorimeter, and Fig. 33b is a diagram of the spectrophotometer.

The Beer–Lambert Law

The principle underlying the Beer–Lambert law is illustrated in Fig. 34. The law states that the intensity of emergent light (I_e) passed through an absorbing solution of thickness L and containing a solute of concentration c is given by

$$I_e = I_i e^{-acL},$$

where I_i = intensity of the incident light,
I_e = intensity of the emergent light,
a = absorption coefficient for the dissolved substance for the wavelength of the incident radiation,
c = concentration of the dissolved substance,
L = thickness of the solution measured along the direction of the light, and
e = 2.71828.

It is important to recognize that a, the absorption coefficient, is wavelength-dependent. Figure 34 illustrates a typical relationship and calls attention to the need to select the appropriate wavelength for measurement.

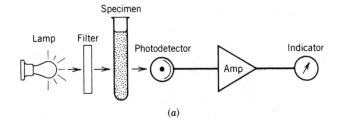

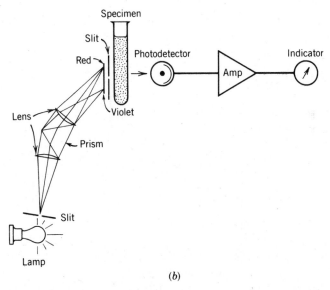

Figure 33 (*a*) The colorimeter; (*b*) the spectrophotometer in both instruments the amount of light emerging from the specimen is measured by a photodetector, the output of which is enlarged by an amplifier (Amp) that drives an indicator.

It is easier to understand the absorption of light resulting from the presence of a dissolved substance by considering the transmission fraction T, which is the ratio of the emergent intensity I_e to the incident intensity I_i:

$$T = \frac{I_e}{I_i} = e^{-acL}.$$

Because it is desired to measure the concentration of the material in solution, this expression is manipulated by taking the natural logarithm of each side as follows:

$$\ln T = \ln(e^{-acL}) = -acL,$$

which yields

$$\ln \frac{1}{T} = acL.$$

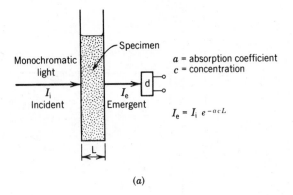

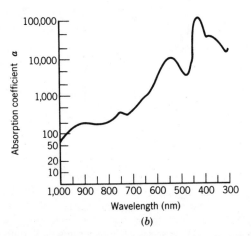

(b)

Figure 34 *(a)* The Beer–Lambert law; *(b)* the absorption coefficient a for hemoglobin. The absorption coefficient a is often called the molecular extinction coefficient. a = absorption coefficients; c = concentration; T = transmission; D optical density.

Now $\ln(1/T)$ is defined as the optical density D; therefore,

$$D = acL.$$

From this expression it is seen that the concentration c of the dissolved substance is proportional to the optical density, i.e.,

$$c = \frac{D}{aL}.$$

In a particular case, the path length L, is the diameter of the test tube or cuvette that contains the specimen. At a given wavelength the absorption coefficient a is constant; consequently,

$$c = KD = K \ln \frac{1}{T} = K' \log \frac{1}{T}.$$

Therefore it can be seen that if the optical density D is measured and the constant K is known, concentration can be determined.

Use of Colorimeters and Spectrophotometers

Prior to describing the use of a colorimeter or spectrophotometer, it is worthwhile examining the arrangement of components in each shown in Fig. 33. Both instruments contain a lamp, a method for obtaining colored light from the light source, a means for directing the colored light through the container that holds the specimen to be measured, and a photoelectric detector. In the colorimeter, a colored filter is used to obtain the colored light that is passed through the specimen to be analyzed. In a typical spectrophotometer, a prism is used to break up the light into its spectral components. The prism is usually linked to a calibrated dial that allows moving the spectrum so that only light of the desired color passes through a slit in front of the colored specimen.

The photodetector is chosen to have a spectral sensitivity that is appropriate for the spectral range of the instrument. Usually spectrophotometers cover the range extending from violet (300 nm) to deep red (700 nm). The vacuum phototube is frequently used to measure light intensity in this spectral range. There are sophisticated spectrophotometers that permit the measurement of absorption in the ultraviolet (below 300 nm) and infrared (above 700 nm ranges).

In using a colorimeter or spectrophotometer to measure the concentration of a dissolved substance, certain important facts about colored solutions should be appreciated. Perhaps the best way of presenting this information is to examine the transmission of light through solutions containing different amounts of a substance that imparts a color to the solution. Figure 35 is such a graph showing the percent transmission through aqueous solutions of different concentrations of Evans blue. Note that there is a wavelength where the transmission is a maximum and a wavelength where it is a minimum. This information can be used to demonstrate how a colorimeter or spectrophotometer is used to determine the concentration of a dissolved substance.

The first step in measuring concentration is to choose a wavelength for the measurement. Although any wavelength can be selected, it is wise to choose one where the transmission is a minimum (optical density is a maximum). The second best choice is where the transmission is a maximum (optical density is a minimum). The use of any other wavelength opens the possibility of low reproducibility if the instrument cannot be set to exactly the same wavelength.

Using the wavelengths for minimum (600 nm) and maximum (430 nm) transmission, graphs of percent transmission and optical density versus concentration have been composed, which are illustrated in Fig. 36. Note that the percent transmission (Fig. 36a) decreases nonlinearly with increasing concentration. Note also (Fig. 36b) that at both wavelengths the optical density is linear with concentration

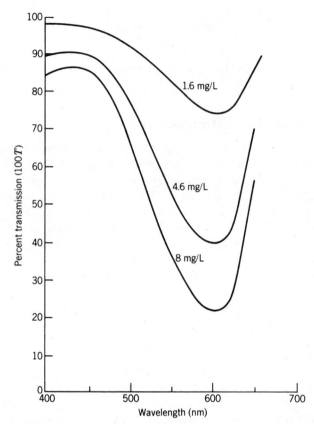

Figure 35   Percent transmission versus wavelength for three solutions containing different concentrations of Evans blue.

c. In practice, if the sensitivity of the instrument will permit, it is better to select the wavelength for minimum transmission because it provides the best opportunity for linearity in the light-intensity-measuring system.

There are other important considerations in using colorimeters and spectrophotometers to measure the concentration of a dissolved substance. For example, the substance is usually dissolved in a clear solvent (e.g., water), which is contained in a test tube placed in the optical path of the instrument. The Beer–Lambert law states that with no material dissolved in the solution (i.e., the concentration $c = 0$), the transmission is 1.0 and the optical density is zero. Although this is true, in practice, introduction of the test tube containing only the solvent decreases the amount of light received by the light-intensity-measuring system. This problem is eliminated by placing what is known as a blank—a test tube full of solvent with no dissolved material—in the light path of the instrument and adjusting the light intensity (or the sensitivity of the light-measuring system) so that the transmission scale reads 1.0 (i.e., the optical intensity is zero). When this is done, it is important to be sure that the "blank" test tube and all other test tubes to be used are free

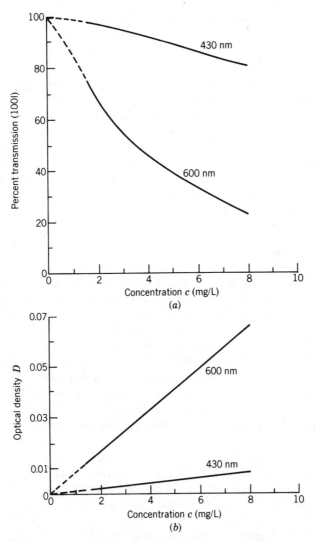

Figure 36   (*a*) Percent transmission and (*b*) optical density versus concentration for solutions of Evans blue measured at (*a*) 430 and (*b*) 600 mm.

from optical flaws by rotating them in the instrument to be sure that the light transmission does not change. There are specially constructed test tubes for colorimetric use, many of which have an index mark that is aligned with an index mark on the instrument.

In practice, the length of the liquid column and the absorption coefficient are unknown. The wavelength is known (or can be selected). Therefore the first step in using a colorimetric instrument is to calibrate it by using a blank containing only solvent to set the instrument to read an optical density of zero. Then a test tube containing a solution of known concentration is placed in the instrument, and the optical density is read. From these two measurements a straight-line graph of optical density versus concentration is constructed. Then when the optical density of a unknown solution is read, the graph will allow identification of its concentration.

Although a two-point calibration technique is often satisfactory, increased accuracy in measuring the concentrations of unknown solutions can be obtained by composing a calibration graph with different known concentrations of solution. A line that is the best fit for these data points provides the best calibration.

It should be recognized that the Beer–Lambert law holds for dilute solutions. Concentrated solutions can be measured by selecting a sample and diluting it with a measured amount of solvent. The concentration of the diluted sample is measured colorimetrically, and the concentration of the original solution can be calculated by multiplying by the dilution factor.

FLAME PHOTOMETER

The flame photometer is a colorimetric device for measuring substances that impart color to a colorless flame. The color spectrum emitted when the substance is placed in the flame is characteristic for each type of substance. The intensity of emitted light is a measure of the concentration of the substance.

When a substance is introduced into a hot colorless flame, its components are ionized by the heat energy of the flame. The return to the ground state results in the emission of light. Each substance emits its own characteristic line spectrum, the most familiar example being that due to sodium (Na). If salt (NaCl) is introduced into a colorless flame, it becomes bright yellow-orange due to the spectrum emitted by sodium. Table 8 lists the principal spectral lines emitted by various elements.

In clinical chemistry, flame photometers are used to measure the concentration of sodium (Na), potassium (K), and lithium (Li). These three substances are easily analyzed because their light spectra are intense and quite different. Moreover, the spectra lie predominantly in the visible range, making it easy to quantitate the intensity of the emitted light.

Figure 37 illustrates the components of a flame photometer used to measure sodium, potassium, and lithium. The essential requirement is the availability of a hot colorless flame of constant intensity. Illuminating gas or frequently propane is used to produce a flame of about 2000°F. The specimen, in an aqueous solution, is aspirated into the flame. When the sample reaches the flame, the spectrum characteristic of the substance in the sample is emitted. In order to detect a single substance, a narrow-band filter or monochromator is placed in front of the photo-detector.

To detect Na, the spectral intensity at 589.2 nm is measured; for K and Li, the radiation at 670.78 and 766.49 nm is measured. Photodetectors connected to amplifiers display the concentrations, which are usually expressed in milliequivalents per liter (meq/L).

TABLE 8 Wavelengths and Relative Intensities of Some Selected Emission Lines in Hydrogen–Oxygen and Acetylene–Oxygen Flames

Element or Molecule	Wavelength (nm)	Relative Intensity[a] H_2-O_2 Flame	$C_2H_2-O_2$ Flame
Ag	338.29	170	50
Al	396.15	1	2
AlO	484.2	3	0.3
Au	267.60	2	1.7
BO_2	547.6	60	15
Ba	553.56	40	10
Ba^+	493.41	25	5
BaO	535.0	20	2
BaOH	830, 873	30	15
BeO	470.9	0.7	0.25
Bi	472.26	0.25	0.05
Ca	422.67	1,000	250
CaOH	622	2,500	500
Cd	326.11	2	0.25
CeO (?)	494	7	0.7
Co	352.8	35	7
Cr	425.43	100	20
Cs	852.11	1,000	1,000
Cu	324.75, 327.40	100	100
Fe	371.99	40	15
Ga	417.21	200	20
In	451.13	350	70
K	766.49	30,000	30,000
Li	670.78	50,000	10,000
Mg	285.21	100	70
MgOH (?)	370.2	100	5
Mn	403.2	1,000	500
MoO_2 (?)	550–600	10	3[b]
Na	589.2	50,000	25,000
Ni	352.45	50	15
Pb	405.78	10	0.3
Pd	363.47	80	10
Pt	306.47	1	0.7
Rb	780.02	3,500	2,000
Rh	369.24	35	15
Ru	372.80	20	30
ScO	607.3	250	30
Sr	460.73	1,000	200
SrOH	605	1,000	100
TiO	544.9, 575.9	45	1.5
TiO	673, 715	20	10
VO	573.7	40	6
VO	710, 800	10	10

[a]Larger numbers indicate more intense lines.
[b]Estimated value.

Source: M. Margoshes, in *Physical Techniques in Biological Research*, Vol. IV. W. Nastuk (ed.). Academic Press, New York, 1962, pp. 215–260.

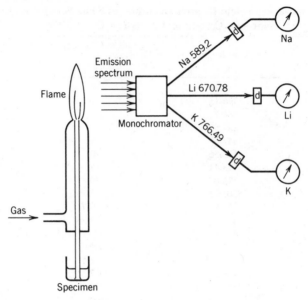

Figure 37   The flame photometer, as used for measuring the concentration of Na, Li, and K in a specimen of solution. Each substance causes a characteristic spectrum to be emitted by the flame. A monochromator selects the desired wavelengths, the intensities of which are measured by photodetectors (d) connected to indicators.

Figure 37 represents a three-channel flame photometer. In most instruments there is only one readout. In some, the lithium channel provides a signal to compensate for any random fluctuations in the intensity of the flame.

Flame photometers are calibrated by introducing a specimen of known concentration of the substance into the specimen chamber. Some instruments have internal standards that allow the aspiration of known concentrations of the substances that the instrument is designed to measure.

RESPIRATORY GASES

Introduction

Oxygen, carbon dioxide, and nitrogen are the respiratory gases; Table 9 presents typical values for inspired and expired air at sea level. Along with measurement of oxygen and carbon dioxide in blood, assessment of respiration involves measurement of the volumes and concentrations of all three gases. Before describing the transducers for the respiratory gases, it is useful to discuss the various lung volumes.

Lung Volumes

The amount of air that enters and leaves the lungs with each normal breath is called the tidal volume (TV). In a typical healthy 70-kg adult this amounts to about

TABLE 9   The Composition of Inspired and Expired Air at Sea Level

Component	Inspired Air %	Inspired Air ρ (mmHg)	Expired Air %	Expired Air ρ (mmHg)
Oxygen	20.8	158	15.3	116
Nitrogen	78.4	596	74.3	565
Carbon dioxide	0.04	0.3	4.21	32
Water vapor	0.75	5.7	6.18	47
Totals	99.9	760	99.9	760

500 mL during quiet breathing. Of course, the respiratory system is capable of moving much more air than the tidal volume. Starting at the resting expiratory level (REL in Fig. 38), it is possible to inhale a volume amounting to about seven times the tidal volume; this volume is called the inspiratory capacity (IC). A measure of the ability to inspire more than the tidal volume is the inspiratory reserve volume (IRV). Starting from the resting expiratory level, it is possible to forcibly exhale an appreciable volume, amounting to about twice the tidal volume; this is the expiratory reserve volume (ERV). However, even with the most forcible expiration, it is not possible to exhale all of the air from the lungs; there remains a residual volume (RV) about equal to the expiratory reserve volume. The sum of the expiratory reserve volume and the residual volume is designated the functional residual capacity (FRC). The volume of air exhaled from a maximum inspiration to a maximum expiration is called the vital capacity (VC). The total lung capacity

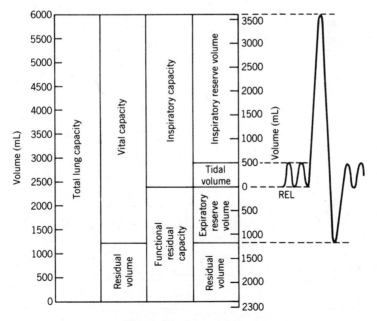

Figure 38   Lung volumes.

(TLC) is the total air within the lungs following a maximum inspiration—the air that can be moved in a vital capacity maneuver plus the residual volume. All lung volumes except the residual volume can be determined with a volume-measuring instrument connected to the airway.

The vital capacity depends on age, height, weight, and sex. There are many nomograms and formulas from which vital capacity and other respiratory volumes can be obtained. Disease alters many of these lung volumes, and their measurement is of diagnostic importance.

Measurement of Lung Volumes

The spirometer (Latin *spirare*, to breathe) is the traditional device used to measure the volume of air moved in respiration. The most popular type of spirometer consists of a hollow cylinder closed' at one end, inverted and suspended in an annular space filled with water to provide an airtight seal. Figure 39 illustrates the method of suspending the cylinder (bell), which is free to move up and down to accommodate the volume of air under it. Movement of the bell, which is proportional to volume, is usually recorded by a stylus applied to a chart that is caused to move with a constant velocity in a direction perpendicular to the movement of the recording stylus (Fig. 39). Below the cylinder, in the space that accommodates the volume of air, are inlet and outlet breathing tubes. At the end of one or both of these tubes is a check valve designed to maintain a unidirectional flow of gas through the spirometer. Outside the spirometer, the two breathing tubes are brought

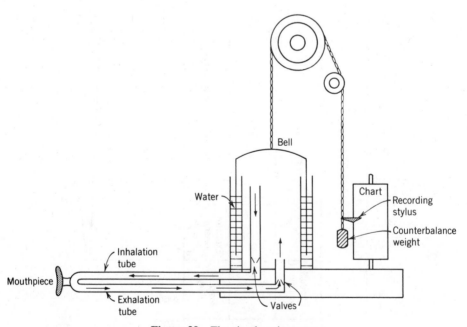

Figure 39   The simple spirometer.

to a Y tube that is connected to a mouthpiece. With a pinchclamp placed on the nose, inspiration diminishes the volume of gas under the bell, which descends, causing the stylus to rise on the graphic record. Expiration produces the reverse effect. Thus, starting with the spirometer half-filled, quiet respiration causes the bell to rise and fall. By knowing the "bell factor," the volume of gas moved per centimeter excursion of the bell, the tidal volume can be measured. A maximal deep inspiration starting from the resting expiratory level will show the maximum gas volume inhaled, which is called the inspiratory capacity. A maximum expiratory effort started from the resting expiratory level will cause the spirometer to display the expiratory reserve volume. Likewise, starting from the maximum expiratory level, a maximum inspiration will allow measurement of the vital capacity. Thus the simple spirometer can be used to measure all of the lung compartments except the residual volume.

Frequency Response of Spirometers

The appearance of dynamic respiratory tests, in which the rate of movement of respiratory gas is measured, drew attention to the matter of frequency response of spirometers. Obviously, if rapid breathing is to be measured accurately, the volume changes indicated by the spirometer must not depend on breathing frequency.

Bernstein was perhaps the first to call attention to the error in the standard metal-bell, water-sealed spirometer with breathing rates in excess of 40 breaths/min (Bernstein and Meindel, 1951). They eliminated this defect and extended the useful range to about 100 breaths/min by using a plastic bell and a silk thread to drive the recording stylus. A comparison between the plastic- and metal-bell types was carried out by Hamilton and Kory (1958), who showed that above a respiratory frequency of 90/min in normal humans the metal-bell spirometer volumes were greater than those indicated by the plastic-bell instrument. Stead et al. (1959) reinvestigated the frequency response of two popular 9- and 13-L water-sealed spirometers by varying sinusoidally both the stroke (tidal) volume and frequency of the delivery of air. They also measured the transient response of the two spirometers. In general they found that the frequency response of the 9-L spirometer was uniform up to about 40/min and exhibited a first resonant peak at 48/min and a pronounced peak at 180/min. The 13-L spirometer exhibited a slight resonant peak at about 70/min. Above 100/min the spirometer indicated a larger volume than was presented to it. At a frequency of 180/min the amplitude was 30% too large. Stead et al. (1959) then tested the same spirometer equipped with a plastic bell and found that the frequency response curve was essentially uniform to about 120/min, with a rise of about 5% at 170/min. At higher frequencies the chain supporting the suspension became dislodged from the pulley. With the stylus mounted directly on the plastic bell and the counterweight eliminated, the sinusoidal frequency response was remarkably uniform to 220/min, and at 360/min it indicated only 13% greater than the volume presented to it. Figure 40 presents the results of Stead's studies on the 13.5-L spirometer.

The best estimate of the frequency response required for spirometers to be used

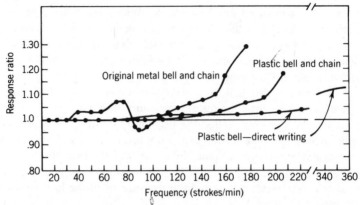

Figure 40 Sine wave frequency response of bell-type water-sealed 13-L spirometers. Stroke volume = 1200 cm^3. [From W. W. Stead et al. *J. Appl. Physiol.* **14:**449 (1959). By permission.]

for dynamic respiratory tests is to be found in a paper by Wells et al. (1959). Using a water-sealed spirometer with a light plastic bell to which a recording pen was attached (no counterbalancing system was used), they first measured the sinusoidal frequency response of the spirometer in a frequency range of 0–30 Hz. Both the frequency response curve and the transient response record indicated that the system did not behave as an ideal system with one degree of freedom with viscous damping. The response was somewhat dependent on the amplitude of the stroke volume used to measure the frequency response. The measured transient response indicated that the system was damped to 0.05 critical with a resonant frequency of about 40 Hz. These data indicated that their spirometer could be used with confidence to measure respiratory volumes with an error of less than 5% at respiratory rates up to 240/min. They then carefully measured a maximum-breathing-capacity record and applied a frequency analysis to it, finding that the amplitude of the fourth harmonic (9.1 Hz) was about 3%. Hence, at least for the subject studied, a uniform sinusoidal frequency response extending up to the fourth harmonic of the respiratory frequency provided faithful registration of the maximum-breathing-capacity spirogram.

The practical significance of using the high-fidelity Stead–Wells spirometer was investigated by Kory and Hamilton (1963), who conducted pulmonary function tests on a series of subjects using conventional 9- and 13.5-L spirometers and the Stead–Wells instrument. In general they found that the data obtained with the conventional 13.5-L spirometer were reliable up to a respiratory frequency of 110 breaths/min, but those obtained with the 9-L spirometer were reliable only to a respiratory rate of 50 breaths/min. With a minor modification in the 13.5-L spirometer, the data were reliable to a respiratory rate of 140 breaths per min.

The foregoing discussion of spirometer frequency response has practical significance. For the measurement of lung volumes in which the flow of air is slow, almost any spirometer can be used. However, if dynamic tests that require rapid breathing or the forceful movement of gas at high velocity are to be performed, the spirometer must be capable of responding rapidly. In such cases, all flow-restricting devices (e.g., valves and CO_2 absorber) must be either specially designed for this purpose or removed. The mass and friction of the moving parts must be low; plastic-bell models appear to be the best for this purpose.

Standardization of Volume

When spirometers are used to measure respiratory volumes, certain corrections must be applied. This is especially true when the volumes measured are to be compared to those in blood.

The volume of gas in the lungs exists at body temperature and atmospheric pressure and is saturated with water vapor (BTPS). Measurement of respired volumes is carried out at ambient temperature and atmospheric pressure, and the gas is saturated (ATPS). Because measurements are made in this way, it is necessary to correct the measured volumes to body temperature (37°C) and a saturated water vapor pressure of 47 mmHg. The following equation, derived directly from the gas laws, permits application of the temperature and pressure corrections:

$$\text{volume (BTPS)} = \left(\begin{array}{c}\text{volume collected}\\\text{at } t°C\end{array}\right)\left[\frac{273 + 37}{273 + t}\right]\left[\frac{P_B - P_{H_2O}}{P_B - 47}\right],$$

where t = temperature of the gas in the spirometer (°C),

P_B = barometric pressure (mmHg), and

P_{H_2O} = water vapor pressure (mmHg) of the gas in the spirometer at $t°C$. (See values in Table 10.)

In practice, use of the above expression is time consuming; the temperature and pressure corrections can be obtained from published tables and nomograms.

TABLE 10   Vapor Pressure of Water (P_{H_2O})

T (°C)	P_{H_2O} (mmHg)	T (°C)	P_{H_2O} (mmHg)	T (°C)	P_{H_2O} (mmHg)	T (°C)	P_{H_2O} (mmHg)
0	4.58	11	9.84	22	19.8	33	37.7
1	4.93	12	10.5	23	21.1	34	39.9
2	5.29	13	11.2	24	22.4	35	42.2
3	5.68	14	12.0	25	23.8	36	44.6
4	6.10	15	12.8	26	25.2	37	47.1
5	6.54	16	13.6	27	26.7	38	49.7
6	7.01	17	14.5	28	28.3	39	52.4
7	7.51	18	15.5	29	30.0	40	55.3
8	8.04	19	16.5	30	31.8	41	58.3
9	8.61	20	17.5	31	33.7	42	61.5
10	9.20	21	18.6	32	35.7	43	64.8

Source: Handbook of Chemistry and Physics, 48th ed. Chemical Rubber Pubishing Co., Cleveland, Ohio, 1967–1968.

OXYGEN UPTAKE AND CONCENTRATION

The simple water-sealed spirometer used for measuring lung volumes can be used to determine oxygen uptake if a CO_2 absorber is included inside the bell. Without such an absorber, the exhaled CO_2 will accumulate and produce hyperventilation, because CO_2 is a potent respiratory stimulant.

The CO_2 absorber incorporated into the spirometer is soda lime, a mixture of calcium hydroxide, sodium hydroxide, and silicates of sodium and calcium. The exhaled carbon dioxide combines with the soda lime and forms solid carbonates. A small amount of heat is liberated by this reaction.

Starting with a spirometer filled with oxygen (or air) and connected to a subject wearing a noseclip to prevent nasal breathing, respiration causes the bell to move up and down, indicating tidal volume, as shown in Fig. 41. Examination of the spirogram shows that with continued respiration the baseline of the recording rises, reflecting the disappearance of oxygen from under the bell. By measuring the slope of the baseline of the spirogram in milliliters per minute, the volume of oxygen consumed per minute can be determined. Figure 42 presents a typical record obtained on a normal subject, which indicates an O_2 uptake of 400 mL/min at ambient temperature and pressure. The method of standardizing this volume to BTPS conditions was explained in the previous section, and sample calculations are included in the legend to Fig. 42.

Paramagnetic Oxygen Analyzer

Oxygen is paramagnetic, that is, it is drawn into a magnetic field; the other respiratory gases are diamagnetic. Table 11 presents the magnetic susceptibilities

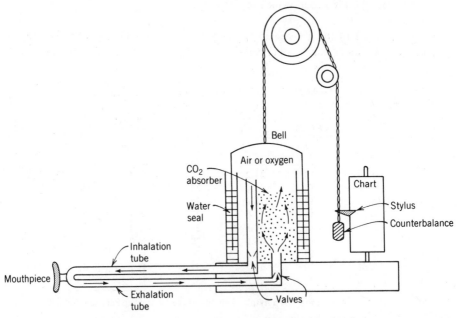

Figure 41   The spirometer with carbon dioxide absorber.

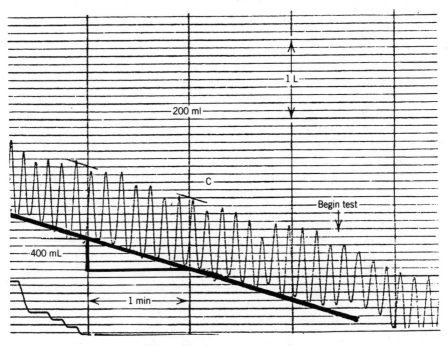

Figure 42   Oxygen consumption.

$$V_{BTPS} = V_{meas} \times F, \qquad F = \frac{273 + 37}{273 + T} \times \frac{P_B - P_{H_2O}}{P_B - 47}$$

$$V_{meas} = 400 \text{ mL at } t = 26°C, \qquad F = \frac{273 + 37}{273 + 26} \times \frac{750 - 25.2}{750 - 47} = 1.069$$

$$(P_B = 750 \text{ mmHg}; P_{H_2O} = 25.2 \text{ (from Table 10)})$$

$$V_{BTPS} = 400 \times 1.069 = 427.6 \text{ mL}$$

of the respiratory gases and shows that oxygen is strongly paramagnetic, while the other respiratory gases are weakly diamagnetic.

The paramagnetic property of oxygen has been used to increase the concentration of oxygen in a tube exposed to a strong magnetic field, thereby causing a change in resistance to flow (Rein, 1944). In another application, the increased concentra-

TABLE 11   Magnetic Susceptibilities of Respiratory Gases

Type of Gas	Susceptibility $\times 10^{-6}$ (cgs units)
Oxygen	+106.2
Nitrogen	−0.342
Carbon dioxide	−0.423

tion of oxygen in a magnetic field displaces a nitrogen-filled dumb-bell suspension (Pauling et al., 1949). Both methods of detecting oxygen will now be described.

Rein (1944) devised what may be called a pneumatic analog of the Wheatstone bridge to measure oxygen concentration in a flowing gas sample; Fig. 43 illustrates Rein's concept. The gas flow is divided into two tubes (A, B) with a manometer (M) between them at their midpoints. Ahead of the manometer in one tube and beyond it in the other, a strong magnetic field (3500 G) was established. Oxygen concentrated in the magnetic fields and changed the resistance to flow. This produced a pressure difference P proportional to oxygen concentration, which was indicated by a turpentine-filled manometer (M).

Rein's instrument worked well, but the pressure difference was extremely small; a microscope was used to make the readings. A differential pressure transducer could be used, but such devices were not available at that time. The tubes carrying the gas sample had to be made very small in diameter to achieve a strong magnetic field. The low flow velocity permissible and the high resistance to flow make it impractical for breath-by-breath respiratory applications. However there are commercially available instruments that use the principle described by Rein. Instead of measuring a differential pressure, flow can be measured using a heated thermistor; the change in resistance will depend on the oxygen concentration. Other methods of arranging the magnetic and pneumatic circuits will undoubtedly be developed.

Pauling et al. (1949) employed the paramagnetic principle to displace a nitrogen-filled dumb-bell mounted on a torsion suspension in a nonuniform magnetic field. Figure 44 illustrates this configuration. The dumb-bell test body is supported by a quartz torsion fiber. Any oxygen admitted to the apparatus will concentrate between the poles of the magnet and, due to its relatively high density, will displace the nitrogen-filled spheres. The force displacing the spheres is proportional to the concentration of oxygen present and is opposed by the torque produced in the quartz fiber. A mirror on the suspension reflects a light beam onto a scale calibrated in percent oxygen.

The Pauling–Beckman oxygen analyzer operates by admitting a sample of gas into the chamber containing the dumb-bell suspension and nonuniform magnetic

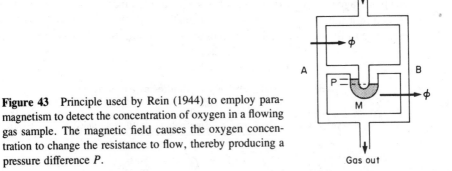

Figure 43 Principle used by Rein (1944) to employ paramagnetism to detect the concentration of oxygen in a flowing gas sample. The magnetic field causes the oxygen concentration to change the resistance to flow, thereby producing a pressure difference P.

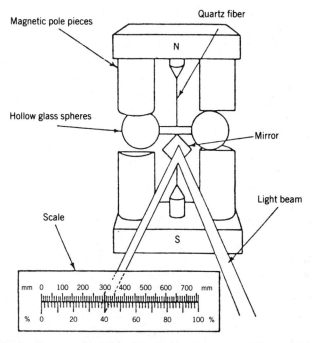

Figure 44   The Pauling paramagnetic oxygen analyzer, commercially available from Beckman Instruments.

field, so it cannot be used as a flow-through device. The suspension is fragile, and, because the paramagnetic property is temperature-dependent (Fig. 45), the instrument requires thermostatic control. The device is very convenient for sampling the concentration of oxygen in a volume of mixed gas.

There are other methods of using the principle described by Pauling; some of these are embodied in commercially available instruments. In one method the dumb-bell assembly is rhodium plated, and an electrostatic field is applied to prevent the dumb-bell suspension from deflecting. The voltage required to hold the suspension in its null position is proportional to the concentration of oxygen admitted to the analyzer.

Electrochemical Oxygen Analyzer

The Mine Safety Appliance (MSA, Pittsburgh, Pennsylvania) analyzer is an electrochemical cell contained in a Lucite cylinder filled with an oxylite (proprietary) solution in which are mounted a zinc electrode and a hollow carbon electrode. Gas to be analyzed is circulated through the inside of the carbon electrode. If oxygen is present, it diffuses through the porous carbon to combine with hydrogen and depolarizes the carbon electrode of the zinc–carbon cell. Removal of the hydrogen in this combination reduces the internal resistance of the cell and increases the current flowing from it. The change in cell output is then directed to an indi-

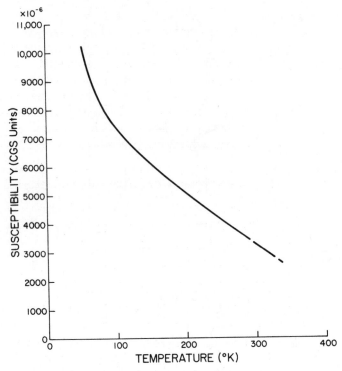

Figure 45   Magnetic susceptibility of oxygen plotted versus temperature.

cating meter that is graduated in percent oxygen. Flexible synthetic rubber tubing is used to convey the sample from the point of measurement to the instrument.

The MSA analyzer indicates the percent oxygen in a gas mixture. The instrument is inexpensive, small, and very slow responding, being designed for environmental monitoring.

Ultraviolet Absorption Oxygen Analyzer

The strong absorption of ultraviolet radiation by O_2 is a property that permits the application of rapidly responding electronic detectors for determining O_2 concentration. In studies of atmospheric absorption of ultraviolet energy, it has been found that at wavelengths below 200 nm the absorption becomes very strong, chiefly owing to the presence of O_2 (Koller, 1952). In addition, CO_2 and N_2 are virtually transparent in the ultraviolet region. Water vapor exhibits only a slight absorption in the ultraviolet (Lyman, 1914). Because of the strong absorption of ultraviolet by O_2, spectral studies are carried out in vacuum; hence the spectral band below 200 nm is often called the vacuum ultraviolet region. Figure 46 summarizes this information.

To date, only one oxygen analyzer based on ultraviolet absorption has been

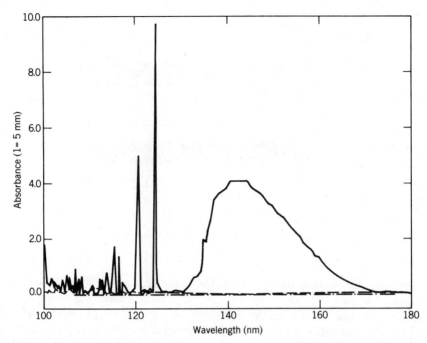

Figure 46   Spectral absorbance of gaseous CO_2 ($- \cdot -$), H_2O (dashed line), and O_2 (solid line). N_2 was also present but produced no line since it is transparent at these wavelengths.

described. Wong (1978) used a broad-band HgI radiator and a filter to pass two ultraviolet bands. After passing through the gas sample, the intensity of the emergent radiation was detected by an ultraviolet-sensitive diode. Although the device worked, it was inefficient, and further work was abandoned because of practical considerations.

Fuel-Cell Oxygen Analyzer

The Westinghouse fuel cell generates a current when oxygen is admitted to it. In normal operation, oxygen or air is fed into one side and hydrogen or other fuel into the other (Fig. 47). A ceramic electrolyte is the basic transducing component of the device. At elevated temperatures (400–1000°C), this material becomes a "sieve" through which oxygen as O^{2-} ions readily passes, migrating through the crystal structure of the electrolyte by activated diffusion. The electrolyte exhibits high ionic conduction and negligible electronic conduction under these conditions. Other gases, such as nitrogen, hydrogen, water vapor, carbon monoxide, and carbon dioxide, cannot penetrate the electrolyte.

To make a fuel cell from this ceramic electrolyte, electrodes are applied to both sides of the ceramic. An oxygen molecule from the gas sample on one side of the electrolyte adsorbs on the electrode, dissociates, acquires four electrons, and enters

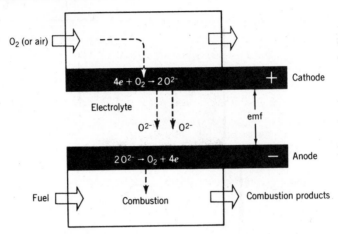

Figure 47 The Westinghouse oxygen fuel cell.

the ceramic electrolyte as two O^{2-} ions. The electrode is positively charged by the process. The two O^{2-} ions pass through the heated ceramic electrolyte to the opposite electrode and give up the four electrons when the oxygen reacts with the fuel to form combustion products. The fuel electrode becomes negatively charged, thus creating a voltage across the electrodes. The fuel cell continues to generate current as long as there is a difference in oxygen concentration on the two sides of the electrolyte. The fuel serves to keep the oxygen pressure low at the anode.

The output voltage is $0.0557 \log (0.2/P)$, where P is the partial pressure of oxygen at the measuring electrode.

The fuel cell requires a gas flow rate of 4 ft^3/hr. The response time is a fraction of a second after the gas enters the cell, which must be kept at a high temperature. Although suitable for measuring the concentration of oxygen in inspired and collected expired gas samples, it does not lend itself to breath-by-breath flow-through operation.

The Westinghouse fuel cell oxygen analyzer was adapted to physiological studies by Weil et al. (1967), who linearized the output signal. They pointed out that the optimal flow through the cell for sampling oxygen was 0.4–0.9 L/min and that the response time was the transit time in the sampling tube plus about 0.2 sec, the latter being the response time of the detector. They advocated calibration using room air and any other gas containing a known concentration of oxygen.

The Lex-O_2-Con Analyzer

Hersch (1965) developed a remarkably efficient oxygen fuel cell in which the current delivered reflects the amount of oxygen presented to it. This device contains two specially designed electrodes separated by a thin porous membrane containing only a tiny quantity of electrolyte. When oxygen gas is admitted to the cell, the oxygen molecules give up their electrons, a voltage is developed and current is delivered. The time integral of the current, therefore, represents the total volume of oxygen admitted to the cell. In reality, all the oxygen molecules passing through the cell are counted, because each provides electrons that appear as current. In fact, the Hersch cell operates on Faraday's law of electrolysis, which states that 96,500 C (A-sec) are required to liberate one chemical equivalent of an element. When applied to the oxygen fuel cell, this means that 8 g of oxygen provide 96,500 A-sec of current. Stated another way, 1 mL of oxygen at 20°C and 1 atm pressure provides 287 mA-min of charge.

The Hersch cell has been incorporated into a very practical oxygen analyzer known as the Lex-O_2-Con (Lexington Instruments, Waltham, Massachusetts). This device provides a quantitative indication of the volume of oxygen in the blood sample that is introduced. The reading is expressed in volume percent, that is, milliliters of O_2 per 100 mL of blood.

The method of using the Hersch cell in the Lex-O_2-Con instrument is illustrated in Fig. 48, where the various valves are in the "Use" (i.e., "measure") position. A carrier gas (nitrogen containing 2% hydrogen and 1% carbon monoxide) is admitted into the gas inlet and passed over a catalyst to remove all traces of oxygen. This oxygen-free carrier gas (with the carbon monoxide) is bubbled into distilled water in the scrubber chamber. The constant bubbling keeps the distilled water circulating. The oxygen-free carrier gas then passes into the Hersch cell and on to a water-filled reservoir, where it escapes. Since there is no oxygen in the carrier gas, the Hersch cell produces no current (although there may be a very small residual current).

The measurement of oxygen in a blood sample is accomplished by filling a 20-μL syringe with the blood to be analyzed. The blood sample is injected into the scrubber solution through the septum. The blood gradually gives up its oxygen because of the partial pressure gradient and because carbon monoxide combines with the hemoglobin, rendering it incapable of carrying oxygen. The carrier gas transports the released oxygen through the Hersch cell, which delivers current that flows until all the electrons have been released by the oxygen. A typical current–time curve is included in Fig. 48. An electronic integrator measures the area under the curve and provides a readout when the oxygen current falls to zero. This reading is expressed in terms of the volume of oxygen in 100 mL of blood.

The relationship between the values of oxygen content provided by the Lex-O_2-Con instrument and those determined by the conventional Van Slyke method was examined by Valeri et al. (1972); these data, presented in Fig. 49, show that the Lex-O_2-Con instrument provides a linear and accurate relationship for oxygen content.

GASEOUS CARBON DIOXIDE ANALYZER

Gaseous carbon dioxide (CO_2) absorbs infrared radiation strongly at 15.4, 4.26, 2.77, and 2.69 μm. Figure 50 illustrates the absorption spectra of CO_2 and water vapor. The other respiratory gases are transparent to infrared energy. Therefore,

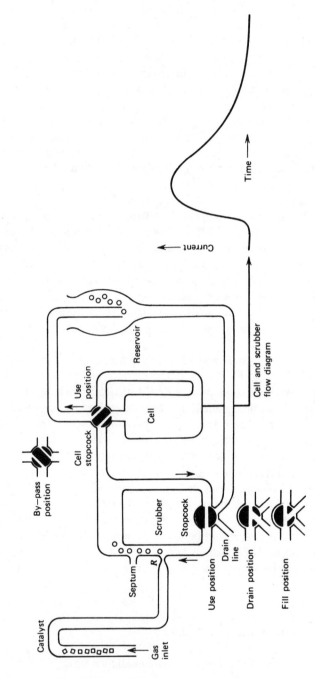

Figure 48 The Lex-O₂-Con oxygen content analyzer and a current–time record illustrating the analysis of a blood sample injected into the apparatus via the septum. (Courtesy of Lexington Instruments, Waltham, Massachusetts.)

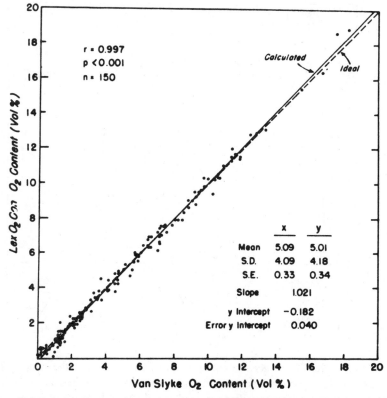

Figure 49   Relationship between the oxygen content in blood as determined by the Lex-O_2-Con instrument and values obtained by the Van Slyke method. [From C. R. Valeri et al., *J. Lab. Clin. Med.* **79**:1035–1040 (1972). By permission.]

radiant energy at any one or more of the CO_2-absorbing wavelengths can be used to measure CO_2. The technique involves measurement of the incident and emergent energy of radiation passing through the gas sample.

Absorption Types

The first rapidly responding gaseous CO_2 analyzer was described by Luft (1943). In it, the transducer was a CO_2-filled differential capacitor (see Chap. 4). Thermopiles have also been used as detectors (Fastie and Pfund, 1947; Fowler, 1949).

Liston (1950) and White and Liston (1950) described a gas microphone CO_2 analyzer that became available commercially as the Liston–Becker CO_2 analyzer.

The first to use a photoconductive cell detector were Bullock and Silverman (1950). In these devices, a broad-band infrared radiator (Nernst glower) emitted the infrared energy. Part of the beam from the glower passed directly to a reference photoconductor; another part of the beam passed through the gas sample to be analyzed. The difference in the signals produced by the two photoconductors was

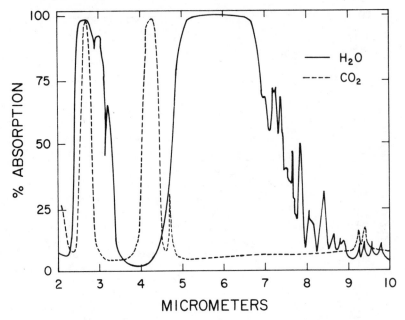

Figure 50   Spectral absorbance of CO_2 and H_2O.

proportional to the CO_2 concentration in the gas flowing through the sample chamber. Baker (1961) used a lead selenide photoconductive infrared detector and a Fabry–Perot type interference filter centered at 4.3 μm. Sinusoidal chopping of the infrared radiation provided sinusoidal reference and absorption signals. Use of this strategy permitted narrow-band, high-gain amplification to provide a low-noise signal dependent on CO_2 concentration. The response time was shorter than that required for breath-by-breath recording of expired CO_2. Such a recording is now called a capnogram (*capnos* = smoke, i.e., CO_2).

In one popular, commercially available (Hewlett-Packard) CO_2 analyzer, the gas sample to be analyzed passes between an infrared source (blackbody) and a detector (photoconductive cell). Sapphire windows (which are transparent to infrared energy) are used in the optical path. Also in the optical path is an infrared bandpass filter to permit measurement of absorption at a wavelength where water vapor does not interfere. A rotating filter wheel is also in the optical path. Figure 51 illustrates the transducer assembly, which is thermostatically controlled to ensure stability of operation.

The filter wheel contains a sealed chamber containing a high known concentration of CO_2, a chamber vented to the transducer's internal environment, and a sealed chamber containing nitrogen (i.e., no CO_2). The rotating filter wheel permits the generation of a train of signals that are used for calibration.

With the transducer applied to the airway adapter, continuous recordings of inhaled and exhaled CO_2 concentration can be recorded. Inspired air contains only

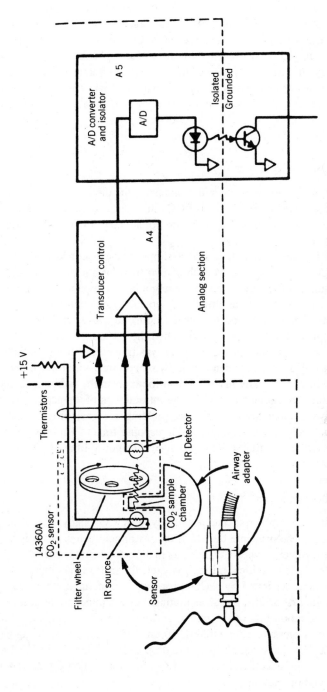

Figure 51 The Hewlett-Packard infrared CO_2 analyzer. (Redrawn from HP Capnometer Manual 47210A. Hewlett-Packard, Waltham, Massachusetts.)

a trace of CO_2; expired air contains about 5% CO_2 (end-tidal). End-tidal CO_2 concentration is very close to arterial pCO_2. At 760 mmHg, 5% CO_2 corresponds to a pCO_2 of $0.05 \times 760 = 38$ mmHg. This feature of displaying end-tidal CO_2 makes the analyzer very useful for metabolic monitoring.

Bergman et al. (1958) called attention to a potential error in using broad-band infrared energy to detect CO_2 in the presence of anesthetic mixtures containing N_2O. This gas has an absorption in the CO_2 band and will cause error. According to Bergman, reducing the pressure in the detector to 10 mmHg virtually eliminates this error.

Thermal Conductivity Types

In the past, and to some extent still in industry, the thermal conductivity method is used to measure the concentration of CO_2 in a gas sample. Because of the long response time of such instruments, they are not suitable for breath-by-breath measurements.

Ledig and Lyman (1927) described a simple thermal conductivity instrument for gaseous CO_2 measurement. In each of two thermostatically controlled sample cells was mounted a resistance element having a large temperature coefficient. The gas sample to be analyzed was dried and separated into two paths—one leading directly to one sample cell, and the other leading to a CO_2 absorber and then to the other sample cell. Thus one cell contained the respiratory gases, and the other contained the same gases minus CO_2. Heat was transferred from the walls of the sample cells to the thermal elements. The two thermoresistors formed two arms of a Wheatstone bridge, initially balanced with room air in the two sample cells. The temperature difference brought about by the introduction of the gas containing CO_2 into the analyzer unbalanced the bridge, yielding a signal proportional to CO_2 concentration. Ledig and Lyman reported a response time of 1 min, while a similar instrument described by Rein (1933) provided a response time of 40 sec.

Critical-Orifice Analyzer

An interesting, simple, and inexpensive type of CO_2 analyzer was developed by Mead (1955). The principle by which the instrument detects CO_2 is the difference in flow encountered when CO_2 appears in the sample and is chemically trapped in an absorber. Called a critical orifice analyzer, the instrument employs two flow-controlling orifices separated by a CO_2 absorber. An inclined manometer is connected across the first orifice, and an aspirating pump is joined to the second orifice. At the basal aspiration rate of the pump, and with no CO_2 in the air admitted to the instrument, a pressure differential of 10 cmH_2O is indicated. A sample of air containing 5% CO_2 increases the pressure drop by 10%. On the inclined manometer, 16 cm of scale is equivalent to 8% CO_2, and the response time is 4 min for this range of carbon dioxide.

THE NITROGEN ANALYZER

The nitrogen analyzer measures the concentration of nitrogen in a volume of gas. In respiratory studies, this instrument is employed to measure the functional residual capacity (FRC) and residual volume (RV) of the lungs.

The nitrogen analyzer operates on the principle of spectral emission. Perhaps the most familiar example of this phenomenon is the color that is imparted to a flame when an ionizable substance is placed in it. For example, sprinkling salt into a Bunsen burner flame causes it to emit a brilliant yellow-orange glow due to the presence of sodium ions. By analyzing the color spectrum emitted by ionized substances, it is possible to identify the type and amount of material present.

Lilly et al. (1943) induced nitrogen gas to emit its characteristic spectrum by drawing the gas sample to be analyzed into a cylindrical glass tube capped by two hollow electrodes and maintained at a low pressure by a vacuum pump; Fig. 52 illustrates the principle. The gas to be analyzed enters through a needle valve, and because of the continuous action of the vacuum pump the admitted gas sample appears in the cell at a pressure of about 1 mmHg. A high voltage derived from a constant-current dc power supply is applied to the electrodes, and the electric field produced thereby causes ionization of all the gases in the tube. The color spectrum emitted by the gases identifies each. Fortunately, with the respiratory gases (oxygen, nitrogen, carbon dioxide, and water vapor), the spectrum of nitrogen is dominant, being pinkish-blue in color. With the appropriate filter in front of the photodetector, only the spectrum of nitrogen is presented to the photodetector. Thus, the output of the photodetector is proportional to the percentage of nitrogen admitted into the spectral emission cell. Amplification and display via a meter or graphic recorder permits continuous recording of the nitrogen concentration presented to the inlet needle valve. Calibration of the nitrogen analyzer is accomplished by presenting known concentrations of nitrogen (in oxygen) to the inlet valve.

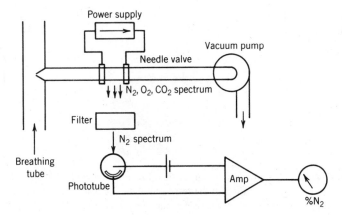

Figure 52   The nitrogen meter.

Certain practical points should be recognized. For example, the vacuum pump must be operated continuously to maintain a constant low pressure in the measuring cell. The current through the measuring cell must also be kept constant. To keep the response time as short as possible, the tube between the inlet needle valve and the measuring cell must be as short as possible and have a thick wall and small bore. The tube between the measuring cell and the vacuum pump can be any convenient length and size.

The Nitrogen-Washout Technique

Because nitrogen does not participate in respiration, it can be called a diluent. Inspired and expired air contain about 80% nitrogen, despite the fact that the concentration of oxygen and carbon dioxide vary according to the subject's metabolism. Between breaths, the functional residual capacity (FRC) of the lungs contains the same concentration of nitrogen as the environmental air, i.e., 80%. If the subject inspires from a spirometer filled with 100% oxygen and exhales into a second collecting spirometer, all of the nitrogen in the FRC can be replaced by oxygen; that is, the nitrogen will be "washed out" into the collecting spirometer. Measurement of the concentration of nitrogen in the collecting spirometer, along with a knowledge of its volume, permits calculation of the amount of nitrogen originally in the FRC and hence allows calculation of the FRC.

Figure 53 illustrates the arrangement of equipment for the nitrogen-washout test. The nitrogen analyzer is connected to the mouthpiece, and valve V is used to switch the subject from breathing environmental air to the measuring system. The spirometer on the left contains 100% oxygen, which is inhaled by the subject via the inspiratory check valve. A nose clip is applied so that all of the respired gases

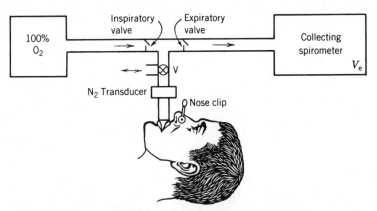

Figure 53   Arrangement of equipment for the nitrogen-washout technique. Valve V allows the subject to breathe room air until the test is started. The test is started by operating valve V at the end of a normal breath: The subject starts breathing 100% O_2 through the inspiratory valve and exhales the N_2 and O_2 mixture into a collecting spirometer via the expiratory valve.

flow through the tube connected to the mouthpiece. It is in this tube that the sampling inlet for the nitrogen analyzer is located. Thus, starting at the resting expiratory level, inhalation of pure oxygen causes the nitrogen analyzer to indicate zero. Expiration closes the inspiratory valve and opens the expiratory valve. The first expired breath contains nitrogen derived from the functional residual capacity (diluted by the oxygen that was inspired); the nitrogen analyzer indicates this percentage. The exhaled gases are collected in the spirometer on the right. The collecting spirometer and all of the interconnecting tubing are first flushed with oxygen to eliminate all nitrogen. This simple procedure eliminates the need to apply corrections and facilitates calculation of the FRC. With continued breathing, the nitrogen analyzer indicates less and less nitrogen because it is being washed out of the FRC and replaced by oxygen. Figure 54 illustrates a typical record from a normal subject of the diminishing concentration of nitrogen during the early part of the test. In most laboratories, the test is continued until the concentration of nitrogen falls to about 1%. The nitrogen recording permits identification of this concentration. In normal subjects, virtually all of the nitrogen can be washed out of the FRC in about 2–3 min.

If the peaks on the nitrogen-washout record are joined, a smooth exponential decay curve is obtained in normal subjects. A semilogarithmic plot of N_2 concentration versus time provides a straight line. In subjects with trapped air or poorly ventilated alveoli, the nitrogen-washout curve consists of several exponentials as the poorly ventilated regions give up their nitrogen. In such subjects, the time taken to wash out all of the nitrogen usually exceeds 10 min. Thus, the nitrogen concentration–time curve provides useful diagnostic information on the ventilatory activity of the alveoli.

If it is assumed that all of the collected (washed-out) nitrogen was uniformly distributed within the lungs, it is easy to calculate the functional residual capacity. If the environmental air contains 80% nitrogen, then the volume of nitrogen in the FRC is 0.8 FRC. Since the volume of gas in the collecting spirometer is known,

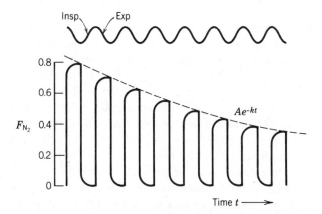

Figure 54   The nitrogen-washout curve.

it is only necessary to determine the concentration of nitrogen in this volume. To do so merely requires admitting some of this gas to the inlet valve of the nitrogen analyzer. Note that this concentration of nitrogen (F_{N_2}) exists in a volume that includes the volume of air expired (V_E) plus the original volume of oxygen in the collecting spirometer (V_0) at the start of the test and the volume of the tubing (V_t) leading from the expiratory collecting valve. It is therefore advisable to start with an empty collecting spirometer ($V_0 = 0$). Usually the tubing volume V_t is negligible compared to the volume of expired gas collected. In this situation the volume of nitrogen collected is $F_{N_2}V_E$, where F_{N_2} is the concentration. Therefore,

$$0.80 \, \text{FRC} = F_{N_2}V_E$$

and

$$\text{FRC} = F_{N_2} \frac{V_E}{0.80}.$$

It is important to note that the FRC so obtained is for lung gases at ambient temperature and pressure and saturated with water vapor (ATPS). In respiratory studies, this value is converted to body temperature and saturation with water vapor (BTPS).

In the example shown in Fig. 54, the washout to 1% N_2 took 44 breaths. With a breathing rate of 12 breaths/min, the washout time was 220 sec. The expired volume collected (V_E) was 22 L, and the concentration of nitrogen (F_{N_2}) in the collecting spirometer was 0.085. Therefore,

$$\text{FRC} = \frac{0.085 \times 22}{0.80} = 2.337 \, \text{L}.$$

MASS SPECTROMETER

The mass spectrometer is an instrument that can be used to analyze the composition of the gases of respiration as well as many encountered in anesthesia. While the instrument has been employed by physicists for some time, its use in physiology and medicine is more recent. Although not a complex instrument in principle, its size, weight, and cost, along with the need for accessory equipment and a trained operator, are probably the reasons for its limited popularity in the biosciences. Now that smaller, less expensive, and simpler instruments are becoming available commercially, their use in respiratory studies is beginning to increase, particularly in anesthesia monitoring, where one mass spectrometer is time-shared by several operating rooms, with sampling lines connecting the patients to the instrument. Perhaps the most valuable feature of the mass spectrometer is its ability to identify the concentration of a single gas species in a complex mixture of gases.

The principle underlying the operation of the mass spectrometer is simple. The gas molecules to be measured are bombarded by electrons to produce positive ions, which are then accelerated by a strong electric field. The rapidly moving ions then pass through a magnetic field which causes them to travel with a curved trajectory that is defined by the mass-to-charge ratio. The curvature of the trajectory is least for the heaviest ions. Therefore by strategic location of an electrode, the individual species of ions can be collected, the ion current being proportional to the number of ionized molecules of that particular species.

In a practical application, the gas mixture to be analyzed is drawn through a small sampling orifice into an ionizing chamber maintained constantly at a very low pressure (e.g., 10^{-4}–10^{-7} torr). In the chamber the gas mixture is bombarded, as shown in Fig. 55, by a stream of high-velocity electrons emitted from a hot cathode. The electron gun configuration is not unlike that found in many cathode ray tubes. The gas molecules, which become ionized and positively charged, are given a high velocity by an accelerating voltage applied to an electrode with a hole. The high-velocity ions then encounter a magnetic field (h, h), which causes them to assume a curved trajectory. The radius of the trajectory of each charged particle depends on its speed, mass, and charge, and the strength of the magnetic field. The radius of curvature r is

$$r = \sqrt{\frac{2V}{h^2} \times \frac{m}{e}},$$

where V is the accelerating voltage, h is the magnitude of the magnetic field, and m/e is the mass-to-charge ratio. If the accelerating and deflecting forces are kept constant, the trajectory will vary with the molecular mass, the heaviest giving the least curvature and the lightest, the greatest. In this way, the ion stream is split up into beams of different molecular masses. Electrodes placed at appropriate locations in the chamber can detect an ion current that is proportional to the amount of the mass component present in the gas mixture admitted to the spectrometer.

It should be obvious that there are at least two ways of using the principle just

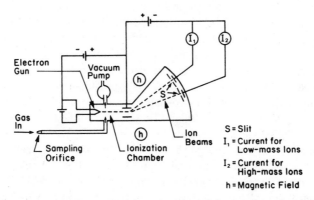

Figure 55   Principle underlying operation of the mass spectrometer.

described. One method is to use multiple electrodes to collect the ion currents produced by each ionic species. Another method employs a fixed electrode, and the accelerating voltage can be varied to cause the ions of different masses to be sequentially collected by a single electrode. Such instruments are called scanning spectrometers. Other methods have been devised and are well described by Khandipur (1981).

Among the earliest to press the mass spectrometer into service in physiology were Hunter et al. (1949). Their instrument continuously analyzed N_2, O_2, and CO_2. Miller et al. (1950) developed a smaller scanning instrument for monitoring respiratory gases. Instead of using multiple electrodes for the several ion beams, they varied the accelerating voltage to cause each beam to impinge on a single ion-collecting electrode; CO_2, N_2O, and O_2 were recorded during anesthesia, one reading for each gas being indicated every 20 sec. Fowler and Hugh-Jones (1957) developed a 25-Hz scanning instrument that analyzed CO_2, O_2, N_2, and argon. Three presentation systems for the data were provided: (1) The mass spectrum showing instantaneous N_2, O_2, CO_2, and Ar was displayed on the face of a cathode ray tube; (2) four meters indicated the amounts of the four gases; and (3) a four-channel pen-writer recorded their concentrations.

Primarily as a result of upper atmosphere research in the space program, O'Halloran (1961) described the Bendix rapidly responding, six-channel, time-of-flight (TOF) mass spectrometer, which is well suited for the detection of the respiratory gases. The output of any of the five channels can be preset for any mass below 500, while the sixth continuously scans masses in the same range. O'Halloran presented continuous breath-by-breath records of CO_2, N_2, H_2O vapor, and O_2. The response time was 60 msec for 0–90% response.

As stated previously, the mass spectrometer is seeing increased use in monitoring during the administration of anesthesia (Sodal and Swanson, 1982). In this application, a single mass spectrometer is connected sequentially to the airways of many patients; thus the device can be time shared. The long sampling lines cause the response times to be long. Sometimes complications arise at the sampling orifice, which can become clogged due to the high vapor/mucous environment at the sampling site. However, this multiple use of a mass spectrometer probably justifies the need for a technician to maintain the system.

Fowler and Hugh-Jones (1957) evaluated the characteristics of mass spectrometers available then. They also provided useful design goals for manufacturers. For example, they advocated a mass resolution $(M/\Delta M)$ of more than 20, i.e., 5% mass discrimination. They also recommended a response time of 0.1 sec or less to accommodate breath-by-breath analysis. They pointed out the difficulties of long sampling lines and advocated a two-stage vacuum system to obtain the shortest response time under these conditions. They also identified improvements needed in the sampling and vacuum systems.

Sodal et al. (1983) also examined the limitations of existing mass spectrometers and developed a unit that eliminated many of them. For example, to control the vacuum, a piezoelectrically controlled sampling valve was developed. The feedback to control the valve was derived from the ion current. They also recommended locating the ion chamber in the respiratory airstream to obtain the shortest response time.

The main advantage of the mass spectrometer is its ability to identify a single gas species in a complex mixture. Incredibly small amounts of a gas can be identified easily. However, the use of a mass spectrometer has several limitations in respiratory physiology. For example, it is unable to distinguish between different gases with the same molecular weights; e.g., CO (12 + 16) and N_2 (2 × 14) are indistinguishable. While this is not a problem in ordinary respiratory studies, when a mass spectrometer is used with anesthetic gases this potential source of error must always be borne in mind. Another drawback is the long response time when a long sampling line is used. For respiratory studies, a breath-by-breath response time is needed. With a long sampling tube, this is not possible. Moreover, the transit time is different for the different gases, which makes it difficult to conduct studies in which appearance and disappearance times are important. Finally, it is difficult to obtain a sampling orifice that maintains a constant-diameter opening in the face of small temperature changes.

VELOCITY-OF-SOUND ANALYZER

One distinguishing property of each of the respiratory and anesthetic gases is the velocity of sound through it. Measurement of this parameter has been used to create detectors for respiratory and anesthetic gases, notably nitrous oxide and ether. Dublin et al. (1939) described the use of a tuning fork and a resonating tube, the length of which could be adjusted by varying the level of water in it, to determine the half-wave resonant length and thus calculate the velocity of sound. With a fixed frequency, the length of the tube for resonance is dependent on the gas mixture filling the tube. At the shortest length for resonance, the length is $\lambda/2$, where λ is the wavelength of the sound wave. The velocity of sound is related to the resonant wavelength by the relationship

$$v = f\lambda,$$

where v = the velocity (m/sec), and
f = the frequency of the sound wave (Hz).

The velocity of sound is intimately related to the gas by the expression

$$v = \gamma P/d,$$

where γ = ratio of specific heats at constant pressure and constant volume and depends on the type of gas,
P = pressure (dyn/cm^2), and
d = density (g/cm^3).

TABLE 12   Velocity of Sound in Gases

Gas	Velocity (m/sec)	Ratio of Specific Heats γ
Air	331.7	—
O_2	317.2	1.401
N_2	337.8	1.404
Ether (vap)	179.2	—
Nitrous oxide	261.8	—
Carbon dioxide	258.0	—
Helium	960.	1.66
Water vapor	404.8	—

Dublin et al. (1939), Faulconer et al. (1943), and Faulconer and Ridley (1950) gave the velocities and ratios of specific heats for the various gases; Table 12 presents a summary. The range of velocities is adequate to permit use of the principle for detecting some of the respiratory and anesthetic gases. The method described by Dublin et al. (1939) was applied to the analysis of mixtures of O_2, N_2, and He. The amount of oxygen present was analyzed by chemical means, and a nomograph was drawn up to show the velocity of sound with varying mixtures of N_2 and He. Faulconer et al. (1943) used the same principle to develop an apparatus for O_2, N_2O, and ether vapor, the ether vapor first being removed by absorption. Instead of a water level to adjust the length of the resonating column, they used a movable piston. The tuning fork was replaced by a sound source energized by an oscillator–amplifier system.

Faulconer (1949) added practicality to the use of the sound-velocity method by eliminating the need to manually adjust the length of the resonating column, thereby permitting continuous monitoring of gas concentration. This he achieved by constructing the resonating chamber with a sound reproducer at one end and a microphone at the other. They were connected by an amplifier having a gain of 1000. Thus the system self-oscillated at a frequency dependent on the length of the resonating tube and the sound velocity of the gas in it. With the tube dimensions fixed, the frequency of oscillations reflected the velocity of the gas, which in turn was related to gas composition. As the gas composition changed, an electronic frequency meter indicated the frequency change. A similar method was reported by Stott (1957).

Faulconer (1949) used the sound-velocity technique to develop an interesting ether meter. He found that different mixtures of ether vapor and air gave slightly different readings. After investigating all of the variables he constructed a calibration curve that corrected for the partial pressure of oxygen. A Pauling paramagnetic oxygen analyzer was employed to determine the oxygen partial pressure. After making all corrections, Faulconer was able to state that, in practice, the ether meter readings were "probably within ±5 mm partial pressure for a partial pressure of ether vapor within the range 0–200 mm." Using a more elaborate instrument of similar design, Faulconer and Ridley (1950) determined the frequency changes for various mixtures of nitrous oxide, oxygen, and ether. They stated that with an auxiliary oxygen analyzer the components of a four-gas mixture could be continuously analyzed when the mixture contained O_2, N_2O, N_2, and ether vapor.

Use of the method based on the velocity of sound to identify a particular gas in a mixture has not been pursued. Although not ideally applicable to respiratory and anesthetic gas mixtures, it may have value when fewer gases are present.

REFERENCES

Albisser, A. M., B. S. Leibel, T. G. Ewart, Z. Davidovac, and W. Zingg. 1974a. An artificial endocrine pancreas. *Diabetes* **23**:389–396.

Albisser, A. M., B. S. Leibel, T. G. Ewart, Z. Davidovac, C. K. Butz, W. Zingg, H. Schipper, and R. Gander. 1974b. Clinical control of diabetes by the artificial pancreas. *Diabetes* **23**:397–404.

Albisser, A. M., B. S. Leibel, B. Zinman, F. T. Murray, W. Zingg, C. K. Botz, A. Denoga, and E. B. Marliss. 1977. Studies with an artificial pancreas. *Arch. Intern. Med.* **137**:639–649.

Baker, L. E. 1961. A rapidly responding, narrow-band, infra-red CO_2 analyzer for physiological studies. *IRE Trans. Biomed. Electron.* **BME-8**:16–24.

Band, D. M., and S. J. G. Semple. 1967. Continuous measurement of blood pH with an indwelling arterial glass electrode. *J. Appl. Physiol.* **22**:854–857.

Bergman, N. A., H. Rarkow, and M. J. Fruman. 1958. Collision broadening effect of nitrous oxide upon infra-red analyzers of carbon dioxide during anesthesia. *Anesthesiology* **19**:19–26.

Bergveld, P. 1970. Development of an ion-sensitive, solid-state device for neurophysiological measurements. *IEEE Trans. Biomed. Eng.* **BME-17**:70–71.

Bergveld, P. 1972. Development, operation, and application of the ion-sensitive, field-effect transistor as a tool for electrophysiology. *IEEE Trans. Biomed. Eng.* **BME-19**(5):342–351.

Bergveld, P., J. Wiersma, and H. Meertens. 1976. Extracellular potential recordings by means of a field effect transistor without gate metal, called OSFET. *IEEE Trans Biomed. Eng.* **BME-23**(2):136–144.

Bernstein, L., and D. Meindel. 1951. The accuracy of spirographic recording at high respiratory rate. *Thorax* **6**:297–309.

Bessman, S. P., and R. D. Schultz. 1972. Sugar electrode sensor for the "artificial pancreas." *Horm. Metab. Res.* **4**:413–417.

Bessman, S. P., and R. D. Schultz. 1973. Prototype glucose-oxygen sensor for the artificial pancreas. *Trans.—Am. Soc. Artif. Intern. Organs* **19**:361–364.

Brems, N. 1962. Measurement of pH electrodes and pertinent apparatus. *Acta Anesthesiol. Scand.* **6**(Suppl. 11):199–206.

Broekhuyse, H. M., J. D. Nelson, B. Zinman, and A. M. Albisser. 1981. Comparison of algorithms for the closeed-loop control of blood glucose using the artificial beta cell. *IEEE Trans. Biomed. Eng.* **BME-28**(10):678–687.

Bronk, D. W., M. A. Larrabee, and P. W. Davies. 1946. The rate of O_2 consumption in localized regions of the nervous system in presynaptic endings in cell bodies. *Fed. Proc.* **5**:11.

Bronk, D. W., F. Brink, C. M. Connelly, F. D. Carlson, and P. W. Davies. 1947. The time course of recovery of oxygen consumption in nerve. *Fed. Proc.* **6**:83–84.

Bull, H. B. 1943. *Physical Biochemistry.* Wiley, New York.

Bull, H. B. 1964. *An Introduction to Physical Biochemistry.* Davis, Philadelphia, PA.

Bullock, B. W., and S. J. Silverman. 1950. A rapid scanning spectrophotometer for oxcillographic presentation in the near infra-red. *J. Opt. Soc. Am.* **40**:608–615.

Carlson, F. D., F. Brink, and D. W. Bronk. 1948. A method for direct measurement of rate of O_2 utilization by nerve. *Fed. Proc.* **7**:18.

Cater, D. B., A. F. Phillips, and I. A. Silver. 1957a. Apparatus and techniques for the measurement of oxidation-reduction potentials, pH and oxygen tension *in vivo*. *Proc. R. Soc. London, Ser. B.* **146**:289-297.

Cater, D. B., A. F. Phillips, and I. A. Silver. 1957b. The measurement of oxidation-reduction potentials, pH and oxygen tension in tumors. *Proc. R. Soc. London Ser. B.* **146**:382-399.

Cater, D. B., A. F. Phillips, and I. A. Silver. 1957c. Induced changes in oxidation-reduction potentials, pH and oxygen tension in the intact lactating mammary gland. *Proc. R. Soc. London Ser. B* **146**:400-415.

Chang, K. W., S. Aisenberg, J. S. Soeldner, and J. M. Hiebert. 1973. Validation and bioengineering aspects of an implantable glucose sensor. *Trans.—Am. Soc. Artif. Intern. Organs* **19**:352-360.

Cheung, P. W., W. H. Ko, D. J. Fung, and S. H. Wong. 1978. Theory fabrication, testing and chemical response of ion-sensitive, field-effect transistor devices. In *Theory, Design and Applications of Solid-State Chemical Sensors*. P. W. Cheung and D. G. Fleming (eds.). CRC Press, Boca Raton, FL, 296 pp.

Clark, L. C. 1956. Monitor and control of blood and tissue oxygen tensions. *Trans.—Am. Soc. Artif. Intern. Organs* **2**:41-48.

Clark, L. C. 1962. Electrode systems for continuous monitoring in cardiovascular surgery. *Ann. N.Y. Acad. Sci.* **102**:29-45.

Clark, L. C. 1970. Membrane polarographic electrode system and method with electrochemical compensation. U.S. Patent 3,539,455, November 10.

Clark, L. C. 1978. The future of enzyme electrodes. In *Theory, Design and Biomedical Applications of Solid State Chemical Sensors*. P. W. Cheung and D. G. Fleming (eds.). CRC Press, Boca Raton, FL, 296 pp.

Clark, L. C. 1979. The hydrogen peroxide sensing platinum electrode. *Methods Enzymol.* **56**(Part G):448-479.

Clark, L. C., and C. A. Duggan. 1982. Implanted enzymatic glucose sensors. *Diabetes Care* **5**(3):174-180.

Clark, L. C., and G. Misrahy. 1957. Chronically implanted polarograph electrodes. *Fed. Proc.* **16**:22-23.

Clark, L. C., and L. K. Noyes. 1984. Theoretical and practical bases for implantable glucose sensors with special reference to the peritoneum. *Proc. Symp. on Biosensors, 1984* pp. 69-74.

Clark, L. C., and G. Sachs. 1968. Bioelectrodes for tissue metabolism. *Ann. N.Y. Acad. Sci.* **148**:133-153.

Clark, L. C., G. Misrahy, and R. P. Fox. 1958. Chronically implanted polarographic electrodes. *J. Appl. Physiol.* **13**:85-91.

Covington, A. K. 1979. *Ion-Selective Electrode Methodology*. CRC Press, Boca Raton, FL, 257 pp.

Davies, P. W. 1946. Rapid bursts of oxygen consumption in stimulated muscle. *Fed. Proc.* **5**:21-22.

Davies, P. W. 1962. The oxygen cathode. In *Physical Techniques in Biological Research*, Vol. IV. W. L. Nastuk (ed.). Academic Press, New York, 410 pp.

Davies, P. W., and F. Brink. 1942a. Direct measurement of brain oxygen concentration with platinum electrode. *Fed. Proc.* **1**:19.

Davies, P. W., and F. Brink. 1942b. Microelectrodes for measuring local oxygen tension in animal tissues. *Rev. Sci. Instrum.* **130**:524-532.

Davies, P. W., W. S. McCulloch, and E. Roseman. 1943-1944. Rapid changes in the O_2 tension of cerebral cortex during induced convulsions. *Am. J. Psychiatry* **100**:825-829.

Davies, P. W., R. G. Grenell, and D. W. Bronk. 1948. The time course of *in vivo* oxygen consumption of cerebral cortex following electrical stimulation. *Fed. Proc* **7**:25.

Dole, M., R. M. Roberts, and C. E. Holley. 1941. The theory of the glass electrode. V. The influence of negative ions. *J. Am. Chem. Soc.* **63**:725–730.

Dublin, W. B., W. M. Boothby, and M. Williams. 1939. Determination of the velocity of sound in gas. Application to analyses of mixtures of oxygen, helium and nitrogen. *Proc. Staff Meet. Mayo Clin.* **14**:588–592.

Dubuisson, M. 1937a. A method for recording pH changes of muscle during activity. *J. Physiol.* **90**:47p–48p.

Dubuisson, M. 1937b. pH changes in muscle during and after contraction. *Proc. Soc. Exp. Biol. Med.* **35**:609–611.

Dusser de Barenne, J. C., W. S. McCulloch, and L. F. Nims. 1937. Functional activity and pH of the cerebral cortex. *J. Cell. Comp. Physiol.* **10**:277–289.

Eisenman, G. 1967. The origin of the glass-electrode potential. In *Glass Electrodes for Hydrogen and Other Cations—Principles and Practice.* G. Eisenman (ed.). Dekker, New York.

Eisenman, G., D. O. Rudin, and J. U. Casby. 1957. Glass electrode for measuring sodium ion. *Science* **126**:831–834.

Fastie, W. G., and A. H. Pfund. 1947. Selective infra-red gas analyzers. *J. Opt. Soc. Am.* **37**:762–768.

Faulconer, A. 1949. A study of physical methods for the determination of the tension of ether vapor in air-ether mixtures. *Anesthesiology* **10**:1–14.

Faulconer, A., and R. W. Ridley. 1950. Continuous quantative analyses of mixtures of oxygen, nitrous oxide and ether with and without nitrogen. *Anesthesiology* **11**:265–278.

Faulconer, A., F. C. Clarke, and A. E. Osterberg. 1943. An apparatus for the clinical determination of percentage constituents of anesthetic gas mixtures. *Proc. Staff Meet. Mayo Clin.* **18**:89–93.

Fowler, K. T., and P. Hugh-Jones. 1957. Mass spectrometry applied to clinical practice and research. *Br. Med. J.* **1**:1205–1211.

Fowler, R. C. 1949. Rapid infra-red gas analyzer. *Rev. Sci. Instrum.* **20**:175–178.

Frant, M. S., and S. W. Ross. 1966. Electrode for sensing fluoride-ion activity in solution. *Science* **154**:1553–1554.

Friedman, S. M., J. D. Jamieson, J. A. M. Hinkle, and C. L. Friedman. 1958. Use of glass electrode for measuring sodium ion in biological mixtures. *Proc. Soc. Exp. Biol. Med.* **99**:727–730.

Friedman, S. M., J. D. Jamieson, J. A. M. Hinkle, and C. L. Friedman. 1959. Drug-induced changes in blood pressure and in blood sodium as measured by glass electrode. *Am. J. Physiol.* **196**:1049–1052.

Fruhling, G., and H. Winterstein. 1934. Registrierung der pH in stromenden Blut. *Pfluegers Arch. Gesamte Physiol.* **233**:475–485.

Gardner, T. R. C., and I. A. Silver. 1979. A simple enzyme polarographic glucose sensor. *J. Physiol.* **295**:6P.

Gesell, R., and A. B. Hertzman. 1926. Regulation of respiration. *Am. J. Physiol.* **78**:206–223.

Glasstone, S. 1946. *The Elements of Physical Chemistry.* Van Nostrand, Princeton, NJ.

Gotoh, F., J. S. Meyer, and S. Ebihara. 1966. Continuous recording of human cerebral blood flow and metabolism: methods for electronic monitoring of arterial and venous gases and electrolytes. *Med. Res. Eng.* **5**(2):13–19.

Hamilton, C. H., and R. C. Kory. 1958. Evaluation of spirometers used in pulmonary function studies. *Physiologist* **1**(4):32–33.

Hersch, P. A. 1965. Method and means for oxygen analysis of gases. U.S. Patent 3,223,597, December 14.

Hertz, C. H., and B. Siesjö. 1959. A rapid and sensitive electrode for continuous measurement of pCO_2 in liquids and tissue. *Acta Physiol. Scand.* **47**:115–123.

Huch, A., and R. Huch. 1976. Transcutaneous noninvasive monitoring of pO_2. *Hosp. Pract.* (June):43–51.

Huch, R., A. Huch, and D. W. Lübbers. 1973. Transcutaneous measurement of blood pO_2. *J. Perinat. Med.* **1**:183–191.

Huch, R., D. W. Lubbers, and A. Huch. 1974. Reliability of transcutaneous monitoring of arterial pO_2 in newborn infants. *Arch. Dis. Child.* **49**:213–218.

Huch, R., A. Huch, M. Albane et al. 1976. Transcutaneous pO_2 monitoring in routine management of infants and children with cardiorespiratory problems. *Pediatrics* **57**:681–690.

Hunter, J. A., R. W. Stacy, and F. A. Hitchcock. 1949. A mass spectrometer for continuous gas analysis. *Rev. Sci. Instrum.* **20**:333–336.

Kadish, A. H. 1964. Automatic control of blood sugar. *Am. J. Med. Electron.* (Apr.–June):81–86.

Kadish, A. H., and D. A. Hall. 1965. A new method for the continuous monitoring of blood glucose by measurement of dissolved oxygen. *Clin. Chem. (Winston-Salem, N.C.)* **11**:869–875.

Khandipur, R. 1981. *Handbook of Modern Analytical Instruments.* Tab Books, Blue Ridge Summit, PA, 580 pp.

Koller, L. R. 1952. *Ultraviolet Radiation.* Wiley, New York.

Kory, R., and L. H. Hamilton. 1963. Evaluation of sprirometers used in pulmonary-function studies. *Am. Rev. Respir. Dis.* **87**:228–238.

Kraegen, E. W., R. Whiteside, D. Bell, Y. O. Chia, and L. Lazarus. 1978. Development of a closed-loop artificial pancreas. In *Feedback Controlled and Programmed Insulin Infusion in Diabetes.* Thieme-Stratton, New York.

Kreuzer, F., T. R., Watson, and J. M. Ball. 1958. Comparative measurements with a new procedure for measuring the blood oxygen tensions *in vitro. J. Appl. Physiol.* **12**:65–70.

Ledig, P. G., and R. S. Lyman. 1927. An adaptation of the thermal conductivity method to the analysis of respiratory gases. *J. Clin. Invest.* **4**:495–505.

Lengyel, B., and E. Blum. 1934. The behavior of the glass electrode in connection with its chemical composition. *Trans. Faraday Soc.* **30**:461–471.

Lilly, J. C., T. F. Anderson, and J. F. Harvey. 1943. Nitrogen meter. *Natl. Res. Counc. Comm. Aviat. Med. Rep.* **299.**

Liston, M. 1950. Performance of a double-beam infra-red recording spectrophotometer. *J. Opt. Soc. Am.* **140**:93–101.

Lubbers, D. W., and N. Opitz. 1975. The pCO_2/pO_2 optode. *Z. Naturforsch., C: Biosci.* **30C**:532–533.

Lubbers, D. W., and N. Opitz. 1976. Quantitative fluorescence photometry with biological fluids and gases. *Adv. Exp. Med. Biol.* **75**:65–69.

Luft, K. F. 1943. Uber ein neue Methode der registrierung Gasanalyse mit Hilfe der absorption ultraroter Strahlen. *Z. Tech. Phys.* **24**:97–104.

Lyman, T. 1914. *The Spectropy of the Extreme Ultraviolet,* Monogr. Phys. Longmans Green, London.

Marshall, C., and L. F. Nims. 1937. Blood pH *in vivo.* II. Effects of acids, salts, dextrose and adrenalin. *Yale J. Biol. Med.* **10**:561–564.

Matsuo, T., and K. Wise. 1974. An integrated field-effect electrode for biopotential recording. *IEEE Trans. Biomed. Eng.* **BME-21**:485–486.

Mattock, G., and D. M. Band. 1967. Interpretation of pH and cation measurements. In *Glass Electrodes.* G. Eisenman (ed). Dekker, New York.

McClendon, J. F. 1915. New hydrogen electrode and rapid method of determining hydrogen ion concentrations. *Am. J. Physiol.* **38**:180–185.

McKinley, B. A., J. Saffle, W. J. Jordan, J. Janata, S. D. Moss, and D. E. Westenskow. 1980. In vivo continuous monitoring of K^+ in animals using ISFET probes. *Med. Instrum.* **14**(2):93–97.

McKinley, B. A., K. C. Wong, J. Janata, W. S. Jordan, and D. R. Westerkow. 1981. In vivo continuous monitoring of ionized calcium ion in dogs using ion-sensitive field effect transistors. *CRC Crit. Care Med.* **9**(4):334–339.

Mead, J. 1955. Critical orifice CO_2 analyzer suitable for student use. *Science* **121**:103–104.

Miller, F., A. Hemingway, A. O. Nier, R. T. Knight, E. B. Brown, and R. L. Vasco. 1950. The development of certain clinical applications for a portable mass spectrometer. *J. Thorac. Surg.* **20**:714–720.

Moss, S. D., J. Janata, and C. C. Johnson. 1975. Potassium ion-sensitive field effect transistor. *Anal. Chem.* **47**(13):2238–2243.

Moss, S. D., C. C. Johnson, and J. Janata. 1978. Hydrogen, calcium and potassium ion-sensitive FET transducers: A preliminary report. *IEEE Trans. Biomed. Eng.* **BME-25**(1):44–59.

Niebauer, M., L. A. Geddes, and C. F. Babbs. 1986. Defibrillator shock-induced K^+ efflux from myocardial cells. *Med. Instrum.* **20**(3):135–137.

Nims, L. F. 1937. Glass electrodes and apparatus for direct recording of pH *in vivo*. *Yale J. Biol. Med.* **10**:241–246.

Nims, L. F., and C. Marshall. 1937. Blood pH *in vivo*. 1. Changes due to respiration. *Yale J. Biol. Med.* **10**:445–448.

Nims, L. F., C. Marshall, and H. S. Burr. 1938. The measurement of pH in circulating blood. *Science* **87**:197–198.

O'Halloran, G. J. 1961. A rapid-response mass spectrometer for respiratory function analysis. *Clinic on Instrumentation Requirements for Psychological for Psychological Research. Lafayette Clinic, Detroit, Michigan. May 16–17, 1961.* Sponsored by Fund for Instrumentation Education and Research, New York.

Olson, R. A., F. S. Brackett, and R. G. Crickard. 1949. Oxygen tension measurement by a method of time selection using the static platinum electrode with alternating potential. *J. Gen. Physiol.* **32**:681–703.

Passey, R. B. et al. 1977. Evaluation and comparison of 10 glucose methods and the reference method recommended in the proposed product class standard. *Clin. Chem. (Winston-Salem, N.C.)* **23**(1):131–139.

Pauling, L., R. E. Wood, and L. H. Sturdevant. 1949. An instrument for determining the partial pressure of oxygen in a gas. *Science* **103**:338.

Peterson, J. L., S. A. Goldstein, R. V. Fitzgerald, and D. K. Buckhold. 1980. Fiberoptic pH probe for physiological use. *Anal. Chem.* **52**:864–869.

Pfeiffer, E. E., C. Thum, and A. H. Clemens. 1974. An artificial beta cell. *Horm. Metab. Res.* **6**:339–342.

Postemak, J. M., M. A. Larrabee, and D. W. Bronk. 1947. Oxygen requirements of the neurones in sympathetic ganglia. *Fed. Proc.* **6**:182.

Rein, H. 1933. Elin Gaswechelschrieber. *Naunyn-Schmiedeberg Arch. Exp. Pathol. Pharmakol.* **171**:363–402.

Rein, H. 1944. Magnetsche O_2 Analyze in *Gasgemischen. Pfluegers Arch. Gesamte Physiol.* **247**:576–592.

Reyes, R. J., and J. R. Neville. 1967. An electrochemical technic for measuring carbon dioxide content of blood. *USAF Sch. Aerosp. Med. Tech. Rep.* **SAM-TR-67-23**.

Ross, J. W. 1967. Calcium-selective electrode with liquid ion exchanger. *Science* **156**:1378–1379.

Santiago, J. V., A. H. Clemens, W. L. Clarke, and D. M. Kipnis. 1978. Closed-loop and open-loop devices for blood glucose control in normal and diabetic subjects. *Diabetes* **28**(1):71–81.

Seitz, W. R. 1984. Chemical sensors based on optical fibers *Anal. Chem.* **56**:16A.

Severinghaus, J. W. 1962. Electrodes for blood and gas pCO_2, pO_2, and blood pH. *Acta Anaesthesiol. Scand.* **6**(Suppl. IX):207–220.

Severinghaus, J. W., and A. F. Bradley. 1958. Electrodes for blood pO_2 and pCO_2 determination. *J. Appl. Physiol.* **13**:515–520.

Shichiri, M., R. Kawamori, Y. Yamasaki, N. Hakui, N. Asakawa, and H. Abe. 1985. Needle-type glucose sensor for wearable artificial endocrine pancreas. In *Implantable Sensors for Closed-Loop Prosthetic Systems*. W. Ko (ed.). Futura Publ. Co., Mt. Kisco, NY.

Siggard-Andersen, O. 1962. The pH–log pCO_2 blood acid–base nomogram revised. *Scan. J. Clin. Lab. Invest.* **14**:598–604.

Siggaard-Andersen, O., and K. Engel. 1960. A new acid-base nomogram an improved method for the calculation of the relevant blood acid-base data. *Scand. J. Clin. Lab. Invest.* **12**:177–186.

Silver, I. A. 1976. An ultra micro glucose electrode. In *Ion and Enzyme Electrodes in Biology and Medicine*. M. Kessler, L. C. Clark, D. W. Lubbers, I. A. Silver, and W. Simon (eds.). Urban & Schwarzenberg, Munich.

Sodal, I. E., and G. D. Swanson. 1982. Making the mass spectrometer an efficient anesthetist's aide. *EMB Mag.* (March):32–35.

Sodal, I. E., G. D. Swanson, A. J. Micco, F. Sprague, and D. G. Ellis. 1983. A computerized mass spectrometer and flowmeter system for respiratory gas measurement. *Ann. Biomed. Eng.* **11**:83–99.

Stead, W. W., H. S. Wells, N. L. Gault, and J. Ognanovich. 1959. Inaccuracy of conventional water-filled spirometer for recording rapid breathing. *J. Appl. Physiol.* **14**:448–450.

Stott, F. D. 1957. Sonic gas analyzer for measurement of CO_2 on expand air. *Rev. Sci. Instrum.* **28**:914–915.

Stow, R. W., and B. F. Randall. 1954. Electrical measurement of pCO_2 in blood. *Am. J. Physiol.* **179**:678.

Stow, R. W., R. F. Baer, and B. F. Randall. 1957. Rapid measurement of the tension of carbon dioxide in blood. *Arch. Phys. Med. Rehabil.* **38**:646–650.

Tobias, J. M. 1949. Syringe oxygen cathode for measurement of oxygen tension in solution and respiratory gases. *Rev. Sci. Instrum.* **20**:519–523.

Tobias, J. M., and R. Holmes. 1947. Observation on the use of the oxygen cathode. *Fed. Proc.* **6**:215.

Towe, B. C., and E. J. Gilbeau. 1985. A glucose sensor using a thin-film thermopile. *Proc. Annu. Conf. Eng. Med. Biol.* **27**:93.

Updike, S. J., and G. P. Hicks. 1967. The enzyme electrode. *Nature* **214**:986–988.

Valeri, C. R., C. G., Zaroulis, L. Marchionni, and K. J. Path. 1972. A simple method for measuring oxygen content in blood. *J. Lab. Clin. Med.* **79**:1035–1040.

Voegtlin, C., F. F. De Eds, and H. Kahler. 1930. *Public Health Rep.* **45**:2222–2233.

Voegtlin, C. F., F. F. De Eds, and H. Kahler. 1935. *N.I.H. Bull.* **164**,(Part II):15–27.

von Lengyel, B., and E. Blum. 1934. The behavior of the glass electrode in connection with its chemical composition. *Trans. Faraday Soc.* **30**:461.

Vurek, G. G., P. J. Feustel, and J. W. Severinghaus. 1983. A fiberoptic pCO_2 sensor. *Ann. Biomed. Eng.* **11**:499–510.

Weil, J. V., I. E. Sodal, and R. P. Speck. 1967. A modified fuel cell for the analysis of oxygen concentration of gases. *J. Appl. Physiol.* **23**(3):419–422.

Wells, H. S., W. W. Stead, D. Rossing, and J. Ognanovich. 1959. Accuracy of an improved spirometer for recording fast breathing. *J. Appl. Physiol.* **14**:451–454.

White, J. W., and M. D. Liston. 1950. Construction of a double beam recording infra-red spectrophotometer. *J. Opt. Soc. Am.* **40**:29–85.

Wong, J. Y. 1978. Measuring gaseous oxygen with UV absorption. U. S. Patent 4,096,388, June 20.

9

Electrodes

INTRODUCTION

Electrodes are used both for the measurement of bioelectric events and to deliver current to living tissue. In the former case, the electrode current density is very low, but in the latter it is quite high. In performing these functions, an electrode may establish ohmic contact with the tissue, or the mode of communication may be capacitive. Capacitive electrodes have been used for measuring bioelectric events and for stimulation. Apart from a few specialized uses (e.g., electrosurgery and diathermy) they are fairly uncommon. The most frequently encountered electrodes establish ohmic contact with tissue via an electrolyte. The properties of these electrodes will receive extensive coverage in this chapter.

Although much is known about the properties of electrode–electrolyte–tissue interfaces, it is not possible at present to predict the electrical properties of this structure with accuracy. The characteristics of capacitively coupled electrodes are also discussed in this chapter. Because of the simpler interface with the tissue, it is possible to predict their electrical properties with fair accuracy. A third type of electrode is covered with a semipermeable membrane and functions as a chemical transducer. These are described in Chapter 8.

ELECTRODE–ELECTROLYTE INTERFACE

When a metallic electrode comes into contact with an electrolyte, an ion–electron exchange occurs. There is a tendency for metallic ions to enter into solution and a tendency for ions in the electrolyte to combine with the metallic electrode. Although the details of the reaction may be complex in a given situation, the net result is the existence of a charge distribution at the electrode–electrolyte interface. The spatial arrangement of the charge depends on the manner in which the electrode and electrolyte react. Several types of charge distribution have been proposed. The simplest was conceived by Helmholtz (1879), who postulated that there exists a layer of charge of one sign tightly bound to the electrode and a layer of charge of the opposite sign in the electrolyte. The separation between the two layers of charges (often called the electrical double layer) is of course measured in ionic dimensions. Figure 1a diagrams this concept. Gouy (1910) and Stern (1924) proposed different charge distributions as illustrated in Fig. 1b, c, and d.

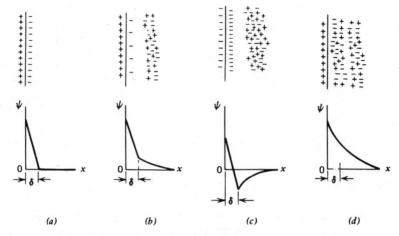

Figure 1 Various configurations of charge distribution and potentials at an electrode-electrolyte interface; (*a*) Helmholtz (1879), (*b*) Gouy (1910), (*c*) Stern (1924), (*d*) pure Gouy.

Parsons (1964) described electrodes in terms of the reactions at the double layer, referring to electrodes in which no net transfer of charge occurs across the metal-electrolyte interface as "perfectly polarized." Those in which unhindered exchange of charge is possible were called "perfectly nonpolarizable." Real electrodes have properties that lie between these idealized limits. MacInnes (1961) stated that the term "electrode polarization" is applied in two ways; first, as just stated and second, as the condition in which the electrode–electrolyte potential is altered by the passage of current.

In a conceptual sense, an electrode–electrolyte interface resembles a voltage source and a capacitor. However, it is well known that current can pass through an electrode–electrolyte interface. Therefore any electrical model for such an interface must include resistance, capacitance, and a potential. Figure 2 summarizes this concept. Although it is easy to identify these three components, it is by no means easy to create an accurate electrical model to include them because their magnitude depends on the electrode metal, its area, the electrolyte, temperature, current density, and the frequency of current used for measurement.

ELECTRODE POTENTIAL

The voltage developed at an electrode–electrolyte interface is designated the half-cell potential. The total voltage between a pair of electrode terminals is therefore the algebraic difference of the two half-cell potentials. Since it is impossible to measure the potential developed at a single electrode, an arbitrary standard electrode has been chosen, and electrode potentials are measured with respect to it. The standard electrode is the hydrogen electrode; it consists of a specially

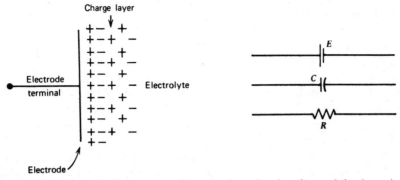

Charge layer

Electrode
terminal

Electrolyte

E

C

R

Electrode

Figure 2 The charge distribution at an electrode–electrolyte interface and the three circuit elements (voltage E, capacitance C, and resistance R) that can be used to describe it in terms of an electrical model.

prepared platinum surface in contact with a solution of hydrogen ions (of unit activity) and dissolved molecular hydrogen; the activity of the latter is specified by requiring it to be in equilibrium with hydrogen at 1 atm of pressure in the gas phase (Janz and Kelly, 1964). The potentials of many of the metals used for electrodes are listed in Table 1. Inspection of this table indicates that an appreciable voltage can be produced when dissimilar metals are employed.

TABLE 1   Electrode Potentials (E^0 values) for Commonly Used Materials in Electrodes

Metal and Reaction	Potential $(E^0_{25°C})$ (V)	Temperature Coefficient (mV/°C)
$Al = Al^{3+} + 3e$	-1.662	$+1.375$
$Zn = Zn^{2+} + 2e^-$	-0.7628	$+0.962$
$Zn(Hg) = Zn^{2+} + Hg + 2e^-$	-0.7627	$-$
$Cr = Cr^{3+} + 3e^-$	-0.744	$+1.339$
$Fe = Fe^{2+} + 2e^-$	-0.4402	$+0.923$
$Cd = Cd^{2+} + 2e^-$	-0.4029	$+0.778$
$Ni = Ni^{2+} + 2e^-$	-0.250	$+0.93$
$Pb = Pb^{2+} + 2e^-$	-0.126	$+0.420$
$Pt(H_2)H^+$	0	$-$
$Ag + Cl^- = AgCl + e^-$	$+0.2225$	$+0.213$
$Cu = Cu^{2+} + 2e^-$	$+0.337$	$+0.879$
$Cu = Cu^+ + e$	$+0.521$	$+0.813$
$2 Hg = Hg_2^{2+} + 2e^-$	$+0.788$	$-$
$Ag = Ag^+ + e^-$	$+0.7991$	-0.129
$Pt = Pt^{2+} + 2e^-$	$+1.2$ approx.	$-$
$Au = Au^{3+} + 3e^-$	$+1.498$	$-$
$Au = Au^+ + e^-$	$+1.691$	$-$

Source: A. J. de Bethune, in *Handbook of Electrochemistry.* C. A. Hampel (ed.). Reinhold, New York, 1964.

ELECTRODE POTENTIAL STABILITY

Table 1 indicates that a pair of electrodes of the same metal, placed in the same electrolyte, should produce no potential difference because the half-cell potentials are equal. In practice, however, it has been found that when this procedure is carried out and a high-gain recording of the potential difference is made, there appears a net potential difference that is not constant. Several investigators have performed such an experiment to evaluate the stability of various pairs of electrodes. Table 2 presents the results.

Inspection of Table 2 shows that zinc and amalgamated (mercury-coated) zinc electrodes exhibit large potential differences. Surprisingly, platinum exhibits a large potential. It would appear that in the practical construction of electrodes something has been overlooked. More will be said on this later; in the meantime, it should be noted that such fluctuating noise potentials have sometimes been eliminated by connecting the electrodes together and allowing them to reach a stable equilibrium with the electrolyte. This technique has been employed by electrophysiologists. A related observation has been that newly prepared electrodes are often noisy when placed in an electrolyte, but with the passage of time the noise decreases.

The subject of electrode potential stability was investigated by Aronson and Geddes (1985). They demonstrated that a pair of electrolytically clean electrodes of the same metal were stable when placed in 0.9% saline. However, the intro-

TABLE 2   Fluctuations in Potential Between Two Electrodes in an Electrolyte

Electrode Metal	Electrolyte	Potential Difference Between Electrodes	Reference
Calomel	Saline	1–20 μV	Greenwald (1936)
Zn–ZnSO$_4$	Saline	180 μV	Greenwald (1936)
Zn	Saline	450 μV	Greenwald (1936)
Stainless steel	Saline	10 mV	Lykken (1959)
Zn	Saline	100 mV	Lykken (1959)
ZnHg	Saline	82 mV	Lykken (1959)
Ag	Saline	94 mV	Lykken (1959)
AgHg	Saline	90 mV	Lykken (1959)
Ag–AgCl	Saline	2.5 mV	Lykken (1959)
Pb	Saline	1 mV	Lykken (1959)
PbHg	Saline	1 mV	Lykken (1959)
Pt	Saline	320 mV	Lykken (1959)
Ag, AgCl sponge	ECG paste	0.2 mV, 0.07 mV drift in 1 hr	O'Connell et al. (1960)
Ag, AgCl (11-mm disk)	ECG paste	0.47 mV, 1.88 mV drift in 1 hr	O'Connell et al. (1960)
Pb (11-mm disk)	ECG paste	4.9 mV, 3.70 mV drift in 1 hr	O'Connell et al. (1960)
Zn, ZnCl$_2$ (11-mm disk)	ECG paste	15.3 mV, 11.25 mV drift in 1 hr	O'Connell et al. (1960)

Source: L. A. Geddes, *Electrodes and the Measurement of Bioelectric Events*. Wiley, New York, 1972. (By permission.)

duction of a minute amount of contaminant of another metal on one electrode produced fluctuating potentials. Removal of the contaminant restored the electrodes to their stable condition.

Figure 3 illustrates the equipment used to record electrode potential fluctuations. Two electrodes of the same metal are connected to a high-gain, high-input-impedance recording system with a time constant of 3.2 sec and a high-frequency response extending to 60 Hz (-3 dB). The left side of Figs. 4 and 5 show the recordings obtained with two identical electrolytically clean electrodes. In the center of these figures are the records made with various metallic contaminants on a single electrode. On the right are the potential recordings after removal of the contaminant.

The foregoing study clearly demonstrates that even a tiny contaminant on a single, electrolytically clean electrode causes fluctuating current to flow in the electrolyte. Note that a foreign metal on a single electrode constitutes a short-circuited cell of dissimilar metals, which causes current to flow in the electrolyte, thereby creating a potential field between the electrodes. Unfortunately, such current flow is not stable and therefore the potential fluctuates.

A useful piece of information derives from the effect of mechanical disturbance. It has been found that electrodes relatively free of movement artifacts are of the recessed type, in which the electrode–electrolyte interface is removed from direct contact with the subject. Because the double layer is a region of charge gradient, which is a source of potential, disturbance of it gives rise to a change in voltage that, although small electrochemically, is often large with respect to the magnitude of bioelectric events. Movement artifacts produced by disturbance of the electrical double layer are in the frequency range of many of these events; hence filtering techniques can seldom be employed with success. Therefore the electrical stability

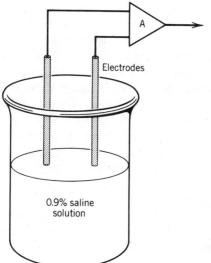

Figure 3 Apparatus for measuring electrode noise.

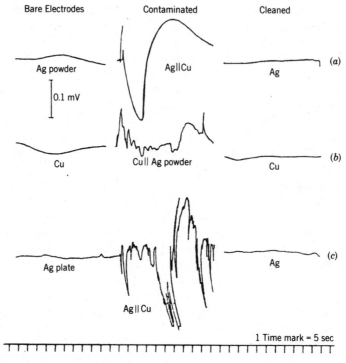

Bare Electrodes   Contaminated   Cleaned

Figure 4   Noise recordings of electrode pairs in saline: (left) bare, (center) one electrode with contaminant, and (right) with the contaminant removed (cleaned) (*a*) Copper electrodes coated with silver powder; copper contaminant introduced by removing a small area of the powder. (*b*) Copper electrodes; silver powder contaminant. (*c*) Silver plated on copper; copper contaminant introduced by removing a small area of silver plate.

of an electrode is considerably enhanced by stabilization of the electrode–electrolyte interface. This phenomenon has been demonstrated practically when attempts have been made to measure bioelectric events on moving subjects. For example, Forbes et al. (1921) were perhaps the first to employ a type of recessed electrode to obtain electrocardiograms and electromyograms on an elephant. When standing, elephants sway from side to side, making it difficult to obtain artifact-free records with plate electrodes. Forbes employed a zinc electrode in the neck of a funnel filled with zinc sulfate. The opening of the funnel was covered with a permeable membrane soaked in saline. Two rubber-gloved assistants held these electrodes against the inner surfaces of the forelimbs of the animal. The electrocardiogram was success-fully recorded by a string galvanometer.

In a study of the electrocardiograms of perspiring miners, Atkins (1961) found that the main source of artifacts was contact variations between the electrode metal and the skin. When the electrodes were separated from the skin by a layer of filter paper or gauze soaked with an electrolyte, electrode artifacts virtually disappeared.

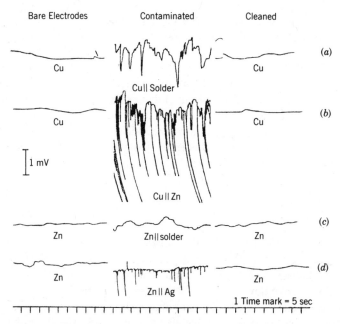

Figure 5   Noise recordings of electrode pairs in saline: (left) bare; (center) one electrode with contaminant; (right) with the contaminant removed (cleaned). (*a*) Copper electrodes with solder contaminant applied with a soldering iron. (*b*) Copper electrodes with zinc contaminant applied by rubbing the zinc onto the electrode. (*c*) Zinc electrodes with solder contaminant. (*d*) Zinc electrodes with silver powder contaminant.

Roman and Lamb (1962), using miniature recessed electrodes applied to the skin over each end of the sternum, presented some truly remarkable records of the ECG in which no artifacts were to be observed when the electrodes were tapped or struck or when the subject was jumping or engaged in vigorous activity. These electrodes were employed for monitoring ECG changes in pilots flying in high-performance aircraft. Lucchina and Phipps (1962) similarly demonstrated that their electrodes were free from artifacts when pressure was applied or when the electrodes were displaced. To prove their point, high-quality electrocardiograms were recorded from ambulatory subjects. Similar recessed electrodes have been employed successfully to record the ECG of astronauts, laborers, swimmers, and a variety of other subjects exercising strenuously.

To record the EEG on moving subjects, Kado et al. (1964) constructed interesting electrodes in which the metal was tin in contact with a tin chloride solution contained in a small ceramic chamber. Contact between the ceramic chamber and the skin was made via a sponge soaked in physiological saline. Other than removing oil from the scalp, no special precautions were required for the installation of the electrodes. When carefully applied, these electrodes produced remarkably stable EEG recordings in subjects who were moving their heads rapidly.

In summary, the electrical stability of an electrode is related to the stability of the regions of charge gradient. With electrodes in which there is a metal–electrolyte interface, stabilization of the interface prevents the development of variable electrochemical voltages. It should not be concluded, however, that all electrode artifacts are due to disturbance of the electrode–electrolyte interface. In the case of skin-surface electrodes, the skin potential that exists across the outer dermal layers is responsible for artifacts when the skin is distorted by electrode movement. This source of artifact can be eliminated by the skin-drilling technique introduced by Shackel (1959). A discussion of this technique will be presented elsewhere in this chapter.

CHLORIDED SILVER ELECTRODES

It was d'Arsonval (1880) who introduced the chlorided silver electrode. His reason for doing so was to create a pair of easily prepared electrodes with no potential difference. The incorrect term nonpolarizable became associated with these electrodes. We now know that what d'Arsonval meant was that the half-cell potentials were equal and that the net voltage from the pair was zero.

d'Arsonval's silver–silver chloride electrode consisted of a chlorided silver wire mounted in the stopper of a glass tube (like a medicine dropper) filled with saline. The saline was prevented from escaping by the mounting stopper at one end and the saline-soaked wick, which protruded from the small end. The saline-soaked wick contacted the tissue from which the bioelectric event was being recorded.

The ability of a chloride coat on silver to achieve stabilization was investigated by Geddes and Baker (1967), who studied the potential difference between a pair of newly prepared silver-ball electrodes made by melting the tip of a silver wire in the flame of a Bunsen burner. The electrodes were then scraped to clean them and placed in saline to record the potential stability. Figure 6a illustrates the result. The noise was diminished by maintaining the electrodes positive by about 3 V with respect to a 1 × 2 in. silver plate in the saline for 2 min and reconnecting them to the recording equipment without changing their position in the saline. This process is known as chloriding. The noise record obtained is shown in Fig. 6b.

To further demonstrate the phenomenon, the electrodes were scraped to remove the coating, and they became noisy again (Fig. 6c). The electroplating current was reapplied, but this time in reverse (electrodes negative by 3 V for 3 min), and much of the electrode noise disappeared (Fig. 6d) after this electrolytic cleaning process. Finally, the electrodes were most effectively quieted by the simple procedure of chloriding them after the electrolytic cleaning. The polarity was then reversed (electrodes positive), and, with a milliammeter in the circuit, the current was turned on and then interrupted when it started to fall. After the electrodes were connected to the amplifier, the noise record shown in Fig. 6e was obtained. To illustrate that all the noise cannot be attributed to the electrodes, Fig. 6f shows the inherent noise level of the amplifying channel under open- and short-circuit conditions.

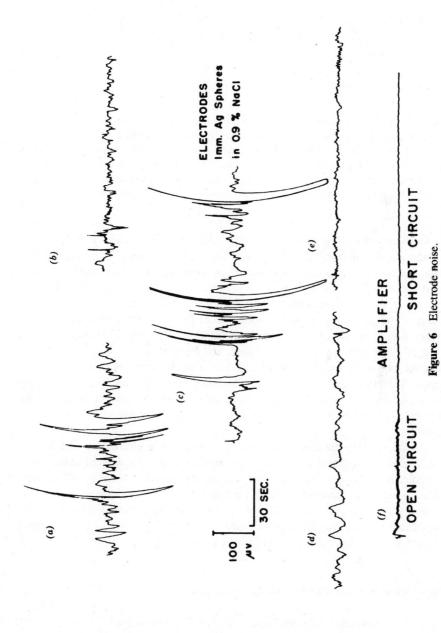

Figure 6   Electrode noise.

323

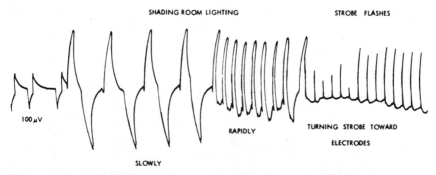

Figure 7   The photosensitivity of a pair of chlorided silver electrodes in 0.9% saline in a lighted room. After the 100 μV calibration, the electrodes were shaded and exposed to light by slowly and rapidly casting a shadow on them by placing the hand above them. Then the light from a flashing stroboscope was directed toward the electrodes to evoke a similar photovoltaic effect due to the action of light on the electrode–electrolyte double layer of charge. [From L. A. Geddes, *Am. J. EEG Technol.* **13**:195–203 1973. By permission.]

An ingenious method of stabilizing chlorided silver electrodes while they are in storage was described by Cooper (1956). The method serves to maintain the electrodes short circuited to each other and at the same time keeps them in a chlorided condition. These two actions are brought about by mounting the electrodes with their silver–silver chloride surfaces immersed in a dish of saline in which is mounted a carbon rod projecting out of the solution. At the tip of the carbon rod, Cooper affixed a stainless steel plate to which all the electrode terminals were connected. Thus all electrodes were joined together, and because carbon is slightly electronegative with respect to silver–silver chloride, a small chloriding current was maintained. Therefore, during storage the electrodes were maintained at the same potential to each other and were continuously chlorided. Cooper reported that electrodes treated in this way were adequately stable for use with high-gain dc amplifiers.

Chlorided silver electrodes can be made very stable electrically and for this reason enjoy widespread popularity. However, they are not without defects. For example, an electrodeposited chloride coating can be removed easily by abrasion. In addition, silver–silver chloride is photosensitive (i.e., it changes its potential slightly when exposed to light). Therefore, if such electrodes are used during photic stimulation studies, they should be shaded from changing light intensity. Figure 7 illustrates the photosensitivity of chlorided silver electrodes.

Potential of a Silver–Silver Chloride Electrode

It is to be noted that the silver–silver chloride electrode is a chloride ion electrode with a potential that reflects the activity (A_{Cl^-}) of the environmental chloride ions; the activity is in turn dependent on the molal concentration m and the activity

TABLE 3   The Potential of Silver–Silver Chloride Electrodes

Electrode | Electrolyte (at 25°C)	Potential (V)	Temperature Coefficient (mV/°C)
Ag–AgCl | 0.001 M KCl	+0.401	+0.77
Ag–AgCl | 0.01 M KCl	+0.343	+0.62
Ag–AgCl | 0.1 M KCl	+0.288	+0.43
Ag–AgCl | 1.0 M KCl	+0.235	+0.25
Ag–AgCl | (A = 1) KCl	+0.222	0.213 (calc.)

Source: Data obtained from A. J. de Bethune, in *Handbook of Electrochemistry*. C. A. Hampel (ed.). Reinhold, New York, 1964. By permission.

coefficient γ. The potential is given by the following expression:

$$E = E_T^0 - \frac{2.303RT}{F} \log A_{Cl^-}. \tag{1}$$

In this expression, E_T^0 is the potential of the silver–silver chloride electrode (Table 3) at the temperature T K, R is the gas constant (8.317 J/cal), F is the faraday (96,500 C). The activity A_{Cl^-} is equal to γm. The foregoing expression can be evaluated to give the potentials under specified conditions.

$$E = 0.2214 - 0.0582 \log \gamma m \qquad \text{at } 20°C$$
$$E = 0.2225 - 0.05915 \log \gamma m \qquad \text{at } 25°C$$
$$E = 0.2251 - 0.06153 \log \gamma m \qquad \text{at } 37°C$$

Very frequently the silver–silver chloride electrode is used in conjunction with potassium chloride solutions having various concentrations expressed in molar concentration M. The data covering this situation from de Bethune (1964) are presented in Table 3; the data are plotted in Fig. 8. Sometimes the silver–silver chloride electrode is used with a saturated potassium chloride solution, which at 25°C is equivalent to about 4.7 M; for this situation Castellan (1964) reported an electrode potential of +0.197 V.

ELECTRODE IMPEDANCE

In addition to developing a half-cell potential, each electrode exhibits an impedance that is dependent on the nature of the electrical double layer. This impedance is often called the polarization impedance. Through the impedance of both electrodes and the input impedance of the recording apparatus flows a small current derived from the bioelectric event. Because the input impedance of most bioelectric recorders is high, the current is very small and the voltage drop caused by the electrode impedance is usually negligible. As pointed out later, however, this situation does not always obtain, and in its absence, besides a loss of amplitude, undesirable waveform distortion of a bioelectric event can occur.

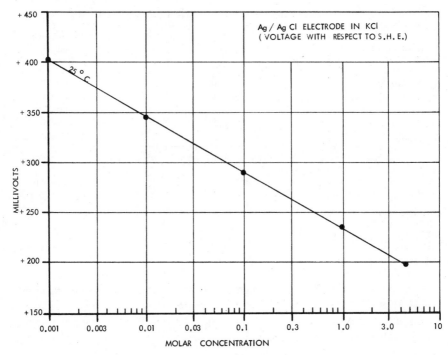

Figure 8 The potential of a silver–silver chloride electrode in contact with potassium chloride solutions of different molar concentrations. The standard hydrogen electrode was used as the reference.

With stimulating electrodes, the electrode–electrolyte impedance can become a very important consideration because of its resistive and reactive nature and both components depend on current density. These facts, along with the nature of the output circuit of the stimulator, can result in the current and voltage waveforms being different. Moreover, with stimulating electrodes, the current density distribution is not uniform across their surfaces. These factors are also discussed in Chapter 10.

Electrode impedances are complex and can be difficult to measure with high accuracy on living subjects. The term electrode impedance really refers to the impedance at each electrode and does not include the impedance of the biological material between the electrodes. Frequently, however, the term is used to describe the total impedance of the circuit between the electrode terminals, which includes the impedance at both electrodes and that of the biological material between them.

Electrode Capacitance and Resistance

The presence of a charge distribution at an electrode–electrolyte interface produces not only an electrode potential but also a capacitance. Conceptually, two layers of charge of opposite sign, separated by a distance, constitute a capacitance.

The distance between the layers of charge is molecular in dimension; therefore the capacitance per unit area is quite large (Grahame, 1941, 1952). In fact, this is one of the properties that allowed the first electrolytic capacitors to exhibit such large capacitances in relatively small packages.

It is difficult to measure the capacitance and resistance of a single electrode–electrolyte interface. The impedances of the electrode–electrolyte interfaces in conductivity cells plagued the early electrochemists who desired to obtain accurate values for the resistivities of electrolytes. Kohlrausch (1897; Kohlrausch and Holborn, 1898) reduced the electrode–electrolyte impedance to a negligible value by using platinum black electrodes, which have a very rough surface and hence large effective area. The large area provides a high capacitance, the reactance of which is negligible at 1000 Hz (the frequency most often used to measure electrolytic resistivity).

Warburg (1899, 1901), a contemporary of Kohlrausch, was one of the first to investigate the components of the electrode–electrolyte interface, and his studies provided a model that equates a single electrode–electrolyte interface to a series resistance and capacitance. It is important to note that the magnitude of each of these components is dependent on electrode type and area (including surface condition), the electrolyte, the frequency, and the current density used to make the measurement. More recently, the Warburg equivalent circuit has been elaborated for conductivity cells by Grahame (1952), Feates et al. (1956), and Robinson and Stokes (1959).

To illustrate the difficulty in determining the capacitance and resistance of a single electrode–electrolyte interface, it is merely necessary to set down the expression for the impedance appearing between the two terminals of a pair of electrodes immersed in an electrolyte of resistivity ρ. For convenience, assume that circular electrodes of area A are applied to the ends of a cylinder of electrolyte of length L and diameter d (see Fig. 9). The terminal impedance Z_{12} is

$$Z_{12} = Z_1 + \frac{\rho L}{A} + Z_2. \tag{2a}$$

In this expression Z_1 and Z_2 are the impedances of the electrode–electrolyte interfaces at electrodes 1 and 2. Using the series-equivalent (Warburg) model for each electrode–electrolyte interface, the terminal impedance Z_{12} is

$$Z_{12} = R_1 + \frac{1}{j\omega C_1} + \frac{\rho L}{A} + R_2 + \frac{1}{j\omega C_2}. \tag{2b}$$

In this expression, R_1, C_1 and R_2, C_2 are the equivalent series resistances and capacitances of the two electrode–electrolyte interfaces. Note that for any given frequency it is possible to use the reactive component of the terminal impedance to obtain the capacitive components C_1 and C_2 if it is assumed that there are no other capacitances present. In fact, there is another capacitive component (C_d), which is the capacitance of the cell itself, consisting of the two electrodes; the

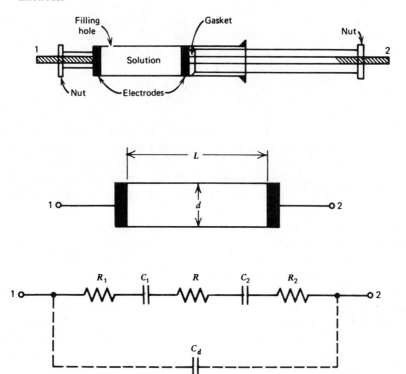

Figure 9   The electrolytic conductivity cell and its series-equivalent representation.

intervening electrolyte is the dielectric. In most cases, in the low-frequency region, C_d can be neglected.

Rearranging the foregoing expression to collect the reactive and resistive components provides

$$Z_{12} = \left(R_1 + \frac{\rho L}{A} + R_2 \right) + \frac{1}{j\omega} \left(\frac{1}{C_1} + \frac{1}{C_2} \right). \tag{3a}$$

Now if at a single frequency an impedance bridge (Fig. 10) with equal resistors R_i is used to provide the series-equivalent values R_b and C_b, then

$$R_b + \frac{1}{j\omega C_b} = \left(R_1 + \frac{\rho L}{A} + R_2 \right) + \frac{1}{j\omega C_1} + \frac{1}{j\omega C_2}. \tag{3b}$$

Equating the resistive and reactive components gives

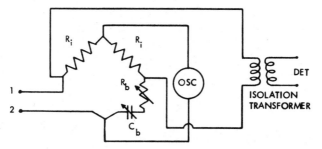

Figure 10 Constant-current comparison impedance bridge for measurement of the components of an electrode–electrolyte interface. The value of R_i is chosen to be many times higher than the impedance appearing between the measuring terminals (1, 2). The bridge-balance values (R_b and C_b) are equal, respectively, to the series-equivalent resistive and capacitive components of the impedance between terminals 1 and 2.

$$R_b = R_1 + \frac{\rho L}{A} + R_2, \qquad (4a)$$

$$\frac{1}{C_b} = \frac{1}{C_1} + \frac{1}{C_2}. \qquad (4b)$$

If it is assumed that the electrode areas are the same, $R_1 = R_2 = R$ and $C_1 = C_2 = C$, where R and C are the equivalent resistance and capacitance of a single electrode–electrolyte interface, then by substitution and rearrangement, the following are obtained:

$$2R = R_b - \frac{\rho L}{A}, \qquad (5a)$$

$$C = 2C_b. \qquad (5b)$$

Recalling that R_b and C_b are the series-equivalent bridge-balance values, it can be seen that if there are no other capacitances present the capacitance of a single electrode–electrolyte interface (at the frequency and current density employed to make the measurement) is twice the bridge-balance capacitance. However, the resistance R of a single electrode–electrolyte interface cannot be obtained by this single measurement. The additional information required is indicated by equation (3), namely, the resistivity ρ of the electrolyte and the length L and area A of the cell. Alternatively, if the resistivity is not known, two measurements can be carried out at the same frequency and with the same current density (I/A). Measurements can be repeated with two known values of electrode area A, which is difficult, or with two different lengths L for the conductivity cell; the latter technique is by far the easiest to carry out, and its use is discussed subsequently.

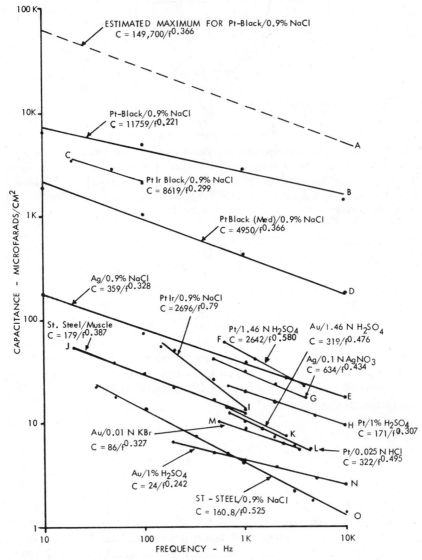

Figure 11 Equivalent series capacitance–frequency data for various electrode–electrolyte interfaces. (From L. A. Geddes, *Electrodes and the Measurement of Bioelectric Events.* Wiley, New York, 1972. By permission.)

The equivalent series capacitance has been measured in the audiofrequency range for a variety of electrode–electrolyte interfaces using a low current density. Figure 11 summarizes the data reported. Inspection of these data reveals that the series-equivalent capacitance decreases with increasing frequency. The magnitude of the capacitance also depends on the surface condition of the electrode. In the illustration, the values for polished metals are the lowest; the values for specially roughened surfaces (e.g., platinum black) are the highest. To obtain the highest capacitance values (curve A) Schwan (1963) sandblasted platinum and then electrodeposited platinum black on this surface. A high electrode–electrolyte capacitance value is, of course, indicative of a low reactive component ($1/2\pi f C$) for the electrode–electrolyte impedance.

It is interesting to note that Warburg (1899, 1901) postulated that the capacitance of an electrode–electrolyte interface varies inversely with the square root of frequency; actually, $C = Kf^{-\alpha}$, where K is a constant depending on the metal species, electrolyte concentration, and temperature. The capacitance C, of course, should be expressed in microfarads per square centimeter with a specified surface and current density. The data in Fig. 11 generally support Warburg's hypothesis; however, Fricke (1932) pointed out that the exponent α is often less than 0.5. A survey of values calculated from the published literature was presented by Geddes (1972) and showed values for α ranging from 0.22 to 0.79, the majority being slightly less than 0.5.

If it is desired to measure the equivalent resistance of a single electrode–electrolyte interface, the variable-length method (Geddes, 1972, 1973) is the easiest to employ and can be carried out by mounting the electrodes so that the length of electrolytic column can be controlled. The conductivity cell (Fig. 9) designed for this purpose uses a disposable syringe with one electrode mounted on the piston and the other on the end of the barrel. An outlet hole in the side at the end permits expulsion of electrolyte to accommodate a decrease in length. With this variable-length conductivity cell, it is only necessary to make measurements at two lengths (L, L') to determine the equivalent resistance and capacitance of a single electrode–electrolyte interface. From the same data, the resistivity of the electrolyte can be determined with high accuracy. The following derivation describes the operation of the variable-length conductivity cell.

Balance condition for length L:

$$R_b + \frac{1}{j\omega C_b} = 2R + \frac{2}{j\omega C} + \frac{\rho L}{A}. \tag{6a}$$

Balance condition for a shorter length L':

$$R_b' + \frac{1}{j\omega C_b'} = 2R + \frac{2}{j\omega C} + \frac{\rho L'}{A}. \tag{6b}$$

Manipulation of these two expressions to separate R, C, and ρ by equating the resistive and the reactive components gives

$$R = \frac{LR_b' - L'R_b}{2(L - L')} = \frac{LR_b' - L'R_b}{2\Delta L}, \tag{7}$$

$$C = \frac{4(C_b C_b')}{(C_b + C_b')} \quad \text{and if} \quad C_b' = C_b, \quad \text{then} \quad C = 2C_b, \tag{8}$$

$$\rho = \frac{A(R_b - R_b')}{L - L'} = \frac{A \, \Delta R_b}{\Delta L}. \tag{9}$$

Using the variable-length conductivity cell, Geddes (1972, 1973) investigated the validity of the Warburg concept, which states that both the equivalent resistance and the capacitance vary inversely with the square root of frequency and that the resistance is approximately equal to the reactance. The data obtained (Fig. 12a) indicate that for stainless steel in contact with 0.9% sodium chloride at room temperature, both the capacitance and the resistance of a single electrode–electrolyte interface decrease with increasing frequency. Figure 12b shows that the reactance of the capacitance $(1/2\pi f C)$ is approximately equal to the resistance.

Perhaps the most remarkable characteristic of the series-equivalent circuit for an electrode–electrolyte interface is the frequency dependence of the values for capacitance and resistance; this condition emphasizes the difficulty of assigning single values for resistance and capacitance for a given electrode area. Another interesting relationship is that the ratio of the reactance to the resistance, which is the tangent of the phase angle ϕ, is approximately unity (i.e., $\tan \phi = X/R = 1$). Schwan called attention to the fact that Fricke had derived a relationship, which Schwan called Fricke's law, that states that the phase angle ϕ is dependent on α, the exponent describing the manner by which capacitance varies with frequency.

$$\phi = \frac{\pi}{2}(1 - \alpha). \tag{10}$$

To a first approximation, $\alpha = 0.5$, and under this condition the phase angle, the tangent of which is the ratio of a reactance to resistance, is 45°. This means that the reactance and the resistance are equal; Fig. 12b shows that this is approximately true, at least for the case cited.

Current-Density Considerations

To illustrate how the series-equivalent resistance and capacitance values depend on the current density used for measurement, Geddes et al. (1971) measured these quantities using stainless steel electrodes in contact with 0.9% saline solution. Figure 13 presents such data and shows that for a given frequency the equivalent resistance decreases and the capacitance increases as current density is increased. Note that the largest change occurs in the low-frequency region. This type of relationship is in agreement with the studies by Schwan and Maczuk (1965) Schwan (1968), and Jaron et al. (1969), who used platinum electrodes and reported that the 20- and 500-Hz capacitance increased and the resistance decreased with increasing current density. They defined the "limit of linearity" at a specified frequency as that current density for which the value of capacitance increased or the resistance decreased by 10% from the value found with very low current density.

Schwan (1968) elaborated on the nature of an electrode–electrolyte interface when operated under high-current-density conditions, namely, that (with his definition) "the limit of linearity shrinks to zero as the frequency decreases to zero."

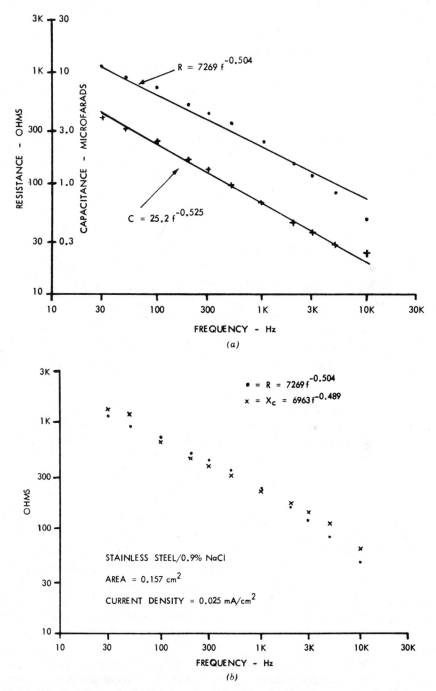

Figure 12 Stainless steel 0.9% saline electrode–electrolyte interface measured with a current density of 0.025 mA/cm² over a frequency range from 20 Hz to 20 kHz. (a) Series-equivalent resistance R and capacitance C; (b) series-equivalent resistance R and reactance $X = \frac{1}{2}\pi fC$. [From L. A. Geddes et al., *Med. Biol. Eng.* **9**:511–521 (1971). By permission.]

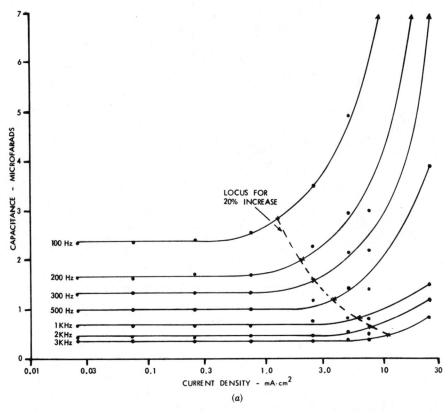

Figure 13   Dependence of (*a*) the series-equivalent capacitance and (*b*) the series-equivalent resistance on current density and frequency; stainless steel electrode (0.157 cm^2) in contact with 0.9% saline. [From L. A. Geddes et al., *Med. Biol. Eng.* **9**:511–521 (1971). By permission.]

This relationship, which is indicated by the dashed lines in Fig. 13, raises some questions regarding the suitability of small-area metal microelectrodes for the measurement of transmembrane potentials. However, since few measurements have been made of electrode properties below 10 Hz, one can only speculate about the equivalent circuit for 0 Hz (i.e., the situation that obtains when direct current is passed through an electrode–electrolyte interface). It is well known that direct current can be passed through an electrode–electrolyte interface, and for this reason the simple Warburg series-equivalent circuit cannot be considered truly representative.

Because it is easier to understand the behavior of an electric circuit by using reactance and resistance values, it is of interest to compare the resistance and reactance at different current densities; Fig. 14 makes this comparison and shows that at low current densities the Warburg equivalent ($R = X$ and both vary approximately as $1/\sqrt{f}$) is reasonably accurate. However, as current density is in-

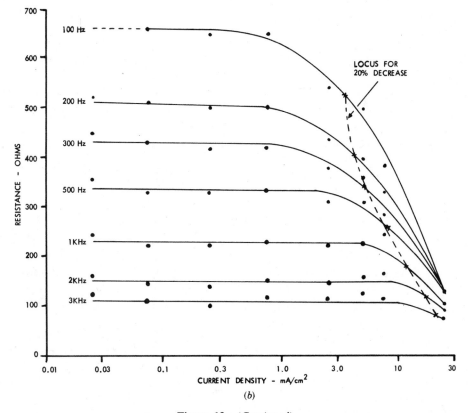

Figure 13　(*Continued*)

creased, both resistance and reactance decrease and the manner in which each varies with frequency does not permit a power function approximation (i.e., one that is linear on a log-log plot).

The foregoing indicates that at a given frequency the magnitude of the series impedance $\sqrt{R^2 + X^2}$ of an electrode–electrolyte interface decreases with increasing current density. In addition, because increasing current density preferentially alters the low-frequency values for resistance and capacitance, it would be expected that the low-frequency impedance would be reduced markedly by an increase in current density. To illustrate this point, the impedance–frequency characteristic of a silver-ball electrode (1.35 mm diameter) immersed in 0.9% saline and paired with a large circular silver disk (3 cm diameter) was measured in the frequency range extending from 20 to 10 kHz using current densities in the range of 0.1–40 mA/cm^2 for the ball electrode. Figure 15, which illustrates the results, shows that the electrode impedance diminishes with increasing current density and that the greatest reduction occurs in the low-frequency region.

In addition to a decrease in impedance with increasing current density, another effect—rectification—occurs. This phenomenon of the electrode–electrolyte inter-

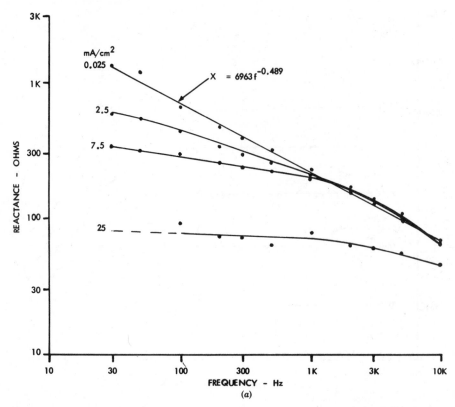

Figure 14 Dependence of (*a*) the series-equivalent reactance *X* and (*b*) the series-equivalent resistance *R* on frequency and current density; stainless steel electrode (0.157 cm^2) in contact with 0.9% saline. [From L. A. Geddes et al., *Med. Biol. Eng.* **9**:511–521 (1971). By permission.]

face was used to construct electrolytic rectifiers before high-current diodes were available. This subject is discussed near the end of this chapter in the section dealing with stimulating electrodes.

It should be apparent now that an electrode–electrolyte interface represents a complex electric circuit and that its impedance depends on the frequency and current density used for measurement. In coupling a bioelectrical event to an amplifier via electrodes, consideration should be given to the nature of the impedance of the electrodes. Every precaution should be taken to pass as little current as possible through the electrode–electrolyte interface so that a minimum of voltage loss and waveform distortion will be introduced by the electrode impedance. The practical method employed to avoid these distortions is to use an amplifier with an adequately high input impedance. This subject, discussed elsewhere in this chapter, verifies the concern reported by Schwan (1968):

"Much work in biological research (for example, studies of membranes with

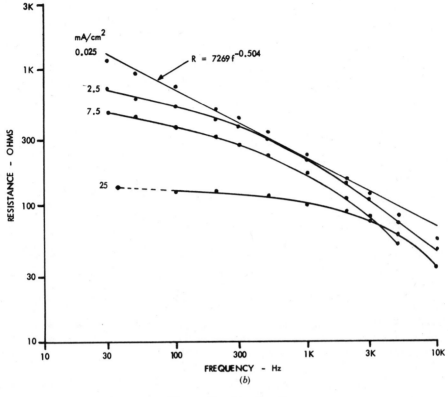

Figure 14   (*Continued*)

transients), and clinical practice (for example, in cardiac pacemaker design), is conducted with microelectrodes where current densities are applied far in excess of the [above reported] limit of current linearity values [a few mA/cm^2]. It appears, therefore, that electrodes often introduce nonlinear characteristics which are erroneously ascribed to the biological system under study.''

Improved Model for the Electrode–Electrolyte Interface

At this point it is useful to summarize the facts that pertain to an electrode–electrolyte interface and to recognize their significance. The simple Warburg model consists of a series resistance R and capacitance C; Fig. 16a illustrates this model. The magnitude of R decreases and that of C increases with increasing electrode area. Both the resistance and reactance ($1/2\pi fC$) decrease with increasing frequency. However, the Warburg model predicts an infinite impedance for direct current (0 Hz). Since it is known that direct current can be passed through an electrode–electrolyte interface, it is necessary to modify the model to bring it into conformity with reality. Electrochemists place a resistance R_f across the equivalent

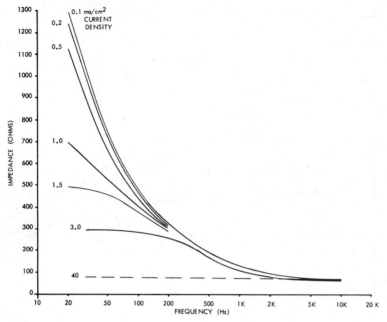

Figure 15 The impedance–frequency characteristics measured between a silver ball (1.35 mm in diameter) and a silver disk (3 cm in diameter) in 0.9% saline using different current densities. The resistance of the intervening saline is 67 Ω.

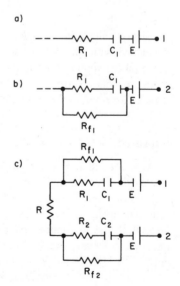

Figure 16 (a) The Warburg equivalent for an electrode–electrolyte interface, including the half-cell potential E. To account for the low-frequency behavior, the faradic leakage R_f is added in (b). (c) An approximate equivalent circuit for two electrodes in an electrolyte of resistance R.

circuit for the double layer, as shown in Fig. 16b. This resistance is called the faradic leakage.

The equivalent circuit for a pair of electrodes (electrodes 1 and 2) in an electrolyte is shown in Fig. 16c. The resistance of the electrolyte is represented by R. Pure electrolytes are resistive in the low-frequency region. Looking into the electrode terminals (1, 2), the low-frequency impedance Z_1 will be

$$Z_1 = R + R_{f1} + R_{f2}. \tag{11}$$

As the frequency is increased, the impedance decreases (due to a decrease in both R and X), and the impedance approaches R asymptotically. If the impedance–frequency characteristic is measured at a higher constant-current density, a similar curve will be obtained, but it will be below that for a curve taken at a lower current density. This occurs because both the resistance and reactance decrease with increasing current density.

ELECTRODES ON A SUBJECT

From the foregoing, it is possible to create a reasonable model to represent the approximate circuit of a pair of electrodes in electrolytic contact with a subject, as shown in Fig. 17a. Looking into the electrode terminals (1, 2), the circuit contains two half-cell potentials (E_1, E_2), two electrode–subject impedances (R_1, C_1, R_{f1} and R_2, C_2, R_{f2}), and a circuit representing the subject (R_s, C_s, R'_s). The bioelectrical event E_b, (when present) is also shown.

Figure 17b demonstrates that the bioelectric signal E_b is in series with two half-cell potentials E_1 and E_2, the sum of which may not be zero or even stable. If the sum is not zero, the bioelectric signal E_b is superimposed on an offset or bias potential.

The impedance of the circuit between terminals 1 and 2 comprises two electrode–electrolyte impedances and that of the living tissue ($R_s C_s R'_s$), which, although represented by a series-parallel circuit, is more complex. Because of the characteristics of the electrode–electrolyte impedance and (to a lesser degree) the nature of the tissue impedance, the low-frequency impedance will be high and the high-frequency impedance will be low, amounting to substantially that of the tissues between the electrodes. Figure 17c illustrates this point. It is to be noted that the skin potential has not yet been included. This subject is discussed in the section dealing with skin abrasion to reduce artifacts.

IMPEDANCE OF CHLORIDED SILVER ELECTRODES

In a previous section in this chapter it was pointed out that one of the advantages of chloriding a silver electrode is stabilization of the electrode potential. The ap-

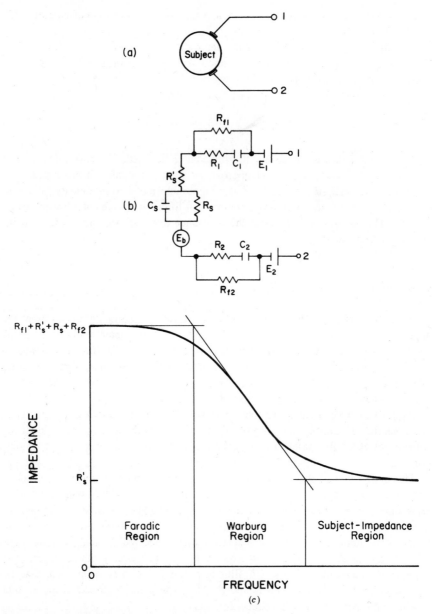

Figure 17 (*a*) Electrolyte-coated electrodes on a subject; (*b*) approximate equivalent circuit; (*c*) typical impedance–frequency characteristic.

plication of a deposit of silver chloride alters the impedance between the electrode and the electrolyte it contacts. The magnitude of the change in impedance depends on the thickness of the chloride deposit. There is, however, substantial variation in the amount of deposit considered adequate. This situation probably arises because there are two distinct groups of users of silver–silver chloride electrodes.

The electrochemists use them as reference electrodes and require a known stable electrode potential; the other group—electrophysiologists—demand a stable electrode potential and a low electrode–electrolyte impedance. It is doubtful that both requirements are fulfilled by the same chloride deposit.

Faraday's law of electrolysis specifies the weight of a material that will be deposited on an electrode in contact with an electrolyte; the important factors are current and time. In fact, the unit of current, the ampere, was first quantified by Faraday's law; the ampere was defined as that steady current which, when passed through a solution of silver nitrate (under conditions in which only siver is deposited), deposits silver at the rate of 1.11800 mg/sec. Thus the unit of current was established by measurement of weight and time.

The unit quantity of electricity is the coulomb (C), which is one ampere-second (A-sec). From careful measurement of electrodepositions in various cells, it has been found (cf. MacInnes, 1961) that a certain number of coulombs of electricity is required to deposit one chemical equivalent (the gram atomic weight divided by the valence) of a substance at a metal–electrolyte boundary. The quantity of electricity is 96,497 C (i.e., ampere-seconds); in practice the figure used is 96,500 C, which is defined as one faraday (F). This means that 1 F will deposit the gram atomic weight of a monovalent element; half that weight will be deposited if the element is divalent. It is to be noted that although Faraday's law specifies the amount of deposit, it says nothing about which ions in an electrolyte will take part in an electrochemical reaction in which a current enters or leaves an electrode.

From Faraday's law it can be seen that it is appropriate to describe the amount of chloride deposit on a silver electrode by specifying the magnitude of the current and the time it flows. With this criterion in mind, it is informative to examine the amount of chloride deposited by various investigators who reported the production of satisfactory chlorided silver electrodes. To make the data comparable, the deposit (mA-sec), has been converted to the deposit per square centimeter of electrode area. Table 4 presents these data along with the density of current (milliamperes per square centimeter of electrode area) that was used in the chloriding process.

From Table 4, it can be seen that chloride deposits ranging from 48 to 168,000 mA-sec/cm^2 have been employed. In order to discover the effect of depositing chloride on silver (Geddes et al., 1969) compared the impedance–frequency characteristic of bare silver electrodes in saline with that obtained after electrolytic deposition of silver chloride (about 500 mA-sec/cm^2). Figure 18a illustrates the impedance–frequency characteristic of the bare electrodes; Fig. 18b shows the same relationship for the chlorided electrodes. Clearly evident is a remarkable decrease in the low-frequency impedance. The relative constancy with increasing frequency of the impedance–frequency characteristic of the chlorided electrodes indicates that the impedance of the electrode–electrolyte interface has become lower and the resistance of the electrolyte now dominates the circuit.

The change in electrode–electrolyte impedance accompanying the chloriding of silver electrodes was studied quantitatively by Geddes et al. (1969). Impedance-frequency characteristics of square and circular silver electrodes of differing areas (225, 100, 78.5, 49, 38.5, 25, 19.6, and 3.14 mm^2) were measured bare and with different amounts of chloriding. Each electrode was mounted on a slide that could

TABLE 4   Parameters Employed for Chloriding Silver Electrodes

Chloride Deposit (mA-sec/cm²)	Chloriding Density (mA/cm²)	Investigator and Year
500–1400	1.7–2.3	MacInnes and Parker (1915)
4000–5600	3.3–4.7	MacInnes and Beattie (1920)
3600	1.0	Carmody (1929)
18,000–21,600	0.2	Afanasiev (1930)
8500	2.4	Carmody (1932)
4800	2.7	Brown (1934)
28,800–43,200	8–12	Smith and Taylor (1938)
18,000–168,000	5.3–31	O'Connell et al. (1960)
432–43,200	0.01–1.0	Bures et al. (1962)
7800	8.7	Goldstein et al. (1962)
48–108	0.4–0.6	Grayson (1962)
300–500	2.5	Cooper (1963)
3600	3	Day and Lippitt (1964)
600	1.0	Skov and Simons (1965)
1000–2000	—	Cole (1962)
—	0.4–10	Janz and Ives (1968)

be fitted into a slot in a rectangular plastic box filled with 0.9% saline solution. A large, heavily chlorided silver electrode (25 × 25 mm) located at the other end of the box was used as the reference electrode for each impedance–frequency measurement. The measurements were carried out over the frequency range of 10 Hz to 10 kHz, using the same current density (0.1 mA/cm²) for each electrode.

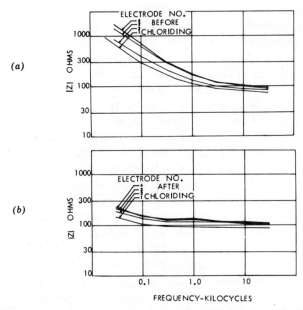

Figure 18   Impedance–frequency curves for bare and chlorided silver electrodes. [From L. A. Geddes and L. E. Baker, *Med. Biol. Eng.* **7**:49–56 (1969). By permission.]

The procedure for investigating the electrode characteristics consisted of first measuring the impedance–frequency characteristic of the bare silver electrode, which had been polished with emery cloth and washed clean of the abrasive material. Then a known amount of chloride was deposited, and the impedance–frequency characteristic was measured again. An additional amount of chloride was then deposited and the impedance–frequency relationship was measured once again. The procedure was repeated until a heavy coat of chloride had been deposited. Chloriding was carried out in room light using a constant-current circuit consisting of a 50-V dc power supply in series with a resistance box and milliammeter. With this arrangement, the chloriding current could be preset to the desired value and then connected to the chloriding bath, which consisted of a rectangular plastic box containing 0.9% saline and a large (25 × 25 mm) bare silver cathode. Fresh saline solution was used to chloride each electrode.

Figure 19 presents a typical family of curves obtained from a single electrode (0.25 cm^2). The impedance–frequency curve of the bare silver electrode (curve A) exhibited capacitive reactance (i.e., the impedance decreased markedly with an increase in frequency). Even with a small chloride deposit, there was a considerable reduction in low-frequency impedance (curve B). As chloriding was increased, there was a further reduction in the low-frequency impedance (curves C, D), and the behavior of the electrode–saline–electrode circuit became much more resistive, as shown by the impedance–frequency curve, which became nearly parallel to the frequency axis. With continued chloriding, both the low- and high-frequency impedances increased (curve E). With additional chloriding, the impedance values at all frequencies were increased and the impedance–frequency curves still indicated a circuit that was mainly resistive. A continuation of chloriding further raised the

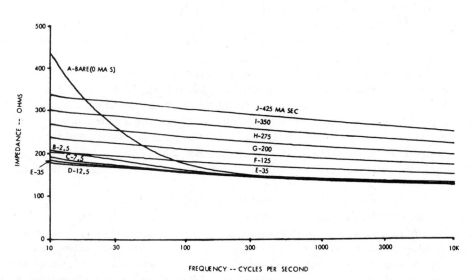

Figure 19 Impedance-frequency curves with different amounts of chloride deposit (mA-sec); electrode area 0.25 cm^2. [From L. A. Geddes and L. E. Baker, *Med. Biol. Eng.* 7:49–56 (1969). By permission.]

impedance at all frequencies, and equal increments of chloriding resulted in parallel, equally spaced curves (curves F–J).

It is of some interest to speculate on the reason for the initial decrease, followed by an increase in the electrode–electrolyte impedance resulting from the continued deposition of silver chloride. Although there is still no complete explanation, it is conceivable that the initial decrease in impedance results from an increase in area because of the manner in which electrolytic deposits are laid down. Although silver chloride is a relatively good insulator, having a resistivity in the range of 0.5×10^5 to 6×10^5 Ω-cm (according to Jaenicke et al., 1955), a very thin deposit may increase the electrode area more than it decreases its capacitance. With an increase in deposition, the area increase may be offset by the effect of an increase in thickness, which in turn would raise resistance and decrease capacitance; both situations would lead to an increase in impedance. That the deposition of silver chloride causes a considerable increase in area was demonstrated by Marmont (1949), who microscopically examined silver chloride deposits. He also showed that when the silver chloride deposit was converted to silver, using photographic developer, the impedance of a silver chloride electrode was dramatically reduced.

Figure 20 was composed to demonstrate that, irrespective of area, there is an optimum amount of chloriding for electrodes to obtain the lowest impedance. In this illustration the 10-Hz (Fig. 20a) and 10-kHz (Fig. 20b) impedances are plotted versus the normalized amount of chloriding (milliampere-seconds per square centimeter of electrode area), calculated by dividing the actual chloriding milliampere-second value used for a particular electrode by the electrode area (in square centimeters). In this manner, the changes produced by chloriding each electrode are more readily seen and compared. Figure 20b illustrates that, in general, chloriding to between 100 and 500 mA-sec/cm^2 provided the lowest values of electrode impedance. Prolongation of chloriding beyond 500 mA-sec/cm^2 increased the impedance of all electrodes at all frequencies. This deposit is somewhat lower than that advocated by Cole and Kishimoto (1962), who stated that the chloride deposit for minimum impedance is 2000 mA-sec/cm^2.

Another series of tests was conducted to identify the limits of interchangeability of current and time to achieve a desired chloride deposit. Using the reduction in low-frequency impedance as an indicator of the attainment of the desired chloride deposit, it was found that if chloriding was carried out with a current density of 5 or more mA-sec/cm^2, milliamperes and seconds could be manipulated for convenience to attain the desired chloride deposit. This value is in fairly good agreement with the current densities used by many of the investigators listed in Table 4.

The study reported by Geddes and Baker (1967) and that reported by Cole and Kishimoto (1962) indicate that a chloride deposit in the range of 100–2000 mA-sec/cm^2 on a silver electrode achieves the lowest electrode–electrolyte impedance. To attain this deposit, by convenient choice of current and time, a chloriding current density in excess of 5 mA/cm^2 should be used. Because the impedance of an electrode–electrolyte interface is altered by passage of current, it is recommended that a constant-current source be used for chloriding. Thus during the chloriding

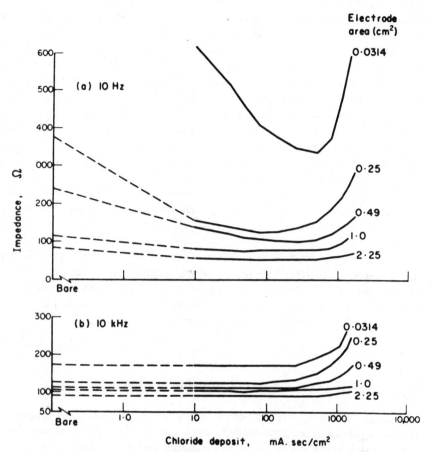

Figure 20 The dependence of the impedance of a silver electrode on the chloride deposit. Note that the lowest impedance was obtained with a deposit of about 500 mA-sec/cm². [From L. A. Geddes and L. E. Baker, *Med. Biol. Eng.* **7**:49–56 (1969). By permission.]

process the current will not vary as the electrode–electrolyte interface changes its properties. A constant-current source can be approximated by connecting a resistor that is high in resistance with respect to the resistance of the electrodes and the chloriding bath in series with a controllable voltage source (e.g., a power supply) having a milliammeter in series with its output.

The first step in chloriding is to carefully clean the electrode to be chlorided; failure to do so will result in a nonuniform deposit of chloride. The electrode is then placed in the chloriding solution (NaCl, KCl, or HCl) and connected to the positive pole of the current source. A large silver electrode is also placed in the solution and is connected to the negative pole of the current source. The two electrodes are connected together (short circuited) before the current is applied. The current is then turned on and adjusted to the desired valule. When the chloriding is to be started, the connection across the electrodes is removed and the current is allowed to pass through the chloriding bath for the desired time.

It must be added that the literature contains a wealth of useful data on chlorided silver electrodes. In particular, the papers cited in Table 4 and the reviews by Janz and Taniguchi (1953) and Janz and Kelly (1964) are recommended to the reader who desires to delve more deeply into this important subject. In addition to the electrolytic method of fabricating a silver chloride electrode, it is important to recognize two other methods. One is due to Burr and Mauro (1948, 1949), who coated a silver wire by dipping it into melted silver chloride; the other consists of compressing a mixture of silver and silver chloride under high pressure to form a pure silver–silver chloride pellet electrode.

Grubbs (1983) described a method of fabricating a silver–silver chloride electrode with a stable impedance lower than that attainable with optimal chloriding, which he found to occur at 75 mA-sec/cm^2. The silver electrode was first etched in aqua regia for 30 sec. Then a heavy chloride coat was deposited (6000 mA-sec/cm^2) at a current density of 50 mA/cm^2. The electrode was dechlorided (by reversing the current) for 30 sec, which removed about one-fourth of the original chloride coat. The result was an electrode with the same low impedance over a frequency range extending from 50 to 50,000 Hz. Not only was the impedance low, but it remained low for a prolonged period.

THE PLATINIZED PLATINUM (PLATINUM BLACK) ELECTRODE

In electrochemistry, and to some degree in electrophysiology, the platinized platinum or platinum black electrode is employed. This electrode was introduced by Kohlrausch in the late 1890s for the measurement of the conductivity of electrolytic solutions; his work is well summarized in his book (Kohlrausch and Holborn, 1898). Since Kohlrausch's time, the platinum black electrode has been used with gaseous hydrogen as the standard reference electrode; it is still the most practical and accurate electrode for electrolytic conductivity cells because the electrode–electrolyte impedance is reduced to a very low value by the platinization process.

Although it was realized at the time that Kohlrausch's method of electrolytically depositing a finely divided deposit of platinum on a bare platinum electrode dramatically reduced the electrode–electrolyte impedance, probably by virtue of the considerable area of electrode in intimate contact with the electrolyte, it was more than a quarter-century later that Jones and Bollinger (1935) conducted studies to quantify the effect of depositing different amounts of platinum black on platinum electrodes. After each deposition they measured the impedance–frequency characteristics in a frequency range extending from 500 to 3070 Hz. They found that a bare (bright) platinum electrode exhibited a decreasing impedance with increasing frequency, which is characteristic of the capacitance of the electrode–electrolyte interface. Even after a thin deposit of platinum black (424 mA-sec/cm^2) the electrode–electrolyte impedance dropped 67-fold, although the deposit was barely vis-

ible. Additional deposition caused a steady but much smaller decrease in imped-
ance; with a deposit of 5950 mA-sec/cm^2, the impedance had dropped 856-fold.
Further deposition did not reduce the impedance proportionally. In fact, Jones and
Bollinger noted a slight increase in impedance when the deposit was doubled.

From these data it would appear that, in round numbers, 500 mA-sec/cm^2
constitutes a light platinum black deposit and 6000 mA-sec/cm^2 is perhaps a more
desirable value. In an earlier paper, Jones and Bollinger (1931) reported that a light
deposit was 750 mA-sec/cm^2 and a heavy deposit was 73,500 mA-sec/cm^2. Cole
and Kishimoto (1962) found that a deposit of 10,000 mA-sec/cm^2 provided an
electrode impedance of 1 Ω (at 1 kHz) for a 1-cm^2 electrode. Schwan (1968) found
that the optimum deposit was about 30,000 mA-sec/cm^2; his studies are discussed
here.

The method advocated by Kohlrausch is still used to produce a platinum black
deposit on a platinum electrode. The electrode is first cleaned thoroughly and placed
in a solution of 0.025 N hydrochloric acid containing 3% platinum chloride and
0.025% lead acetate. Such solutions are available from many laboratory supply
houses. Failure to include the lead acetate yields a flaky gray deposit; inclusion of
the lead acetate results in a stronger deposit having a velvety black appearance. A
direct current is passed through the solution via a large-area platinum anode, and
the electrode to be blackened is made the cathode. There is no unanimity on the
current density to be employed; Kohlrausch employed 30 mA/cm^2. Jones and
Bollinger used 6 mA/cm^2 for a light deposit and 27 mA/cm^2 for a heavy deposit.
Schwan (1963) carried out important studies which indicated that there is an optimum current density to obtain the lowest electrode–electrolyte impedance. He
studied the change in the series-equivalent electrode–electrolyte capacitance with
different platinizing current densities and different amounts of platinum deposit,
which he expressed in coulombs (i.e., ampere-seconds) per square centimeter of
electrode surface area. His data, which appear in Fig. 21, illustrate that sandblasting
is the best method of cleaning a platinum electrode and that the maximum capacitance, which is synonymous with the lowest electrode–electrolyte impedance, occurs when a current density of 10 mA/cm^2 is used to platinize the electrode and
the optimum deposit is 33 A-sec/cm^2. Jones and Bollinger (1935) obtained a
maximum capacitance with 64.3 A-sec/cm^2 platinum black deposit. Schwan pointed
out that his parameters apply for electrodes with an area greater than 1 mm^2; smaller
electrodes require the use of a higher current density for optimum platinizing. In
summary, with the above-mentioned restriction reported by Schwan, it would appear that the optimum parameters for platinizing a platinum electrode are a current
density of 10 mA/cm^2 of electrode area and a deposit of about 30–60 A-sec per
square centimeter of electrode area.

The impedance of the platinum–platinum black electrode has been studied extensively by Schwan (1963, 1968), Schwan and Maczuk (1965), Jaron et al. (1969),
and Onaral and Schwan (1982, 1983), These papers contain a wealth of information
on the behavior of the platinum black electrode under a range of current densities.
Time-domain information was provided by Onaral and Schwan (1983). Although
this electrode has a low electrode–electrolyte impedance, it exhibits the same characteristics as shown by other metal–electrolyte interfaces.

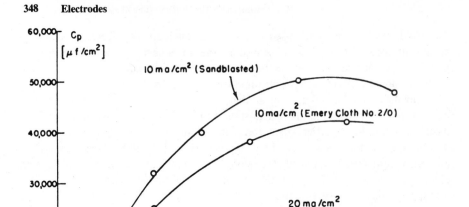

Figure 21 The increase in the capacitive component of the impedance of a platinum electrode with platinization (coulombs per square centimeter of electrode area). The effect of platinizing on different surfaces with different current densities is shown. From these data, measured at 20 Hz, the maximum capacitance (and hence the lowest impedance) was obtained by using a platinizing current of 10 mA/cm^2 and obtaining a deposit corresponding to about 33 A-sec. [From H. P. Schwan, in *Physical Techniques in Biological Research*, Vol. VI, Part B. W. L. Nastuk (ed.). Academic Press, New York, 1964. By permission © Academic Press.]

ELECTRODES FOR MEASURING BIOELECTRIC EVENTS

As stated previously there are two types of bioelectrodes. One establishes ohmic (electrolytic) contact with the excitable tissue; the other establishes capacitive communication. The latter type is often called an insulated electrode. The characteristics of such electrodes will be discussed later in this chapter.

Bioelectrodes range in area from perhaps 100 cm^2 to a few square micrometers. The impedance appearing between a pair of electrodes will depend primarily on the inverse of the area of the smallest electrode. The electrode–electrolyte interface is a complex structure that contains both resistive and reactive components, the magnitudes of which depend on the frequency and intensity of the current used to make the measurement. Moreover, it should be recognized that irrespective of the area of the smallest electrode of the pair, the goal is to measure the potential of the bioelectric generator without drawing current. Therefore, matching a measuring device (e.g., amplifier) to the electrodes requires that the amplifier have an input impedance that is high with respect to the impedance of the circuit between the electrode terminals over the entire frequency spectrum of the bioelectric event.

Amplifier Input Impedance

Devices for measuring bioelectric events are recording voltmeters that display the voltage presented to them via the electrode terminals. To record a bioelectric event faithfully, the input impedance of the bioelectric recorder must be much higher than the impedance appearing between the electrode terminals. This point will be developed in a simplified manner; the consequences of not meeting this requirement will be discussed also.

The problem of measuring a bioelectric event is analogous to that of measuring the voltage of a cell with a high resistance in series with it. Figure 22a illustrates such a cell having a voltage E and a series resistance r (which is analogous to the

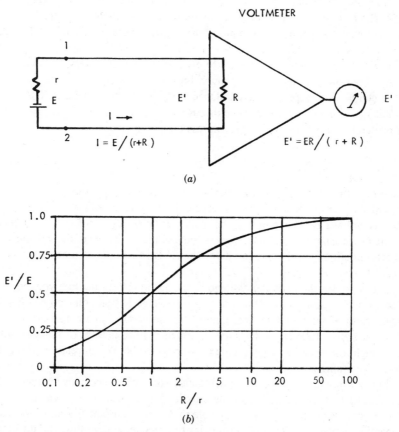

(a)

(b)

Figure 22 (a) The measurement of a voltage E in series with a resistance r using a voltmeter with an input resistance R. (b) A graph of the ratio of measured voltage E' to true voltage E versus the ratio R/r.

electrode impedance). Access to the voltage E is through terminals 1 and 2, and its measurement requires the connection of a voltmeter. All voltmeters have an internal resistance, which, although high, is not infinite. The voltmeter illustrated in Fig. 22a is a calibrated meter driven by an amplifier (the triangle) so that only the smallest possible current is drawn from the voltage source being measured. It must be recognized that the voltmeter merely displays the magnitude of the voltage across its terminals. In Fig. 22a this value is E' when the voltmeter is connected across the terminals.

The voltage $E' = IR$, the product of current I flowing in the voltmeter through its internal resistance R. The current that flows is equal to the voltage available E divided by the total resistance in the circuit $(r + R)$; thus $I = E/(r + R)$. Therefore, the voltage appearing across the voltmeter terminals is

$$E' = ER/(R + r).$$

Note that the indicated voltage E' will be equal to the true cell voltage E if the ratio $R/(r + R)$ is equal to 1, a condition that is approached if R, the input resistance of the voltmeter, is much higher than r, the resistance of the voltage source to be measured.

It is of more than passing interest to examine the effect of varying the ratio R/r. A good question to ask is, How much higher should the input resistance of the voltmeter be with respect to the resistance of the source being measured? An answer to this question can be given by letting $R/r = n$; any value can be chosen for n. Substituting for $R/r = n$ into the expression above gives

$$E'/E = n/(n + 1).$$

Note that this expression shows that when the ratio of the voltmeter resistance to that of the voltage source (cell) is larger, the measured voltage E' is very nearly the true voltage E. This point can be made very clear by choosing $n = 1$, the case where the resistance of the voltmeter is equal to the resistance of the voltage source. In this circumstance, the measured voltage E' is equal to one-half the true voltage. That is, when $R = r$, $E' = E/2$.

If $R/r = 10$, the indicated voltage is $10/11$ or 91% of the true voltage. Figure 22b presents a plot of the ratio of indicated voltage to true voltage (E'/E) versus n, the ratio of the voltmeter resistance R to the voltage source resistance r. Note that when $R = 100r$ ($n = 100$) the indicated voltage is 99% of the true voltage. How high n is made depends on the usefulness of the data in relation to the dollar cost of attaining a high ratio.

In the example just given, r is analogous to the impedance between the electrode terminals and R is the analog of the amplifier input impedance, which should be 100 or more times as high as r to enable measuring substantially all of the voltage appearing across the electrode terminals. In practice, every effort should be made to make the input impedance as high as possible. Input impedances on the order of 2–10 MΩ are used in many bioelectric recorders. Such amplifiers are more than adequate for use with electrodes as small as needle electrodes. Special amplifiers with a very high input impedance are used with the very small diameter electrodes that are employed for transmembrane potential recording.

If the amplifier input impedance is not high with respect to the impedance of the electrode–subject circuit, the measured signal is distorted in two ways: (1) It is reduced in overall amplitude and (2) its waveform is distorted. The first type of distortion is obvious from the preceding discussion; the reason for the second type of distortion will now be explained.

Recall that the electrode–electrolyte interface contains a capacitive element; it is this component, along with the amplifier input resistance (and the other resistances in the input circuit), that can produce waveform distortion. Examples of this type of distortion, which is really electrical differentiation, will be presented later in this chapter.

Plate and Disk Electrodes

Among the largest recording electrodes are those formerly used for electrocardiography (Fig. 23a), which consist of two rectangular (3.5 × 5 cm) or circular (4.75 cm) plates of German silver, nickel–silver, or nickel-plated steel. When these electrodes are applied to a subject with electrode jelly, typical dc resistance values are in the range of 2–10 kΩ; the high-frequency impedance amounts to a few hundred ohms. Figure 24 illustrates a typical impedance–frequency characteristic for such electrodes.

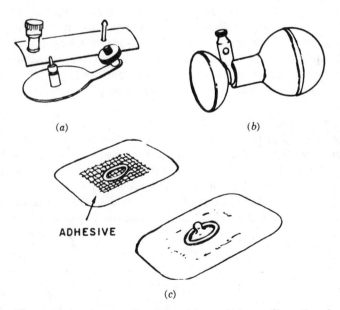

(a)   (b)

ADHESIVE

(c)

Figure 23   Electrodes for electrocardiography: (a) metal plates; (b) suction electrode; (c) screen.

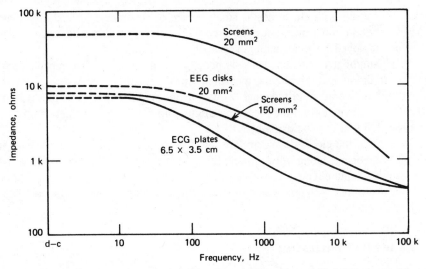

Figure 24   Impedance–frequency characteristics of electrodes applied to human subjects.

` In 1910 James and Williams reported that such plate electrodes replaced the more cumbersome immersion (bucket) electrodes traditionally used for recording the ECG. The metal-plate electrodes were separated from the subject by cotton or felt pads soaked in concentrated saline. Pardee (1917a, b) indicated that the electrodes used then were 12 × 25 cm, and the saline was described as "strong." The plate electrodes and the electrolytes developed were so practical for electrocardiography that they quickly displaced the immersion electrodes, which had been observed to have serious practical defects that made the taking of an ECG a time-consuming procedure: the subject had to remove his boots; the subject had to be seated (hence the ECGs of many bedridden patients could not be obtained), and spillage of the electrolytes made it difficult to keep the subject insulated from ground.

In electroencephalography, solder pellets a few millimeters in diameter are sometimes applied to the cleaned scalp and contact is established via electrode paste. Small needles inserted subcutaneously are also used. In most studies, however, small silver disks approximately 7mm in diameter, such as those in Fig. 25, are employed. Sometimes the disks are chlorided, and occasionally they are separated from the scalp by a washer of soft felt (Jasper and Carmichael, 1935). In both cases contact with the cleaned scalp is made by way of an electrolytic paste.

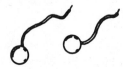

Figure 25   EEG scalp electrodes.

In practice, the dc resistance measured between a pair of these electrodes on the scalp varies between 3 and 15 kΩ.

The impedance measured between pairs of the electrodes just described was determined by Geddes and Baker (1966) in the frequency range extending from 0 to 100 kHz. The measurements were made with the same current density at each frequency. Often there were appreciable differences between individual electrodes of the same type. When this occurred, many electrodes were tested and the data were averaged. The values plotted in Fig. 26 include the impedance of the electrodes and that of the subject between them. In each case dc resistance was mea-

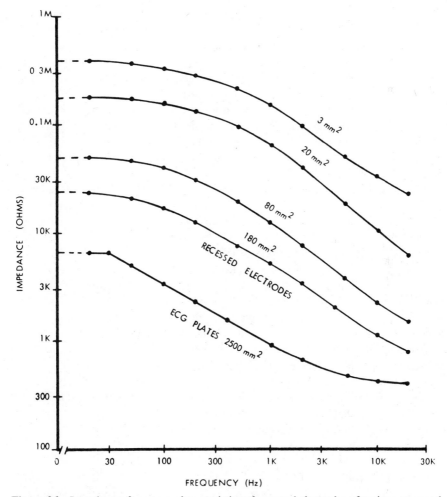

Figure 26 Impedance–frequency characteristics of recessed electrodes of various areas and conventional ECG electrodes applied to the human thorax. [From L. A. Geddes and L. E. Baker, Electrocardiology **1**:51–56 (1968). By permission.]

sured, using a low-current ohmmeter. Figure 26 also presents the impedance–frequency characteristics of several other types of electrodes. In general, for all electrodes the dc resistance is greater than the high-frequency impedance, indicating that if a low-current ohmmeter is used to measure the resistance, the value obtained, although indicative of circuit continuity, only approximates the low-frequency impedance of the circuit. In the 10–100-Hz region, the impedance approximates the dc resistance. Above 100 Hz the impedance decreases progressively, reaching values many times smaller than the magnitude of the dc resistance.

Although the figures given for the impedances of large-surface electrodes can be called typical, considerable variation that is dependent on the quality of application to the subject may be encountered. To demonstrate this point, Schmitt et al. (1961) measured the 60-Hz impedance between standard ECG plate electrodes on subjects before taking routine electrocardiograms. Although a median value of 2400 Ω was obtained, even under well-controlled conditions impedances 40 times this large were encountered. In this investigation, which employed technicians familiar with attaching electrodes to human subjects, impedances as high as 100,000 Ω were occasionally measured.

Although the physical size of the electrode most directly determines its impedance, it is noteworthy that the effective area of the electrode is increased by wetting the skin with electrolytic solutions (e.g., electrode paste or perspiration). Blank and Finesinger (1946) directed attention to the importance of this factor when measuring the resistive component of the galvanic skin reflex. Effective area can also be increased by special treatment of the electrode metal. Electrodeposition of a spongy layer of metal greatly increases the area and reduces the impedance. Use of this technique was described by Marmont (1949), Svaetichin (1951), and Dowben and Rose (1953).

A very useful type of electrode is the suction-cup electrode (Fig. 23b), the forerunners of which were described by Roth (1933–1934) and Ungerleider (1939). Such an electrode is extremely practical as an ECG chest electrode and is well suited for temporary attachment to flat surfaces of the body and to regions where the underlying tissue is soft. Although physically large, this electrode has a small area because only the rim is in contact with the skin.

A variant of the plate electrode that permits quick application is contained in a strip of adhesive tape. This electrode (Fig. 23c) consists of a lightweight metallic screen backed by a pad for electrolytic paste. Measuring approximately 1.5 in. square, it adheres well to the skin and exhibits a relatively low resistance. The adhesive backing holds the electrode in place and retards evaporation of the electrolyte. This electrode is infrequently used today.

Recessed Electrodes

It was gradually recognized that an electrode in which the electrode–electrolyte interface was protected from movement exhibited superior stability. It appears that

Forbes et al. (1921) were the first to develop such a skin-surface electrode. They employed a fluid-filled funnel with a zinc rod in its neck; the mouth of the funnel was covered with a permeable membrane soaked in saline and the funnel was also filled with saline. Pairs of these electrodes were applied to elephants to record their electrocardiograms. Baudoin et al. (1938) described a similar electrode consisting of a small rubber cup, which was cemented to the skin. The cup was filled with electrolyte into which a chlorided silver wire was dipped. Baudoin et al. used their electrode for a variety of purposes, including recording the EEG.

Other versions of the recessed electrode were described by Haggard and Gerbrands (1947) and Clark and Lacey (1950). Shackel (1958) embodied the principle in an interesting suction-cup electrode consisting of a silver–silver chloride rod mounted centrally in the rubber cup, which was filled with electrode jelly. This electrode was found to have remarkably high electrical stability despite movement of the cup on the skin. The dc resistance between a pair of these electrodes applied to the forearm was 2000–7000 Ω. Another highly stable recessed electrode, consisting of a silver–silver chloride sponge in a small enclosure resembling a top hat, was described by O'Connell et al. (1960). This electrode was designed for skin-resistance measurement. Hendler and Santa Maria (1961) described a recessed electrode in which the metallic conductor was mounted in a flat rubber or plastic washer, which was cemented to the skin by special adhesives, such as Eastman 910 (Eastman Kodak Co., Rochester, New York) or Stomaseal (3M Manufacturing Co., St. Paul, Minnesota). The washer held the electrode away from the skin, and contact was established via a thick film of electrolytic paste.

Many different types of metal have been used as the electrode material in recessed electrodes. Monel wire screens (Hendler and Santa Maria, 1961), tinned copper wires (Rowley et al., 1961), stainless steel screens (Roman and Lamb, 1962; Mason and Likar, 1966), silver disks (Boter et al., 1966), chlorided silver screens and plates (Day and Lippitt, 1964; Skov and Simons, 1965), and disks of a compressed mixture of silver and silver chloride (Lucchina and Phipps, 1962, 1963; Kahn, 1964) have been employed with considerable success. With these electrodes applied to the human thorax, the dc resistance varies with the method of preparing the skin and the type of conducting electrolyte as well as the area of the electrodes. In practice a dc resistance varying from about 2 to 50 kΩ is typical. Figure 26 presents the impedance–frequency characteristics of several recessed electrodes of different areas.

There are many modern versions of the recessed electrode. Most are disposable and use a thinly chlorided silver electrode in a plastic washer that holds the electrode metal a short distance from the skin. The intervening space is filled with an electrolytic gel. The edge of the washer that contacts the skin is coated with an adhesive that is protected by a peel-off cover that also prevents the electrolyte from drying in storage. Figure 27 is a typical example of such an electrode, which is supplied with a small abrader pad to clean the skin prior to application. When used for electrocardiography, their performance is specified by the AAMI/ANSI (1984) Standard for Conducting Electrodes.

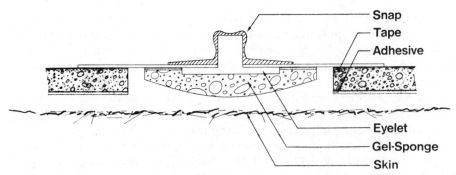

Figure 27 Recessed electrode consisting of an eyelet (electrode), gel sponge (which contains the electrolyte), and tape washer with an adhesive that holds the electrode to the skin. (Courtesy of 3M Manufacturing Co., St. Paul, Minnesota.)

Conducting-Adhesive Electrodes

Figure 28 illustrates the newest type of electrode, the metal-foil-backed conducting-adhesive electrode. It combines the electrode paste, electrode, and adhesive into a single structure. In storage, the conducting adhesive is covered with a peel-off plastic cover. Such electrodes are used for recording the ECG; they are also used for transcutaneous electrical nerve stimulation (TENS).

Conducting-adhesive electrodes consist of a metal foil coated with conducting adhesive about 1 mm thick. Both potassium and sodium salts are used as the electrolyte in the adhesive. The metal foil is often tin, which is very flexible and establishes good electrolytic communication with the conducting adhesive.

Aluminum is typically used when conducting-adhesive electrodes are used as the dispersive (ground-pad) electrode for electrosurgery. Aluminum forms a low high-frequency (capacitive) impedance communication with the conducting adhesive, which makes it ideal for this application. However, the low-frequency impedance is extremely high. Consequently, aluminum-foil conducting-adhesive electrodes are unsuitable for recording bioelectrical events.

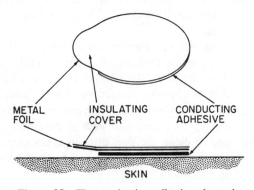

Figure 28 The conducting-adhesive electrode.

Radiotranspartent Electrodes

Occasionally while a subject is being fluoroscoped or X rayed, it is desirable to record the electrocardiogram. In many instances the electrodes and the connecting wires are in the X-ray field, consequently obscuring the area of interest. To overcome this problem, Castillo and Marriott (1974) developed recessed electrodes that cannot be detected during X-ray visualization. Their electrodes (Fig. 29) consist of a foam rubber container (corn plaster) 3 mm thick, saturated with electrode paste. A vinyl feeding tube (also filled with electrode paste) is connected to the electrode. At the other end of the vinyl tube is a chamber containing electrode paste and a chlorided silver disk, 15 mm in diameter. The wire from the disk is connected to the electrocardiograph. The electrodes are transparent to X rays because only an electrolytic fluid column is in the X-ray field. Electrode pastes, like tissue fluids, are transparent to X rays.

Castillo and Marriott reported that the use of vinyl tubes of electrolytic paste adds only 5000 Ω to the electrode impedance. They also stated that these electrodes had been applied to the precordium to record electrocardiograms during 25 cardiac catheterization procedures.

Low-Mass Electrodes

When recordings are to be made on subjects experiencing large vibration or acceleration forces, it is impotant to make the electrodes as small and light as possible. Thompson and Patterson (1958), Sullivan and Weltman (1961), Roman and Lamb (1962), Lucchina and Phipps (1962), and Simons et al. (1965) described such electrodes and demonstrated their value. Sullivan and Weltman's electrode weighed 2 mg and consisted of mylar 0.001 in. thick on which was deposited a metallic film. The center was filled with electrode jelly, and Eastman 910 adhesive was employed to cement the electrode to the subject. Remarkably clean electromyograms were obtained on exercising subjects. Thompson's electrodes consisted of small pieces of silvered nylon applied to an area of skin that had been lightly sanded. The electrodes were applied with a special conducting adhesive. Although the electrodes were small and performed remarkably well during vigorous movement, the dc resistance between pairs was in the vicinity of 100,000 Ω, a characteristic that demanded the use of an amplifier with a very high input impedance.

Dry Electrodes

With the increasing availability of solid-state amplifiers with high input impedances, it is becoming recognized that bare conducting surfaces applied directly to the unprepared skin can be used as electrodes to detect bioelectrical events from human subjects. Such "dry" electrodes seldom remain dry when they are placed on skin that is endowed with sweat glands because perspiration usually accumulates and provides an electrolytic connection with the subject. It is therefore important to recognize that the impedance appearing between the electrode terminals will be high initially and will remain so if no perspiration accumulates to render the stratum

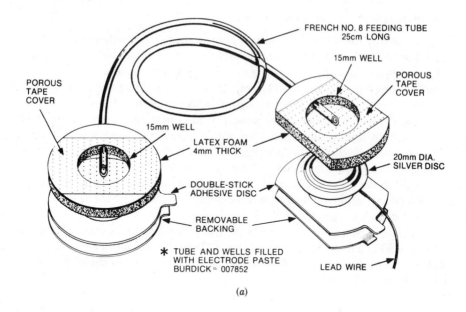

FRENCH NO. 8 FEEDING TUBE
25cm LONG

15mm WELL

POROUS
TAPE
COVER

POROUS
TAPE
COVER

15mm WELL

LATEX FOAM
4mm THICK

20mm DIA.
SILVER DISC

DOUBLE-STICK
ADHESIVE DISC

REMOVABLE
BACKING

* TUBE AND WELLS FILLED
WITH ELECTRODE PASTE
BURDICK ⓒ 007852

LEAD WIRE

(a)

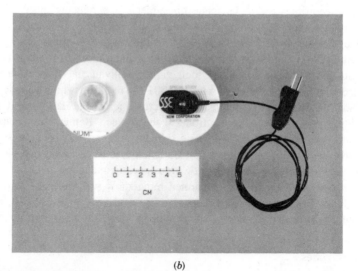

(b)

Figure 29 Radiotransparent electrodes for electrocardiography. [From H. Castillo and
H. Marriott, 1974. Radio transparent ECG electrodes for use during cardiac catheterization
Med. Instrum. **8:**116. By permission.]

corneum (the outer dry layer of the skin) conductive. In fact, if the sweat glands
are blocked by drugs (such as atropine), or if the skin is devoid of sweat glands,
or if it is thick and dry as in hypothyroidism, the electrodes may function largely
as capacitors and exhibit the characteristics of insulated electrodes, which capacitively couple the subject to the recording apparatus.

Johnson and Allred (1968) reported using dry silver-screen electrodes connected to a FET differential amplifier (with an input impedance of 10^7 Ω and a common-mode rejection ratio of 80 dB) to record the human electrocardiogram. They measured a range of electrode–subject impedances extending from 20 kΩ to 10 MΩ (for very dry skin). In another study, Bergey et al. (1971) applied bare metal electrodes (2.5 cm diameter) to unprepared human skin to record the electrocardiogram. They made measurements using several different metals and chose stainless steel as the optimum. However, a similar decrease in impedance with time was seen with all metals. After a few minutes the low-frequency impedance with stainless steel electrodes was in the range of 20–60 kΩ.

Bergey et al. (1971) investigated the impedance–frequency characteristics of dry 2.5-cm disks of anodized aluminum, stainless steel, gold, and silver applied to the unprepared inner surface of the forearm with Micropore adhesive tape. The current employed was 2 μA (peak to peak.) They measured the effect of perspiration on the impedance–frequency characteristics. The data for dry skin were obtained by placing the electrodes on the forearm; those for moist skin were obtained by placing the electrodes on the palm. The data they obtained appear in Fig. 30a.

Bergey et al. pointed out that the presence of perspiration lowered the impedance of the electrodes (Fig. 30b). They also noted that although silver exhibited the lowest impedance, they chose stainless steel for their electrode, because the least amount of movement artifact was obtained with this metal in a series of electrocardiographic tests with the various electrodes mounted directly on source-follower amplifiers.

The statement that the accumulation of perspiration under dry conducting surfaces, used as electrodes, results in a gradual decrease in the impedance measured between the electrode terminals is documented in Fig. 31. The initial value of impedance depends on the type of skin, its thickness, and the area of the electrode. The rate of decrease in impedance is quite variable and depends on a variety of environmental factors and the nature of the subject to whom the electrodes are applied. The following paragraphs provide some quantitative data on these points. In general, there is little change in impedance after about 30 min.

The electrooculogram has been recorded by Geddes and Valentinuzzi (1973) using dry coin-silver electrodes (1.7 cm in diameter) applied bitemporally. The initial impedances ranged from 5.1 to 230 kΩ. After about 20 min, the average impedance had dropped by about one order of magnitude.

One of the first practical clinical applications of dry electrodes was described by Wolfe and Reinhold (1973); they employed a dry conducting elastomer ¼ in. thick and measuring 2⅛ × ⅞ in. These electrodes were placed in the axillae of humans to acquire the ECG for aural monitoring and telemetry by a frequency-modulated tone transmitted by telephone. The impedance of these dry electrodes ranges from 2.5 to 60 kΩ, averaging 12.7 kΩ; these values were attained within a minute after application. Wolfe's electrodes were designed for emergency application by unskilled personnel to provide early diagnostic information on myocardial infarction.

Geddes et al. (1976b) described a dry silver suction electrode (18 mm in diameter) in a plastic housing containing an annulus (2.5 mm wide), to which neg-

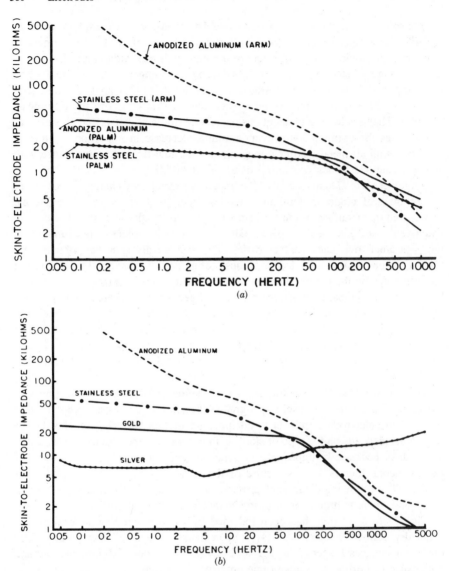

Figure 30 (*a*) Impedance–frequency characteristics of single disks (2.5 cm in diameter) of different metals placed on the inner aspect of the forearm; no skin preparation or electrode paste was employed. Measurements were made within 10 min of application; a peak-to-peak current of 2 μA was employed. (*b*) The effect of perspiration on the impedance–frequency characteristics.

ative pressure could be applied to hold the electrode against the skin. Figure 32 (inset) shows a sketch of the electrode and the force required to pull the electrode off (let-go force), versus negative pressures ($-P$) applied to different subjects.

The approximate impedance of a pair of the dry silver suction electrodes was measured by first recording the ECG with an amplifier having an input impedance

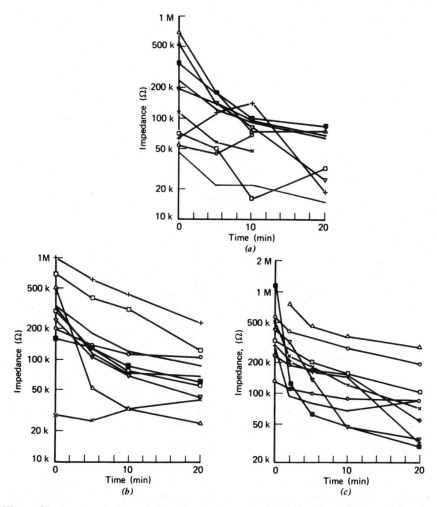

Figure 31 Temporal change in impedance encountered with dry electrodes supplied to the right arm and left leg to record the electrocardiogram: (*a*) silver electrodes (3.9 × 6.2 cm); (*b*) stainless steel electrodes (3.9 × 6.2 cm); (*c*) German silver electrodes (3.3 × 5.1 cm). [From L. A. Geddes and M. E. Valentinuzzi, *Ann. Biomed. Eng.* **1**:350–367 (1973). By permission.]

of 4000 MΩ. The input impedance was then reduced by placing a variable resistance across the input terminals and adjusting its value until the amplitude of the ECG was reduced by one-half. This resistance value was taken as the approximate electrode–subject impedance. The procedure was repeated at 2, 5, 10, and 20 min; Fig. 33 illustrates the results in 20 subjects. Initially impedances ranged from 0.18 to 10 MΩ (average 2.2 MΩ). The impedance decreased with time in most subjects. The impedance at 20 min ranged from 0.25 to 1.7 MΩ, with an average value of 0.68 MΩ. Placing a drop of tap water under each electrode dramatically decreased the average initial impedance to 0.449 MΩ (range 0.12–0.76 MΩ).

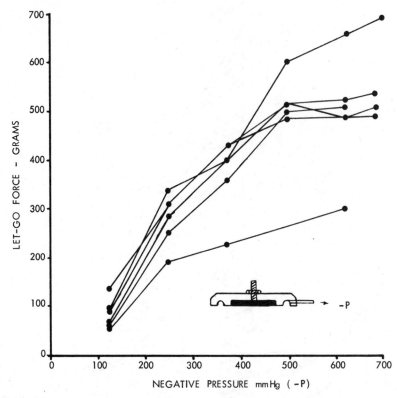

Figure 32 Let-go force versus negative pressure applied to the annulus surrounding the dry suction electrode on different subjects. [Redrawn from L. A. Geddes et al., *J. Electrocardiol.* **9**(2):155–159 (1976).]

The dry suction electrode is ideal for rapid screening of electrocardiograms. Prolonged application results in a red ring on the skin, which soon disappears after the electrode is removed. The width of the annulus and its diameter both determine the let-go force. These quantities can be selected to suit a particular application. The prior application of water to the skin not only reduces the initial impedance but also increases the let-go force.

Active Cables for Dry Electrodes. When dry electrodes, with their inherently high electrode–subject impedance, are used to measure bioelectric events, power-line interference is usually encountered. This undesirable event can be dramatically reduced by locating an amplifier at the dry electrode. A convenient method of achieving this goal was described by Bourland et al. (1978), who devised the active cable, which consists of a unity-gain amplifier located in a small housing behind an alligator clip (Fig. 34a). The alligator clip is affixed to the dry electrode, and three conductors (in a shield) connect the active cable to the recording apparatus. Two of the conductors and the shield provide operating voltage for the unity-gain

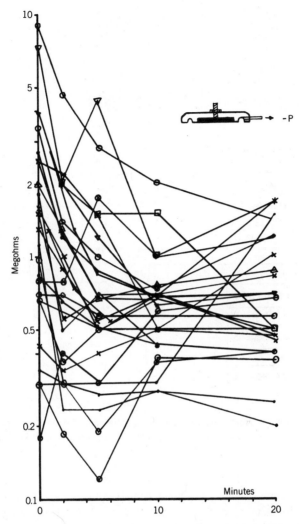

Figure 33   Impedance versus time for the dry silver (18-mm diameter) suction electrode applied to different subjects. [Redrawn from L. A. Geddes et al., *J. Electrocardiol.* **9**(2):155–159 (1976).]

amplifier; the third carries the output back to the recording apparatus, as shown in Fig. 34*b*. The same power supply (±9 V) can be used to energize multiple active cables. Because the output signal appears across the low output impedance of the unity-gain amplifier, there is little restriction on the length of the conductors. The input circuit of the active cable resembles a 1000-MΩ resistance shunted by 6 pF. The amplification is about 0.999. The common-mode rejection ratio of a pair of active cables with 10,000-Ω source impedance is typically more than 10,000 at 60 Hz.

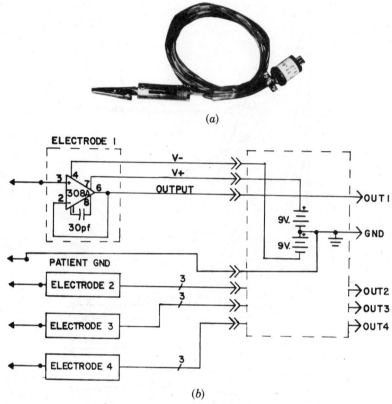

(a)

(b)

Figure 34 (a) Active cables and (b) their circuit diagram. In the plastic housing behind the alligator clip is located the operational amplifier. [Redrawn from J. D. Bourland et al., *J. Electrocardiol.* **11**(1):71–74 (1978).]

Figure 35 illustrates an ECG obtained with conventional electrodes and one obtained with dry metal-plate electrodes (6 × 3.8 cm). The two tracings were taken simultaneously from the arms of a human subject.

The active cables perform very well with a wide variety of dry electrodes. In fact, it is possible to record the ECG from anesthetized animals by pinching a fold of skin between the jaws of the alligator clips and placing a single drop of water on each clip–tissue interface.

Electrodeposited Electrodes. Edelberg (1963) described an efficient dry electrode made by electrodeposition of silver into the layers of the skin. The resistance between a pair of silver depositions was remarkably low, and no electrolytic paste was required; the silver spots were virtually terminals on the subject. The only drawback to these remarkable electrodes is their relatively short life. As time passes, the silver undergoes chemical changes and the spot eventually disappears. Nonetheless, because of their obvious advantages, use of these electrodes will continue to be investigated.

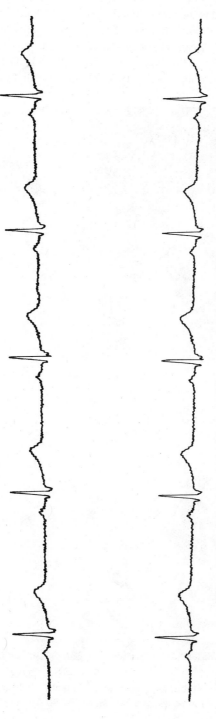

Figure 35 Electrocardiogram from the forearms of a human subject using (top) standard gelled electrodes and (bottom) dry metal plates. The tracings were made simultaneously. [Redrawn from J. D. Bourland et al., *J. Electrocardiol.* **11**(1):71–74 (1978).]

Spray-on Electrodes. An interesting low-mass dry electrode (Fig. 36) designed for aerospace research was described by Roman (1966), and technical details were presented by Patten et al. (1966). This electrode, which exhibits many desirable characteristics for human use, can be applied to the skin in only a few minutes. With a pair of these electrodes on the thorax, remarkably clean ECG and impedance respiration recordings can be obtained. By 1966 500 hr of in-flight and 700 hr of

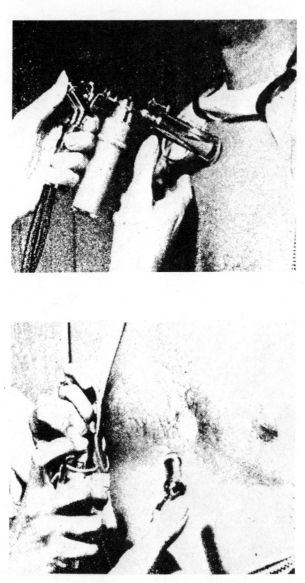

Figure 36 Spray-on electrode. [From J. Roman, and L. Lamb, Flight research program III. High impedance electrode techniques, *Aerosp. Med.* **37**:790–795 (1966). By permission.]

ground recording of the ECG had been logged successfully on Air Force personnel. The electrodes are applied by first rubbing electrode jelly into the skin with a toothbrush and then wiping the skin dry with gauze. Next a film of conducting adhesive [consisting of 43 g of Duco Household Cement (Dupont S/N 6241), 23 g of silver powder (Handy and Harman Silflake 135), and 125 mL of acetone] is painted or sprayed on the skin, forming a conducting spot about 20 mm in diameter. Then a silver-plated copper wire is placed in the conducting adhesive glue and is captured as drying occurs. When dry, the assembly is coated with insulating cement to cover the electrode (see Fig. 36). The impedance of these electrodes is dependent on their area. In the sizes customarily used, the low-frequency impedance is in the range of 50 kΩ, so that an amplifier with an input impedance of 2 MΩ or more is required if distortion-free ECGs are to be recorded.

ELECTRODE ELECTROLYTES

When metallic electrodes are placed on the surface of the body, contact is made via electrolytic solutions. If the electrodes are to be left in place for extended periods, evaporation of the solution takes place. To prevent such an occurrence, it is sometimes possible to locate the electrodes in body cavities and use the fluids in these regions as electrolytic conductors; sometimes the cavities can serve as containers for the electrolytes. Although not all the body cavities can be employed in unanesthetized subjects, consideration should be given to using the nose, ear, mouth, axilla, navel, rectum, vagina, and urethra. Often electrodes in these and other areas can be combined with other transducers, such as electrical thermometers or acoustic pickups. Sometimes the metallic cases of these devices can serve as active, indifferent, or ground electrodes.

Electrode jellies and pastes were developed during the early string-galvanometer days of electrocardiography when investigators were anxious to eliminate the cumbersome immersion electrodes, which required that the subject be seated with both hands and feet in saline-filled buckets. Study was begun of the behavior of electrodes consisting of sheets of metal wrapped in saline-soaked bandages and applied to the skin. Since the string galvanometer was activated by the electrical current that would flow as a result of the potential differences appearing on the body surface during cardiac activity (ECG), large electrodes and strong electrolytes were needed to obtain a low-resistance contact with the subject.

About 1935, when electrode pastes and jellies began to replace the saline-soaked pads, the characteristics of several of the earliest electrode jellies were investigated by Bell et al. (1939). Using lead electrodes (14 × 5 cm) on human subjects, they measured the dc resistance and 300-Hz impedance with the following substances under the electrodes: (a) 1% saline; (b) a paste of saline, glycerine, water, and pumice; (c) soft green soap; and (d) electrode jelly that contained crushed quartz. They found that when the electrodes were wrapped in gauze, soaked in 1% saline, and applied to the subjects, the dc resistance was highest (3080 Ω). With the other three preparations in direct contact with the electrodes and skin, the resistances were 2010, 2040, and 1100 Ω, respectively. By analyzing their results, Bell and his colleagues quickly found that the presence of an abrasive reduced the resistance considerably. They were able to show that the resistance with green soap was reduced by a factor of 3 when crushed quartz was added and the mixture rubbed into the skin. They also found that by lightly rubbing the dry skin with glass paper (fine sandpaper) and applying the electrolyte, they could obtain very low and extremely stable dc resistance and impedance values. This early observation demonstrated the need for abrasives in electrode pastes and jellies.

A modern reappraisal of traditional electrode jellies for recording the ECG was presented by Lewes (1965a, b), who called attention to the fact that strong electrolytes were essential in the string-galvanometer days, when the electrode–subject resistance had to be in low-kilohm range, but with the advent of electronic instruments with high input impedance the need for a low electrode resistance had disappeared. To prove his point he recorded more than 4000 ECGs with instruments of high input impedance (2–4 MΩ), using a remarkable variety of substances as electrode jellies. The recordings made with each substance were compared with those obtained with standard electrode jelly. The substances used were lubricating compounds (K-Y jelly, Lubrifax), culinary compounds (mayonnaise, French mustard, tomato paste), and toilet preparations (hand cream and tooth paste). All these substances are poor conductors, and all produced ECGs indistinguishable from those taken with standard electrode jelly.

From studies such as those jsut reported, it can be seen that two types of electrode preparation are now in use. One has low resistivity and originated in the days when it was necessary to obtain a low-resistance contact with the subject. Such preparations are still used for recording bioelectric events and must be used when electrodes are used to pass current, as in the case of stimulation or defibrillation. The other type of electrode electrolyte that is available is high in resistivity and resembles skin lotion. Such preparations are suitable for recording bioelectric events with modern equipment, which has an adequately high input impedance. Such preparations should never be used with stimulating or defibrillating electrodes. Table 5 presents the resistivity values for various electrode electrolytes.

The electrodes, and the electrolytes used with them, must not be considered to be independent of the recording equipment to which the electrodes are connected. Presented elsewhere in this chapter are additional studies relative to the type of distortion encountered when high-impedence electrodes are employed with amplifiers having input impedances that are not high enough.

Although most of the commercially available electrode pastes are satisfactory for recording a variety of bioelectric events, various authors have presented their own recipes. Among these are Jenks and Graybiel (1935), Bell et al. (1939), Marchant and Jones (1940), Thompson and Patterson (1958), Shackel (1958), Lykken (1959), Edelberg and Burch (1962), Asa et al. (1964), and Fascenelli et al. (1966).

TISSUE RESPONSE TO ELECTROLYTES

When recording bioelectric events with surface electrodes, attention should be given to the choice of the metal and electrolyte employed, since each may produce

TABLE 5   Resistivities of Electrode Electrolytes

Preparation and Supplier	Resistivity[a] (Ω-cm)
Redux Electrode Paste	9.4
Sanborn Div., Hewlett Packard: Waltham, Mass.	
Electrode Cream EC-2	30.0
Grass Instrument Co.: Quincy, Mass.	
Cambridge Electrode Jelly	10.4
Cambridge Instrument Co., Inc.	
Ossining, N.Y.	
Beckman-Offner Paste	5.9
Offner Division, Beckman Instruments, Inc.	
Chicago, Ill.	
EKG-Sol	200.0
Burton, Parsons & Co., Washington, D.C.	
Burdick Electrode Jelly	10.0
Burdick Co., Milton, Wis.	
Cardiopan	120.0[b]
Leichti: Berne, Switzerland	
Cardette Electrode Jelly	313.0[b]
Newmark Instrument Co., Croydon, Surrey, England	
Electrode Jelly	118.0[b]
Smith and Nephew Res. Ltd., Harlow, Essex, England	
Cardioluxe Electrode Jelly	84.0[b]
Philipps Electrical Ltd., Balham, London	
Electrode Jelly	196.0[b]
Data Display, Ltd., Liverpool, England	
NASA Flight Paste	13.0
National Aeronautics and Space Administration (NASA), Houston, Tex.	
Electrode Cream	82.0[b]
National Aeronautics and Space Administration (NASA), Houston, Tex.	
K-Y Lubricating Jelly	323.0[b]
Johnson & Johnson: Slough, Buckinghamshire, England	
0.9% (physiological) saline solution	70

[a]At room temperature
[b]From Hill and Khandpur, *World Med. Instrum.* 7:12–22 (1969) (By permission.)
Source: L. A. Geddes, *Electrodes and the Measurement of Bioelectric Events*. Wiley New York, 1972. (By permission.)

its own physiological effects. The constituents of some electrode pastes can cause allergic reactions, erythema, or discoloration of the skin. Some species of ions stimulate cells; others are toxic. For example, a high concentration of calcium chloride, such as was used in the older electrode jellies and pastes, causes sloughing of the skin. Seelig (1925) showed that subcutaneous injections of calcium chloride solutions with concentrations greater than 1% produced sloughing.

When recording the GSR, the ionic composition of electrolytes merits special consideration. For example, Edelberg and Burch (1962) conducted a series of ingenious experiments in which the responses at test and control sites were compared; they found that (1.0 M) solutions of calcium chloride, ammonium chloride, and potassium sulfate potentiated the GSR by 100–300%. Aluminum chloride potentiated by 1000%, and zinc chloride (0.5 M) approximately doubled the response. Very dilute acids, alkalis, and detergents decreased the response. A solution of 0.05 M sodium chloride had negligible effect on the GSR, and Edelberg recommended its use for this purpose. Thus in the routine recording of a bioelectric event from skin surfaces containing sweat glands, what may appear as an artifact may actually be an enhanced GSR. On the other hand, if one is attempting to record the GSR, the electrolyte may enhance or diminish the response. Scarification of the region under the electrode can produce unwanted voltages. Edelberg and Burch (1962) reported that although cuts or skin punctures lower skin resistance, they also reduce the GSR.

ARTIFACT REDUCTION BY SKIN ABRASION

Perhaps one of the most demonstrated facts in bioelectrical recording is the reduction in artifacts when the skin is abraded before application of the electrolytic gel and electrode. This desirable result is worthy of note because of its practical importance. Skin abrasion accomplishes two desirable goals: (1) reduction in electrode–subject impedance and (2) a reduction in artifacts due to electrode displacement (motion artifacts).

A novel method for obtaining a low resistance, which Shackel (1959) called the skin-drilling technique, is painless when properly employed. The area of skin where the electrode is to be placed is first cleaned with an antiseptic solution. The region is then abraded with a dental burr in a hand tool. Only the epidermis is eroded, and no blood is drawn. The amount of abrasion required depends on the type of skin. Kado (1965) reported that deeply pigmented skin requires more abrasion. In a few seconds, tissue fluid can be seen seeping into the drilled depression. The area is then cleaned with alcohol or with acetone (which is less popular today). If the skin has been drilled to the proper depth, the subject should feel a slight tingling sensation when the region is cleaned with either of these solutions. The electrode jelly is then applied and the electrode secured.

To test the value of the technique, Shackel compared the resistance values obtained with and without skin drilling. The drilled sites consistently exhibited values one-fifth to one-tenth of those of undrilled areas. When the electrodes are removed, the drilled site is again cleaned with antiseptic solution. Lanolin cream is then rubbed in, and the site soon becomes invisible.

Edelberg (1973) reported that the skin potential that appears across the granular layer of the skin is altered by skin deformation. This potential, which is affected by psychic stimuli, underlies the two components of the galvanic skin reflex, (1) a change in potential and (2) a change in resistance. Skin abrasion abolishes both responses.

To the equivalent circuit for electrodes on a subject (Fig. 17.), we can add the skin potential (E_p), as shown in Fig. 37. The other components in the circuit are the same as those in Fig. 17. Thus it can be seen that deformation of the skin by

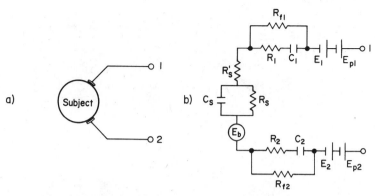

Figure 37   Equivalent circuit (including skin potential (E_p)), for electrodes on the skin of a subject for biopotential recording. (See Fig. 17 for identification of the other components.)

displacement of an electrode will change the skin potential and give rise to a motion artifact. Tam and Webster (1977) showed that the application and removal of a 500-g load to a skin-surface electrode produces a change of about 5 mV in skin potential. By abrading the skin with about 100 light strokes of very fine sandpaper (SN2 flint), the potential change was reduced to a negligible value.

Burbank and Webster (1978) showed that the change in potential due to skin deformation could be reduced to a negligible value by using a skin-puncture technique that consists of using a lancet protruding 0.5 mm from its holder. Only 10 punctures under the electrode site reduced the skin-deformation potential 25- to 50-fold. Tam and Webster (1977) pointed out that when skin abrasion was used with some standard, commercially available skin-surface electrodes, the electrolytes in them produced a mild skin irritation. When skin abrasion is to be used, they recommended that a mild electrolytic gel be used.

An interesting dry electrode (Fig. 38a) described in 1965 by Lewes (1965b) produces multiple-point punctures of the strateum corneum and should provide the characteristics of electrodes used with skin abrasion. This "multipoint" electrode consists of a 6 × 5 cm segment of a standard nutmeg grater made of stainless steel or tin-plated soft iron. It is slightly curved to fit over fleshy parts of the body; the abrasive side is placed against the skin. Approximately 1000 fine, active contact points are obtained when the electrode is applied to the skin with a very slight rotary movement that causes the multipoints to penetrate the stratum corneum, the layer responsible for the major part of skin resistance. When penetration occurs, a low-resistance contact is established with the subject. Lewes reported that the multipoint electrode resistance was similar to that obtained with plate electrodes and jelly. The impedance–frequency curves (Fig. 38b) obtained by Lewes and Hill (1966) over a frequency range of 1 Hz to 1 kHz closely resemble those produced with conventional plate electrodes and electrode jelly. With a smaller 1-in. circular chest electrode, the dc resistance was slightly higher (6 kΩ).

Multipoint electrodes are of special value in some unusual recording circumstances. For example, for screening the ECG in large numbers of human subjects, the short time required for application and removal is a most attractive feature. In

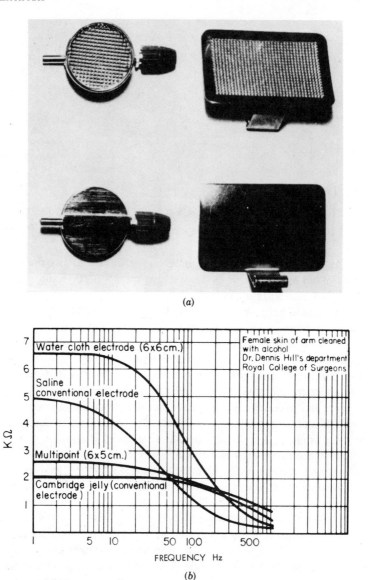

(a)

(b)

Figure 38 (*a*) Multipoint electrodes and (*b*) their impedance–frequency characteristics. (Courtesy of D. Lewes and D. Hill.)

a demonstration on one of the authors by Lewes, installation, recording three standard leads, and removal of the electrodes required only 80 sec. When it is not possible to prepare the skin for conventional electrodes, multipoint electrodes are ideal. For example, with hairy animals, when it is not permissible to remove the hair, coarse multipoint electrodes can be readily employed. Using such electrodes applied directly to the unprepared skin of the horse, Hill (1967) recorded the ECG and impedance respiration. Multipoint electrodes also see useful service in extreme environmental conditions. In situations of low temperature and barometric pressure, it is difficult to store electrode pastes and jellies in their containers. The use of multipoint electrodes eliminates the need for these substances and permits easy recording under field conditions.

In summary, it is now possible to identify the major sources of potential change that contribute to motion artifacts when skin-surface electrodes are used to measure a bioelectric event. Referring to Fig. 37, it can be seen that in addition to the bioelectric event E_b, there are four other potentials. Two (E_1 and E_2) are due to the electrode–electrolyte potentials, and two (E_{p1} and E_{p2}) are due to the skin potential under each electrode. Stabilization of E_1 and E_2 is accomplished by protecting the electrode–electrolyte interface from movement. The silver–silver chloride recessed electrode appears to be the best to date in this regard. Minimization of skin-potential changes, which give rise to the majority of the motion artifacts, can be achieved by skin abrasion, which effectively shunts the skin potential, reducing it to a low value.

CAPACITIVE ELECTRODES

A capacitive electrode consists of a conductor completely covered by an insulator (dielectric). Since there is no ohmic connection, coupling to the subject is capacitive. Such electrodes were described by Richardson (1967a, b), Richardson and Coombs (1968), Richardson et al. (1968), and Lopez and Richardson (1969). Their electrodes consisted of an aluminum plate (2.5 × 2.5 cm) anodized on the surface and placed in contact with the skin. On the back of the electrode was mounted a field-effect transistor (FET) with the gate terminal connected to the electrode. Surrounding the anodized electrode was a block of insulating potting compound, contained by a circular metal ring that acts as an electrostatic shield (Fig. 39a). The FET was connected as a source follower (Fig. 39b). To protect the FET from acquiring a high electrostatic voltage, a high-resistance leakage path was provided by using two diodes (IN3600) placed in series opposition. The diodes can be omitted if a higher input impedance is desired. Richardson reported that the resistance of the anodized electrode, measured between the gate of the transistor and the subject, is between 1000 and 30,000 MΩ.

According to the various investigators who have used capacitive electrodes, the high input impedance of the FET provides a time constant long enough (about 3 sec) for reproduction of the human ECG. In use, two electrodes are applied to the subject with no skin preparation. The outputs of the source followers (or unity-gain amplifiers), can be connected to a conventional electrocardiograph. Figure 40 is an example of recordings taken with insulated electrodes and conventional plate electrodes to which electrode jelly has been applied.

Following Richardson's lead, Wolfson and Neuman (1969) developed a small insulated electrode consisting of a chip of N-type silicon (6 × 6 mm, 0.23 mm thick) on which was thermally deposited a circular layer of silicon dioxide (0.2 μm thick, 4.5 mm in diameter). The region outside the circle and on the edges of the chip were insulated with a layer of silicon dioxide 1.5 μm thick. The electrode

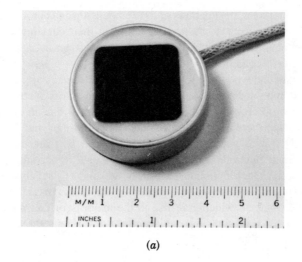

(a)

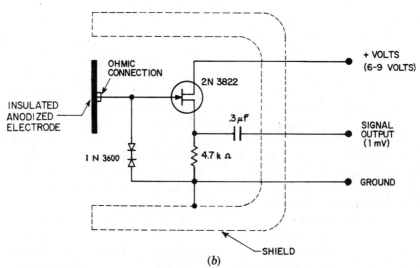

(b)

Figure 39 Insulated electrodes. (*a*) Richardson's insulated electrodes; (*b*) source-follower circuit for use with the insulated electrode. (Courtesy of P. C. Richardson, personal communication, 1969.)

was connected and mounted to an ultrahigh-input impedance amplifier that employed a metal oxide semiconductor field-effect transistor (MOSFET) as the input stage arranged in a source–follower configuration. A second MOSFET was used as an electronic switch to protect the input transistor from damage caused by stray electrostatic voltages. The input impedance attained was 10^{10} Ω, and the sinusoidal frequency response, measured from the subject to the output of the source follower, extended to 0.005 Hz, which indicates a capacitive coupling to the subject of 3200 pF and provides an input time constant of 32 sec.

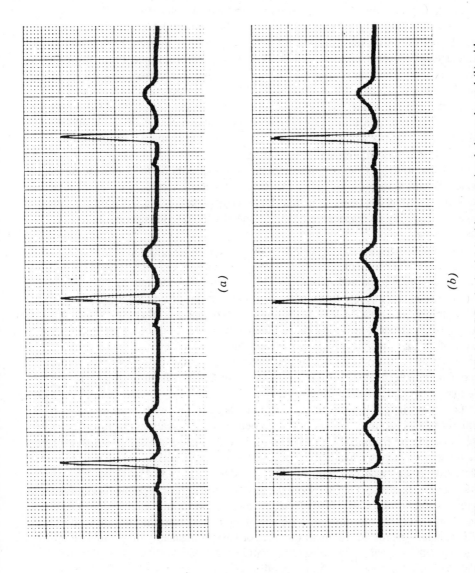

(a)

(b)

Figure 40 Simultaneously recorded ECGs obtained (a) with conventional electrodes and (b) with insulated electrodes. (Courtesy of P. C. Richardson, personal communication, 1969.)

Although capacitive electrodes showed initial promise, they did not gain wide acceptance, probably because they were rather sensitive to electrostatic discharges. Their application to hairy skin usually produces artifacts and reduces the coupling capacitance. However, certain of the interesting characteristics can be identified. Like any dry electrode, a capacitive electrode can be applied quickly without skin preparation, eliminating all danger of tissue response, which accompanies the long-term use of some conventional electrolytes. There is no doubt that under ideal circumstances the amount of capacitive coupling and input impedance attainable is adequate for the measurement of a variety of bioelectric events. From the data given by the various authors and by Rylander (1970), it appears that the capacitances attained range from about 5000 to 20,000 pF per square centimeter of electrode area. In using such capacitively coupled electrodes with FETs, it is necessary to take precautions to prevent electrostatic puncture of the insulation (dielectric). When completely isolated instruments (e.g., battery-operated telemeters) are used, this requirement is less stringent.

With the insulated electrode, although there is no electrode–electrolyte interface, which is one source of artifacts with conventional electrodes, another type of movement artifact can be encountered. Displacement on the skin will alter the skin potential and vary the capacitive coupling, thereby altering the charge distribution and potential.

At present there are attempts to provide ultrathin films of insulating materials having high dielectric constants and strengths so that a high electrode-to-subject capacitance will be attained and the insulation will not be punctured by the voltages that insulated electrodes may acquire. Heroic efforts in this direction may not be amply rewarded, because it must be remembered that the other "plate" of the capacitive electrode is in reality constituted by the tissue fluids below the older dry layer of the skin, which varies in thickness. Initially, the dielectric consists of the dry outer layer of skin plus the insulating film on the electrode. As time passes, perspiration will accumulate and hydrate the skin; then the dielectric thickness will be that of the dielectric film.

Lagow et al. (1971) called attention to the fact that the insulation deposited on some insulated electrodes is permeable to perspiration. In particular, films of aluminum oxide are corroded by exposure to saline; this results in a dramatic reduction in resistance, thereby invalidating use of the term "insulated" to describe the electrode. To eliminate this problem, they first demonstrated that oxidized tantalum is saline-resistant; they then anodized this material to fabricate capacitive electrodes with a stability much in excess of that encountered with aluminum oxide. David and Portnoy (1972) recommended the use of saline-resistant films of silicon dioxide, tantalum pentoxide, titanium dioxide, or barium titanate, which could be applied by radiofrequency sputtering. They fabricated capacitive electrodes with these dielectrics and demonstrated their capabilities for recording the electrocardiogram.

ELECTRODES FOR EXPOSED TISSUE

When the electrical activity of the exposed cortex is recorded, it is customary to employ silver-ball electrodes approximately 1 mm in diameter, bare or chlorided,

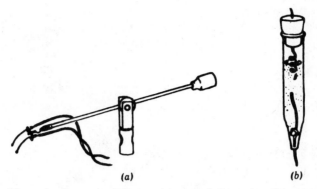

(a)   *(b)*

Figure 41   Electrodes for exposed tissues: *(a)* cortical electrodes; *(b)* wick electrode.

and sometimes covered with a small cotton pad. Geddes (1948–1949) described the preparation and use of these electrodes, one type of which is illustrated in Fig. 41*a*. The dc resistance between a pair of these electrodes spaced a few centimeters apart on the human brain is in the 10–50-kΩ range.

In some studies it is necessary to employ the wick electrode illustrated in Fig. 41*b*, which is often made from a medicine dropper. A cotton wick is placed in the tapered end, and a cork in the large end holds a chlorided silver wire in contact with the electrolyte in the dropper. These electrodes were described and thoroughly investigated by Burr (1944, 1950). They are frequently used for dc recording because a pair can be made having a voltage difference as small as 10 μV or less. The dc resistance of two cotton-wick electrodes in saline is in the 10–50-kΩ range. Kahn (1965) described electrodes of this type in which the metal consisted of a compressed mixture of silver and silver chloride. The electrolyte employed was saline and in some instances plasma. The voltage difference between a saline-filled pair varied between 5 and 10 μV.

A similar type of medicine dropper electrode, developed for total implantation, was described by Rowland (1961). The stem of his electrode measured 15 mm long and 6 mm in diameter, and in it he placed a coiled-coil electrode made from 30-gauge silver wire that was in contact with saline. The coiled coil was made by first winding 5 in. of wire around a 20-gauge needle and then removing and stretching the coil slightly so that the individual turns did not contact each other. The coil was then wrapped around a needle of the same size and inserted into the stem of the small medicine dropper. This technique permits obtaining a large electrode-electrolyte junctional area in a small space. Rowland reported that the dc resistance range of such electrodes was 30–50 kΩ with a potential difference in the millivolt range between pairs. He demonstrated their value in recording six channels of EEG in the cat.

PERCUTANEOUS ELECTRODES

Collar-Button Electrodes

Mooney et al. (1974) described a most ingenious method of creating a percutaneous vitreous carbon terminal in human subjects; one part is above the skin,

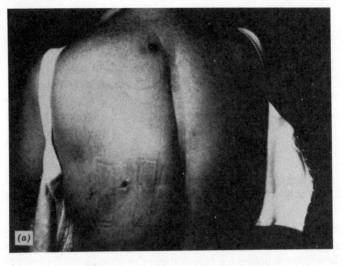

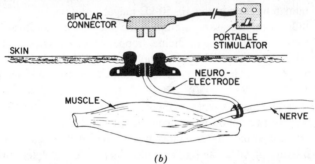

(b)

Figure 42 (a) Vitreous carbon percutaneous implants applied to the human subject; (b) implants used as cable connector for electrodes applied to a nerve. [From V. Mooney et al., *Arch Surg. (Chicago)* **108**:148–153 (1974). By permission.]

and the other is below; Fig. 42 illustrates these devices, which resemble a collar button made of vitreous carbon. Using local anesthesia, the devices can be implanted surgically with the larger part of the collar button below the skin and the smaller part protruding. Healing, without reddening, occurs around the protruding portion in a manner that resembles the skin surrounding the base and sides of finger nails.

Vitreous carbon, which is surprisingly well tolerated by living tissue, is made by firing an organic polymer in an inert atmosphere at about 1800°C. The firing time is adjusted so that all elements other than carbon are eliminated. The resulting hard material is very smooth and retains the shape of the original polymer, except that a shrinkage of about 40% has occurred. The vitreous material can be polished with a diamond polishing compound.

Figure 42a illustrates a typical percutaneous "collar button" and the appearance of the skin surrounding it 26 months after implantation. Mooney and Hartmann reported implantation of 23 vitreous carbon implants into 11 persons. The implants can be used as cable connectors, as in Fig. 42b, or as stimulating or recording electrodes. They have also been used for skeletal attachment for limb prostheses. Rarely has there been any difficulty with healing or infection; however more research is needed to verify these observations.

Depth Electrodes

Because electrodes placed on the scalp or cortex detect mainly the electrical activity of the neurons in the superficial layers of the brain, the need has arisen to find a method of detecting the electrical activity of subcortical nerve cells. Two types of depth electrodes have been developed; one, due to Delgado (1955, 1964) (see Figs. 43a, b), the other due to Ray (1966) (see Figs. 43c, d). Delgado's electrode consists of a bundle of Teflon-insulated stainless steel wires (0.005 in. in diameter) of differing lengths bonded to a central supporting wire (0.007 in. in diameter) by an insulating varnish. The end of the supporting wire is rounded for ease of insertion into the brain. The ends of the individual wires are staggered 3 mm, and their 1-mm exposed surfaces constitute the individual electrodes. The active area of each electrode is in the vicinity of 0.5 mm^2. The end of the central supporting wire often serves as an indifferent electrode.

Ray's electrode consists of a bundle of 18-gauge insulated wires bonded to a length of 24-gauge stainless steel needle tubing with a high-temperature varnish. Each wire is platinum (90%)–iridium (10%) and is 0.0035 in. in diameter; the active electrodes are made by scraping the varnish from the wires at the desired places. The scraped area is then platinized to reduce the tissue–electrode impedance by about a hundredfold. The contact area employed by Ray was 0.075 × 1.00 mm.

The depth electrodes described by Delgado and Ray have been implanted into the brains of animals and humans and left there for prolonged periods to record the electrical activity of subcortical neurones under a variety of normal and abnormal states. Ray reported that the central stainless steel needle that supports the electrodes could be used for the injection of materials into the brain or the passage of a guarded microelectrode. He also stated that his electrodes could serve to measure localized impedance changes; with application of the proper polarizing voltage, moreover, the electrodes are suitable for the continuous recording of oxygen tension.

Needle Electrodes

Electromyographers often find it convenient to use a variety of electrodes; some are placed on the skin, whereas others are inserted directly into the muscle being examined. For precise localization, steel needle electrodes are inserted directly into the muscle. Usually the electrodes are coated with an insulating varnish and are bare only at the tip. Frequently one needle electrode is paired with a metallic plate on the surface of the skin. Figure 44a illustrates this type of needle electrode,

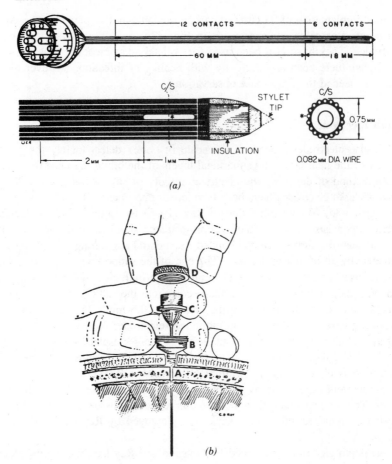

(a)

(b)

Figure 43 (*a*) Delgado's depth electrode; (*b*) method of insertion. [From J. M. R. Delgado, *EEG Clin. Neurophysiol.* **7**:637–644 (1955). By permission.] (*c*) Ray's depth electrode (now available from Medical Applications Dept. 249, IBM Corp., Rochester, Minnesota). (*d*) method of insertion. [From C. D. Ray, *J. Neurosurg.* **24**:911–921 (1966). By permission.]

which was described by Jasper et al. (1945). When the shaft of the needle electrode is coated with insulating varnish, the area of the electrode in contact with active tissue is quite small. In the case of Jasper's needle electrode, the area was approximately 0.2 mm^2.

There is a need for EMG electrodes that can be left in place for prolonged periods. To meet this requirement, many interesting electrodes have been developed. The main goals have been ease of insertion, freedom from pain during insertion, mechanical and electrical stability during muscular contraction, minimal interference with muscular movement, and freedom from pain while in situ. Although few types have attained all these goals, some very promising electrodes have been constructed. For example, Basmajian and Stecko (1962) developed a

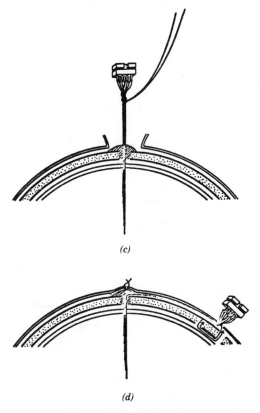

(c)

(d)

Figure 43 (*Continued*)

bipolar fine-wire (25 μm in diameter) electrode that is easily inserted and remains well anchored in the muscle. The steps in construction of this electrode are shown in Fig. 44*b*. In the lower right-hand corner of the figure, the electrode is ready for insertion into the muscle by advancing the hypodermic needle. When the desired depth is reached, the hypodermic needle is withdrawn, leaving the electrode in the muscle. The bent ends serve as hooks to prevent the electrode from coming dislodged.

In a similar fine-wire electrode described by Scott (1965), the insulated wire (Karma) is passed through the lumen of the hypodermic needle and bent back to pass along the outside of the needle [Fig. 44*c*(1)]. The hypodermic needle and wire are then inserted to the desired depth in the muscle [Fig. 44*c*(2)]. With the outside wire held firmly, a pair of forceps is applied to the inner wire, and the wire is cut by winding it on the forceps [Fig. 44*c*(3)] so that it contacts the sharp edge of the hypodermic needle. Then the needle is withdrawn, leaving the outer wire in the tissue [Fig. 44*c*(4)]. The active surface of the electrode is approximately the cross-sectional area of the wire.

Another method of inserting fine-wire electrodes was developed by Parker

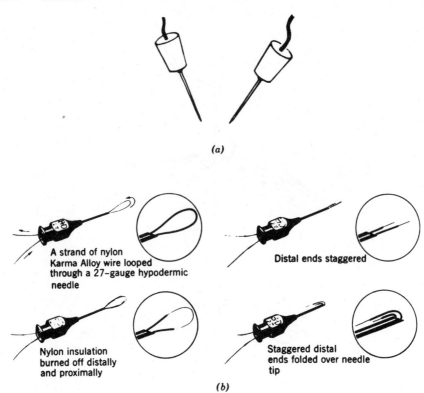

Figure 44a, b   Electrodes for electromyography. (*a*) Needle electrodes; (*b*) steps in making a bipolar electrode assembly before sterilization. [From J. V. Basmajian and G. Stecko, *J. Appl. Physiol.* **17**:894 (1962). By permission.]

(1966). A short length at the end of a fine wire is bent back upon itself. The bent-back portion is then inserted into the tip of the hypodermic needle [Fig. 44*d*(1)] and the needle and wire are advanced into the muscle [Fig. 44*d*(2)]. At the desired depth the hypodermic needle is withdrawn, leaving the electrode hooked into the muscle [Fig. 44*d*(3)]. With this technique, monopolar or bipolar electrodes can be installed. The active surface of the electrode is the cross-sectional area of the wire. Hook electrodes are removed by a brisk pull, which straightens the wire so that it exits without tissue damage.

Geddes and Baker (1966) measured the impedance–frequency characteristics of a variety of pairs of stainless steel needle electrodes similar to those illustrated in Fig. 44*a*. The electrodes were insulated down to the tip, which was left bare. The area of each pair of electrodes was carefully measured before insertion into the left hind limb and right forelimb of an anesthetized dog. After 5 min, impedance–frequency curves were determined. The procedure was repeated for each pair of electrodes. Current density was maintained at the same level at each frequency.

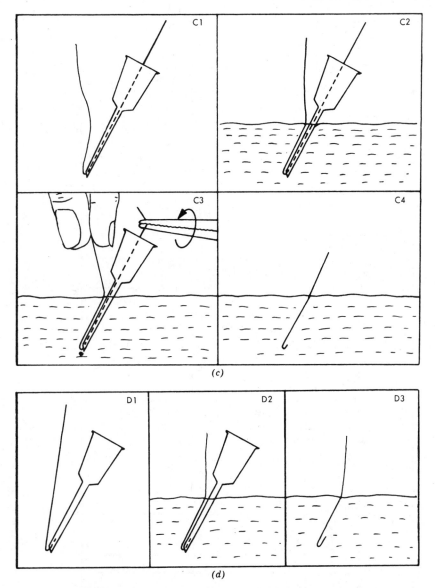

Figure 44c, d   (c) Scott's electrode. (d) Parker's electrode.

The impedance–frequency curves for the various pairs of needle electrodes are presented in Fig. 45. Clearly evident at all frequencies is the inverse relationship between electrode area and impedance. Also apparent is a decrease in impedance with increasing frequency. The contours of the impedance–frequency curves of the various electrodes examined are similar to those predicted by the nature of the electrode–electrolyte interface.

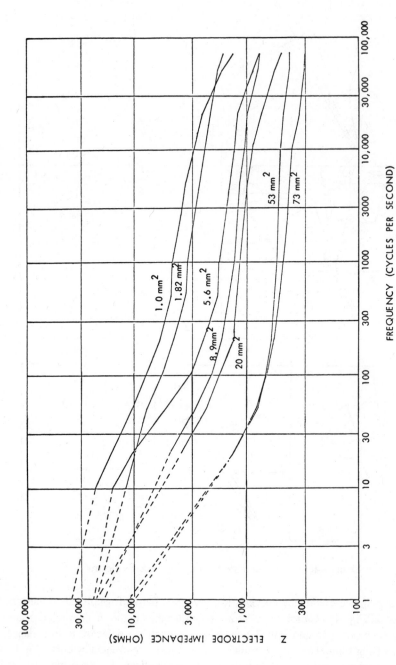

Figure 45 Impedance–frequency curves for needle electrodes.[From L. A. Geddes and L. E. Baker, *Med. Biol. Eng.* **4**:439–450 (1966). By permission.]

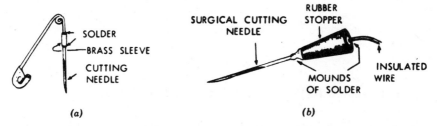

Figure 46 Cutting electrodes: (a) safety pin electrodes; (b) needle electrodes. [From L. A. Geddes et al., *Southwest. Vet.* **18**:56–57 (1964). By permission.]

Cutting Electrodes

Occasionally it is necessary to record from animals with thick dry hides and conventional needle electrodes cannot be easily inserted. To solve this problem, Geddes et al. (1964) developed two types of cutting electrodes (Fig. 46). These electrodes are made from surgical cutting needles, and their beveled, sharpened shanks permit easy insertion through the hide.

When cutting electrodes are used, movement artifacts can be minimized by inserting the needles in a manner such that the area of the bare metal electrode in contact with the tissues is constant. The safety-pin electrode should be inserted through a pinch of skin and fastened. When the pinch is released, the skin will press against the head and spring of the safety pin. The connecting wire is soldered to the brass sleeve, and the sleeve and solder connection are covered with insulation to prevent their contact with body fluids. To provide strain relief for the solder joint, the connecting wire is passed through the coils of the spring and tied. Similarly, with the needle electrode it is advisable to insulate the soldered portions of the electrode and the part of the shank above the cutting edge and to insert the electrode into the animal far enough that no bare needle protrudes.

Hypodermic Needle Electrodes

To record the electrical activity of small groups of cells, monopolar and bipolar hypodermic electrodes are often used. Such types, first described by Adrian and Bronk (1929), are shown in Fig. 47. The monopolar electrode was made with 36-

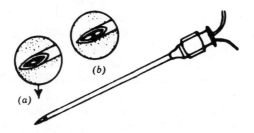

Figure 47 (a) Monopolar and (b) bipolar hypodermic needle electrodes.

gauge wire (190 μm in diameter), and the bipolar electrode contained two 44-gauge wires (80 μm in diameter). These electrodes exhibit dc resistances in the range of tens of kilohms.

TISSUE RESPONSE TO IMPLANTED ELECTRODE METALS

In many recording situations, electrodes must remain in direct contact with body tissues and fluids for prolonged periods. For example, when electrodes are implanted in muscle and brain tissue to record the bioelectric signals of these structures for periods of months, special consideration must be given to the type of metal employed. There were only a few studies of the relative toxicity of the various species of metallic ions in the early days of depth electrode recording in the human brain. Dodge et al. (1955) had the opportunity to study the tissue response to two electrodes, each consisting of six strands of Formvar-insulated copper wire (97.5 μm in diameter), which had been in situ for 6 days. Nineteen months later the brain was examined histologically. Tissue changes were seen at the points of entry of the electrodes. Minimal tissue changes were found along the tracks of the electrodes.

Faced with the problem of recording the electrical activity of structures deep within the brains of human and animal subjects, Fischer et al. (1957) studied the response of the brains of cats to 1-cm lengths of 24-gauge wires left in situ for periods up to 4 weeks. The wires employed were of chlorided silver, bare copper, and stainless steel. Both bare and insulated wires were employed. After 1 week, histological studies showed tissue responses to all of the materials used. The responses were dependent on the type of metal employed; the insulating compounds were virtually without tissue response. Silver and copper wires proved to be the most toxic to brain tissue. After 3 weeks a narrow ring of necrotic tissue surrounded the silver wire. Around this ring was a circular edematous region 2 mm in diameter. The reaction to the copper wire after 3 weeks was similar except that an increase in vascularity had also occurred. The copper wire was encircled by necrotic tissue and an edematous region. The diameter of the lesion varied between 1.5 and 7 mm. With the stainless steel wire, the size of the lesion was determined by the extent of the mechanical trauma produced by its introduction into the brain. Only minimal edema was found. Fischer and co-workers therefore concluded that the electrode material of choice for such studies is stainless steel.

In another study, carried out by Collias and Manuelidis (1957), bundles of six stainless steel electrodes (125 μm in diameter) were inserted into the brains of cats. Describing the histological changes that occurred over periods extending up to 6 months, the investigators found that an orderly sequence of changes took place in the tissue surrounding the electrode track. At the end of 24 hr there was a zone of hemorrhage, necrosis, and edema extending to about 1 mm from the electrode. After 3 days there was less hemorrhage and necrotic debris, and by the seventh day a 0.1-mm layer of capillaries occupied the necrotic zone. By the fifteenth day the capillaries had almost completely replaced the necrotic region, and connective tissue had started to form. After the passage of a month the necrotic debris had disappeared, and a well-defined capsule surrounded the electrode track. Capsule formation was virtually complete after 4 months, at which time a thick, dense capsule completely encircled the electrode.

Robinson and Johnson (1961) carried out studies similar to those just described. They implanted wires (125 μm in diameter) of gold, platinum, silver, stainless steel, tantalum, and tungsten into cat brains and studied the tissue responses at various times over a period extending to 6 months. Responses similar to those previously described were observed. After about a week the differences between the metals in regard to the reaction produced began to be detectable. Gold and stainless steel evoked the least tissue response; tantalum, platinum, and tungsten produced more. Silver precipitated a vigorous tissue reaction. Encapsulation of all electrodes was evident at 15 days, with thicker capsules around the metals that provoked the greatest tissue response.

It is important to emphasize that these tissue changes were studied in cat brains with electrodes that carried no current. Studies on the responses of other tissues to other electrode materials and on tissue responses to current-carrying electrodes are now being made. It is anticipated that the tissue response to current-carrying electrodes will be different in view of the many electrolytic reactions that can occur.

WAVEFORM DISTORTION DUE TO INPUT IMPEDANCE OF THE BIOELECTRIC RECORDER

When recording bioelectric events, it is necessary to make the input impedance of the bioelectric recorder many times larger than the impedance appearing between the electrode terminals. When this technique is employed, only a small current flows through the electrode impedance, and there is a minimal loss of voltage at the electrode–electrolyte interface. However, if the bioelectric recorder has an input impedance that is not high with respect to the impedance of the smallest-area electrode, there can occur a distortion in the waveform of the bioelectric event. Because of the resistive and reactive components of the electrode–electrolyte impedance, the various components of the bioelectric event will not be presented to the bioelectric recorder with the same relative amplitudes they initially possessed. Moreover, phase distortion accompanies such amplitude–frequency distortion, and the time relations between the various frequency components will be altered. In addition, it is known that the resistive and reactive components of the impedance decrease when high current densities are encountered. If the input impedance of the bioelectric recorder is so low that high current densities result, it is possible for the electrode impedance to become dependent on the amplitude of the bioelectric event. If this occurs, small- and large-amplitude signals will be injected differently into the input of the bioelectric recorder. It is thus apparent that the use of an input stage whose impedance is not very high with respect to the electrode–subject impedance virtually guarantees that the bioelectric event will be distorted. A high electrode current density can occur when the electrode area is small (as it is with metal microelectrodes) and a conventional amplifier is employed.

It has already been demonstrated that waveform distortion of clinical significance occurs when high-resistance electrodes are employed with recorders having a low resistive input impedance. In the early days of electrocardiography, when string galvanometers with their relatively low resistance (5–20 kΩ) were used, Lewis (1914–1915) showed that a normal ECG was distorted when recorded with polarizable platinum electrodes. In such cases attenuated P and T waves and enhanced S waves were obtained. Similarly, Pardee (1917a, b), using a string galvanometer and German silver electrodes applied to a bandage soaked in saline, showed that the rectangular wave calibration signal was distorted when the area of each electrode was decreased from 300 to 8 cm^2. With the smaller electrodes, the calibration signal, instead of rising rapidly and exhibiting a flat top, showed a sharp overshoot and an R-C decay to a sustained plateau. On turning off the calibrate signal, there was an undershoot and R-C decay to the baseline. Pardee (1917a, b) observed a similar type of distortion when electrodes were applied to patients with thick, dry skin or when the blood vessels under the electrodes were constricted. The distortion disappeared when an electrolyte was rubbed into the skin. It often disappeared as time passed and the electrolyte penetrated the dry, horny layers of the skin. Although Pardee did not investigate the phenomenon thoroughly, his observations are in agreement with those of previous and later workers, notably Einthoven (1928), who demonstrated that the electrode–subject interface impedance introduced a time constant into the circuit that electrically differentiated the P and T waves.

The practical importance of these facts in recording the ECG was again made evident by Sutter (1944) and Roman and Lamb (1962). These investigators applied small-area electrodes to the chest of a human subject and used them first with an amplifier having a high input impedance to obtain control records. They then lowered the input impedance of the amplifier by connecting different resistances across it. The distortions in the ECG were what would be called clinically significant, consisting of a displacement of the S-T segment and a slight depression in the latter part of the T wave.

Studies focusing attention on the relationship between recorder input impedance and electrode impedance were carried out by Geddes and Baker, who investigated the relationship between resistive input impedance and electrode area in recording the ECG (1966) and the EMG (1967). By using electrodes of differing areas and shunting the amplifier input with various resistors (loading), the effect of electrode interface impedance was made to manifest itself.

Figure 48, showing a lead II ECG in an anesthetized dog, illustrates the type of distortion encountered when this technique was employed. Stainless steel needle electrodes such as those in Fig. 44a were used. The needles were insulated to within 1 mm of the tip. The geometric area in contact with the body tissues and fluids was approximately 1 mm^2. To illustrate the nature of the distortion, a square pulse was inserted in series with the electrodes. Figure 48b shows the control ECG and square pulse recorded with an amplifier having a 4-MΩ resistive input impedance. Figures 48c–e reveal the changes produced by placing resistors of successively lower values across the input of the amplifier. During the various trials the electrodes were not disturbed. In Figs. 48b–d, the recording sensitivity was the same. In Fig. 48e the recording sensitivity was doubled for clearer comparison with Fig. 48b.

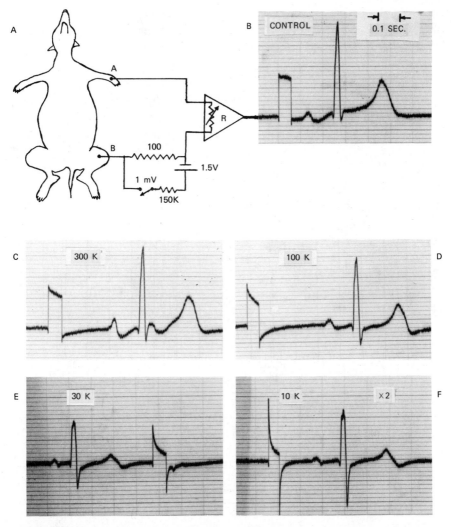

Figure 48 Distortion in the ECG produced by lowering input impedance. [From L. A. Geddes and L. E. Baker, *Med. Biol. Eng.* **4:**439–450 (1966). By permission.]

The outstanding changes seen in these records are those expected in a system that is deficient in low-frequency response. Such a situation can be predicted on the basis of the general nature of the impedance–frequency curves of electrodes. With 300 kΩ across the input terminals, there were recognizable P and T wave changes, and a noticeable tilt appeared on the square pulse. With 100 kΩ, and especially with 30 kΩ, across the input terminals, the P and T waves and the square pulse were dramatically changed, all becoming diphasic. As loading was increased, there was a continued loss of overall amplitude, and in Figs. 48*d* and *e* the resemblance to the control record was all but lost. In Fig. 48*f*, recorded with twice the amplification, the ECG is vastly different from that in Fig. 48*b*. The outstanding

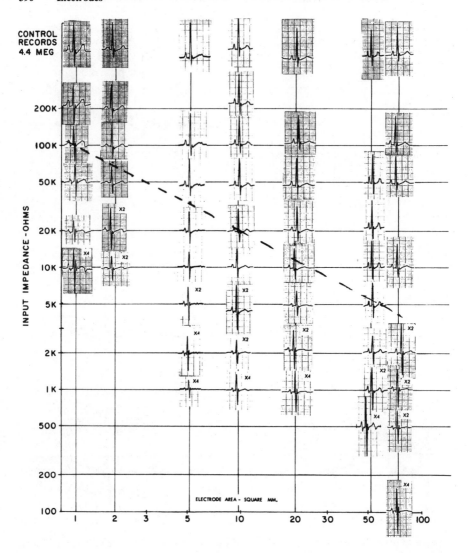

Figure 49a   Relationship between input impedance and electrode area for recording the ECG with needle electrodes. The distortion can be easily identified below the dashed line. [Redrawn from L. A. Geddes and L. E. Baker, *Med. Biol. Eng.* **4**:439–450 (1966).]

differences are the loss of P and T wave amplitudes and the addition of diphasic components to each. The QRS complex has similarly been changed by exaggeration of the S wave.

The manner in which this type of distortion is related to electrode area is shown in Fig. 49a. In this illustration, ECGs of anesthetized dogs were recorded with various pairs of needle electrodes connected in lead II configuration. The control records, shown along the top of each column, were all obtained with an input impedance of 4.4 MΩ. The changes that occurred as the input impedance of the amplifier was lowered can be appreciated by reading from top to bottom of any column; for example, for the 1-mm^2 electrodes, noticeable distortion occurred when the input impedance was reduced to 100 kΩ. For the 10-mm^2 electrodes, detectable distortion occurred when the input impedance was 20 kΩ. Clearly evident in this illustration is the relationship between distortion, amplifier input impedance, and electrode area.

Figure 49*b* shows the relationship between input impedance and electrode area in recording evoked muscle action potentials and a square wave in series with the electrodes. Along the top of the figure are the control records obtained with an input impedance of 1000 MΩ. Reading from top to bottom it is seen that distortion is produced when the input impedance is reduced sufficiently. The waveforms above the dashed curve exhibit little distortion; those below are noticeably distorted. Note that there is an inverse relation between electrode area and input impedance to avoid distortion.

From the foregoing, it can be seen that for a given bioelectric event, the smaller the electrode area, the higher the input impedance must be to avoid distortion of the bioelectric event. This statement constitutes the rule for recording bioelectric events. In a particular case, the relationship will depend on the waveform of the bioelectric event. Figure 50 shows the relationship for recording frog muscle action potential and the dog ECG with needle electrodes of different areas and for recording the human ECG with recessed electrodes of different areas. Note, however, that these relationships identify resistive input impedances for detectable distortions. Obviously an input impedance many times higher should be used in practice.

The relationship between amplifier input impedance and electrode area is not the same for all metals. Cooper (1963) compared the distortions encountered when silver–silver chloride, platinum, silver, copper, gold, and stainless steel electrodes, all of the same area (0.1 mm^2), were connected to an amplifier with a 750-kΩ input impedance. The test consisted of passing a square wave of current through a saline bath in which the electrode pairs were immersed. The types of waveforms detected by the various electrode pairs are presented in Fig. 51. Clearly evident is the same kind of distortion that appeared in Figs. 48–50, electrical differentiation or, stated differently, a loss of low-frequency response. Interestingly enough under these circumstances, the silver–silver chloride electrodes reproduced the waveform most accurately, and the stainless steel electrodes provided the poorest reproduction of the test signal. This does not mean that stainless steel electrodes cannot be used with success; it does indicate that an amplifier having high input impedance is required with stainless steel electrodes of small surface area.

These results, which are consistently reproducible, are in agreement with those described by other investigators. They call attention to the need to use an input stage with an input impedance many times larger than that of the bioelectric generator–electrode system.

The distortion illustrated in Figs. 48, 49, and 51 is caused by two factors. First, with loading (i.e., the use of an amplifier input circuit in which the input impedance

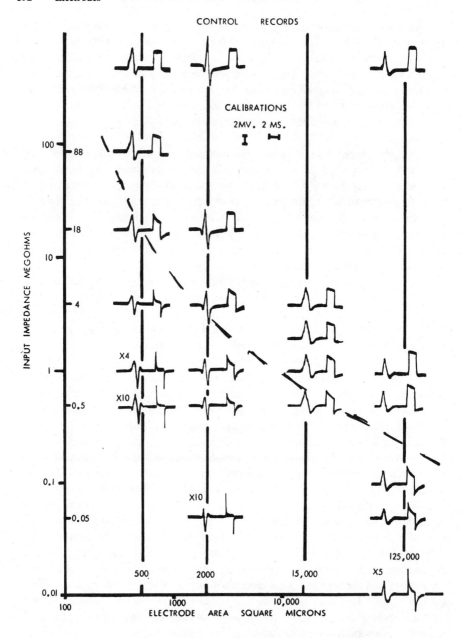

Figure 49b   The relationship between input impedance and electrode area for recording muscle action potentials and a square wave in series with the electrodes. The distortion is clearly apparent in the recordings below the dashed curve. [Redrawn from L. A. Geddes and L. E. Baker, *Med. Biol. Eng.* **5**:561–569 (1967).]

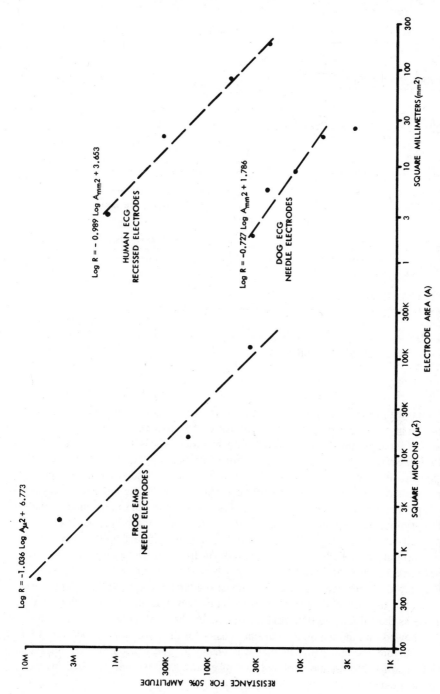

Figure 50 The relationship between resistive input impedance and electrode area for identifiable distortion when recording frog muscle action potential and the dog ECG with needle electrodes and the human ECG with recessed electrodes.

393

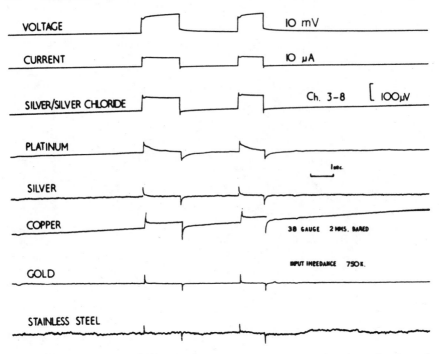

Figure 51   Relationship between surface type and constant input impedance for electrodes of various metals. [From R. Cooper, *Am. J. EEG Technol.* **3**:91–101 (1963). By permission.]

is not high with respect to the electrode–bioelectric generator system) the electrode–electrolyte impedance becomes a dominant part of the input circuit, and the voltage across the input terminals of the bioelectric recorder is less than that under the electrodes. Second, the amount of phase shift is different for the various frequency components of the bioelectric event. With loading, the electrode current density is increased, and the resistive and reactive components of the electrode–electrolyte impedance become nonlinear. Because of this nonlinearity, the magnitude of the electrode impedance becomes a function of the amplitude of the bioelectric event. Thus small- and large-amplitude signals will encounter different impedances. The exact contribution of each of the two sources of distortion is as yet unknown for the various electrodes employed in recording bioelectric events.

Not only does an increase in current density alter the electrode impedance, it also changes the half-cell potential. Even with such a relatively nonpolarizable electrode as the calomel cell, current flow alters the half-cell potential. Rothschild (1938) showed that the maximum current density for this type of electrode was 15 $\mu A/cm^2$ before the half-cell potential was changed. The exact limits of current densities permissible for the various types of electrodes have not yet been investigated adequately.

MICROELECTRODES

When it is desired to examine the electrical activity of a single cell, it is necessary to construct an electrode with dimensions that are small with respect to the cell so that insertion of the electrode can be accomplished without destruction of the cell. Two types of electrodes are used for this purpose; one is metal, and the other is the micropipet, an electrolyte-filled glass tube drawn down to a fine hollow microtip. Metal microelectrodes are fabricated in many different ways: mechanical sharpening, electrolytic sharpening (electropointing), heat pulling, electrodeposition, vapor deposition, and the use of integrated-circuit techniques. All of these methods will be described along with the electrical properties of metal and micropipet microelectrodes.

Mechanical Sharpening

Because of the small tip sizes desired, it is difficult to mechanically sharpen metal rods or wires. Nonetheless, Grundfest and Campbell (1942) described a method of grinding steel needles to produce 5–10-μm points. The needle is mounted in a rotating chuck and the tip is sharpened with a high-speed counterrotating grinding wheel, which permits attainment of a high cutting speed despite the small tip diameter.

Electropointing

In most instances it is possible to point the end of a metal wire by electrolytically removing material; this technique was introduced by Grundfest et al. (1950), who employed it to fabricate stainless steel electrodes having 1-μm tips. They placed the end of a stainless steel wire (0.25 mm in diameter, hard-drawn 18-8 type) in an acid bath consisting of

"34 cc concentrated sulfuric acid (sp. gr. 1.84), 42 cc of *ortho*-phosphoric acid (sp. gr. 1.69), and 24 cc of distilled water to total 100 cc of solution. A portion of this solution is placed in a small metal beaker which is connected to the negative side of a 6-V dc source. The wire to be electropointed is made the anode. A switch, variable resistance, and a milliammeter are included in the circuit. A microscope of low magnification is fitted in front of the beaker so that the stage of the electrolytic pointing may be observed at any time by raising the needle out of the acid solution."

A current of 30 mA was first employed to form the taper of the needle. During this part of the procedure the end of the wire was gradually withdrawn. When the taper was formed, the current was reduced and the needle was withdrawn more slowly to allow the etching process to provide the final taper and tip diameter desired. Following the pointing process, the authors recommended dipping the tip in 10% hydrochloric acid, then washing and thoroughly drying it and giving it a coat of insulating compound.

Use of the electrolytic technique to point tungsten wire was also described by Hubel (1957), who fabricated needles having tip diameters ranging from 0.5 to 0.05 μm. Starting with tungsten wire (0.125 mm in diameter), he found that the slope of the taper could be controlled by raising and lowering the wire during all but the final stage in fabrication. After electrolytic pointing was completed, a final polishing step was added in which the terminal few millimeters was immersed in a saturated aqueous potassium nitrate (KNO_3) solution and a 2-6-V alternating current was passed between the wire and a nearby carbon rod; the current could be conveniently obtained from a 6.3-V transformer fed by a Variac (General Radio Co.). The optimum voltage is not critical, but currents that are too low or too high tend to cause pitting. Hubel (1957) stated:

"If the polishing is allowed to continue until all bubbling ceases, a rather abrupt pencil-like point is obtained which has a tip of ultramicroscopic dimensions (from 0.5 to 0.05 μm in diameter). Such a result is explained by the fact that the meniscus height depends on the diameter of the wire, which decreases as the polishing proceeds."

An ingenious automatic method of using the electropointing technique to produce a batch of 20 stainless steel or tungsten electrodes with tip diameters ranging from 1 to 10 μm was described by Mills (1962). The only difference in the fabrication techniques for the two metals was the type of solution used for the etching.

Mill's method consisted of mounting 20 lengths ($1\frac{1}{2}$-2 in.) of the material to be pointed on a metal shaft that rotated at about 5 rpm. As the shaft turned, the electrodes dipped into and out of the electropointing solution, which was composed of equal parts of sulfuric acid, phosphoric acid, and water for stainless steel needles and 0.5 M sodium hydroxide for tungsten wires (0.010 in. in diameter). The rotating shaft was connected to the positive pole of a 3-V battery with the negative terminal connected to a 2-cm^2 platinum electrode mounted to the side of the electrolytic bath, which contained 500 mL of solution. The current that flowed when the electrodes were in the solution was about 200 mA. Mills started with stainless steel pins having tip diameters of 30-50 μm; after about 6 hr of electropointing, during which the direction of rotation was reversed every half hour, 85% of the electrodes had tip diameters ranging between 1 and 6 μm. They were made ready for recording by washing, drying, and coating with several layers of insulating varnish (Formvar). After each coat was applied, the electrode was allowed to air dry (tip upward); the insulation was then hardened by baking in an oven at 150°C for 30 min.

The use of alternating current for electropointing was described by Wolbarsht et al. (1960). These investigators placed the end of a length of 8-10 mil platinum–iridium (70%, 30%) wire "in a solution of 50% sodium cyanide and 30% sodium hydroxide, added to prevent the formation of hydrogen cyanide." Alternating current (60 Hz) was passed between the wire to be pointed and a nearby carbon electrode in the solution. The taper was formed by connection of a 6-10-V (rms) source, and, while current flowed, the solution was stirred and the wire was slowly withdrawn. The tip, which measured about 1 μm, was formed by reducing the voltage from 8 to 0 V; agitation of the solution was not necessary at this stage of the procedure. The electrode was coated with glass insulation, and the tip was platinized to lower its resistance. (Making the microelectrode negative with respect to a platinum wire in a 1% platinous chloride solution accomplished the platinization.) The current was provided by a 15-V power supply in series with a 1-MΩ resistor; the platinization process required passage of the current for 15–30 sec.

The method of using alternating current for electropointing was further developed by Guld (1964), who etched 0.25-mm platinum–iridium (70%, 30%) wires to produce electrodes having tip diameters of 1 μm. Guld presented considerable quantitative data on his technique for obtaining a desired taper and tip diameter. In general, an electrode was etched by the application of 12 V (rms) to the platinum–iridium wire and a nearby carbon electrode (10 cm^2 in area); the solution employed was 100–500 mL of sodium cyanide (8 M); enough sodium hydroxide was added to prevent the formation of hydrogen cyanide. Current was passed for about 3 min; the rate of withdrawal determined the taper. The tip was formed by etching at 12 V (rms) in a slightly unsaturated sodium cyanide solution and stopping the current when it reached 30% of its initial value. The electrode was then coated with glass using Wohlbarsht's method, and the tip was exposed by the platinizing process, employing 0.1% platinous chloride solution. Platinization was accomplished by using 10-msec current pulses; the electrode was made the negative pole of an 8–15-V source. After each current pulse, the electrode impedance was measured and the process was stopped when the "desired impedance" (1–20 MΩ) was reached.

The first thought that occurs when alternating-current etching is proposed is that the method will not work. With alternating current, theoretically, as much current flows in one direction as in the opposite; and according to Faraday's law of electrolysis, the net effect on each electrode would be zero. However, as will be shown later in this chapter, operation of an electrode–electrolyte interface at a high current density results in rectification.

Insulating Metal Microelectrodes

No matter how metal electrodes with small-diameter tips are fabricated, it is necessary to place insulation on all but the tip. Grundfest et al. (1950) advocated withdrawing the needle from the insulating compound and allowing drying to take place with the tip upward. Hubel (1957) coated his electrodes with E53 Insul-X (Insul-X Co., Ossining, New York) or with clear vinyl lacquer (S-986S, Stoner-Mudge, Inc., Pittsburgh, Pennsylvania). An electrode was slowly withdrawn from the insulating compound, and when the tip emerged from the insulating material, a bead ran up the tapered portion of the electrode. At this time the tip was quickly reimmersed and withdrawn slowly until no bead formed. Then the insulating compound was allowed to dry at room temperature; no baking was advocated.

A technique for placing glass insulation on a small metal electrode was described by Wohlbarsht et al. (1960). Starting with an electropointed platinum–iridium (70%, 30%) electrode, they were able to insulate it by advancing it through a melted bead of glass (Corning glass 7570) having the same thermal coefficient of expansion as the metal [8.5 × 10^{-6}/°C]. The bead was formed by heat in an electrically energized V-shaped platinum–iridium element. During passage of the electrode through the melted glass, the tip was also covered by a very thin layer of glass; this was ruptured by passage of current through it by the platinizing process. The appearance of gas bubbles at the tip indicated that the thin glass covering had been removed.

A glass covering provides a very durable low-leakage insulation. However, successful use of it requires that the chosen glass have exactly the same thermal coefficient of expansion as the metal electrode. If the coefficients are different, the glass will crack during cooling and the insulation will be imperfect.

Heat-Pulled Metal Microelectrodes

Taylor (1925) reported that a 35-gauge platinum wire placed in a quartz capillary could be heat pulled in a microburner to produce a glass-insulated platinum electrode having an exposed tip of 1 μm. Presumably the type of quartz used had nearly the same thermal coefficient of expansion as the platinum wire (8.99 × 10^{-6}/°C), because Taylor did not mention any breakage during cooling. Interestingly enough, in the same paper he reported making a micromagnet by heat pulling an iron wire (thermal coefficient 12.1 × 10^{-6}/°C) in a quartz capillary. Because of success with metals having different coefficients of expansion, it would appear that a slight mismatch in coefficients can be tolerated.

A low-cost, high-quality metal microelectrode was developed by Svaetichin (1951), who first melted silver solder in a 1-cm diameter soda glass tube, then pulled the tube to obtain a long length of 5-mm diameter glass-covered conductor of silver solder. Because silver solder and glass melt at nearly the same temperature and both have similar thermal expansion coefficients, a uniformly insulated and mechanically stable structure was obtained. Segments of this material were then heat pulled in a microburner to produce glass-insulated electrodes with tip diameters in the range of 1–90 μm. To reduce the impedance of the small metal tip, it was first plated with rhodium and then covered with platinum black. Considering the tip diameters obtained, the resistance of the electrodes was remarkably low.

A slightly different procedure for producing metal-filled glass capillary electrodes was described by Dowben and Rose (1953). These investigators melted a mixture of gallium (50%) and indium (50%), or pure indium, and sucked the melted metals (melting points 110 and 150°C, respectively) halfway up into a 5-in. length of 0.5-mm i.d. Pyrex tube having a thermal coefficient of expansion of 3.3 × 10^{-6}/°C. The alloy, which wetted the glass tubing, was then allowed to cool. At a point 2 mm beyond the level of the alloy, the glass tube was heat-pulled to form the empty glass taper and the tip of the electrode. After the tip had formed, the electrode was heated on a hot plate until the alloy melted, whereupon a sewing needle was inserted into the tubing and used as a piston to force the melted metal into the empty end and out the tip so that a bead (~ 30–50 μm diameter) formed beyond the tip. When the electrode cooled, the bead was blown off and the exposed metal tip (2–4 μm in diameter) was gold plated and, then platinized. For gold plating, they stated:

"A gold cyanide solution (0.2% Au) is used for plating, with a 1.5 V dry cell in series with a 5–10 megohm resistor as a source of current. The microelectrode is connected to the negative pole. For an electrode with a 2–4 μ tip, the plating time is 30–45 sec. On the chemically inert and impervious gold base, platinum black is electrodeposited from a bath of 0.4% platinum chloride. The plating time and current are the same as those for gold plating."

The technique of heat pulling a metal in a quartz or glass tube is simple to use and produces insulated electrodes with exposed metallic tips ranging from 1 to 90 μm in diameter. The application of platinum black to such electrodes is highly desirable to reduce the electrode–electrolyte impedance. The electrical characteristics of these electrodes are described later.

The two requirements that should be recognized for successful use of this technique are the use of a metal and insulation with about the same melting points and the same thermal coefficients of expansion. From the reports presented, it would appear that not all investigators took care to use a metal with the same thermal expansion coefficient as the insulating covering. Omitting to do this causes stresses to develop as the electrode cools. There is thus the danger of producing microcracks and sudden fracture if the electrode is tapped gently. However, since such failures did not occur, some degree of mismatch in thermal coefficients of expansion may be tolerable in practice. The data in Table 6 may be of value to those who are contemplating use of this simple process.

Electrodeposited Metal-Filled Micropipet

To overcome the high resistance of the electrolyte-filled micropipet, Weale (1951) devised a method of filling a micropipet with silver, which was deposited electrolytically. Starting with an empty glass micropipet, he advanced a pointed silver wire into it. The silver wire (60 μm in diameter) was pointed by drawing it until it broke, whereupon a piece of platinum wire was soldered to the opposite end. With the pointed silver wire in the taper of the micropipet, the large end was sealed to the platinum wire by melting the glass. Then the electrode was placed in boiling distilled water, and some of the air in the micropipet was expelled by the increased temperature. The submerged electrode was then allowed to cool, which caused water to enter the capillary tip and establish contact with the silver wire. Then the tip of the micropipet was filled with silver by electroplating with a saturated solution of silver nitrate. The platinum wire (soldered to the silver wire in the micropipet) was connected to the negative pole of a 12-V battery in series with a variable resistance and a microammeter; the positive side of the battery was connected to a silver electrode in the silver nitrate solution. The plating process was carried out using 30 μA for about $\frac{1}{2}$ hr, the time necessary to fill the tip with

TABLE 6   Melting Points and Thermal Expansion Coefficients

Material	Melting Point (°C)	Expansion Coefficient $\times 10^{-6}/°C$
Pyrex glass	1245	3.3
Vycor glass	1550	0.8
Soda glass	1000	12.0
Quartz crystal		5.21
Quartz fused	1500	0.256
Silver solder		
(10% Ag, 52% Cu, 38% Zn)	870	
(45% Ag, 15% Cu, 15% Zn, 25% Cd)	620	
Corning 7570 solder glass		8.5
Silver	960	17.04
Platinum	1773	8.99
Platinum–iridium		8.84
Gallium	30	
Indium	156	41.7
Tin	232	22.57
Antimony	630	12.0
Gold	1063	13.2
Iron (soft)	1535	9.07
Iron (stainless steel)	1400–1450	10–20
Flame temperatures		
Natural gas–air	1950	—
Acetylene–air	2325	—
Acetylene–oxygen	2900–3000	—

silver. Weale employed an automatic device to determine when this point had been reached; a sudden drop in the resistance, which was continually measured during the plating process, indicated that the tip was filled with silver. Weale stated that he was able to make electrodes with tip diameters of 10 μm and resistances on the order of 1500 Ω. Smaller-diameter electrodes exhibited considerably higher resistance. No additional processing was carried out.

Vapor-Deposited Metal-Film Microelectrode

Two interesting types of small vapor-deposited metal electrodes are available commercially (Transidyne General Corp., Ann Arbor, Michigan). One type is solid, and the other is hollow like a micropipet; both are made from glass stock 0.75 or 1 mm in diameter. In both types (called Microtrodes), the glass is covered with a thin layer of platinum applied by vapor deposition. Several of the geometric arrangements available are shown in Fig. 52. The exposed platinum tip beyond the insulation is about 1–2 μm; tip diameters are in the range of 1–20 μm.

Integrated Circuit Fabrication Technique

Another method of constructing small-area electrodes was developed by Wise and Starr (1969), who applied integrated-circuit technology to make single and

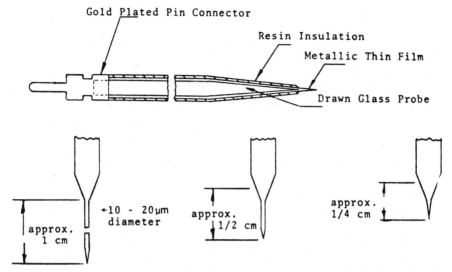

Figure 52   Vapor-deposited metal film microelectrodes. (Courtesy of Transidyne General Corp., Ann Arbor, Michigan.)

multiple electrodes from gold strips that are bonded to a film of silicon dioxide on a substrate of silicon (Fig. 53). The gold was then covered with a 0.4-μm layer of silicon dioxide, which was etched off to form the exposed tip. Wise and Starr have fabricated electrodes with exposed tips having areas of 15 μm^2. An illustration (Fig. 53) presented by the authors shows a linear array of three electrodes that occupies less than 50 μm. The capacitive coupling to the silicon support (ground) is given as 0.5 pF per millimeter of electrode length.

The electrodes described by Wise and Starr have the advantage of precise control of dimensions. However, in their present state of development, they can only be used extracellularly or placed into relatively large cells. Nonetheless, there is no doubt that a slight improvement in technology will permit fabrication of much smaller electrodes.

The next step in the use of integrated-circuit technology will be the incorporation of a source follower (or operational amplifier) directly on the substrate that carries the metal microelectrodes. In this way, the bioelectric event will be coupled to an input stage having a high input impedance. The output, which is derived from the low output impedance of the headstage, could be led to the measuring apparatus without the many practical difficulties of capacitive loading and 60-Hz interference.

Measurement of the Exposed Area of Metal Microelectrodes

With the insulating procedures described earlier, it is often difficult to see the extent of the exposed tip, because the layer of insulating material is usually so thin near the tip that microscopic examination fails to uncover the boundary of the insulation. Under such circumstances, the tip area can often be determined by using

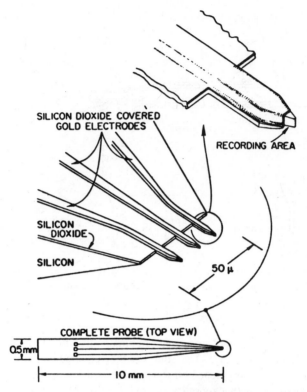

SILICON DIOXIDE COVERED GOLD ELECTRODES

RECORDING AREA

SILICON DIOXIDE

SILICON

50 μ

COMPLETE PROBE (TOP VIEW)

0.5 mm

10 mm

Figure 53 Integrated-circuit technology microelectrodes. (From K. D. Wise and A. Starr, *Proc. 8th Int. Conf. Med. Biol. Eng., 1969* Sect. 14–5. By permission.)

the method described by Hubel (1957). A drop of saline on a glass slide is viewed with a microscope. A small wire is then placed in the drop and connected to the positive pole of a battery; the other pole is connected to the metal microelectrode. The electrode is advanced into the drop, and the tip is viewed in the microscope. The active area can be estimated by observation of the area from which hydrogen bubbles are evolved. This method is very convenient to apply and has been used successfully by Geddes and Baker (1966) and others to measure the area of a variety of large and small needle electrodes.

Electrical Properties of Metal Microelectrodes

Impedance. The high impedance of a metal microelectrode is due to the characteristics of the small-area metal–electrolyte interface. By knowing the electrical parameters of such a structure, it is possible to estimate the impedance of an electrode of a known area. It was pointed out earlier that, over a considerable frequency range, the series-equivalent reactance X and resistance R for many metal–

electrolyte interfaces are approximately equal and that each varies approximately as $1/f^\alpha$, where f is the frequency and α is approximately 0.5. Assuming that $R = X$, then the magnitude of the impedance Z will be

$$Z = \sqrt{R^2 + X^2} = \sqrt{2}\,X = 1.41X = \frac{1.41}{2\pi fC}. \tag{12a}$$

Therefore, if the series capacitance–frequency (C-f) relationship is known for a given area of electrode–electrolyte interface, it will be possible to calculate the approximate impedance.

Because electrode capacitance varies with area, it is possible to use the data in Fig. 11 to estimate the impedance–frequency characteristic for a small-area metal microelectrode within the constraint that reactance and resistance are equal and both vary as $1/f^\alpha$. In order to use the data in Fig. 11 and equation (11) to calculate the approximate impedance–frequency relationship for a metal microelectrode of area a, it is necessary to modify the constant K, which was derived using the units of microfarads and square centimeters, to allow its use with electrodes whose area is measured in square micrometers ($1\ \mu m^2 = 10^{-8}\ cm^2$) and capacitances measured in farads ($1\ \mu F = 10^{-6}\ F$). Performing this adjustment gives the following expression for the series capacitance C (in farads) for an electrode of area a (in square micrometers):

$$C = 10^{-14}\frac{Ka}{f^\alpha}. \tag{12b}$$

The impedance–frequency relationship can be obtained by substitution of this expression into equation (11). Performing this substitution gives the following for the magnitude of the impedance Z (Ω):

$$Z = \frac{1.41}{2\pi f(10^{-14}Ka/f^\alpha)} = \frac{0.225 \times 10^{14}}{Kaf^{(1-\alpha)}}, \tag{13}$$

where Z = impedance in ohms

$\quad K$ = capacitance/cm^2 coefficient for the electrode–electrolyte interface (Fig. 11, $C = K/f^\alpha$)

$\quad a$ = electrode area in square micrometers

$\quad \alpha$ = coefficient of capacitance versus frequency (Fig. 11)

$\quad f$ = frequency in hertz

It is of interest to use this expression to calculate the impedance–frequency relationship for a particular electrode area and to compare the data with those in the published literature. A useful electrode size would be 10 μm^2, which is equivalent to the surface of a conical electrode 1 μm in diameter and 6.35 μm high (i.e., the tip angle is 9 degrees). Inspection of Fig. 11 reveals that the highest impedance would be expected with bare metals because of the low values for the capacitance–frequency relationship; conversely, the lowest impedance would be expected from platinum black because it exhibits the highest value for the capacitance–frequency relationship. Using an average value of $C = 350/f^{0.5}$ for bare metal and $C = 149,700/f^{0.366}$ for heavy platinum black, the expected impedance–frequency characteristics for a 10-μm^2 electrode of each of these surfaces have been calculated. The plots obtained (Fig. 54, dashed lines) also show the values obtained by Gray and Svaetichin (1951–1952) for their 5-μm-diameter glass-insulated platinum black electrode (19.4 μm^2), by Gesteland et al. (1959) for their 3-μm platinum black electrode (28 μm^2) and 50 μm^2 silver–silver chloride electrode, and by Hubel for his 8-μm tungsten electrode.

Inspection of Fig. 54 reveals that the impedance–frequency values reported in the literature cited are in fairly good agreement with those predicted by equation

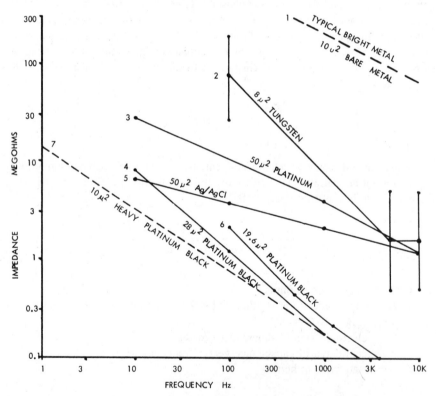

Figure 54 Impedance–frequency characteristics of metal microelectrodes: (1) bare metal (calculated from $C = 350/f^{0.5}$ and $X = R$); (2) tungsten (Hubel, 1957); (3) platinum (Gesteland et al., 1959); (4) platinum black (Gesteland et al., 1956); (5) silver–silver chloride (Gesteland et al., 1959); (6) platinum black (Gray and Svaetichin, 1951–1952); (7) heavy platinum black (calculated from $C = 149,000\,f^{0.366}$ and $X = R$).

(13), using the data in Fig. 11. Perhaps the most important point made by Fig. 54 is that electrolytically prepared electrodes (e.g., platinum black and silver–silver chloride) have quite low impedances. Likewise, Hubel's 8-μm^2 electrolytically pointed electrode has an impedance considerably lower than was predicted on the basis of a bare metal surface slightly larger in area, probably because electrolytically formed surfaces have quite large areas.

From the foregoing it can be seen that the deposition of a coat of platinum black offers an excellent means of reducing the impedance at all frequencies to values well below those exhibited by bare platinum. Although the platinizing process has been specified for large-area electrodes, the values obtained may not be directly scaled for the platinization of microelectrodes. Robinson (1968) pointed out that the current density value obtained by scaling on an area basis are such that platinization will not occur; he therefore advocated the use of a current density 10 times that found to be optimum for large-area (cm^2) electrodes.

The impedance–frequency characteristic for a small-area (50-μm^2) silver–silver chloride surface in contact with saline illustrates that this surface has a much lower impedance than bare silver but somewhat higher than platinized platinum. Attractive as the relatively low impedance of the silver–silver chloride surface may be, it is not well suited mechanically for metal microelectrodes; the chloride coat is friable and easily damaged. In addition, there are no data available regarding the current density and time for optimum chloriding of silver–silver chloride microelectrodes; existing data can only serve as a starting point. The curves in Figs. 19 and 20 for an optimum chloride coat for large-area silver chloride electrodes indicate that it may well be necessary to increase the chloriding current density to achieve an adequate chloride deposit.

Because of its mechanical strength and inertness in living tissue, stainless steel is frequently used for microelectrodes. It should be noted that the price paid for these two desirable qualities is high impedance, since stainless steel exhibits a low value of capacitance at all frequencies.

From the foregoing it is apparent that metal microelectrodes exhibit a very high low-frequency impedance. Thus it is very difficult to use them to measure resting membrane potentials. On the other hand, their lower high-frequency impedance permits their easy use to measure action potentials; with amplifiers with only moderately high input impedances, they are particularly well suited for the extracellular measurement of action potentials. This subject is discussed in the following section.

Equivalent Circuit. Having established that the impedance of a metal microelectrode is high, it is appropriate to develop a simple equivalent circuit to identify all the voltages and impedances that exist between the terminals of a metal microelectrode A and its reference electrode B; Fig. 55a shows a metal electrode located in the environment of an irritable cell. Tracing out the path between terminals A and B, the first item encountered is the resistance of the connecting wire and the metal used for the microelectrode; the former is obviously negligible. Many metal microelectrodes are made from metal rods about 0.25 mm in diameter; the resistance of a 1-cm length depends on the resistivity of the metal employed (most

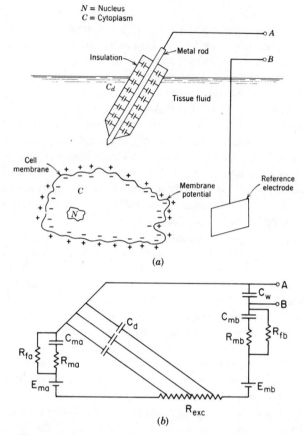

Figure 55   (a) Extracellular metal microelectrode; (b) equivalent circuit.

frequently platinum, tungsten, and stainless steel). The resistances per centimeter of an 0.25-mm rod of these metals are 20, 11, and 130 Ω, respectively; thus the resistance of the metallic portion of the microelectrode is negligible.

Because the shaft of a metal microelectrode is covered with an insulating material (e.g., glass or insulating varnish), which is in turn in contact with a conducting fluid environment, a coaxial capacitor is created. With an insulating coating amounting to 10% of the diameter of the shaft of the microelectrode, the distributed capacitance C_d of the shaft can be calculated from the expression for the capacitance of a coaxial cable with inner and outer conductors of diameters d and D, respectively, and the space between filled with material of dielectric constant k. The capacitance C_d per millimeter is given by

$$C_d = \frac{0.024\,k}{\log D/d}, \text{pF/mm}.$$

With 10% insulation, $D/d = 110/100 = 1.1$, and with glass or insulating varnish as the dielectric, the dielectric constant will be between 3 and 5, with perhaps 4 as an average value. Under these conditions, the capacitance per millimeter of shaft is

$$C_d = \frac{0.024 \times 4}{\log 1.11} = 2.1 \text{ pF/mm}.$$

Note that although the capacitance depends on the length of the microelectrode surrounded by fluid, it does not depend on the diameter of the microelectrode but rather on the ratio of the diameter (plus insulation) to the shaft diameter. The distributed capacitance C_d exists between the shaft of the metal microelectrode and the extracellular fluid R_{exc} and forms a circuit as shown in Fig. 55b.

The next item to be encountered in tracing the circuit between terminals A and B is the small-area metal–electrolyte interface at the tip of the microelectrode; this can be represented by a Warburg equivalent, consisting of a series capacitance C_{ma} and resistance R_{ma}, shunted by the faradic leakage R_{fa}, all in series with the potential E_{ma} of the electrode–electrolyte interface.

Because the microelectrode is outside the cell, the next item to be encountered is the resistance of the extracellular fluid, R_{exc}. Ignoring the distributed capacitance C_d for the moment, the reference electrode potential E_{mb} and impedance, consisting of the Warburg series resistance R_{mb} and capacitance C_{mb} shunted by the faradic leakage R_{fb}, complete the circuit. Because the area of the reference electrode is so much larger than that of the tip of the microelectrode, the impedance of C_{mb}, R_{mb}, and R_{fb} can be neglected. However, the potential E_{mb} of the reference electrode is not area-dependent and cannot be ignored.

Thus it can be seen that with the metal microelectrode outside a cell, the circuit between the electrode terminals consists of a series circuit of two electrode potentials and impedances and the resistance of the extracellular fluid. The distributed coaxial capacitance of the microelectrode is in parallel with a part of the circuit. Another capacitance C_w is due to the wires connected to the reference and microelectrode; it exists in parallel with the electrode terminals, and its value depends on the length and spacing of the wires used to connect the electrodes to the measuring instrument. Because some of the components in the equivalent circuit are more important than others, simplification of the circuit can be carried out. (A description of such a simplification is reserved for the case of the microelectrode in the cell.)

When the cell becomes active and recovers with the microelectrode outside the cell, the cyclic depolarization and repolarization cause current to flow in the extracellular fluid. Hence, a potential will appear across R_{exc} in the equivalent circuit of Fig. 55b. The amount of this voltage that appears across terminals A and B depends on the distance of the electrodes from the cell, their orientation with respect to the direction of spread of excitation and recovery, the electrode impedances (and C_w), and the magnitude of the impedance of the measuring instrument connected

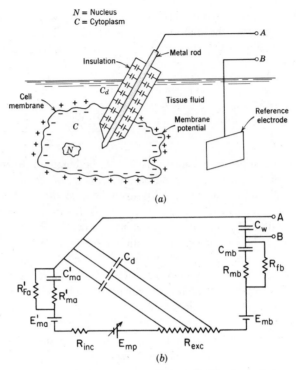

Figure 56 Intracellular metal microelectrode: (*a*) metal microelectrode inserted into a cell; (*b*) equivalent circuit.

across terminals A and B. As stated previously, the circuit is simplified to identify only the most important of these impedances.

When a metal microelectrode is advanced into a cell, as in Fig. 56*a*, the potential appearing between the terminals A and B is the sum of three potentials: the metal–electrolyte potential of the microelectrode E'_{ma}, which now depends on the metal species and the composition of the intracellular fluid; the cell membrane potential E_{mp}; and the potential of the metal–electrolyte interface of the reference electrode E_{mb}. When the membrane potential is being measured, it is assumed that E'_{ma} and E_{mb} are constant. Note, however, that the potential of the microelectrode tip has changed from that which existed when it was in contact with extracellular fluid to its potential when it was in contact with intracellular fluid. Although small, this difference should be recognized; however, it is usually ignored. Because metal microelectrodes are seldom used for the measurement of resting membrane potentials, this difference will not be discussed here.

In addition to the potentials just identified, there are several impedances of importance, and the complete equivalent circuit for a metal microelectrode in a cell can be assembled by tracing out the circuit between the electrode terminals A and B. Referring to Fig. 56*b*, the first component encountered is the Warburg series equivalent R'_{ma} and C'_{ma}, shunted by R'_{fa}, the faradic leakage at the tip of the metal microelectrode which is in contact with intracellular fluid. Because the tip area is so small, R'_{fa} is high and can be omitted. At the tip there is also the half-cell potential E'_{ma}. Neglecting the distributed capacitance for the moment, the next item to be encountered is the resistance of the intracellular fluid R_{inc} and then the membrane potential E_{mp}. The circuit is completed by the resistance R_{exc} of the extracellular fluid and the impedance (R_{mb}, C_{mb}, R_{fb}) and potential E_{mb} of the reference electrode B. Between terminal A and the extracellular fluid appears the distributed capacitance C_d of the insulated shaft of the metal microelectrode. In addition, there is a capacitance C_w between the wires used to connect the electrodes to the instrument that measures the cell potential. To keep C_w as low as possible, these wires are kept as short as possible.

Fortunately, some of the components in the equivalent circuit in Fig. 56b are small with respect to others and can be neglected. Therefore it is possible to synthesize a simple electric circuit that mimics the electrical behavior of the actual circuit. For example, in comparison to the impedance of the microelectrode tip, the resistances of the intracellular and extracellular fluids, R_{inc} and R_{exe}, can be neglected. Because the area of the reference electrode is many times greater than that of the microelectrode tip, the impedance of the former can be neglected. The distributed capacitance C_d between the microelectrode shaft and the extracellular environment can be collected together with that of the wiring C_w to form a single capacitance $C_d + C_w$.

The electrochemical potentials of nonbioelectric origin E'_{ma}, E_{mb} can likewise be collected to form E, and the equivalent circuit reduces to that of Fig. 57. In practice, $C_d + C_w$ is small and can often be neglected. The impedance of the microelectrode tip, constituted by C'_{ma} and R'_{ma} is inversely dependent on the area of the tip.

Figure 57 reveals that when an intracellular metal microelectrode is used to measure the transmembrane potential of a cell, the bioelectric phenomenon is coupled to the measuring instrument by a circuit that has an impedance that increases with decreasing frequency. The zero-frequency impedance (i.e., dc resistance) for small-area metal electrodes is always very high because the faradic leakage R_{fa} is

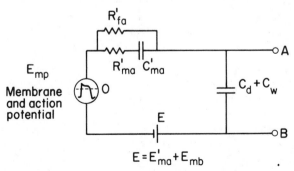

Figure 57   Approximate equivalent circuit for a metal microelectrode used to measure the potential of a cell membrane.

very high. For this reason it is not always possible to obtain a potential-measuring instrument with a high enough input resistance to measure the resting membrane potential with adequate accuracy.

The effect of the circuit of Fig. 57 on the waveform of an action potential is determined by the input impedance of the amplifier to which it is connected. With an adequately high input impedance (e.g., 100–1000 times that of the electrode circuit for the frequency spectrum of the action potential), no waveform distortion will be encountered. However, if the input impedance is not high enough, the low-frequency components of the action potential will be attenuated as in Figs. 48 and 49.

ELECTROLYTE-FILLED MICROPIPET

When transmembrane resting and action potentials are to be measured accurately, it is customary to employ a micropipet (Fig. 58), which resembles a small

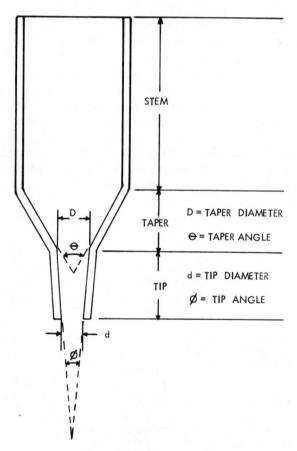

Figure 58 The micropipet.

medicine dropper with a tip drawn down to 1 μm or less in diameter. A terminology has been developed to describe the various parts of a micropipet. The upper part is called the stem or shaft. The region where the stem encounters the tapered portion is called the shoulder or shank. The term tip is usually reserved for the region of the pipet that enters the cell. In this book, the terms stem, taper, and tip along with the taper angle θ and tip angle ϕ, as in Fig. 58, are employed.

A suitable electrolyte is used to completely fill the tip, taper, and stem, and a well-chlorided silver electrode dipping into the filling solution serves as the electrical terminal. The important consideration regarding the micropipet (in addition to use of the proper measuring instrument) is its tip diameter, which should be small with respect to the size of the cell into which it is to be placed.

An interesting study relating the magnitude of the measured membrane potential with the tip diameter of the intracellular electrode was conducted by Woodbury et al. (1951). Using the frog ventricle, which is composed of cells approximately 20 μm in diameter, they measured the membrane potential with micropipets having different tip diameters. Their data (Fig. 59) illustrate that the larger the tip diameter, the less the potential that was measured. The voltage measured with a tip diameter on the order of 1 μm (5% of the cell diameter) was taken as 100%, since this was the smallest diameter electrode used. Extrapolation of their data (Fig. 59), indicates that an electrode with a slightly smaller tip diameter might have measured a slightly larger membrane potential. Therefore, their data lend support to the rule of thumb that 1–10% of the size of a cell is the appropriate range of an electrode diameter.

Micropipets suitable for measuring transmembrane potentials have been avail-

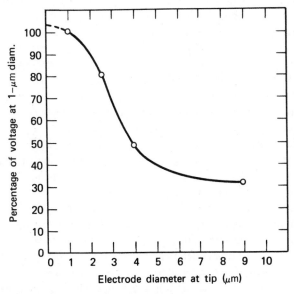

Figure 59   The relation between the measured membrane potential (%) and electrode diameter (μm). The data were obtained from frog cardiac muscle approximately 20 μm in diameter. [From L.A. Woodbury et al., *Am. J. Physiol.* **164**:307–318 (1951). By permission.]

able sincd 1925, when Ettisch and Peterfi described the use of a 2-mm-wide flame to pull 1-mm glass tubing to points about 10 μm in diameter. These electrodes were filled with 0.1 N potassium chloride in agar and were employed with calomel half-cells to measure the (membrane) potentials of plant and animal cells in conjunction with a polarized electrostatic electrometer. In the same year Gelfan used an oxygen flame to draw 0.5-mm glass tubing to make micropipets having tips with openings in the range of 1–2 μm; he also filled his micropipets with 0.1 N potassium chloride. Very shortly thereafter, machines for making micropipets appeared. Du Bois (1931) described the first of these; it employed a spring to apply tension to a glass tube that was softened using an electrically energized platinum heater. As the glass softened, the tube was automatically removed from the vicinity of the heater during the final pull. This technique of using an initial gentle pull followed by a sudden forceful one while the heat is reduced has been employed in almost all subsequent micropipet makers; descriptions of some of these were presented by Livingston and Duggar (1934), Benedetti-Pichler and Rachele (1940), Alexander and Nastuk (1953), Winsbury (1956), Lux (1960), Byzov and Chemystov (1961), and Chowdhury (1969). In the instrument made by Alexander and Nastuk, an initial force of 100 g, followed by 1700 g, produced tips with outside diameters of 0.4–0.5 μm. In Winsbury's machine, an initial force of 0.8 lb was followed by 1–5 lb to produce tips with diameters in the range of 0.5–10 μm. Lux found that cooling a small area of the glass while it was being drawn permitted attainment of a sharper taper. The instrument devised by Byzov and Chemystov, which employed a sharp blow to provide the second force, produced 10–15 degree tips with diameters in the range of 0.1–0.08 μm. Chowdhury's instrument yielded micropipets having tip diameters as small as 0.05 μm by the use of a two-stage pull combined with cooling from two tiny jets of compressed air controlled by solenoid valves. This process yielded tip angles in the range of 11 degrees.

Not all who employed micropipets used automatic machines for their fabrication; Hodgkin and Huxley (1939) and Curtis and Cole (1938, 1942) used simple techniques to construct micropipets 10–100 μm in diameter that were used with squid giant axons 500–1000 μm in diameter. Similarly, Ling and Gerard (1949) were able to draw micropipets down to less than 1 μm in diameter for recording transmembrane potentials in frog skeletal muscle cells.

From the foregoing it is apparent that the basic steps in the fabrication of a small-tip micropipet consist of the circumferential application of heat to a small area of suitable tubing that is placed under an initial tension. When the glass softens, the tension is increased as rapidly as possible and the heat is turned off; sometimes active cooling is added. Careful timing and adjustment of the amount of heat, as well as the initial and final tensions and cooling, permit the production of micropipets with controlled dimensions. An excellent account of how these factors interact to control tip diameter and taper was presented by Frank and Becker (1964). Although many micropipet makers are commercially available, and most provide a means for controlling tension and temperature, each investigator must learn the technique of adjustment to obtain micropipets with the desired tip characteristics.

THE FLOATING MICROPIPET

The tip of a conventional micropipet often breaks during the first contraction when transmembrane potentials from contracting muscle cells are being recorded. To solve this problem, Woodbury and Brady (1956) developed a micropipet that moves along with contracting and relaxing muscle cells. Their micropipet was constructed by placing an 0.001-in. tungsten wire in a conventional 3 M KCl-filled micropipet and breaking the stem to leave a segment about 1 cm long attached to the tip. If the movement is slight, a straight wire a few inches in length is adequate; if the movement is large, it is advisable to use a 3–4-in. length of tungsten wire, later bending it with a right angle near the middle. The broken part is slipped off the tungsten wire, which is then affixed to the preamplifier mounted in a convenient manipulator (Fig. 60). The micropipet is gently lowered so that the tip comes into contact with the muscle. When the muscle contracts, the springiness of the tungsten wire allows the micropipet to move along with the muscle. The record shown in Fig. 60 was made with such an electrode placed on the surface of a turtle ventricle; in this position the conventional ECG was recorded. As the ventricle continued to contract and relax, the tip of the micropipet entered a cell, revealing the membrane and monophasic action potential.

Using a short tungsten wire, Woodbury and Brady reported success in recording resting membrane and action potentials from the cardiac pacemaker of the frog, turtle, rat, guinea pig, rabbit, and monkey, the canine ventricle, frog skeletal muscle, and the uterus of the pregnant guinea pig and rabbit. Geddes and Baker had considerable success using this electrode in the teaching laboratory to record the membrane and action potentials of frog and turtle atria and ventricles.

FILLING MICROPIPETS

The filling of a micropipet with a chosen electrolyte does not come about by filling the shaft or by placing the micropipet tip downward in the electrolyte; special techniques must be used to coax the fluid into the microtip. In general, the difficulty in filling increases as the tip diameter decreases. Frank and Becker (1964) reported that micropipets having tip diameters larger than 5 μm can be filled by applying pressure with a syringe and a blunt-ended needle placed snugly in the tapered portion of the micropipet. Micropipets with tip diameters as small as 0.5 μm or less have been successfully filled using a variety of the techniques to be described. However, there also appears to be a finite time over which filled micropipets can be stored. (Storage of dry empty micropipets is inadvisable because dust particles tend to gain access and block the tip.) If micropipets are filled but not immersed in the electrolyte (usually 3 M KCl), crystals soon appear at the microtip, rendering the micropipet useless. Kennard (1958) reported that even when filled micropipets are stored by immersion in the filling electrolyte, deposits and growths capable of occluding the tip often appear after about a week. To solve this problem, he advocated storage in the dark at reduced temperature and the addition of a bac-

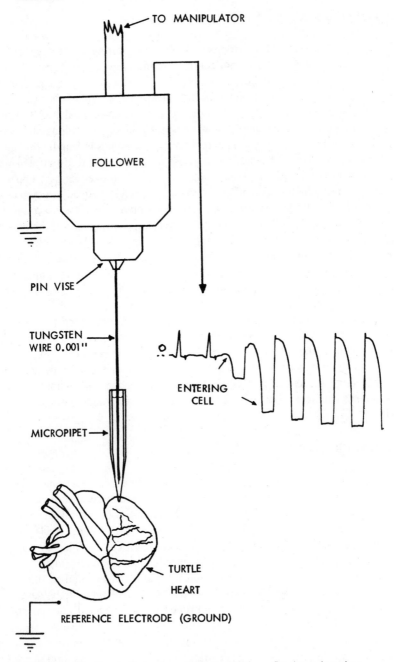

Figure 60   Penetration of a ventricular cell by a floating micropipet.

teriostatic agent to the surrounding solution. Prolonged storage is also inadvisable because repeated handling of the pipets (to remove one or several for an individual experiment) damages the microtip. To avoid these difficulties most investigators fabricate a batch of about 10–50 micropipets, fill them immediately, check several for resistance and electrical stability, and use them all as soon as possible.

When a micropipet is immersed tip upward in an electrolyte, the fluid enters the stem but does not fill the tip; when immersed tip downward, only a very small amount of fluid enters the tip. To cause the electrolyte to fill the tip, taper, and shaft, investigators have replaced entrapped air bubbles with vapor from the electrolytic solution or removed them by the use of positive or negative pressure or boiling.

The filling procedure developed for Geddes and Baker by Cantrell consists of mounting a batch of about 50 micropipets tip downward in a Teflon rack (Fig. 61), which is mounted to a cover that forms an airtight seal on the top of a thick-walled glass vessel 6 in. high and 4 in. in diameter; in the cover there is a tube for the application of negative pressure. The vessel is two-thirds filled with ethyl alcohol, and the cover is carefully placed on it, thereby totally immersing the electrodes in alcohol. Negative pressure is applied using a water-faucet suction device and is maintained for 24 hr; the negative pressure can be maintained by evacuating the

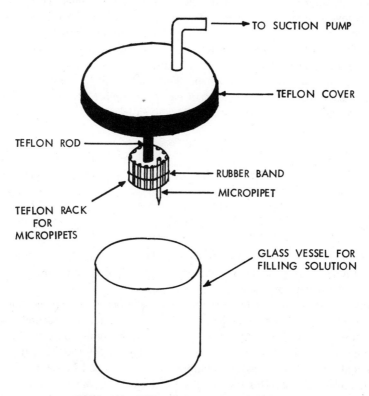

Figure 61   Filling apparatus for micropipets.

vessel and clamping off the tube leading to the suction pump. If any of the electrodes contain air bubbles, after 24 hr they can easily be filled by applying and releasing the negative pressure a few times. The alcohol in the vessel is then replaced with distilled water; when the cover is replaced, the micropipets are immersed in distilled water. Vacuum is again applied, and the micropipets are allowed to stand for 24–48 hr to replace the alcohol with distilled water. The distilled water in the vessel is then replaced by the filling electrolyte (usually 3 M KCl) and the vacuum is reapplied and maintained for 24 hr. The electrodes are now filled and ready for use. A final test of adequacy of filling is the failure of a hard vacuum to produce bubbles in the micropipets. Filling can also be judged from the measurement of resistance; an unusually high resistance for a known micropipet tip diameter indicates the presence of either a bubble or particulate matter.

ELECTROLYTES FOR MICROPIPETS

Because the tip of a micropipet is filled with an electrolyte, it constitutes an electrolytic conductor of small cross-sectional area. It is this property that gives a micropipet its high resistance, not the electrode–electrolyte interface in the stem (which is low in impedance compared with tip resistance); the resistance of the electrolyte in the tapered portion of the micropipet contributes very little resistance. Actually the tip of the micropipet is a truncated conducting cone in which the internal tip diameter d, the angle ϕ (in radians) of the sides (at the tip), and the resistivity ρ (in ohm-centimeters) of the fluid used to fill it constitute the most important factors determining the resistance of a micropipet. By simple integration it is easy to show that the tip resistance R_t is given by

$$R_t = 4\rho / \pi\phi d.$$

If the angle ϕ is larger than 0.17 rad (i.e., 10 degrees) the following general expression should be used:

$$R_t = 4\rho / \pi d \cot \phi.$$

Examination of these expressions shows that the use of an electrolyte with low resistivity ρ and a steep angle ϕ at the tip favor holding the resistance down if a small diameter d must be used.

It was soon learned that the use of filling solutions that were isotonic with intracellular fluids produced micropipets with high resistance. Nastuk and Hodgkin (1950) showed that if their micropipets were filled with isotonic potassium chloride (118 mM), they exhibited resistances in the range of 50–150 $M\Omega$; the values encountered when 3 M potassium chloride was used varied between 10 and 30 $M\Omega$, a fivefold decrease. This reduction is not consistent with the resistivity values for 0.118 mM potassium chloride ($\rho = 75$ Ω-cm at 20°C) and 3 M potassium chloride ($p = 3.7$ Ω-cm at 20°C); here the ratio is about 20—slightly larger than the approximate values reported. Nonetheless, the remarkable reduction in impedance is worthwhile.

Various investigators have measured the resistances of their micropipets, and there is general agreement among the values presented for the various tip diameters and electrolytes used to fill the micropipets. For example, Curtis and Cole (1942), using isotonic potassium chloride as the filling electrolyte, listed the resistance range for 10–60-μm electrodes as 1–25 MΩ. Renshaw et al. (1940) reported a resistance range of 0.5–1 MΩ for their 40-μm electrodes filled with mammalian Ringer's solution. Graham and Gerard (1946) measured resistance values between 7 and 10 MΩ for tip diameters slightly smaller than 5 μm, filled with potassium chloride isotonic with frog muscle. Ling and Gerard (1949), using electrodes about 1 μm in tip diameter, found the resistance to be in the vicinity of 20 MΩ when filled with KCl isotonic with frog muscle. Nastuk and Hodgkin's (1950) micropipets of 0.4-μm tip diameter filled with 3 M potassium chloride exhibited a resistance of 50–150 MΩ. The automatic machine developed by Alexander and Nastuk (1953) produced 0.5-μm micropipets with resistances in the range of 10–13 MΩ when filled with 3 M potassium chloride. The electrodes used by Frank and Fuortes (1955), with tip diameters of 0.5 μm and filled with 3 M potassium chloride, were found to have resistances in the range of 15–50 MΩ. Grundfest (1955) reported that the resistance range of KCl-filled micropipets, having tip diameters from a few μm to 0.1 μm, is from a few megohms to 100 MΩ; Eccles (1955) gave values of 10–20 MΩ for 3 M KCl-filled micropipets 1–0.5 μm in diameter. Hence it is seen that a micropipet with a tip diameter of about 1 μm filled with 3 M potassium chloride, would be expected to have a tip resistance of about 10 MΩ. This value is not inconsistent with that predicted by the foregoing expression. For example, substituting these values [0.5 μm internal tip diameter, $p = 3.7$ Ω-cm for 3 M KCl at 20°C, and tip angle $\phi = 1°$ (0.017 rad)] into the expression gives a tip resistance of 5.5 MΩ. Thus the use of a concentrated potassium chloride solution to fill a micropipet reduces its resistance considerably and thereby imposes less stringent requirements on amplifier input impedance for measuring membrane and action potentials.

When a micropipet is filled with 3 M potassium chloride and the tip is advanced into a cell, there exists a concentration gradient (e.g., 3 M KCl versus intracellular ions). Thus the electrolyte will diffuse from the micropipet into the cell. Initially the diffusion rate will be high, and, according to Nastuk and Hodgkin (1950), with an 0.4-μm tip in a frog muscle cell the diffusion rate is on the order of 6×10^{-14} mol/sec. Coombs et al. (1955a, b) reported that the diffusion of 3 M potassium chloride from a micropipet is on the order of 4×10^{-14} mol/sec. Whether such diffusion fluxes significantly alter cellular function during a measurement remains to be seen.

MEASUREMENT OF RESTING MEMBRANE POTENTIAL

When the potential difference that exists across a cell membrane is measured with a micropipet, it is customary to call the potential between the electrode ter-

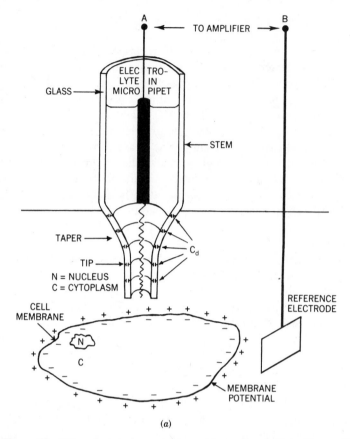

A   ← TO AMPLIFIER →   B

GLASS →

ELEC | TRO-
LYTE | IN
MICRO | PIPET

← STEM

TAPER →

C_d

TIP →
N = NUCLEUS
C = CYTOPLASM

CELL
MEMBRANE

N

C

REFERENCE
ELECTRODE

MEMBRANE
POTENTIAL

(*a*)

Figure 62   Micropipet tip located (*a*) outside a cell and (*b*) inside a cell.

minals A and B zero before the micropipet is advanced into the cell; this situation is diagramed in Fig. 62*a*. When the micropipet is advanced through the cell membrane (Fig. 62*b*), the potential that suddenly appears between electrodes A and B is usually taken as the membrane potential. In fact, the sudden appearance of this potential indicates that the tip of the micropipet has entered the cell. Because an apparent zero potential has been established as described previously, it is possible to identify the overshoot or reverse polarization that occurs when the cell becomes active and recovers; a typical representation appears in Fig. 60.

The procedure just described is eminently practical, but it incorporates a small error that should be identified, particularly in view of the serious efforts now being made to account for the magnitude of membrane and action potentials. The error can be found by examination of Fig. 62*a* for the purpose of identifying all the potentials between the electrode terminals A and B. Starting with electrode terminal A, there is a potential difference between the metallic electrode and the electrolyte filling the micropipet; this potential will be designated E_{ma}. If the fluid in the micropipet is different from that constituting the environment of the cell and if the

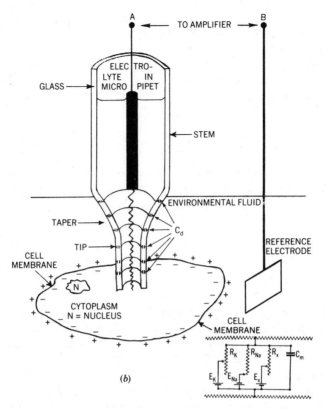

A — TO AMPLIFIER → B

ELEC|TRO-
LYTE | IN
GLASS → MICRO | PIPET

← STEM

ENVIRONMENTAL FLUID

TAPER →

C_d

TIP →

CELL MEMBRANE

REFERENCE ELECTRODE

N

CYTOPLASM
N = NUCLEUS

CELL MEMBRANE

R_K R_{Na} R_x C_m

E_K E_{Na} E_x

(b)

Figure 62   (*Continued*)

mobilities of the ions in each solution are different, there will arise a liquid-junction or diffusion potential at the tip of the micropipet; this potential will be designated E_t. The next potential to be encountered in the extracellular path is the potential between the reference electrode and the environmental fluid; this potential will be designated E_{mb}. Therefore the potential E_{AB} between electrodes A and B before the tip of the micropipet enters the cell is

$$E_{AB} = E_{ma} + E_t + E_{mb}.$$

The potential E_{AB}, measured before the tip of the micropipet is advanced into the cell, is usually assigned the value zero, regardless of what it is. The potential E_{ma} between the metal electrode in the micropipet and the potential E_{mb} between the reference electrode and the environmental fluid depend on the type of metal used for each and the activities (which depend on the concentration and temperature) of the ions in the fluids they contact. Fortunately, these potentials remain the same whether the tip of the micropipet is outside or inside the cell. The tip potential E_t between the fluid filling the micropipet and the environmental fluid depends on the concentrations and mobilities of the ions in each solution.

When the tip of the micropipet penetrates the cell membrane (Fig. 62b), not only does the membrane potential E_{mp} appear in the circuit, but the liquid-junction potential changes slightly because the fluid filling the micropipet is now in contact with that which constitutes the cytoplasm; this tip potential is designated E_t'. Thus the potential E_{AB}' between electrodes A and B after the tip of the micropipet has passed through the cell membrane is

$$E_{AB}' = E_{ma} + E_t' + E_{mb} + E_{mp}.$$

By this procedure, what has been called the membrane potential is the difference between the potential between the electrode terminals with the tip of the micropipet inside the cell, E_{AB}', and that measured before the tip penetrated the cell membrane. The measured membrane potential is

$$E_{AB}' - E_{AB} = E_{ma} + E_t' + E_{mp} + E_{mb} - (E_{ma} + E_t + E_{mb})$$

$$= E_t' - E_t + E_{mp}.$$

As long as $E_t' - E_t$ is small, the potential difference that suddenly appears between the electrode terminals (when the micropipet tip enters the cell) can be taken as the membrane potential. (The use of KCl as a filling solution for micropipets aids in minimizing $E_t' - E_t$ because K^+ and Cl^- ions have very nearly equal mobilities.)

Only a few investigators have concerned themselves with the error in membrane potential that can be contributed by junction potentials; this subject is discussed presently. Because of the difficulty and uncertainty in calculating liquid-junction potentials, Curtis and Cole (1942) wrote that "it seems advisable to report only the measured values of potential." With the techniques routinely employed it would appear that the measured resting membrane potentials are slightly low due to the liquid-junction potential, which may amount to a few millivolts.

EQUIVALENT CIRCUIT

Having identified all the potentials between a reference electrode and a micropipet with the tip located within a cell, it is useful to summarize them and synthesize an equivalent circuit for the micropipet. Starting from terminal A and tracing out the circuit (Fig. 62b), the first potential encountered is E_{ma}, the potential between the electrode metal and the electrolyte filling the micropipet. If the fluid in the cell is different from that in the microelectrode, there will be a tip potential E_t'. Next to appear in the circuit is the membrane potential E_{mp} and then the potential between the reference electrode and the extracellular fluid, E_{mb}.

Neglecting for the moment the potentials and examining the impedances in traversing the circuit, there are the resistance of the connecting wire, which is negligible, then the impedance of the electrode–electrolyte junction in the stem of the micropipet R_{ma}, C_{ma}, R_{fa}, followed by the resistance R_t of the electrolyte filling

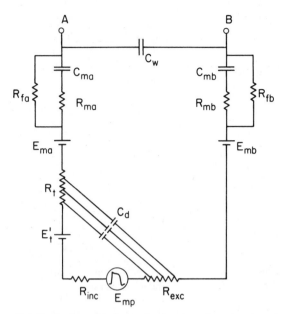

Figure 63 Equivalent circuit for the tip of a micropipet inside a cell.

the tip of the micropipet, the resistance of the electrolyte inside (R_{inc}) and outside (R_{exc}) the cell, the impedance of the reference electrode–electrolyte interface (R_{mb}, C_{mb}, R_{fb}), and finally the negligible resistance of the wire connecting the reference electrode to terminal B. These impedances form a series circuit in conjunction with the four potentials previously identified; they are collected along with the potentials and presented in Fig. 63.

In addition to the components just identified, there is a distributed capacitance C_d existing between the fluid in the micropipet and the extracellular fluid. The magnitude of this important capacitance, along with the tip resistance, determines the response time of the micropipet. As early as 1950, Nastak and Hodgkin recognized that the important part of the capacitance is that which is outside the cell, because there is a potential difference across it.

Since in many measurement situations the relative magnitudes of the various impedances are known, it is possible to simplify the equivalent circuit considerably. For example, the resistances of the connecting wires amount to a fraction of an ohm and therefore can be neglected. In the whole circuit, the resistance R_t of the tip of the micropipet is by far the highest, amounting to about 10–200 MΩ for typical micropipets. The area of the electrode–electrolyte interface in the stem is usually large, or can be made large, which results in the impedance of R_{ma}, C_{ma}, R_{fa} being negligible with respect to the 10–200-MΩ tip resistance. Likewise, the resistance of the intracellular (R_{inc}) and extracellular (R_{exc}) fluids and the reference electrode–electrolyte impedance (R_{mb}, C_{mb}, R_{fb}) can also be ignored; the distributed capacitance C_d cannot be neglected. With reasonable accuracy the circuit can be reduced to that of Fig. 64a. This first simplification shows that the membrane

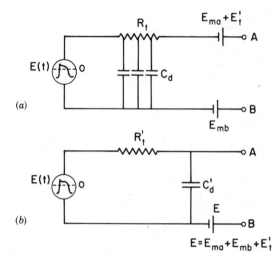

Figure 64 (a) Simplified equivalent circuit for a micropipet used to measure the trans-membrane potential $E(t)$; (b) the lumped equivalent circuit.

potential E_{mp} is connected to the amplifier input terminals A and B via R_t, the 10–200 MΩ resistance of the tip of the micropipet; the resistance is shunted by the distributed capacitance C_d, which amounts to about 0.5 pF per millimeter of tip length. A voltage then appears across the terminals that is the sum of the membrane potential E_{mp}, the potential of the electrode–electrolyte interface in the stem E_{ma}, the tip potential E_t', and the potential of the reference electrode–electrolyte junction E_{mb}.

In many circumstances, E_{ma}, E_t', and E_{mb} are stable and can be corrected for in determining the membrane potential. Therefore, they can be summed to form a single potential E. In addition, it is customary to replace a circuit consisting of distributed parameters with one with lumped parameters in accordance with the known electrical behavior of the circuit; thus the distributed capacitance C_d and tip resistance R_t can be represented as in Fig. 64b, in which R_t' and C_d ($\simeq C_d'$) are the single resistance and capacitance values that simulate the response of R_t with its distributed capacitance C_d.

In Fig. 64b, the membrane potential ($E(t)$) is coupled to the amplifier terminals A and B via a high series tip resistance R_t' and a moderate tip shunt capacitance C_t'. The effect of this particular combination of circuit elements places a limit on the ability of the micropipet to respond to a sudden change in potential; this characteristic is described as the response or rise time. Failure to achieve a response time shorter than the rising phase of the action potential ($E(t)$) will prevent faithful reproduction of the action potential.

Because it is not possible to calculate accurately the resistance and distributed capacitance of the tip of the micropipet, two simple techniques are used to measure them; the circuit arrangements are diagramed in Fig. 65. Both methods can be applied with the tip of the micropipet in the environmental fluid or in the cell.

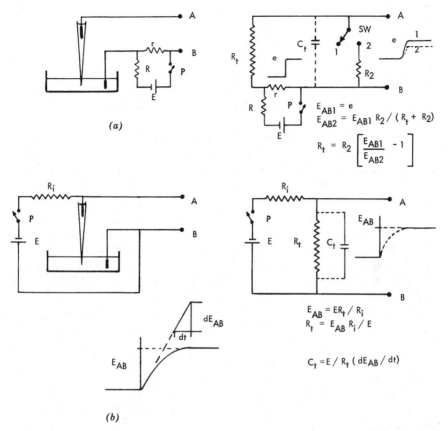

Figure 65 Measurement of tip resistance and capacitance: (*a*) constant-voltage method; (*b*) constant-current method.

MEASUREMENT OF TIP RESISTANCE AND CAPACITANCE

When a micropipet is used with its reference electrode to measure transmembrane resting and action potentials, it is necessary to know the resistance and capacitance of the tip. The resistance, which is determined by the diameter and the angle of the tip and the type of electrolyte filling it, identifies the magnitude of the amplifier input impedance required; that is, for measurement of the true potential difference between the micropipet tip and the reference electrode, the amplifier input impedance must be many times larger than the tip resistance. For a given size of micropipet, tip resistance is often used as a measure of the acceptability of the electrode. For example, if the tip is clogged, the resistance becomes high; if it breaks, the resistance is low. Tip resistance and capacitance, which also depend on tip dimensions, determine the rise time or the ability of the micropipet to reproduce the rapidly changing portion of an action potential.

Tip Resistance

Two methods are used to measure tip resistance. With one, a constant voltage is applied in series with the reference electrode, and the voltage across the electrode terminals is measured without and with a known resistance placed across them. With the other method, a constant-current source is placed in parallel with the micropipet and reference-electrode terminals, and the voltage increase is measured.

Constant-Voltage Method. With the constant-voltage method, a known voltage is suddenly inserted in series with the reference electrode; the technique for carrying this out (Fig. 65a), is used in many commercially available headstages. Often the inserted voltage serves to calibrate the sensitivity of the measuring system. In Fig. 65a, a step of voltage e is caused to appear across a low value of resistance r by closing the switch P. The resistors r and R together constitute a voltage divider, which reduces the large voltage E such that $e = Er/(R + r)$. The actual value for e is chosen so that the cell will not be stimulated when voltage is applied with the electrode tip in the cell. Another reason for using a low voltage is to avoid decomposition of the electrolytes or heating of the fluid in the tip of the micropipet.

When the switch SW is in position 1, the voltage E_{AB1}, which appears when switch P is closed, will be equal to e if measured by an amplifier with a very high input resistive impedance. With the switch in position 2, a resistor R_2 is placed across the terminals A and B, and the voltage E_{AB2}, measured when switch P is closed, will be less. Voltage E_{AB2}, is equal to iR_2; the current i is equal to the voltage applied e divided by the total circuit resistance $R_t + R_2$. If R_t is greater than all the other resistances in the electrode circuit, which is nearly always the case, then

$$E_{AB2} = iR_2 = \frac{eR_2}{R_t + R_2},$$

$$E_{AB1} = e, \text{ and}$$

$$E_{AB2} = \frac{E_{AB1} R_2}{R_t + R_2}.$$

Manipulation of these equations gives a value for the tip resistance R_t in terms of the voltage without (E_{AB1}) and with (E_{AB2}) the resistor R_2 across the terminals A, B; thus

$$R_t = R_2 \left(\frac{E_{AB1}}{E_{AB2}} - 1 \right).$$

Note that the magnitude of the voltage e is unimportant and that in this derivation the tip capacitance and electrode impedances are neglected. The values E_{AB1} and

E_{AB2} are those that persist as long as the switch P is depressed. Note also that if $R_t = R_2$, $E_{AB2} = 0.5\ E_{AB1}$.

Constant-Current Method. With the constant-current method, both tip resistance R_t and effective capacitance C_t can be measured; the former will be discussed first. Referring to Fig. 65b, the procedure consists of passing a very small step of constant current through the micropipet; this is accomplished by connecting a voltage source E, which is in series with a resistor R_i, across the electrode terminals. The value for R_i is chosen to be many times larger than the highest value expected for the tip resistance R_t; in practice, resistance values of 1000–10,000 MΩ are not uncommon for R_i. Thus the current i in the circuit when the switch P is closed will be $E/(R_i + R_t)$. Because R_i is much greater than R_t the current will be very close to E/R_i and virtually independent of R_t. When P is closed, the voltage appearing across the electrode terminals will increase by a value equal to the current $(i = E/R_i)$ multiplied by the tip resistance R_t (i.e., $E_{AB} = ER_t/R_i$). Therefore, the voltage across the electrode terminals is proportional to the resistance of the tip of the micropipet. By knowing the value of the voltage E and the resistance R_i and by calibrating the sensitivity of the measuring apparatus connected to the electrode terminals, the tip resistance can be calculated as

$$R_t = \frac{E_{AB}}{E}\ R_i.$$

Tip Capacitance

After tip resistance has been measured, it is possible to determine the effective capacitance C_t of the tip by the procedure described for the constant-current method. The method consists of determining the initial rate of rise of the voltage dE_{AB}/dt when switch P is closed (Fig. 65b). Solving the differential equation to obtain the manner in which E_{AB} rises with time to its final value $ER_t/(R_i + R_t)$ gives

$$E_{AB} = \frac{ER_t}{R_i + R_t}\left[1 - \exp\left(-\frac{t(R_i + R_t)}{R_i R_t C_t}\right)\right].$$

If R_i is much greater than R_t, the initial slope dE_{AB}/dt becomes

$$\frac{dE_{AB}}{dt} = \frac{E}{R_i C_t}.$$

Rearrangement of the equation isolates C_t to give

$$C_t = \frac{E}{R_i(\text{initial slope})}.$$

Thus by knowing E and R_i, and measuring the initial slope (V/sec), the tip capacitance can be calculated.

In summary, the constant-current method is approximated by applying a voltage in series with a resistance (many times higher than the resistance of the micropipet tip) across the terminals of the reference electrode and micropipet. This produces a voltage that rises exponentially to a final value E_{AB} from which the resistance of the tip can be calculated as follows:

$$R_t = \frac{E_{AB} R_i}{E}.$$

From the initial rate of rise of the voltage dE_{AB}/dt, the capacitance of the tip of the micropipet can be calculated as

$$C_t = \frac{E}{R_i(\text{initial slope})}.$$

NEGATIVE-CAPACITY (POSITIVE-FEEDBACK) COMPENSATION

The effective distributed capacity at the tip of a micropipet and at the input of a headstage can be markedly reduced by the use of a negative-capacity (positive-feedback) amplifier. Figure 66 diagrams a micropipet and reference electrode connected to a typical negative-capacity amplifier created by using a field-effect transistor (FET) as a source follower. The micropipet signal is connected to the non-inverting terminal (+) of an operational amplifier A, whose gain is specified by the ratio of the feedback resistors R_2/R_1; in practice the gain should be only slightly greater than unity. The output, which reflects the bioelectric event detected by the

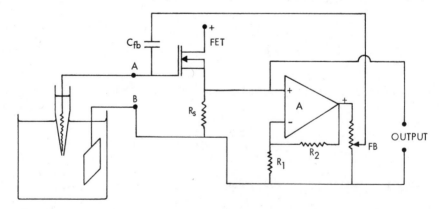

Figure 66 The negative-capacity (positive-feedback) amplifier used to cancel the effective tip capacitance. The feedback is adjusted by the potentiometer FB.

micropipet, is obtained from the ends of the source resistor R_s. Capacity neutralization is provided by feeding a selected fraction of the output of the operational amplifier to the input, in phase, via a coupling condenser C_{fb}, which is a few picofarads. The feedback fraction is selected by use of a potentiometer FB across the output of the operational amplifier; an alternative method consists of connecting the feedback coupling capacitor C_{fb} directly to the output of the operational amplifier and controlling the gain of the latter by varying the ratio of the feedback resistors R_2/R_1. Considerable care must be exercised in adjusting the amount of feedback so that the loop gain—the ratio of the input to the source follower to the output signal fed back—is less than 1.0; sustained oscillations will occur with no input if the feedback fraction exceeds 1.0. Even with slightly less feedback, distortion will be added to a bioelectric event.

In practice, it is never possible to calculate the required feedback because the values of tip resistance and total input capacitance are unknown and moreover vary from micropipet to micropipet. For this reason, a test signal is applied, and the feedback is adjusted for best reproduction of the test signal. At present there are three ways to apply a test signal; with all, the optimum feedback is that which provides the best reproduction of a square wave. The three methods—the square-wave constant-voltage and constant-current methods and the capacitively coupled triangular-wave method—are illustrated in Fig. 67.

With the square-wave constant-voltage method (Fig. 67a), a low resistance r is placed in series with the lead wire to the reference electrode B; across the resistor, a square wave of amplitude e is caused to appear by connecting a square-wave generator (of voltage E) in series with a resistance R that is many times larger than r. The voltage e is therefore equal to $Er/(r + R)$ as shown in Fig. 67a. The frequency of the square wave is chosen so that its period (1/frequency) is long with respect to the rise time of the input circuit, which is determined by the tip resistance and total capacitance at the input circuit. On application of the test signal, an exponentially rising and falling wave (Fig. 68b) appears at the output of the source follower; this is due to the tip resistance and the total capacitance of the input circuit. With an increasing amount of feedback, the rising and falling phases of the reproduced wave become steeper (Fig. 68c); with more feedback, a slight overshoot appears (Fig. 68d); and with excessive feedback, the overshoot becomes much larger and a series of damped oscillations (Fig. 68e), i.e., ringing, appear. Obviously the optimum feedback adjustment is shown in Fig. 68d.

With the square-wave constant-current method (Fig. 67b), the test signal (provided by a square-wave generator) is connected to a resistance R_i, which is much higher in value (e.g., 100–1000 times) than the micropipet tip resistance; the series combination (R_i and the square-wave generator of voltage E) are connected via a switch across the micropipet and reference electrode terminals. The procedure for adjustment of the feedback is the same as with the square-wave constant-voltage method: increase the feedback to obtain the best reproduction of the square-wave test signal.

The triangular-wave, capacitively coupled method is illustrated in Fig. 67c. This method, suggested to Freygang (1958) by Lettvin, employs a triangular-wave gen-

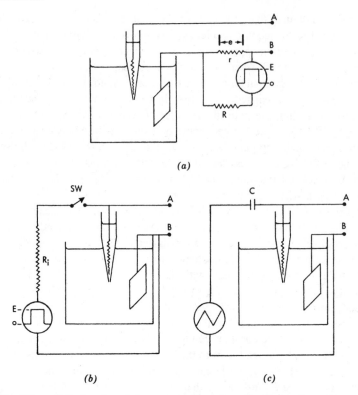

(a)

(b)   (c)

Figure 67   Three methods of applying a test signal for adjustment of negative-capacity (positive-feedback) headstages used with micropipets; (a) Square-wave constant-voltage method; (b) square-wave constant-current method; (c) triangular-wave capacitively coupled method.

erator coupled via a capacitance C that is a few picofarads in value. The amount of feedback is increased until the best square wave is reproduced at the output of the headstage. A square wave results when the proper feedback is obtained because the resistance of the tip of the micropipet, in series with C, constitutes a differentiating circuit. True differentiation of a triangular wave (i.e., one in which the slope is constant) produces a square wave.

The ability of each of the three methods to provide perfect compensation for all the capacitances associated with the micropipet and input circuit of the headstage is subject to question because in each case the circuit facing the bioelectric event at the tip of the micropipet differs from that for which the compensation methods are adjusted. Nonetheless, the three methods offer the best means of adjusting the feedback to compensate for input capacitance. However, as pointed out by Amatneik (1958), the input circuit is more complex and consists of many distributed, rather than lumped, components; complete neutralization is therefore impossible. To clarify this point, the equivalent circuit for a micropipet in a cell is presented in Fig. 63.

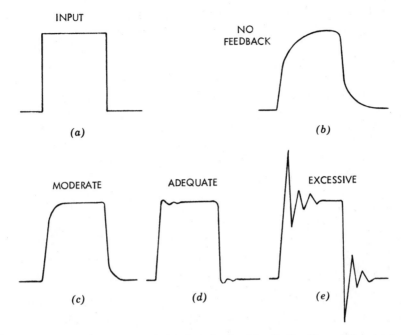

Figure 68 Adjustment of the negative-capacity (positive-feedback) amplifier: (*a*) input; (*b*) no feedback; (*c*) moderate; (*d*) adequate; (*e*) excessive.

COMPARISON OF METAL MICROELECTRODES AND MICROPIPETS

Both metal and micropipet type microelectrodes are used for the measurement of membrane and action potentials. However, it is worthwhile to compare the suitability of each for these two quite different tasks. Because the electrical properties of each type of electrode differ substantially, it might be suspected that each is suitable for one particular task; this is indeed so.

The metal microelectrode is characterized by a small-area metal–electrolyte junction that exhibits an impedance that is extremely high at low frequencies and decreases with increasing frequency. This impedance–frequency characteristic makes it difficult to obtain a potential-measuring device with a high enough input resistance to measure resting membrane potentials with a small-area metal microelectrode. The impedance–frequency characteristic of an electrolyte-filled micropipet is resistive (i.e., not frequency-dependent) in the low-frequency region and has a finite, although high, zero-frequency (dc) resistance. With this type of electrode it is relatively easy to provide a measuring instrument with an input resistance high enough for the accurate measurement of resting membrane potentials.

Both types of electrodes can be used to measure action potentials, provided a high input impedance measuring device is employed; if the impedance is not high enough, distortion results. In the case of a metal microelectrode, if the input impedance of the measuring device is too low, the microelectrode behaves like a high-pass filter (i.e., the low-frequency components of the action potential are attenuated and the waveform is electrically differentiated). Even with a high input impedance device connected to an electrolyte-filled micropipet, the distributed capacitance at the tip causes the electrode to behave like a low-pass filter (i.e., the high-frequency components of the action potential are attenuated, and the waveform lacks sharpness and detail). Although the metal microelectrode has a distributed tip capacitance, the low high-frequency impedance of the metal–electrolyte junction makes the effect of the tip capacitance negligible. In the case of the micropipet, the tip capacitance is extremely bothersome, and, even after all practical steps have been taken to reduce it, further reduction of its effect can be achieved only by the use of a negative-capacity amplifier.

The metal microelectrode and the micropipet can also be compared on the basis of their noise voltages. Because the metal microelectrode has a lower resistance component of its impedance with increasing frequency, its noise voltage is considerably lower than that of the micropipet, which has a uniformly high resistive impedance over a broad frequency spectrum. For this reason, if high-gain recording of action potentials with a wide bandwidth is to be employed, the lower noise of the metal microelectrode is an attractive feature.

For the reasons just given, metal microelectrodes see most service in the measurement of action potentials. Electrolyte-filled micropipets are routinely used to measure resting membrane potentials; with suitable precautions they can measure action potentials. Thus the two types have complementary characteristics, and the statement, attributed to Svaetichin by Gesteland et al. (1959), that metal microelectrodes resemble high-pass filters and micropipets resemble low-pass filters, remains valid.

STIMULATING ELECTRODES

Electrodes for stimulating excitable tissue differ from recording electrodes only in the current density at the electrode–electrolyte interface. Although it is possible to employ insulated (capacitive) electrodes for stimulation, their use is uncommon. Figure 69 illustrates a few types of the commonly encountered stimulating electrodes. However, in addition to these, many of the recording electrodes described earlier can be used for stimulating; the metal-plate electrode is often used as an indifferent, dispersive, or reference electrode.

A very common stimulating electrode is the bipolar hand-held type illustrated in Fig. 69A. It is made from two stiff wires, each insulated and held together with heat-shrink tubing. The ends of the wires are rounded and bent outward to achieve the desired spacing.

Catheter-borne electrodes (Fig. 69B) are very commonly used for cardiac pacing. One or two electrodes are mounted on the catheter (about 1–2 mm in diameter). The first electrodes of this type were about 1 cm long with an area in the vicinity of 30–60 mm^2. However, it was soon realized that current density is what stimulates, and the area was reduced to a few square millimeters to achieve cardiac

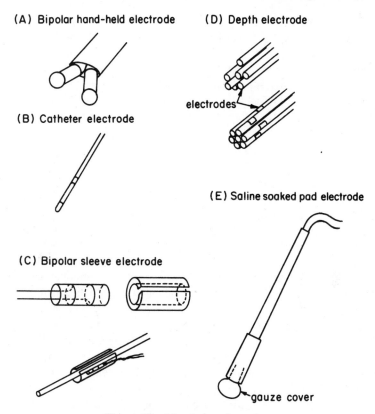

Figure 69   Stimulating electrodes.

pacing with less current, thereby prolonging the life of the battery in the pacemaker. The catheter electrode is passed down the superior vena cava into the right ventricle. When monopolar stimulation is used, the metallic case of the pacemaker becomes the reference electrode (anode). The active electrode (cathode) is small and is located at the catheter tip for both monopolar and bipolar stimulation.

The monopolar or bipolar sleeve electrode, illustrated in Fig. 69C, is easily fabricated and ideally suited for stimulating nerve trunks. It consists of one or two wires wrapped around a short segment of plastic tubing. The leads are brought out through the lumen of the plastic tube (Hoff and Geddes, 1971). The electrode is placed against the nerve trunk and held there by a slitted sleeve of gum-rubber tubing as shown in Fig. 69C.

A variety of electrodes are used for cutaneous stimulation. Often a saline-soaked pad wrapped around a metal ball is used as the active (cathode) electrode. Figure 69E illustrates such an easily fabricated electrode, consisting of a hollow insulating tube and a threaded rod with a metal ball mounted on the end. The ball is covered with gauze, which is held in place by the insulating tube that forms the handle. The nut at the opposite end of the electrode allows drawing the ball to the end of the handle, thereby securing the gauze, which is then soaked in saline.

As stated at the beginning of this chapter, the electrode–electrolyte impedance decreases with increasing current density. Therefore, the impedance exhibited by stimulating electrodes will be much lower than that exhibited by the same pair of electrodes when they are used to record a bioelectric event. Moreover, the current-density distribution under stimulating electrodes is not uniform, a fact that is not generally recognized. The situation for a current-carrying plate electrode on the skin can be used to illustrate this point.

ELECTRODE CURRENT-DENSITY DISTRIBUTION

When an electrolytically coated plate electrode is placed on the skin and used to deliver current, the current density is higher under the perimeter than under the center (Nelson et al., 1975; Overmeyer et al., 1979; Caruso et al., 1979; Wiley and Webster, 1982). Figure 70a illustrates this concept. The reason for the high perimeter current is that all the current that flows beyond the electrode must leave by the perimeter. Similarly, if a needle electrode is used for stimulating, the current density at the tip and where the insulation begins will be higher than over the rest of the exposed surface. The significance of a nonuniform current-density distribution relates to the fact that stimulation occurs in the region of highest current density. It is for this reason that it is not strictly accurate to specify a stimulus in terms of average current density by dividing the current by electrode area.

Evidence for the nonuniform current density under an electrode is seen following ventricular defibrillation with chest-surface electrodes. After delivery of the current pulse (typically 40–50 A, 5 msec), there can be seen red rings on the chest that identify the perimeters of the electrodes. Likewise, with conductive electrosurgical dispersive electrodes, the skin under the center of the electrode is cooler than that under the perimeter. Figure 70b is a thermogram of the temperature distribution under a circular electrode applied to the thigh of a human subject using a low-resistivity electrode paste. The white circle identifies the hot perimeter. It is useful to recall that the temperature rise is proportional to the square of the current density.

IMPLICATIONS OF ELECTRODE–SUBJECT IMPEDANCE FOR STIMULATION

As stated earlier in this chapter, the impedance of an electrode–electrolyte interface decreases with an increase in current density. In addition, the impedance of living tissue decreases slightly with increasing current density. Although there is a paucity of information on this subject, the implications of these facts are apparent.

Chapter 10 discusses the constant-voltage and constant-current output stimulator circuits. It is pointed out that due to the reactive nature of the electrode–subject circuit the current and voltage waveforms will differ for any waveform other than the sinusoidal. Moreover, due to the nonlinear nature of the circuit, the relationships

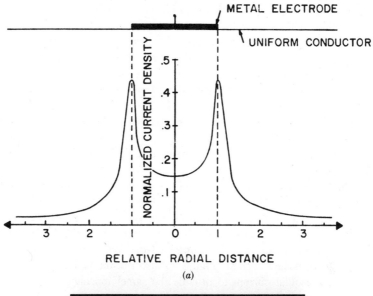

RELATIVE RADIAL DISTANCE

(a)

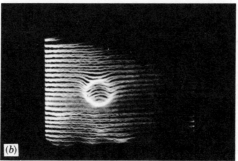

Figure 70   (a) Theoretical current density distribution under an electrode delivering current to the skin. (Redrawn from Overmeyer et al., 1979). (b) Thermogram illustrating skin temperature under circular disk electrodes on the thigh after passage of 1 A of 500-kHz current for 1 min. The white area shows the increased temperature corresponding to the perimeter of the electrode (Courtesy J. A. Pearce.)

will depend on current density. Even with sinusoidal current, the voltage and current waveforms will differ slightly.

With complex waves, it is technically incorrect to express impedance as the ratio of voltage to current. If the voltage and current waveforms differ, the meaning of their ratio is obscure. However, the ratio does identify something about the conducting path for current, and for this reason it is used by many. Perhaps a better term for the ratio of voltage to current is "apparent impedance."

A situation in which there is an easily recognized reduction in apparent impedance with increasing current density is in ventricular defibrillation. To illustrate the nature of the electrode–electrolyte impedance to pulses of defibrillating current (damped sine wave, 5 msec), Geddes (1975) measured the apparent impedance of typical 9-cm-diameter defibrillating electrodes in contact with a 1-cm-thick column of low-resistivity electrode paste. Figure 71 illustrates the current–voltage and apparent impedance versus current relationships. Note the decrease in apparent impedance with increasing current (Fig. 71b). Next the electrodes were applied to the chest of an 81-kg sheep and the procedure was repeated. Figure 72a illustrates the current versus voltage relationship and Figure 72b illustrates the apparent impedance versus current relationship. Note that the apparent impedance decreases with increasing current.

Because it is desirable to know the apparent impedance to be encountered by defibrillating current applied to chest-surface electrodes, Geddes et al. (1976a) proposed the use of a low-intensity, high-frequency sinusoidal current to measure the impedance of the circuit. In a study using dogs, it was found that the impedance measured with about 30 kHz sinusoidal current provided a good measure of the apparent impedance at threshold defibrillating current. Figure 73 is a plot of the apparent impedance versus thoracic current. Note that the apparent impedance decreases with increasing current. Figure 73 also illustrates the frequencies for a low intensity sinusoidal current to provide the same impedance. At present this technique has been applied by one defibrillator manufacturer to permit identification of the quality of application of the defibrillating electrodes to the chest prior to delivery of the defibrillating current.

It was reported by Geddes et al. (1976a) and Dahl et al. (1976) that the apparent impedance to defibrillating shocks decreased with each successive shock. Figure 74 summarizes these data. It is speculated that the reason for the decrease in apparent impedance is an increasing breakdown of the dielectric of the membranes of the living cells in the current path, particularly those immediately under the electrodes. To date, there is only a limited amount of information on the breakdown of cell membranes exposed to high-intensity field strengths. Coster and Zimmerman (1975a,b, 1979) used transmembrane electrodes to study the breakdown of membranes of valonia with 0.5–1-msec pulses. They found that the breakdown was local and recovery occurred in less than 5 sec. Gauger and Bentrup (1979) investigated membrane breakdown in brown alga using pulses of 1–1760-μsec in duration and field strengths of 50–400 V/cm. They too found that the breakdown was local and recovery occurred in less than 3 sec.

There is not much information available on the change in resistivity of living tissue exposed to high current density. Tacker et al. (1982) measured the resistivity of blood samples with single 30-msec rectangular-wave shocks with field strengths ranging from 30 to 403 V/cm. Packed-cell volumes ranging from 0 (plasma) to 98% were tested. Plasma exhibited virtually no change in resistivity; the higher packed-cell volume samples exhibited a decrease in resistivity with increasing field strength. However, the decrease was not large; the 98% packed-cell volume sample decreased from 2040 to 1509 Ω cm for field strengths ranging from 30 to 403 V/cm.

DeGaravilla et al. (1981) studied the effect of 30-msec rectangular-wave shocks on the resistivity of cardiac muscle. Fifteen shocks ranging from 33 to 405 V/cm

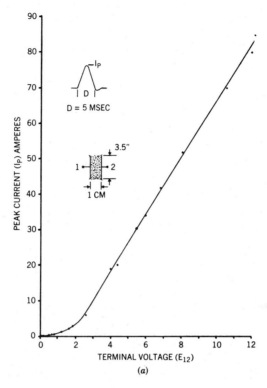

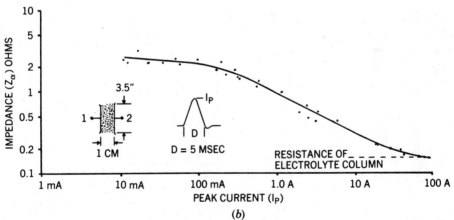

Figure 71   (*a*) Current-voltage relationship and (*b*) apparent impedance versus current for a pair of 9-cm defibrillating electrodes in contact with a 1-cm-thick column of electrode paste. The current pulses were delivered by a typical damped sine wave defibrillator. [From L.A. Geddes, *Eng. Ext. Ser.* (*Purdue Univ.*) No. 147 (1975).]

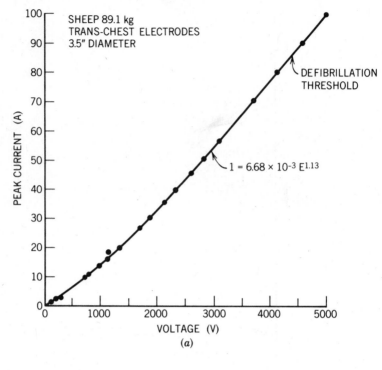

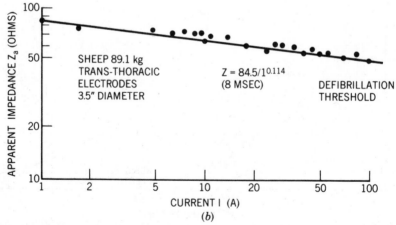

Figure 72   (*a*) Current–voltage relationship and (*b*) apparent impedance versus current for a pair of 9-cm defibrillating electrodes on the chest of an 81-kg sheep. The current pulses were delivered by a typical damped sine wave defibrillator. [From L.A. Geddes, *Eng. Ext. Ser. (Purdue Univ.)* No. 147 (1975).]

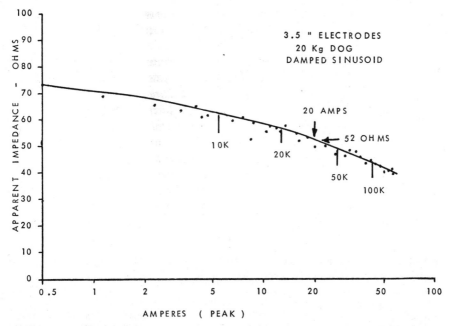

Figure 73 Apparent impedance offered to defibrillating current for 9-cm defibrillating electrodes on the chest of a dog. [Redrawn from L.A. Geddes et al., *Med. Instrum.* **10**(3):159–162 (1976).]

were delivered to different specimens of cardiac muscle. In general, the resistivity decreased with successive shocks, the decrease being slight for the 33-V/cm shocks and more for the shocks having higher field strengths.

Tacker et al. (1984) measured the decrease in resistivity of skeletal muscle, skin, and fat exposed to 30-msec rectangular pulses with field strengths of 50–400 V/cm. The decrease in resistivity was most for skeletal muscle, less for skin, and least for fat.

The foregoing studies indicate that tissue resistivity decreases with increasing current density. Moreover, at the same current density, the resistivity decreases with successive shocks. These decreases in resistivity depend on the type of tissue; plasma and fat appear to exhibit the least decrease in resistivity.

Many phenomena occur at an electrode–electrolyte interface that carries current. Most of the fundamental characteristics of the electrode–electrolyte interface have been described in this chapter and in Chapter 8. Sometimes the electrode phenomena are beneficial, but at other times they present problems. Any comprehensive discussion of electrode properties must distinguish between the application of a constant voltage (direct current), a unidirectional pulse, and sinusoidal voltage. Moreover, attention must be paid to the type of current source, that is, whether it is of the constant-voltage or constant-current type. Obviously, the types of electrolyte and electrode are also very important. Often noble-metal electrodes are used;

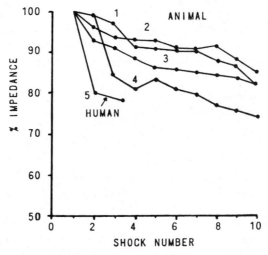

Figure 74 Apparent impedance versus shock number for defibrillating electrodes on the chests of animals and man. The energy levels used are as follows:

Curve Number	Energy (J)	Subject, Weight	Electrode Location	Electrode Size	Investigator, Year
1	320	Sheep, 61 kg	Precordial	3.5 in.	Geddes et al. (1976a)
2	245	Dogs, 16–27 kg	Precordial	8.0 cm	Dahl et al. (1976) (15 sec intervals)
3	245	Dogs, 16–27 kg	Precordial	8.0 cm	Dahl et al. (1976) (1 minute intervals)
4	800	Pigs	Precordial	3.5 in.	Geddes et al. (1976a)
5	100	Humans	Precordial		Chambers (1977)

noble metals are those that do not contribute their ions to or combine with the electrolyte. The electrode properties also depend on the duration and frequency of a pulse of current and the frequency when alternating current is employed. This time-domain component arises because the mobilities of the ions in the electrolyte are participants in the electrode processes.

ELECTROLYSIS AND ARCING

The simple electrolytic cell, consisting of a small-area (bare or membrane-covered) metal electrode paired with a large-area electrode in an electrolyte, forms the basis of polarography. With a slow ramp of direct voltage derived from a constant-voltage source, the current that flows as the voltage is increased shows a series of plateaus, the nature of which depends on the electrolyte species and on what is dissolved therein. Such current–voltage curves are called polarograms; examples are presented in Chapter 8. With about -0.6 V dc applied to the small-area electrode, the current that flows is dependent on the partial pressure of dissolved oxygen. In the peroxide–glucose sensor, the polarity is the opposite, and the current is proportional to the concentration of hydrogen peroxide, one of the products of glucose oxidation. Polarography is an important technique in analytical chemistry.

Everyone is familiar with the high school chemistry demonstration in which direct current is passed through two noble-metal electrodes in acidulated water. At the anode, oxygen bubbles appear and can be collected; at the cathode, twice the volume of hydrogen is liberated. This is the well-known phenomenon of electrolysis that obeys Faraday's law, namely 1 gram equivalent of an element is released by 93,500 C (ampere-seconds). In electroplating, another example of electrolysis, a metal is plated on one electrode and removed from the other; the electrolyte is a salt of the metal that is plated out of solution. In such applications, the direct-current density is typically 5–10 mA/cm^2.

A series of interesting phenomena occur when a unidirectional pulse of current is passed through an electrode–electrolyte interface. At a low current density, the current that flows is determined by the area of the electrode, the nature of the electrode–electrolyte circuit, and the type of current source (e.g., constant voltage or constant current). As the current density is increased, electrolysis will occur during the pulse and gas bubbles will be seen at the electrode surface. The type of gas in the bubbles depends on the electrolyte and whether the electrode is the anode or cathode. In an aqueous solution, oxygen is liberated at the anode and hydrogen is liberated at the cathode. Now, if the current in the pulse is increased, more gas bubbles form, and with further current the gas becomes ionized, emitting a flash of light and creating a shock wave in the electrolyte. This is the principle employed in the lithotripter, a device for destroying kidney stones (see Chap. 13).

Bourland et al. (1977) studied the behavior of a catheter electrode (1.25 cm^2) in 0.9% saline (versus a large indifferent anode electrode) to which rectangular pulses were applied from a constant-voltage source. Figure 75a illustrates the appearance of the electrode with no current. Figure 75b shows the electrode 11 msec after application of a 500-V, 1.8-A current pulse and demonstrates bubble formation. In Fig. 75c is shown the arc that appeared at 17 msec. Just before the arc formed, the current density was on the order of 14.4 A/cm^2. The current pulse was terminated at 20 msec. Figure 75d presents the voltage E and current I waveforms.

Wessale et al. (1987) investigated the current-carrying capability of electrodes of different areas of the type shown in Fig. 75a. The threshold current for arcing was determined for rectangular voltage pulses having durations ranging from 2 to 30 msec. Figure 76a illustrates the results and reveals that for each electrode size there is a strength–duration curve for arc formation. The arcing current (I) threshold is higher for larger area electrodes. In Fig. 76b, the threshold current density J for arcing for each of the four electrodes is plotted versus pulse duration, revealing that under these special circumstances, where efforts were made to obtain as uniform a current density as possible, the current-carrying capacity of an electrode is dependent on current density and pulse duration.

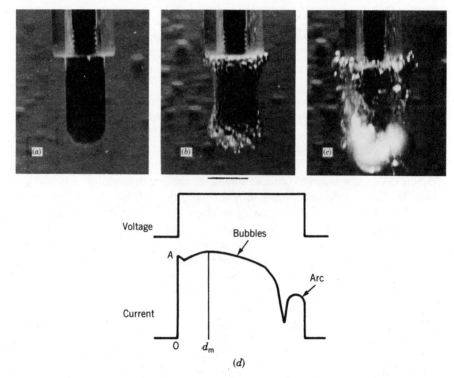

Figure 75   (*a*) Catheter-tip electrode (1.25 cm^2) in 0.9% saline. (*b*) The electrode (cathode) 11 msec after the application of a 500-V, 10.8-A current pulse; note the gas bubbles. (*c*) An underwater arc that formed 17 msec after current application. The voltage source was removed at 20 msec. (*d*) Voltage and current waveforms for a catheter electrode in saline. The small transient at A is probably due to the Warburg capacitance. The slight current increase from 0 to d_m is due to heating of the saline immediately adjacent to the catheter electrode. Following d_m the current decreases due to bubble formation, which culminates in the arc when the gas in the bubbles becomes ionized.

RECTIFICATION

A little-recognized property of an electrode–electrolyte interface is rectification. In the early days of electricity, electrolytic rectifiers were used to charge storage batteries (accumulators). The usual configuration of an electrolytic rectifier consisted of a large-area electrode and a small-area electrode in an electrolyte. Rectification occurred at the small-area electrode. Such rectifiers were sold commercially and were discussed in books by Jolley (1928) and Gunther-Schultze (1929). In 1913 Hill found that the polarity of such rectification could be reversed by making the small-area electrode larger.

A variety of electrolytic rectifiers were available in the 1920s. The Phywe rectifier consisted of a cylindrical iron container filled with ammonium carbonate solution into which an aluminum rod was dipped. The most successful electrolytic

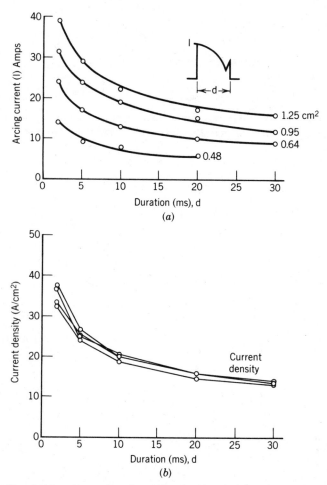

Figure 76 Threshold arcing current *I* versus pulse duration for electrodes of 1.2, 0.95, 0.64, and 0.45 cm²; (*b*) current density versus pulse duration for the same electrodes. [Redrawn from J.L. Wessale et al., *Pace* **10**:427 (1987).]

rectifier consisted of a large-area lead electrode and a smaller area tantalum electrode in a dilute solution of sulfuric acid containing about 0.8% ferrous sulfate. A film of oil on the surface of the electrolyte prevented evaporation and corrosion of the electrodes where they emerged from the electrolyte (Fansteel Co., Chicago, Illinois). Interestingly, there was a circuit symbol for the electrolytic rectifier; it consisted of a bar and a small circle (to represent the electrodes) placed inside a large circle.

When an electrolytic rectifier was connected to the domestic power line (115 V 60 Hz) and a load resistor, current and voltage waveforms such as those shown in Fig. 77 were obtained. Note that there is a slight current flow in the direction opposite to that for rectification.

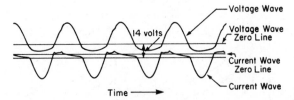

Figure 77 Current and voltage waveforms from a typical electrolytic rectifier. (Redrawn from A. Gunther-Schultze, *Electric Rectifiers and Valves.* Wiley, New York, 1929, 212 pp.)

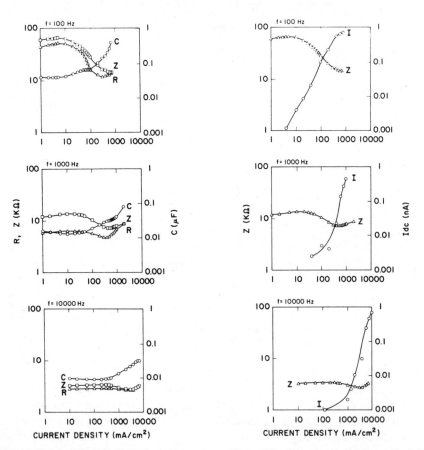

Figure 78 Series-equivalent capacitance *C*, resistance *R*, and impedance *Z* for an 0.01-in.-diameter stainless steel–saline interface versus sinusoidal current density at 100, 1000, and 10,000 Hz. (From *IEEE Trans. Bio-Med. Eng.* 1987, **BME** 34(9):669–672; by permission.)

Figure 79 Impedance *Z* and rectified direct current *I* versus sinusoidal alternating current density for an 0.01-in.-diameter stainless steel–saline interface at 100, 1000, and 10,000 Hz. (From *IEEE Trans. Bio-Med. Eng.* 1987, **BME** 34(9), 669–672; by permission.)

Geddes et al. (1988) investigated the rectifying properties of a single stainless steel–saline interface over a range of sinusoidal current densities and frequencies. In this study, the series-equivalent resistance R, capacitance C, and impedance Z of an 0.01-in.-diameter stainless steel–saline interface were measured at room temperature. A large indifferent stainless steel electrode (of negligible impedance compared to that of the 0.01-in.-diameter electrode) was used to complete the circuit. The small-area electrode was heavily insulated except at the cross section that constituted the interface. A comparison bridge was operated in the constant-current mode; i.e., the value of the resistors used in the ratio arms was equal and high with respect to the impedance of the electrode–electrolyte interface. A sine wave generator with a high output voltage was used to select the frequency and desired current density. To perform the study, a frequency was chosen (100, 1000, or 10,000 Hz), and the series-equivalent resistance R and capacitance C were measured for a current density ranging from 1 to 10,000 mA/cm^2. From the sinusoidal voltage across the electrodes and the current, the series-equivalent impedance Z was calculated. The magnitudes of Z, R, and C were measured versus sinusoidal current density for each of the three frequencies.

To determine the rectifying properties of the electrode–electrolyte interface, the direct current was measured. A frequency was selected (100, 1000, or 10,000 Hz), and the current was increased incrementally by increasing the output of the oscillator. The rectified direct current and the alternating current impedance were measured versus current density for the three frequencies.

Figure 78 illustrates the series-equivalent R, C, and Z versus current density for 100, 1000, and 10,000 Hz. For all frequencies, there was a critical current density where the impedance was lowest; this point occurred at a higher current density with a higher frequency.

The rectifying properties of the stainless steel electrode–electrolyte interface are shown in Fig. 79. When rectification occurred, the small-area electrode became negative. For all frequencies, rectification started to occur about where the impedance started to decrease with increasing current density. The most sensitive indicator of approaching rectification was the increase in capacitance (see Figs. 78 and 79). Rectification occurred at a higher current density as the frequency was increased. To illustrate this point more clearly, the rectified direct current versus sinusoidal alternating current density curves for 100, 1000, and 10,000 Hz are plotted in Fig. 80.

Although there has been much speculation about the mechanisms underlying electrolytic rectification, the intimate details have not been investigated adequately. However, there is speculation that the transient formation of an oxide layer and micro gas bubbles are important ingredients. That gas bubbles are a factor was demonstrated by Jolley (1928), who showed that the rectifying action was reduced when high pressure was applied to an electrolytic rectifier. That there is ionization in the gas bubbles is evident from the faint glow emitted, a phenomenon that is clearly seen in a darkened room. Gunther-Schultze (1929) believed that the high voltage gradient across the bubbles at the electrode–electrolyte interface pulled electrons from the metal and that this effect was responsible for the rectification.

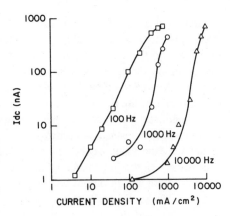

Figure 80 The rectified direct current *I* and peak-to-peak sinusoidal alternating current density for an 0.010-in.-diameter stainless steel–saline interface at 100, 1000, and 10,000 Hz. (From *IEEE Trans. Bio-Med. Eng.* 1987, **BME 34**(9):669–672; by permission.)

However, there is still no satisfactory theory to account for electrolytic rectification, which is a well-established property of electrode–electrolyte interfaces.

REFERENCES

Adrian, E. D., and D. W. Bronk. 1929. Impulses in motor nerve fibers. Part II, *J. Physiol.* **67**:119–151.

Afanasiev, A. I. 1930. Influence of the solvent on the electromotive force of silver halide cells. *J. Am. Chem. Soc.* **52**:3477–3483.

Alexander, J. T., and W. L. Nastuk. 1953. An instrument for the production of microelectrodes used in physiological studies. *Rev. Sci. Instrum.* **24**:528–531.

Amatneik, E. 1958. Measurement of bioelectric potentials with microelectrodes and neutralized input capacity amplifiers. *IRE Trans. Med. Electron.* **PGME-10**:3–14.

Aronson, S., and L. A. Geddes. 1985. Electrode potential stability. *IEEE Trans. Biomed. Eng.* **BME-32**(11):987–989.

Asa, M. M., A. H. Crews, E. L. Rothfield, E. S. Lewis, I. R. Zucker, and A. Berstein. 1964. High fidelity radioelectrocardiography. *Am. J. Cardiol.* **14**:530–532.

Association for the Advancement of Medical Instrumentation (AAMI). 1984. *Standard for Conducting Electrodes.* AAMI, Arlington, VA.

Association for the Advancement of Medical Instrumentation (AAMI). 1985. *General Standard for Blood Pressure Transducers.* AAMI, Arlington, VA.

Atkins, A. R. 1961. Measuring heart rate of an active athlete. *Electron. Eng.* **33**:457.

Basmajian, J. V., and G. Stecko. 1962. A new bipolar electrode for electromyography. *J. Appl. Physiol.* **17**:849.

Baudoin, A. H. Fischgold, and J. Lerique. 1938. Une nouvelle électrode liquide. *C. R. Seances Soc. Biol.* **127**:1221–1222.

Bell, G. H., J. A. C. Knox, and A. J. Small. 1939. Electrocardiography electrolytes. *Br. Heart J.* **1**:229–236.

Benedetti-Pichler, A. A., and J. R. Rachele. 1940. Limits of identification of simple confirmatory tests. *Ind. Eng. Chem., Anal. Ed.* **12**:233–241.

Bergey, G. E., R. D. Squires, and W. C. Sipple. 1971. Electrocardiogram recording with pasteless electrodes. *IEEE Trans. Biomed. Eng.* **BME-18**:206–211.

Blank, I. H., and I. G. Finesinger. 1946. Electrical resistance of the skin. *Arch. Neurol. Psychiatry* **54:**544–557.

Boter, J., A. den Hertog, and J. Kuiper. 1966. Disturbance-free skin electrodes for persons during exercise. *Med. Biol. Eng.* **4:**91–95.

Bourland, J. D., J. L. Wessale, W. A. Tacker, W. E. Schoenlein, J. T. Jones, and L. A. Geddes. 1977. Bubble formation, arcing and waveform distortions produced in human blood by trapezoidal defibrillation current. *Proc. 12th Annu. Meet. Assoc. Adv. Med. Instr.* p. 20.

Bourland, J. D., L. A. Geddes, G. Sewell, R. Baker, and J. Kruer. 1978. Active cables for use with dry electrodes for electrocardiography. *J. Electrocardiol.* **11**(1):71–74.

Brown, A. S. 1934. A type of silver chloride electrode for use in dilute solutions. *J. Am. Chem. Soc.* **56:**646–647.

Burbank, D. P., and J. G. Webster. 1978. Reducing skin potential motion artifact by skin abrasion. *Med. Biol. Eng. Comput.* **16:**31–38.

Bures, J., M. Petran, and J. Zacher. 1962. *Electrophysiological Methods in Biological Research.* Academic Press, New York.

Burns, R. C. 1950. Study of skin impedance. *Electronics* **23:**190, 196.

Burr, H. S. 1944. In *Medical Physics*, Vol. 1, O. Glasser (ed.). Yearbook Publ., Chicago, IL.

Burr, H. S. 1950. In *Medical Physics*, Vol. 2, O. Glasser (ed.). Yearbook Publ., Chicago, IL.

Burr, H. S., and A. Mauro. 1948–1949. Millivoltmeters. *Yale J. Biol. Med.* **21:**249–253.

Byzov, A. L., and V. L. Chemystov. 1961. Machine for making microelectrodes. *Biophysics* **6:**79–82.

Carmody, W. R. 1929. A study of the silver–silver chloride electrode. *J. Am. Chem. Soc.* **51:**2901–2904.

Carmody, W. R. 1932. Studies on the electromotive force in dilute aqueous solutions. II. The silver chloride electrode. *J. Am. Chem. Soc.* **54:**188–192.

Caruso, P. N., J. A. Pearce, and D. P. DeWitt. 1979. Temperature and current density distributions at electrosurgical dispersive electrode sites. *Proc. N. Engl. Bioeng. Conf.* **7:**373–376.

Castellan, G. W. 1964. *Physical Chemistry.* Addison-Wesley, Reading, MA, 717 pp.

Castillo, H., and H. Marriott. 1974. Radio transparent ECG electrodes for use during cardiac catheterization. *Med. Instrum.* **8:**116.

Chambers, W., R. Miles, and R. Stratbucker. 1977. Human chest resistance during successive countershocks. *Circulation* Supp III, 183–1.

Chowdhury, T. K. 1969. Fabrication of extremely fine glass micropipette electrodes. *J. Sci. Instrum.* **2:**1087–1090.

Clark, L. C., and R. J. Lacey. 1950. An improved skin electrode. *J. Lab. Clin. Med:* **35:**786–787.

Cole, K. S., and U. Kishimoto. 1962. Platinized silver chloride electrode. *Science* **136:**381–382.

Collias, J. C., and E. E. Manuelidis. 1957. Histopathological changes produced by implanted electrodes in cat brains. *J. Neurosurg.* **14:**302–328.

Coombs, J. S., J. C. Eccles, and P. Fatt. 1955a. The electrical properties of the motoneurone membrane. *J. Physiol.* **130:**291–325.

Coombs, J. S., J. C. Eccles, and P. Fatt. 1955b. The specific ionic conductances and the ionic movements across the motoneuronal membrane that produce the inhibitory postsynaptic potential. *J. Physiol.* **130:**326–373.

Cooper, R. 1956. Storage of silver chloride electrodes. *EEG. Clin. Neurophysiol.* **8:**692.

Cooper, R. 1963. Electrodes. *Am. J. EEG Technol.* **3:**91–101.

Coster, H. G. L., and U. Zimmerman. 1975a. The mechanism of electric breakdown in the membranes of valonia utricularis. *J. Membr. Biol.* **22:**73–90.

Coster, H. G. L., and U. Zimmerman. 1975b. Dielectric breakdown in the membranes of valonia utricularis. *Biochim. Biophy Acta* **382:**410–418.

Curtis, H. J., and K. S. Cole. 1938. Transverse electric impedance of the squid giant axon. *J. Gen. Physiol.* **21**:757–765.

Curtis, H. J., and K. S. Cole. 1942. Membrane resting and action potentials from the squid giant axon. *J. Cell. Comp. Physiol.* **19**:135–144.

Dahl, C. F., G. A. Ewy, and E. D. Thomas. 1976. Transthoracic impedance to direct current discharge. *Med. Instrum.* **10**(3):151–154.

d'Arsonval, A. 1880. Electrodes impolarizables et excitateur électrique. *C. R. Acad. Biol.* **38**:228–229.

David, R. M., and W. M. Portnoy. 1972. Insulated electrocardiogram electrodes. *Med. Biol. Eng.* **10**:742–751.

Day, J., and M. Lippitt. 1964. A long term electrode system for electrocardiography and impedance pneumography. *Psychophysiology* **1**:174–182.

de Bethune, A. J. 1964. In *Handbook of Electrochemistry.* C. A. Hampel (ed.). Reinhold, New York.

DeGaravilla, L., W. A. Tacker, L. A. Geddes, J. D. Bourland, and C. F. Babbs. 1981. In vitro resistivity of canine heart to defibrillator shocks. *Proc. AAMI 16th Annu. Meet.* p. 28.

Delgado, J. M. R. 1955. Evaluation of permanent implantation of electrodes within the brain. *EEG Clin Neurophysiol.* **7**:637–644.

Delgado, J. M. R. 1964. Electrodes for extracellular recording and stimulation. In *Physical Techniques in Biological Research.* W. L. Nastuk (ed.). Academic Press, New York, 460 pp.

Dodge, H. W., C. Petersen, C. W. Sem-Jacobsen, G. P. Sayre, and R. G. Bickford. 1955. The paucity of demonstrable brain damage following intracerebral electrography: Report of a case. *Proc. Staff Meet. Mayo Clin.* **30**:215–221.

Dowben, R. M., and J. E. Rose. 1953. A metal-filled microelectrode. *Science* **118**:22–24.

Du Bois, D. 1931. A machine for pulling glass micropipets and needles. *Science* **73**:344–345.

Eccles, R. M. 1955. Intracellular potentials recorded from a mammalian sympathetic ganglion. *J. Physiol.* **130**:572–584.

Edelberg, R. 1963. Personal communication.

Edelberg, R. 1973. Local electrical response of the skin to deformation. *J. Appl. Physiol.* **34**:334–340.

Edelberg, R., and N. R. Burch. 1962. Skin resistance and galvanic skin response. *Arch. Gen. Psychiatry* **7**:163–169.

Einthoven, W. 1928. Die Aktionsstrome des Herzens. *Handbuch der Normalen und Pathologischen Physiologie.* Julian Springer, Berlin, pp. 758–862.

Ettisch, G. H., and T. Peterfi. 1925. Zur Methodik der Elektrometric der Zelle. *Pfluegers Arch. Gestamte Physiol.* **208**:454–466.

Fascenelli, F. W., C. Cordova, D. G. Simons, J. Johnson, L. Pratt, and L. E. Lamb. 1966. Biomedical monitoring during dynamic stress testing. 1. *Aerosp. Med:* **37**:911–922.

Feates, F. S., D. J. G. Ives, and J. H. Pryor. 1956. Alternating current bridge for measurement of electrolytic conductance. *J. Electrochem. Soc.* **103**:580–585.

Fischer, G., G. P. Sayre, and R. G. Bickford. 1957. Histologic changes in the cat's brain after introduction of metallic and plastic coated wire used in electroencephalography. *Proc. Staff Meet. Mayo Clin.* **32**:14–22.

Forbes, A., S. Cobb, and McK. Cattell. 1921. An electrocardiogram and an electromyogram in an elephant. *Am. J. Physiol.* **55**:385–389.

Frank, K., and M. Becker. 1964. Microelectrodes for recording and stimulation. In *Physical Techniques in Biological Research,* Vol. V, Part A. Academic Press, New York, 460 pp.

Frank, K. and Fourtes, G. F. 1925. Potentials recorded from the spinal cord with microelectrodes. *J. Physiol.* **130**:625–654.

Freygang, W. H. 1958. An analysis of extracellular potentials from single neurons in the lateral geniculate nucleus of the cat. *J. Gen. Physiol.* **41**:143–564.

Fricke, H. 1932. The theory of electrolyte polarization. *Philos. Mag.* (Ser. 7) **14**:310–318.

Gauger, B., and W. Bentrup. 1979. A study of dielectric membrane breakdown in the fucus egg. *J. Membr. Biol.* **48**:249–264.

Geddes, L. A. 1948–1949. Cortical electrodes. *EEG Clin. Neurophysiol.* **1**:523 (illustrated on cover of *Sci. Am.* **179**, No. 4, 1948).

Geddes, L. A. 1972. *Electrodes and the Measurement of Bioelectric Events.* Wiley, New York, 364 pp.

Geddes, L. A. 1973. Measurement of electrolytic resistivity and electrode-electrolyte impedance with a variable-length conductivity cell. *Chem. Instrum.* **4**:157–168.

Geddes, L. A. 1975. Characteristics of defibrillating electrodes and living tissue. *Eng. Ext. Ser.* (Purdue Univ.) **147**:45–53.

Geddes, L. A., and L. E. Baker. 1966. The relationship between input impedance and electrode area in recording the ECG. *Med. Electron. Biol. Eng.* **4**:439–450.

Geddes, L. A., and L. E. Baker. 1967. Chlorided silver electrodes. *Med. Res. Eng.* **6**:33–34.

Geddes, L. A., and M. E. Valentinuzzi. 1973. Temporal changes in electrode impedance while recording the electrocardiogram with "dry" electrodes. *Ann. Biomed. Eng.* **1**(3):356–367.

Geddes, L. A., J. D. McCrady, H. E. Hoff, and A. Moore. 1964. Electrodes for large animals. *Southwest. Vet.* **18**:56–57.

Geddes, L. A., L. E. Baker, and A. G. Moore. 1969. Optimum electrolytic chloriding of silver electrodes. *Med. Biol. Eng.* **7**:49–56.

Geddes, L. A., C. P. Da Costa, and G. Wise. 1971. The impedance of stainless-steel electrodes. *Med. Biol. Eng.* **9**:511–521.

Geddes, L. A., J. D. Bourland, G. Wise, and R. Steinberg. 1973. Dry electrodes and holder for electro-oculography. *Med. Biol. Eng.* **11**:69–72.

Geddes, L. A., W. A. Tacker, W. Schoenlein, M. Minton, S. Grubbs, and P. Wilcox. 1976a. The prediction of the impedance of the thorax to defibrillating current. *Med. Instrum.* **10**(3):159–162.

Geddes, L. A., A. G. Moore, R. Baker, and R. Mack. 1976b. An easily applied and removed dry annular suction electrode. *J. Electrocardiol.* **9**(2):155–159.

Geddes, L. A., K. S. Foster, J. Reilly, W. D. Voorhees, J. D. Bourland, T. Ragheb, and N. E. Fearnot. 1988. The rectification properties of an electrode-electrolyte interface generated at high current density. IEEE Trans. Bio-Med. Eng. 1987, BME 34(9):669–672.

Gelfan, S. A. 1925. Non-polarizable microelectrode. *Proc. Soc. Exp. Biol. Med.* **23**:308–309.

Gesteland, R. C., B. Howland, J. Y. Lettvin, and W. H. Pitts. 1959. Comments on microelectrodes. *Proc. IRE* **47**:1856–1862.

Goldstein, A. G., W. Sloboda, and J. B. Jennings. 1962. Spontaneous electrical activity of three types of silver EEG electrodes. *Psychophysiol. Newsl.* **8**:10–16.

Gouy, M. 1910. Sur la constitution de la charge électrique à la surface d'un électrolyte. *J. Phys.* (*Paris*) **9**:457–468.

Graham, J., and R. W. Gerard. 1946. Membrane potentials and excitation of impaled single muscle fibers. *J. Cell. Comp. Physiol.* **28**:99–117.

Grahame, D. C. 1941. Properties of the electrical double layer at a mercury surface. *J. Am. Chem. Soc.* **63**:1207–1214.

Grahame, D. C. 1952. Mathematical theory of the faradic admittance. *J. Electrochem. Soc.* **99**:370C–385C.

Gray, J. A. G., and G. Svaetichin. 1951–1952. Electrical properties of platinum tipped microelectrodes. *Acta Physiol. Scand.* **24**:278–284.

Grayson, J. 1962. Silver silver-chloride electrode using optical silver chloride crystals. *J. Electrochem. Soc.* **109**:745–746.

Greenwald, D. U. 1936. Electrodes used in measuring electrodermal responses. *Am. J. Psychol.* **48**:658–662.

Grubbs, D. S. 1983. New technique for reducing the impedance of silver, silver-chloride electrodes. *Med. Biol. Eng. Comput.* **21**(2):232–234.

Grundfest, H. 1955. Instrument requirements and specifications in bioelectric recording. *Ann. N.Y. Acad. Sci.* **60**:841–859.

Grundfest, H., and B. Campbell. 1942. Origin, conduction and termination of impulses in dorsal spino-cerebellar tracts of cats. *J. Neurophysiol.* **5**:275–294.

Grundfest, H., R. W. Sengstaken, and W. H. Oettinger. 1950. Stainless steel microneedle made by electro-pointing. *Rev. Sci. Instrum.* **21**:360–361.

Guld, C. 1964. A glass-covered platinum microelectrode. *Med. Electron. Biol. Eng.* **2**:317–327.

Gunther-Schultze, A. 1929. *Electric Rectifiers and Valves* (translated by N. A. De Bruyne). John Wiley, New York, 212 pp.

Haggard, E. A., and R. Gerbrands. 1947. An apparatus for the measurement of continuous changes in palmar skin resistance. *J. Exp. Psychol.* **37**:92–98.

Helmholtz, H. 1879. Studien über electrische Grenzschichten. *Ann. Phys. (Leipzig)* (Ser. 3) **7**:337–382.

Hendler, E., and L. J. Santa Maria. 1961. Response of subjects to some conditions of a simulated orbital flight pattern. *Aerosp. Med.* **32**:126–133.

Hill, A. V. 1913. The rectification of alternating current by unequal or unequally dirty electrodes. *J. Physiol.* **46**:XVII–XVIII.

Hill, D. 1967. In Hales, Marey, and Chauveau, Report on 1966 course *Classical Physiology with Modern Instrumentation,* NIH Grant Rep. HE 05125.

Hodgkin, A. L., and A. F. Huxley. 1939. Action potentials recorded from inside a nerve fiber. *Nature* **144**:710–711.

Hoff, H. E., and L. A. Geddes. 1971. *Experimental Physiology,* 4th ed. Narco Bio-Systems, Houston, TX.

Hubel, D. H. 1957. Tungsten microelectrode for recording from single units. *Science* **125**:549–550.

Jaenicke, W., R. P. Tischer, and H. Gerischer. 1955. Die anodische Bildung von Silberchlorid Deck-schicten Umlagerungschicten nach ihrer kathodischen Reduktion zur Silber. *Z. Elektrochem.* **59**:448–455.

James, W. B., and H. B. Williams. 1910. The electrocardiogram in clinical medicine. *Am. J. Med. Sci.* **140**:408–421.

Janz, G. J., and D. J. C. Ives. 1968. Silver silver-chloride electrodes *Ann. N. Y. Acad. Sci.* **148**:210–221.

Janz, G. J., and F. J. Kelly. 1964. Reference electrodes. In *Encyclopedia of Electrochemistry.* C. A. Hampel (ed.). Reinhold, New York, 1206 pp.

Janz, G. J., and H. Taniguchi. 1953. The silver-silver halide electrodes. *Chem. Rev.* **53**:397–437.

Jaron, D., S. A. Briller, H. P. Schwan, and D. B. Geselowitz. 1969. Nonlinearity of cardiac pacemaker electrodes. *IEEE Trans. Biomed. Eng.* **BME-16**:132–138.

Jasper, H. H., and L. Carmichael. 1935. Electrical potentials from the intact human brain. *Science* **81**:51–53.

Jasper, H. H., R. T. Johnson, and L. A. Geddes. 1945. The RCAMC electromyograph. *Can. Army Med. Rep.* **C6174.**

Jenks, J. L., and A. Graybiel. 1935. A new simple method of avoiding high resistance and overshooting in taking standardized electrocardiograms. *Am. Heart J.* **10**:683–695.

Johnson, J. B., and J. E. Allred. 1968. *High Impedance Electrocardiogram Amplifier-transmitter for Use with Dry Electrodes,* Tech. Rept. SAM TR-68-55. School of Aerospace Medicine, Brooks AFB, TX.

Jolley, L. B. W. 1928. *Alternating Current Rectification and Allied Problems.* Wiley, New York.

Jones, G., and G. M. Bollinger. 1931. The measurement of the conductance of electrolytes. *J. Am. Chem. Soc.* **53**:411–451.

Jones, G., and G. M. Bollinger. 1935. The measurement of the conductance of electrolytes. VII. On platinization. *J. Am. Chem. Soc.* **57**:280–284.

Kado, R. T. 1965. Personal communication.

Kado, R. T., W. R. Adey, and J. R. Zweizig. 1964. Electrode system for recording EEG from physically active subjects. *Proc. Annu. Conf. Eng. Med. Biol.* **6**:1–129.

Kahn, A. 1964. Fundamentals of biopotentials and their measurement. Biomedical Sciences Instrumentation, 1964. (Dallas). *Am. J. Pharm. Educ.* **28**:805–814.

Kahn, A. 1965. Motion artifacts and streaming potentials in relation to biological electrodes. *Dig. 6th Int. Conf. Med. Biol. Eng.* pp. 562–563.

Kennard, D. W. 1958. Glass microcapillary electrodes. In *Electronic Apparatus for Biological Research.* P. E. K. Donaldson (ed.). Butterworth, London, Chap. 35.

Kohlrausch, F. 1897. Über platinirte Elektroden und Widerstandsbestimmung. *Ann. Phys. (Leipzig)* (Ser. 3) **60**:315–332.

Kohlrausch, F., and L. Holborn. 1898. *Das Leitvermogen der Elektrolyte.* Teubner, Leipzig, 211 pp.

Lagow, C. H., R. J. Sladek, and P. C. Richardson. 1971. Anodic insulated tantalum oxide electrocardiograph electrodes. *IEEE Trans. Biomed. Eng.* **BME-18**:162–164.

Lewes, D. 1965a. Electrode jelly in electrocardiography. *Br. Heart J.* **27**:105–115.

Lewes, D. 1965b. Multipoint electrocardiography without skin preparation. *Lancet* **2**:17–18.

Lewes, D., and D. Hill. 1966. Personal communication.

Lewis, T. 1914–1915. Polarisable as against non-polarisable electrodes. *J. Physiol.* **49**:l–lii.

Ling, G., and R. W. Gerard. 1949. The normal membrane potential of frog sartorius fibers. *J. Cell. Comp. Physiol.* **34**:383–396.

Livingston, L. G., and B. M. Duggar. 1934. Experimental procedures in a study of the location and concentration within the host cell of the virus of tobacco mosaic. *Biol. Bull. (Woods Hole, Mass.)* **67**:504–512.

Lopez, A., and P. Richardson. 1969. Capacitive electrocardiographic and bioelectric electrodes. *IEEE Trans. Biomed. Eng.* **BME-16**:99.

Lucchina, G. G., and C. G. Phipps. 1962. A vectorcardiographic lead system and physiologic electrode configuration for dynamic readout. *Aerosp. Med.* **33**:722–729.

Lucchina, G. G., and C. G. Phipps. 1963. An improved electrode for physiological recording. *Aerosp. Med.* **34**:230–231.

Lux, D. 1960. Microelectrodes of high stability. *EEG Clin. Neurophysiol.* **12**:928–929.

Lykken, D. T. 1959. Properties of electrodes used in electrodermal measurement. *J. Comp. Physiol. Psychol.* **52**:629–634.

MacInnes, D. A., and J. A. Beattie. 1920. The free energy of dilution. *J. Am. Chem. Soc.* **4**:1117–1128.

MacInnes, D. A. 1961. *The Principles of Electrochemistry.* Reinhold, New York; Dover, New York, 478 pp.

MacInnes, D. A., and K. Parker. 1915. Potassium chloride concentration cells. *J. Am. Chem. Soc.* **37**:1445–1461.

Marchant, E. W., and E. W. Jones. 1940. The effect of electrodes of different metals on the skin current. *Br. Heart J.* **2**:97–100.

Marmont, G. 1949. Studies on the axon membrane. *J. Cell. Comp. Physiol.* **34**:351–382.

Mason, R. E., and I. Likar. 1966. A new system of multiple lead electrocardiography. *Am. Heart J.* **71**:196–205.

Maxwell, J. 1957. Preparation of the skin for electrocardiography. *Br. Med. J.* **2**:942.

Maxwell, J. 1958. *Br. Med. J.* **1**:41.

Mills, L. W. 1962. A fast inexpensive method of producing large quantities of metallic microelectrodes. *EEG Clin. Neurop.* **14**:278–279.

Mooney, V., D. B. Hartman, and D. McNeal. 1974. The use of pure carbon for permanent percutaneous electrical connector systems. *Arch. Surg.* **108**:148–153.

Nastuk, W. L., and W. L. Hodgkin. 1950. The electrical activity of single muscle fibers. *J. Cell. Comp. Physiol.* **35**:39–73.

Nelson, J. A., L. C. Gagliano, and D. D. Clements. 1975. Current distribution at electrosurgical ground sites. *Proc. Annu. Conf. Exp. Med. Biol.* **17**:134.

O'Connell, D. N., B. Tursky, and M. T. Orne. 1960. Electrodes for recording skin potential. *Arch. Gen. Psychiatry* **3**:252–258.

Onaral, R., and H. P. Schwan. 1982. Linear and nonlinear properties of platinum electrode polarization. Part I. *Med. Biol. Eng. Comput.* **20**:299–306.

Onaral, R., and H. P. Schwan. 1983. Linear and nonlinear properties of platinum electrode polarization. Part II. *Med. Biol. Eng. Comput.* **21**:210–216.

Overmeyer, K. M., J. A. Pearce, and D. P. DeWitt. 1979. Measurement of temperature distributions at electrosurgical dispersive electrode sites. *Trans. ASME, J. Biomech. Eng.* **101**:66–72.

Pardee, H. E. B. 1917a. Concerning the electrodes used in electrocardiography. *Am. J. Physiol.* **44**:80–83.

Pardee, H. E. B. 1917b. An error in the electrocardiogram arising in the application of the electrodes. *Arch. Intern. Med.* **20**:161–166.

Parker, T. G. 1966. Personal communication. V. A. Hospital, Houston, TX.

Parsons, R. 1964. Electrode double layer. In *The Encyclopedia of Electrochemistry.* C. A. Hampel (ed.). Reinhold, New York, 1206 pp.

Patten, C. W., F. B. Ramme, and J. Roman. 1966. Dry electrodes for physiological monitoring. *NASA Tech. Note* **NASA TN D-3414**:1–32.

Ray, C. D. 1966. A new multipurpose human brain probe. *J. Neurosurg.* **24**:911–921.

Renshaw, B., A. Forbes, and B. R. Morison. 1940. Activity of isocortex and hippocampus. *J. Neurophysiol.* **3**:74–105.

Richardson, P. C. 1967a. The insulated electrode: A pasteless electrocardiographic technique. *Proc. Annu. Conf. Eng. Med. Biol.* **9**:15.7.

Richardson, P. C. 1967b. Progress in long-term physiologic sensor development. *Proc. San Diego Symp. Biomed. Eng.* **6**:39–44.

Richardson, P. C., and F. K. Coombs. 1968. New construction techniques for insulated electrocardiographic electrodes. *Proc. Annu. Conf. Eng. Med Biol.* **10**:13A.1.

Richardson, P. C., F. K. Coombs, and R. M. Adams. 1968. Some new electrode techniques for long-term physiologic monitoring. *Aerosp. Med.* **39**:745–750.

Robinson, D. A. 1968. Electrical properties of metal microelectrodes. *Proc. IEEE* **56**:1065–1071.

Robinson, F. R., and M. T. Johnson. 1961. *Histopathological Studies of Tissue Reactions to Various Metals Planted in Cat Brains,* ASD Tech. Rept. 61-397. USAF Wright-Patterson AFB, Ohio, 13 pp.

Robinson, R. A., and R. H. Stokes. 1959. In *Electrolyte Solutions,* 2nd ed. Academic Press, New York.

Roman, J. 1966. Flight research program. III. High impedance electrode techniques. *Aerosp. Med.* **37**:790–795.

Roman, J., and L. Lamb. 1962. Electrocardiography in flight. *Aerosp. Med.* **33**:527–544.

Roth, I. 1933–1934. A self-retaining skin contact electrode for chest leads in electrocardiography. *Am. Heart J.* **9**:526–529.

Rothschild, Lord. 1938. The polarization of a calomel electrode. *Proc. R. Soc. London, Ser. B* **125**:283–290.

Rowland, V. 1961. Simple non-polarizable electrode for chronic implantation. *EEG Clin. Neurophysiol.* **13**:290–291.

Rowley, D. A., S. Glasgov, and P. Stoner. 1961. Fluid electrodes for monitoring the electrocardiogram during activity and for prolonged periods of time. *Am. Heart J.* **62**:263–269.

Rylander, H. G. 1970a. Capacitive electrocardiograph electrodes. M. S. thesis, University of Texas, Austin.

Schmitt, O. H. M. Okajima, and M. Blaug. 1961. Skin preparation and electrocardiographic lead impedance. *Dig. IRE Int. Conf. Med. Electron.* 288 pp.

Schwan, H. P. 1963. Determination of biological impedances. In *Physical Techniques in Biological Research*, Vol. VI, Part B. W. Nastuk (ed.). Academic Press, New York, 425 pp.

Schwan, H. P. 1968. Electrode polarization impedance and measurements in biological materials. *Ann. N. Y. Acad. Sci.* **148**:191–209.

Schwan, H. P., and J. G. Maczuk. 1965. Electrode polarization impedance: limits of linearity. *Proc. Annu. Conf. Eng. Biol. Med.* **7**:1–270.

Scott, R. N. 1965. A method of inserting wire electrodes for electromyography. *IEEE Trans. Biomed. Eng.* **BME-12**:46–47.

Seelig, M. C. 1925. Localized gangrene following the hypodermic administration of calcium chloride. *JAMA* **84**:1413–1414.

Shackel, B. 1958. A rubber suction cup surface electrode with high electrical stability. *J. Appl. Physiol.* **13**:153–158.

Shackel, B. 1959. Skin drilling: A method for diminishing galvanic skin potentials. *Am. J. Physiol.* **72**:114–121.

Simons, D. G., W. Prather, and F. K. Coombs. 1965. *Personalized Telemetry Medical Monitoring and Performance Data-gathering for the 1962 SAMMATS Fatigue Study*, SAM-TR-65-17. USAF Brooks AFB, TX.

Skov, E. R., and D. G. Simons. 1965. *EEG Electrodes for In-flight Monitoring*, SAM-TR-65-18. USAF Brooks AFB, TX.

Smith, E. R., and J. K. Taylor. 1938. Reproducibility of the silver silver-chloride electrode. *J. Res. Natl. Bur. Stand.* **29**:837–847.

Stern, O. 1924. Zur Theorie der elektrolytischen Doppelschicht. *Z. Elektrochem.* **30**:508–516.

Sullivan, G. H., and G. Weltman. 1961. A low mass electrode for bioelectric recording. *J. Appl. Physiol.* **16**:939–940.

Sutter, von C. 1944. Ueber die Beeinflussung der Ekg-kurve durch elektrische Eigenschaften der Aufnahmeanordnung. *Cardiologia* **8**:246–262.

Svaetichin, G. 1951. Low resistance microelectrode. *Acta Physiol. Scand.* **24**:(Suppl. 86)pp. 1–13.

Tacker, W. A., L. DeGaravilla, C. F. Babbs, L. A. Geddes, and J. D. Bourland. 1982. Resistivity of blood to defibrillator-strength shocks. *Proc. 17th Annu. Meet. AAMI* p. 121.

Tacker, W. A., J. Mercer, P. Foley, and S. Cuppy. 1984. Resistivity of skeletal muscle skin, fat and lung. *Proc. 19th Annu. Meet. AAMI* p. 81.

Tam, H. W., and J. G. Webster. 1977. Minimizing electrode motion artifact by skin abrasion. *IEEE Trans. Biomed. Eng.* **BME-24**(1):134–139.

Taylor, C. V. 1925. Microelectrodes and micromagnets. *Proc. Soc. Exp. Biol. Med.* **23**:147–150.

Telemedics, Inc. 1961. *Med. Electron. News* **1**(4):9.

Thompson, N. P., and J. A. Patterson. 1958. *Solid Salt Bridge Contact Electrodes—System for Monitoring the ECG During Body Movement*, Tech. Rept. 58-453 (ASTIA Doc. AD215538).

Ungerleider, H. E. 1939. A new precordial electrode. *Am. Heart J.* **18**:94.

Warburg, E. 1899. Über das Verhalten sogenannter unpolarisierbarer Elektroden gegen Wechselstrom. *Ann. Phys. (Leipzig)* (Ser. 3) **67**:493–499.

Warburg, E. 1901. Über die Polarizationscapacität des Platins. *Ann. Phys. (Leipzig)* (Ser. 4) **6**:125–135.

Weale, R. A. 1951. A new micro-electrode for electrophysiological work. *Nature* **167**:529–530.

Wessale, J. L., J. D. Bourland, L. A. Geddes, and G. M. Ayers. 1987. Arcing threshold and electrode surface area for catheter electrical ablation. *Pace* **10:**427.

Wiley, J. D., and J. G. Webster. 1982. Analysis and control of current distribution under circular dispersive electrodes. *IEEE Trans. Biomed. Eng.* **BME-29:**381–389.

Winsbury, G. J. 1956. Machine for the fast production of microelectrodes. *Rev. Sci. Instrum.* **27:**514–516.

Wise, K. D., and J. B. Angell. 1969. An integrated circuit approach to extracellular microelectrodes. *Proc. 8th Int. Conf. Med. Biol. Eng., 1969* Paper No. 14-5.

Wise, K. D., and A. Starr. 1969. An integrated circuit approach to extracellular microelectrodes. *Proc. 8th Int. Conf. Med. Biol. Eng., 1969* Sect. 14-5.

Wolbarsht, M. L., E. F. MacNichol, and H. G. Wagner. 1960. Glass insulated platinum microelectrode. *Science* **132:**1309–1310.

Wolfe, A. M., and H. E. Reinhold. 1973. A flexible quick-application ECG electrode system. In *Biomedical Electrode Technology.* H. A. Miller and D. C. Harrison (eds.). Academic Press, New York, 447 pp.

Wolfson, R. N., and M. R. Neuman. 1969. Miniature Si-SiO$_2$ insulated electrodes based on semiconductor technology. *Proc. 8th Int. Conf. Med. Biol. Eng., 1969* Paper No. 14-6.

Woodbury, J. W., and A. J. Brady. 1956. Intracellular recording from moving tissues with a flexibly mounted ultramicroelectrode *Science* **123:**100–101.

Woodbury, L. A., J. W. Woodbury, and H. Hecht. 1950. Membrane and resting action potentials of single cardiac fibers. *Circulation* **1:**264–265.

Woodbury, L. A., H. Hecht, and A. R. Christopherson. 1951. Membrane resting and action potentials of single cardiac muscle fibers of the frog ventricle. *Am. J. Physiol.* **164:**307–318.

10

Stimulators and Stimulation

INTRODUCTION

A variety of physical and chemical agents can be used to stimulate excitable tissue; however, electrical stimuli are perhaps the most controllable. With this in mind, a stimulator may be defined as a device for producing pulses of current or voltage of controlled duration, intensity, and waveform. Single or multiple pulses are usually provided by a typical stimulator. This chapter will discuss stimulation and the various types of electrical stimulators, the basic concept of which is shown in Fig. 1.

A typical stimulator consists of a frequency-generating circuit, a waveform-generating circuit, and an output circuit. The frequency-generating circuit often allows the genesis of either single, manually initiated or repetitive pulses of controlled frequency. Occasionally a prestimulus pulse is provided to trigger an oscilloscope sweep before the stimulus is delivered. The waveform generator provides a pulse of predetermined waveform in response to each triggering pulse from the frequency-controlling circuit. Often the waveform-generating circuit can be triggered by an external frequency generator. Some sophisticated stimulators provide twin waveforms or a train of stimulus waveforms in response to a single triggering pulse; the separation between the waveforms is usually selectable.

It is the function of the output circuit to supply the current or voltage to the electrodes on the excitable tissue. The output circuit may provide a constant voltage or constant current to the tissue, irrespective of its resistance. The properties of these circuits are discussed elsewhere in this chapter.

STIMULATION

An effective stimulus is an environmental change that produces a characteristic and reversible response in a tissue. The response occurs after initiation of the stimulus and usually outlasts it.

Empirical Strength–Duration Curve

The factors that underlie stimulation of an excitable tissue were determined empirically; however, it is now possible to derive the law of excitation analytically,

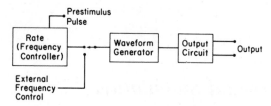

Figure 1   Components of a stimulator.

as will be done subsequently. Lapicque (1909), using capacitor-discharge stimuli, discovered that the current I required to excite a variety of irritable tissues increased as the duration d decreased. He proposed the following expression for the current:

$$I = k/d + b, \tag{1}$$

where k is a constant and d is the duration of the current pulse (i.e., in his studies, the time constant of the current pulse). The quantity b is the current for stimulation with a pulse of infinitely long duration and is known as the rheobase; b depends on electrode size and location with respect to the excitable tissue. Note that b is duration-independent.

Lapicque (1926) defined a point on the strength–duration curve that identifies the duration for a pulse of twice rheobasic intensity; this duration is called the chronaxie (c); Fig. 2a illustrates this concept. He found that the chronaxie is specific for each type of tissue; it is about 3 msec for (denervated) skeletal muscle and about 0.1 msec for mammalian motor nerve. Figure 2b is a log–log plot of the strength–duration curves for various excitable tissues reported by Lapicque (1926). Note that it is the chronaxie that identifies how the current required rises above the rheobase with decreasing stimulus duration. Lapicque pointed out that the chronaxie for a rapidly responding tissue (frog gastrocnemius muscle) is shorter than that for a slowly responding tissue (*Spirogyra*, a blue-green alga). Table 1 presents typical chronaxie values.

The Lapicque strength–duration curve for current $(I = b + k/d)$ can be re-written in terms of the chronaxie by putting $I = 2b$ and $d = c$. Performing this substitution yields $k = bc$, which when placed into the Lapicque expression yields

$$I = b(1 + c/d). \tag{2}$$

This expression illustrates that c, the tissue-dependent property, determines the manner in which the current required for stimulation increases as the duration d is decreased.

The Lapicque strength–duration curve for current can be plotted in normalized form by expressing duration as d/c. Figure 3 presents this relationship, which constitutes a universal strength–duration curve.

Before Lapicque investigated the current strength–duration curve, Weiss (1901),

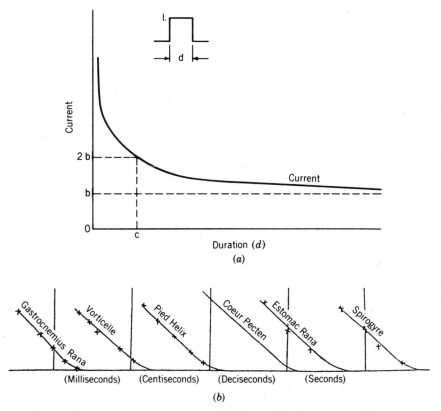

Figure 2 (*a*) The Lapicque strength–duration curve illustrating the concept of chronaxie *c*. (*b*) A log–log plot of the strength–duration curves for different excitable tissues as presented by Lapicque in 1926.

using constant-current rectangular pulses, discovered that the charge–duration relationship was linear. For a rectangular pulse, charge Q is the product of current and duration. For other waveforms, charge is the area under the current pulse. Weiss showed that

$$Q = k + bd. \tag{3}$$

Parenthetically, it should be noted that the slope of the charge–duration line is b, the rheobase. In addition, dividing the Weiss charge–duration expression by d provides the Lapicque strength–duration curve for current.

The Weiss charge–duration expression can be written in terms of chronaxie c as

$$Q = Id = b(d + c). \tag{4}$$

TABLE 1   Chronaxie Values

Tissue Type	Chronaxie (msec)	Temp. (°C)	Reference
Nerve			
Human (motor)	0.01[a]	Body	Ritchie (1944)
Cat A fiber (saphenous)	0.02[a]	29.5	Li and Bak (1976)
Cat C fiber (saphenous)	1.8	29.5	Li and Bak (1976)
	0.80[b]	27.5	Koslow et al. (1973)
	0.66[b]	37	Koslow et al. (1973)
Human (motor)	0.08–0.6	Body	Adrian (1919)
Pain			
Human (skin receptors)	0.8	Body	Notermans (1966)
Human (glans penis)	0.25	Body	Adrian (1919)
Sensation			
Human (skin sensation)	0.35	Body	Ayers et al. (1986)
Human (sensory nerve)	0.12–0.3	Body	Adrian (1919)
Skeletal muscle			
Human (denervated)	3[b]	Body	Ritchie (1944)
Cardiac muscle			
Dog (ventricle)	1.5	Body	Pearce et al. (1982)
Sheep (purkinje)	4.0	37	Fozzard and Schoenberg (1972)
	3.0	37	Dominguez and Fozzard (1970)
Turtle (ventricle)	10	Room	Pearce et al. (1982)
Smooth muscle			
Frog (stomach)	100	Ambient	Brazier (1951)

[a]Recent studies provide larger values.
[b]Estimate.

The linear form of normalized charge–duration line is presented in Fig. 3a. Note that its slope is b and its intercept is bc. Therefore, the ratio of the intercept to the slope is the chronaxie, c.

It follows that the energy U for a rectangular current pulse is the square of the current multiplied by the duration and the resistance r through which the current flows:

$$U = I^2\,rd = b^2 rd \left(1 + \frac{c}{d}\right)^2. \qquad (5)$$

The normalized energy–duration curve is also presented in Fig. 3. It is interesting to observe that the duration for minimum energy is equal to the chronaxie, c, a fact not recognized by Lapicque.

The Weiss–Lapicque strength–duration relationships provide a reasonably good fit for experimentally obtained data and identify the important factors that underlie stimulation. Irnich (1980) found that the chronaxie values for cardiac muscle obtained with small pacing electrodes of different areas are not the same. How this arises is not explained. However, it is important to recall that the current density

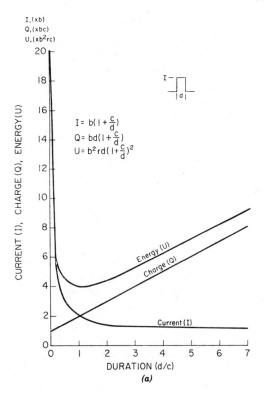

(a)

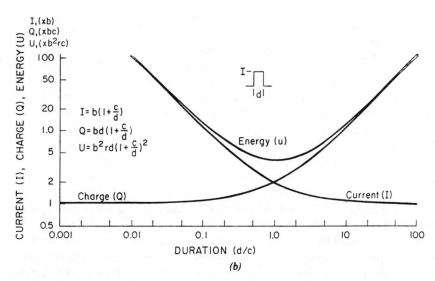

(b)

Figure 3 The normalized empirical (Weiss–Lapicque) strength–duration curves for current, charge, and energy, expressing duration in terms of chronaxie *c*. (*a*) Linear form; (*b*) log–log form.

under typical stimulating electrodes is not uniform; therefore it is difficult to compare thresholds on the basis of average current density (milliamperes per unit electrode area). Whether or not nonuniform current density plays a part in the determination of chronaxie with macroelectrodes has not been investigated.

Analytical Strength–Duration Curve

It is possible to derive the strength–duration curve for the current from the basic components of the cell membrane, i.e., its capacitance C and resistance R. Such an analytical derivation will now be presented. However, it is important to note that the resulting expression derives from equating the cell membrane to a single RC circuit, which is an oversimplification. This information was used by Blair (1932), Plonsey (1969), and Pearce et al. (1982) to derive the strength–duration curve.

Since excitable tissues are enclosed by a charged dielectric membrane, the following derivation for the properties of a stimulus is applicable to a wide variety of excitable cells. Figure 4a illustrates a segment of the surface of the membrane of an excitable cell, such as muscle or nerve. Metabolic activity maintains ionic gradients across the membrane, resulting in a high concentration of potassium (K^+) ions inside the cell and a high concentration of sodium (Na^+) ions in the medium bathing the cell; there are lesser gradients for other ions. The net result of the ionic gradient is a transmembrane potential that is largely dependent on the potassium ion gradient. In many cells, the resting membrane potential (RMP) is slightly less than 100 mV (E_m), with the outside being positive with respect to the inside.

To stimulate an excitable cell, it is only necessary to reduce the transmembrane potential by a critical amount. A reduction in transmembrane potential can be achieved by placing the negative (cathode) stimulating electrode on or near the cell surface. The other stimulating electrode (anode), is made large and is usually placed at a distance from the small-area (active) electrode. The large-area electrode is called the indifferent, reference, or dispersive electrode. Current delivered to the active electrode will reduce the transmembrane potential by an amount that depends on the current intensity I. With an adequate intensity, the membrane potential will be reduced by an amount ΔV, reaching the critical or threshold potential (TP); Figure 4b illustrates this concept. When the threshold potential (TP) is reached, a regenerative process takes place: sodium ions enter the cell, potassium ions exit the cell, and the transmembrane potential falls to zero (depolarizes), reverses slightly, and then recovers or repolarizes to the resting membrane potential (RMP). Thus, to stimulate, it is only necessary to reduce the transmembrane potential slightly, usually by about one-third.

For a stimulus to be effective in producing an excitation, it must have an abrupt onset, be intense enough, and last long enough. These facts can be drawn together by considering the delivery of a suddenly rising cathodal constant-current stimulus of duration d to the cell membrane as shown in Fig. 4b.

It is now well established that cell membranes can be reasonably well represented by a capacitance C, shunted by a resistance R (Fig. 4c); the product RC is the

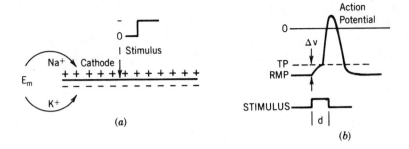

(a)

(b)

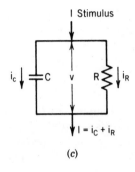

(c)

$$I = i_C + i_R = C\frac{dV}{dt} + \frac{V}{R}.$$

Integrating,

$$V = IR(1 - e^{-t/RC}) = IR(1 - e^{-t/\tau}),$$

where $\tau = RC$, the membrane time constant.

Let Δv be the change in RMP required to stimulate. Then

$$\Delta v = IR(1 - e^{-t/\tau}).$$

When $t = d = \infty$, $I = \Delta v/R = b$ = rheobase. Therefore,

$$I = b/(1 - e^{-d/\tau}).$$

Figure 4   The mechanism of stimulation of excitable tissue. (a) Typical membrane. (b) TP, threshold potential; RMP, resting membrane potential; d, duration. (c) Membrane equivalent circuit.

membrane time constant τ. The stimulating current I will divide between the membrane resistor R and capacitor C, as shown in Fig. 4c. Integration of the differential equation yields the following expression for the current I:

$$I = \frac{V}{R(1 - e^{-t/\tau})},$$ (6a)

where V is the stimulus voltage, R is the membrane resistance, and τ is the membrane time constant (RC).

Now let the threshold current intensity (I) required to reduce the transmembrane potential by an amount ΔV that is needed to excite the cell; therefore,

$$I = \frac{\Delta V}{R(1 - e^{-t/\tau})}. \tag{6b}$$

Letting the duration of the stimulus be infinite, the stimulus current required will be $\Delta V/R$; this current value is the rheobase and is usually assigned the symbol b. Entering this information and putting d equal to the stimulus duration, the expression for the current strength–duration curve becomes

$$I = \frac{b}{1 - e^{-d/\tau}}, \tag{7}$$

where d is the duration of the stimulus and b is the rheobasic current, i.e., the threshold current for a stimulus of infinitely long duration; τ is the membrane time constant, which is dependent on the type of cell.

A log–log plot of the strength–duration curve for current I is shown in Fig. 5 for various values of the membrane time constant τ. Note that as the duration d becomes shorter, the intensity of the current required for stimulation is increased for all membrane time constants. With this exponential form of the strength–duration curve, it is the cell membrane time constant τ that defines the duration where

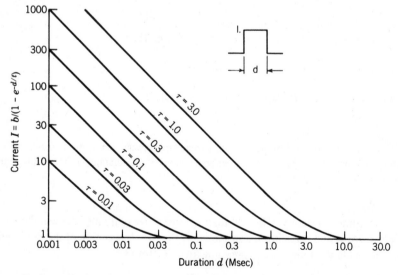

Figure 5 Strength–duration (d) curves for current (I) for excitable tissues with different membrane time constants (τ).

the current required starts to increase as the duration decreases. Observe also that the manner in which the current rises with decreasing duration is similar for all tissues. Table 2 presents typical values for membrane time constants. Ranck (1975) presented a discussion on the time constants of neural tissues. It should be noted that the time constant derived from the strength–duration curve is different from the passive value.

Charge Q and energy U are two other electrical quantities used to describe a stimulus. For a rectangular current pulse, charge Q is the product of current I and duration d:

$$Q = Id = \frac{bd}{1 - e^{-d/\tau}}. \tag{8}$$

Figure 6 illustrates the relationship between charge and duration, normalized in terms of d/τ. Also shown in Fig. 6 is the normalized strength–duration curve for current.

For a rectangular current pulse, energy U is the square of the current I multiplied by the resistance r through which the current flows and the duration d of the

TABLE 2   Membrane Time Constants

Tissue Type	Time Constant (msec)	Temp. (°C)	Investigator and Year
Nerve			
Human (motor)	0.015[a]	Body	Ritchie (1944)
Cat (A fiber)	0.022	29.5	Li and Bak (1976)
Cat (C fiber)	3.1	29.5	Li and Bak (1976)
Cat (C fibers)	0.80[b]	37	Koslow et al. (1973)
Cat (C fibers)	0.85[b]	27.5	Koslow et al. (1973)
Pain fibers			
Human (skin receptors)	1.0	Body	Notermans (1966)
Human (glans penis)	0.28	Body	Adrian (1919)
Sensory receptors			
Human (skin)	0.33	Body	Ayers et al. (1987)
Human (sensory nerve)	0.12–0.36	Body	Adrian (1919)
Skeletal muscle			
Human (denervated)	2[b]	Body	Ritchie (1944)
Cardiac muscle			
Dog (ventricle)	2.2[c]	37	Geddes et al. (1987)
Dog (ventricle)	13.2[c]	25	Geddes et al. (1987)
Dog (ventricle)	2.14 (± 0.97)	37	Pearce et al. (1982)
Sheep (purkinje)	4.3	37	Dominguez and Fozzard (1970)
Sheep (purkinje)	3.75	37	Fozzard and Schoenberg (1972)
Turtle (ventricle)	7.3 (±2.22)	Room	Pearce et al. (1982)

[a]Recent studies provide larger values.
[b]Estimate.
[c]Same animal.

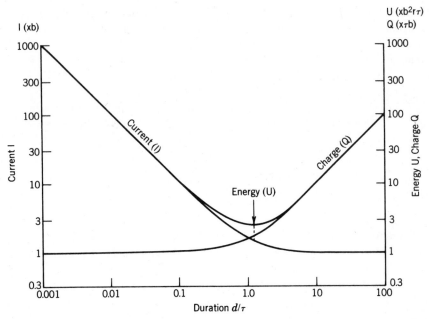

Figure 6 Strength–duration curves for current I, charge Q, and energy U versus normalized duration d divided by τ, the membrane time constant.

stimulus:

$$U = I^2rd = rd \left(\frac{b}{1 - e^{-d/\tau}} \right)^2 . \qquad (9)$$

The strength–duration curve for energy is also plotted in Fig. 6, normalized for duration terms of d/τ.

Observe in Fig. 6 that the three electrical quantities current, charge, and energy are quite different, there being no single duration for a minimum for all three. Minimum current occurs with an infinitely long duration (rheobasic) stimulus.

The tables that list chronaxie values (Table 1) and membrane time constants (Table 2) show some differences for the same excitable tissue. In many instances the temperature was not specified by the various investigators, and it is known that both chronaxie values and membrane time constants depend on temperature. Although there is little published information on this point, Geddes and Bourland (1985), investigated the relationship between cardiac muscle membrane time constant and temperature. They first measured the membrane time constant for canine ventricles at 37°C, finding a value of 2.2 msec. The animal was cooled to a body temperature of 23°C, and the membrane time constant was found to be 12.97 msec. The temperature coefficient is therefore −5.9% per degree Celsius. It is expected that the other chronaxie values would have a similar temperature coefficient.

Comparison of Empirical and Analytically Derived Strength–Duration Curves

Comparison of the Weiss–Lapicque (empirically derived) and the analytically derived (exponential) strength–duration curves reveals many interesting similarities. For example, the long-duration current asymptote b, i.e., the rheobase, is the same for both. Also, the current increases with decreasing duration for both. The energy minimum for the empirical strength–duration curve occurs with a duration equal to the chronaxie c. For the analytically derived curve, the time constant τ corresponds to the duration for $I/b = 1.59$. The energy minimum occurs when the duration is 1.255τ. The short-duration charge asymptote for the empirically derived strength–duration curve is bc; for the analytically derived curve, it is τb. These relationships indicate that the chronaxie c is an analog of the membrane time constant τ; both describe the excitability characteristic of tissues. However, it is not legitimate to equate c and τ.

One method of comparing the Weiss–Lapicque curves and the analytically derived curves is to examine the situation where $I = 2b$; at this point the duration is equal to the chronaxie. Putting $d = c$ into the analytically derived expression for the current, $I = 2b$, and solving for c in terms of τ provides the alternative relationships

$$c = 0.693\tau, \tag{10}$$

$$\tau = 1.443c. \tag{11}$$

Using this fact it is possible to compare the Weiss–Lapicque and analytically derived curves for current, energy, and charge in a single illustration in which duration is normalized in terms of d/τ. Figure 7 makes this comparison. Table 3 presents

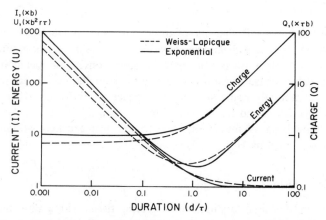

Figure 7 Comparison of the normalized Weiss–Lapicque and analytically derived strength–duration curves, based on solving for τ in terms of c for the point where $I = 2b$.

TABLE 3   Summary of Strength–Duration Data

Item	Weiss–Lapicque	Exponential
Current I	$I = b(1 + c/d)$	$I = b/(1 - e^{-d/\tau})$
b = rheobase	c = chronaxie	τ = membrane time constant
Duration d	When $I = 2b$, $d = c$	When $I = 1.59b$, $d = \tau$
Charge Q	$Q = Id = bd(1 + c/d)$	$Q = bd/(1 - e^{-d/\tau})$
Duration for min Q	$d \ll c$, $Q_{min} = bc$	$d \ll \tau$, $Q_{min} = \tau b$
Energy U	$U = b^2rd(1 + c/d)^2$	$U = b^2rd/(1 - d^{-d/\tau})^2$
r = resistance		
Duration for min U	c	1.255τ
Minimum energy	$U_{min} = 4b^2rc$	$U_{min} = 2.45b^2r\tau$

a summary of the important quantities described by the Weiss–Lapicque and analytically derived strength–duration curves for rectangular pulses.

At this time, it is not known which expression best fits experimentally obtained
data. To date, only one comparison (Ayers et al., 1986) has been made in which
data for skin sensation have been fitted to both the empirical and exponential
strength–duration curves for current. The result was that the correlation coefficients
were quite similar in both cases. A slightly better fit was obtained for the expression

$$I = b \left(1 + \frac{c}{d^\alpha} \right), \tag{12}$$

where α is a constant. Much remains to be done to identify the best expression for
the strength–duration curve.

Accommodation

It was stated previously that one of the requirements for an effective stimulus
is an abrupt onset. It is well known, however, that a slowly rising stimulus can
excite tissue. If a stimulus does not have an abrupt onset, the metabolic activity
of the tissue can increase its threshold during the stimulus, which has to be more
intense than an abruptly rising stimulus to produce an excitation. This process is
called accommodation and has its own time constant. In practice, the threshold
increase, although easily measured, is not large. An excellent account of this
subject was presented by Hill (1935).

Stimulation of Deep-Lying Tissue

It is frequently desired to stimulate deep-lying tissue with a skin-surface electrode while at the same time minimizing stimulation of the overlying tissues. Between the surface electrode and the deep-lying target tissue there may be sensory

receptors; motor, sensory, and autonomic nerves; and skeletal muscle through which the stimulating current must flow. Analysis of a simple two-tissue model will provide guidance in the selection of the optimum electrode location and stimulus duration.

Figure 8 is a sketch showing an active electrode (cathode) over excitable tissue having a membrane time constant τ_1, overlying excitable tissue with a membrane time constant τ_2 that is to be stimulated. It is assumed that the indifferent (anode) electrode is large and distant. The rheobasic currents for stimulating the two types of tissue will, of course, be different; that for the superficial tissue (b_1) will be less than that for the deep-lying tissue (b_2), because the former is closer to the surface electrode than the latter. The current I_1 required to stimulate the superficial tissue with a membrane time constant τ_1 is

$$I_1 = \frac{b_1}{1 - e^{-d/\tau_1}}.\tag{13}$$

The current I_2 required to stimulate the deep-lying tissue with a membrane time constant τ_2 is

$$I_2 = \frac{b_2}{1 - e^{-d/\tau_2}}.\tag{14}$$

It is obviously desirable to choose stimulus parameters that result in a minimum for the ratio I_2/I_1, which can be expressed as

$$\frac{I_2}{I_1} = \frac{b_2(1 - e^{-d/\tau_1})}{b_1(1 - e^{-d/\tau_2})}.\tag{15}$$

The first step in choosing stimulus parameters is to consider stimulation with a stimulus of infinitely long duration, in which case

$$\frac{I_2}{I_1} = \frac{b_2}{b_1}.\tag{16}$$

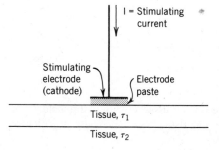

Figure 8 Stimulation of deep-lying tissue having a membrane time constant τ_2, over which lies another excitable tissue having a membrane time constant τ_1.

It is obvious that the only method available for making b_2/b_1 a minimum is to locate the active electrode so that stimulation of the deep-lying target tissue is achieved with the least rheobasic current b_2. Thus the first step in optimizing stimulation of a deep-lying target tissue is to choose the site for the skin-surface electrode to achieve stimulation with the lowest rheobasic current.

The ratio I_2/I_1 depends on stimulus duration d, as well as the two membrane time constants τ_1 and τ_2. Choice of the optimum duration depends on the ratio of the two time constants. Two cases can be selected to illustrate that the optimum duration depends on whether τ_2 is larger or smaller than τ_1.

Case 1: τ_2 Larger Than τ_1. It is desired to pace the cardiac ventricles with the least sensation using a skin-surface electrode over the apex-beat area, the site where b_2 is minimum (Geddes et al., 1984). The time constant for cardiac muscle (τ_2) is about 2 msec (Pearce et al., 1982), and that for sensory receptors (τ_1) is about 0.5 msec. Therefore,

$$\frac{I_2}{I_1} = \frac{b_2(1 - e^{-d/0.5})}{b_1(1 - e^{-d/2})}. \tag{17}$$

Figure 9a is a plot of the ratio of pacing current I_2 to sensation current I_1 versus stimulus duration d. Note that the ratio decreases with increasing duration. There-

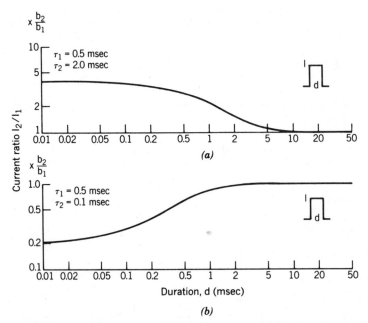

Figure 9 Ratio of threshold current I_2 for deep-lying tissue to current threshold I_1 for overlying tissue for stimulation when the deep-lying tissue has a time constant (a) longer and (b) shorter than that of the overlying tissues.

fore for minimum sensation, the optimum duration would be 10 msec or longer. This duration is presently used in closed-chest cardiac pacers. Thus, when τ_2 is larger than τ_1, a long-duration stimulus is optimum to minimize stimulating tissue 1.

Case 2: τ_2 Less Than τ_1. It is desired to stimulate a subcutaneous nerve with the least skin sensation using a skin-surface (cathode) electrode placed over the site for the minimum rheobasic current b_2. Using membrane time constants of about 0.1 sec for the subcutaneous nerve and 0.5 msec for the superficial receptors, the current ratio becomes

$$\frac{I_2}{I_1} = \frac{b_2(1 - e^{-d/0.5})}{b_1(1 - e^{-d/0.1})}. \tag{18}$$

Figure 9b is a plot of the ratio of the nerve-stimulating current to sensation current versus stimulus duration. Note that the ratio is a minimum for durations shorter than 0.02 msec. This fact is in agreement with the present use of skin-surface electrodes in physical therapy and a stimulus duration less than 50 μsec to stimulate large motor nerves with minimum skin sensation.

Summary. Several important generalizations derive from the foregoing analysis of a two-tissue model. For example, the skin-surface electrode should be placed so that minimum current is required to excite the deep-lying tissue. If the membrane time constant of the target deep-lying tissue is longer than that of the overlying tissue, a long-duration stimulus is optimal. If the membrane time constant of the deep-lying target tissue is shorter than that of the overlying tissue, a short-duration stimulus is optimal. In the latter case, the current ratio I_2/I_1 for a very short duration stimulus is asymptotic to $b_2\tau_2/b_1\tau_1$.

Waveform Considerations

Weiss used single rectangular (square) current pulses (Fig. 10A) to derive the linear relation between charge and pulse duration. Lapicque used single capacitor discharge current pulses (Fig. 10B) to create his hyperbolic strength–duration curve for current, expressing the stimulus strength in terms of peak current I_i, and the duration d was the time constant of the discharge circuit; he later used single rectangular pulses and obtained the same form for the strength–duration curve. The time constant for a capacitor discharge pulse is the time for the current to fall from its peak value I_i to $0.37I_i$.

In a variety of devices, such as cardiac pacemakers, nerve and muscle stimulators, and ventricular defibrillators, the truncated exponential (trapezoidal) wave (Fig. 10C) is used. The term tilt T is usually employed to describe the truncated exponential wave, tilt being defined as the fractional decrease in the current during the pulse: $T = (I_i - I_f)/I_i$, where I_i and I_f are the initial and final values of the current, respectively. Percent tilt is numerically equal to $100T$.

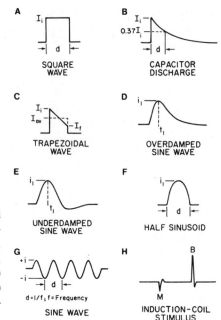

Figure 10 Typical current waveforms used for stimulating excitable tissue. (*A*) Rectangular (square) wave, (*B*) capacitor discharge, (*C*) trapezoidal (truncated exponential) wave, (*D*) critically or overdamped sine wave, (*E*) underdamped sine wave, (*F*) half-sinusoid, (*G*) sinusoidal alternating current, and (*H*) induction-coil stimulus; M, make; B, break.

Critically and overdamped (Fig. 10*D*) or slightly underdamped (Fig. 10*E*) sine waves are used for ventricular defibrillation and tissue stimulation, the latter delivered by the inductorium (induction-coil) stimulator. In the case of critically or overdamped pulses, the current decays to zero without reversal of direction. Because of this, the effective duration *d* is often taken as the time from the onset of current to the point where the current has fallen to 5% of peak I_i. Occasionally a half (rectified) sine wave (Fig. 10*F*) is used for stimulation; such a wave is usually repeated with an interval equal to the duration *d*, which is equal to the reciprocal of twice the frequency ($d = 1/2f$). Similarly, sinusoidal current (Fig. 10*G*) (often derived from the power line), is used in inexpensive stimulators. The current waveform from the inductorium is shown in Fig. 10*H*; *M* identifies the make shock, and *B* identifies the break shock.

In view of the multiplicity of waveforms that can stimulate, there naturally arises an interest in determining how the different waveforms conform to the strength–duration curve. It turns out that if single rectangular, trapezoidal, half sinusoid, and critically damped or overdamped sine waveforms are used to stimulate the same excitable tissue with the same electrodes, the plots of charge versus duration describe straight lines are almost superimposed (Bourland et al., 1978; Geddes and Bourland, 1985). Charge is the area under the current pulse; it is also the average current multiplied by the duration. Thus, it would appear that for at least these waveforms, the critical factor in achieving stimulation is the attainment of a critical average current for a given duration of stimulus pulse. For the rectangular wave, the average current is the peak current, since it is the same during the pulse. For the capacitor discharge, the charge is the capacitance multiplied by the initial voltage, which is equal to the product of initial current and resistance of the circuit. For the truncated exponential wave, the average current (I_{av}) is

$$I_{av} = \frac{TI_i}{\ln[1/(1 - T)]},\qquad(19)$$

where T is the tilt (fractional decrease in current during the pulse), and I_i is the initial current. The average current for the damped sine wave depends on the degree of damping; values ranging from 0.2 to 0.4 of the peak current are typical.

From the foregoing, the strength–duration curve is probably best represented in terms of average current, i.e.,

$$I_{av} = b(1 + c/d)\qquad(20)$$

$$I_{av} = b/(1 - e^{-d/\tau}),\qquad(21)$$

where I_{av} = the average current during the pulse of duration d,
$\phantom{where I_{av}}$ b = the rheobase (the threshold for an infinitely long duration pulse),
$\phantom{where I_{av}}$ τ = the membrane time constant, and
$\phantom{where I_{av}}$ c = the chronaxie of the tissue being stimulated.

Thus for a given tissue and an abruptly rising current pulse, the strength–duration curves for average current should be similar for many different waveforms. However, such comparisons have not been carried out.

Monopolar and Bipolar Stimulation

A stimulus is applied to excitable tissue to produce depolarization; therefore, the cathode is the active electrode and the anode is the reference electrode. In many instances, stimulation is accomplished with the monopolar technique, which consists in making the active electrode (cathode) small in area and local, with the reference electrode (anode) large and usually distant from the stimulating site. It is the high current density that produces stimulation under the active electrode. The low current density under the reference electrode prevents stimulation at this site. Sometimes, however, bipolar stimulation is used with identical electrodes. Then both stimulating electrodes are on, or near, the excitable tissue. Although the current densities are the same under both electrodes, at threshold, stimulation occurs under the negative (cathode) electrode.

An important subtlety arises regarding stimulation with other than a small-area (point) electrode. As discussed in Chapter 9, the current density distribution under skin-surface electrodes and around typical subcutaneous electrodes is not uniform. Stimulation will occur at the electrode site where the cathodal current density is the highest. It is for this reason that it is inappropriate in a typical case to standardize stimulation in terms of average current density.

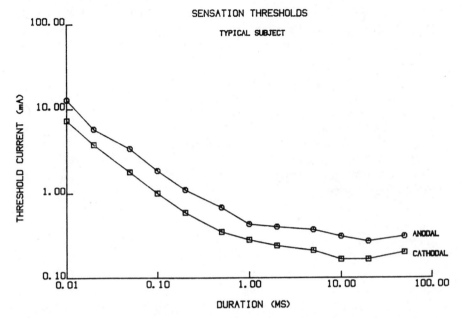

Figure 11   Threshold for sensation on the forearm using a 5-mm-diameter electrode (paired with a large indifferent electrode) for cathodal and anodal current. (Courtesy of J. L. Wessale.)

Cathodal and Anodal Stimulation

Because excitation requires local hypopolarization of the positively charged external membrane of a cell, it is obvious that the active (small-area) electrode nearest the cell should be made the negative electrode (cathode) with respect to the (large-area) dispersive anode. If the active electrode is made positive (the anode), the stimulus will hyperpolarize the region of the cell closest to it. However, the side of the cell facing the dispersive electrode sees the cathode and will be hypopolarized. Because it is local current density that stimulates, and because the cathode is slightly farther from the active electrode, the current density will be slightly less. Therefore, to achieve excitation, the current intensity must be increased. Consequently, the threshold for stimulation with extracellular electrodes will be slightly higher for anodal current than for cathodal current. Figure 11 makes this point.

Stimulation with Repetitive Pulses

The foregoing discussion of excitation and the strength–duration curve dealt with a single stimulus. To understand the response to repetitive stimuli, it is necessary to recognize the role of the refractory period—that period during excitation and early recovery during which a cell cannot be excited. As shown in Fig. 4b, the delivery of a threshold stimulus results in a response, i.e., an action potential, the time course of which depends on the type of cell stimulated.

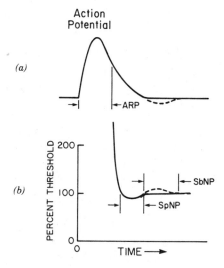

(a)

(b)

Figure 12 (*a*) Action potential; (*b*) excitability during the action potential. During the upstroke and early downstroke of the action potential, the cell is completely unexcitable; this period is called the absolute refractory period (ARP). After the ARP, the cell regains its excitability, first to a suprathreshold stimulus and then to a subthreshold stimulus. The period of increased excitability is called the supernormal period (SpNP), and that of decreased excitability, due to a positive after-potential if present (dashed curve), is called the subnormal period (SbNP).

Figure 12*a* illustrates a typical action potential evoked by a single threshold stimulus. During depolarization and during early repolarization, and well beyond the peak of the action potential, the cell is incapable of being excited; i.e., it is refractory. Only during the descending limb of the action potential has the membrane potential recovered adequately to permit excitation. In this recovery phase, after the absolute refractory (inexcitable) period, the cell becomes responsive, first to a suprathreshold stimulus then to a subthreshold stimulus and finally to a threshold stimulus, Thus, there is a cyclic recovery of excitability following the absolute refractory period. (See Fig. 12*b*.) The end of the absolute refractory period (ARP) is marked by the time when the cell will respond to a very strong stimulus. After the end of the ARP, the stimulus intensity required for excitation decreases. Beyond this point, and to the point of restoration of the full resting membrane potential (RMP), the cell is excitable with a subthreshold stimulus. This feature identifies the supernormal period (SpNP). Figure 12*b* illustrates the current required for excitation during the various phases of recovery. Such a curve is called a strength–interval curve.

From the foregoing it is obvious that the capability of a cell to be restimulated depends on the duration of its action potential and refractory period. Thus, if the stimuli have a frequency that is higher than the reciprocal of the absolute refractory period, the cell will not be excited by each pulse in the train of stimuli. This is illustrated in Fig. 13 for a sinusoidal alternating current as the stimulus.

Stimulation with Sinusoidal Current

It is well recognized that sinusoidal alternating current can be perceived when applied to skin-surface electrodes. Using the concpet that such current can be viewed as a train of short-duration pulses, the strength–duration curve predicts that the current required for stimulation should rise with increasing frequency. The

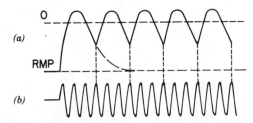

Figure 13 (*a*) Action potentials initiated by (*b*) a sinusoidal stimulus having a period (1/frequency) shorter than the absolute refractory period of a cell. Note that the cell responded to the first sinusoid at an intensity less than the peak. For the pulses that followed, the responses occurred with higher intensity. In this case, the number of action potentials is less than the number of stimuli.

refractory period dictates that if the stimulating pulses have a period shorter than the refractory period of the excitable tissue, only a submultiple number of pulses will produce excitation that will still be perceived, even with a high-frequency sinusoidal current, provided the intensity is sufficient. To examine these concepts, the threshold for sensation was first determined using single rectangular cathodal and anodal stimuli applied to skin-surface electrodes; the result is shown in Fig. 14. Using the same electrodes on the same subject, the sensation threshold was determined for sinusoidal current over a wide frequency range. The threshold current was plotted versus the reciprocal of frequency ($d = 1/f$; see Fig. 14). Thus, the concept of viewing sinusoidal current as a train of pulses of duration equal to the period ($1/f$) seems valid, at least over a limited frequency range.

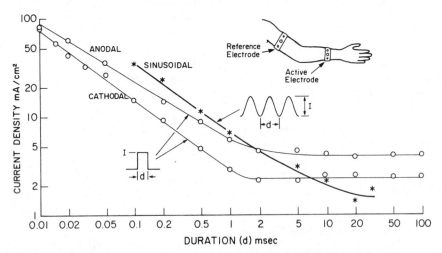

Figure 14 Threshold current *I* for sensation for single rectangular anodal and cathodal pulses of different durations and sensation threshold for sinusoidal current, expressing duration *d* as the reciprocal of frequency.

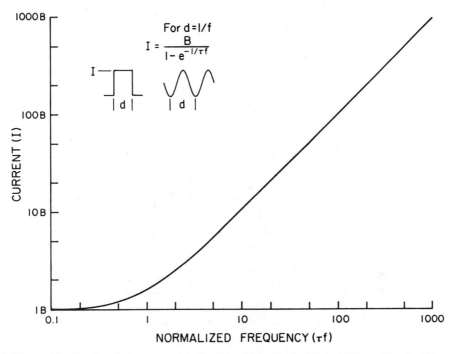

Figure 15 Current–frequency curve for sinusoidal stimulation based on pulse duration being equivalent to the period $(1/f)$; τ is the membrane time constant.

For sinusoidal current, it is more traditional to plot the current required for stimulation versus frequency. If the effective duration d of such current is equated to the period $1/f$, then it would be expected that the strength–frequency curve would have the form

$$I = \frac{B}{1 - e^{-1/\tau f}},$$

where τ is the membrane time constant of the excitable tissue, f is the sinusoidal frequency, and B is the low-frequency current asymptote. Figure 15 is a plot of this equation, which shows that the current I required for stimulation has a low-frequency asymptote B and increases as frequency is increased. In the high-frequency region, the current increases tenfold for a tenfold increase in frequency. The sensation data in Fig. 16b demonstrates this type of relationship.

Perception Threshold and Tolerance to Sinusoidal Current

The perception of and tolerance to sinusoidal current of different frequencies attracted considerable attention at the dawn of the twentieth century when it became necessary to choose a frequency for the distribution of electrical energy.

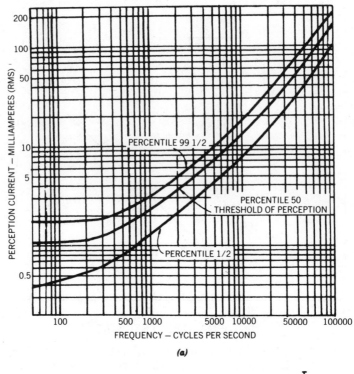

(a)

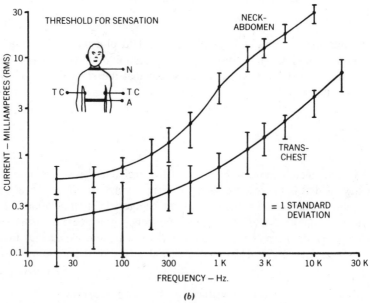

(b)

Figure 16 (*a*) Effect of frequency on perception threshold for current, using hand-held electrodes. [From C. F. Dalziel, *IRE Trans. Med. Electron.* **5**:48 (1956). By permission.] (*b*) Threshold of sensation for sinusoidal current applied to neck–abdomen (¼-in. metal ribbon) and transchest (11-mm circular disks) electrodes. [From L. A. Geddes and L. E. Baker, *J. Assoc. Adv. Med. Instrum.* **5**:13–18 (1971). By permission.]

D'Arsonval (1893a,b, 1896, 1897), of galvanometer fame, showed that when current was passed through the human body, no sensation was perceived as the frequency was increased beyond 2500–5000 Hz. At much higher frequencies, even with a high intensity, there was no perception of the current. To prove his point in a most dramatic manner, d'Arsonval connected two human subjects (arm to arm) and a 100-W light bulb in series with a high-frequency spark coil that delivered enough current (1 A) to cause the bulb to burn brilliantly. The subjects through whom the 1-A, 0.5–1-MHz current flowed reported no sensation. In a later study, d'Arsonval passed 3 A through his own body. These demonstrations, of course, paved the way for the use of high-frequency current for heating living tissues and in reality initiated medical diathermy.

When ac generators capable of providing substantial electrical energy with frequencies up to 0.1 MHz became available, further studies were performed to determine the ability of human subjects to perceive and tolerate alternating current. Kennelly and Alexanderson (1910) reported on a series of experiments in which current was passed through subjects via buckets filled with 3% saline into which the hands were immersed. Using the limit of tolerance as the criterion, they plotted graphs of current versus frequency for five subjects. They found that the tolerance to current increased with rising frequency. At 60 Hz the tolerance current varied between 4 and 100 mA. At 11 kHz the tolerance current was 30 mA, and at 100 kHz it varied between 450 and 800 mA. Even with these high currents the subjects reported only a slight tingling and a sensation of heat at the wrists.

Dalziel (1956) reported that the tip of the tongue is the most sensitive part of the body and determined the threshold for sensation on 115 subjects as 45 μA for both direct current and 60-Hz alternating current. In another series of experiments he measured the ability of more than 100 male subjects to perceive current flowing in the body through electrodes held in the hands. The threshold for sensation was 5.2 mA for direct current and 1.1 mA for 60-Hz alternating current. Dalziel found that the threshold of sensation for women was two-thirds that of the value for men. In another series of studies using hand-held electrodes, Dalziel measured the threshold for sensation for several frequencies of sinusoidal current. The data he obtained are plotted in Fig. 16a.

In a study of the choice of frequency for impedance respiration, Geddes and Baker (1969,1971) determined the threshold of sensation for sinusoidal current with electrodes placed on the human thorax. The data obtained (see Fig. 16b) are in general agreement with those of Anderson and Munson (1951) and Dalziel (1956); that is, above about 300 Hz the threshold of perception rises as frequency is increased. Recently, Lacourse et al. (1985) demonstrated that rat nerve and muscle exhibited a smooth sinusoidal current–frequency curve of the type shown in Figs. 15 and 16 for frequencies up to 1 MHz.

The Effects of Sinusoidal Current Passing through the Thorax

When the intensity of sinusoidal current passing through the thorax is increased to a level well above the threshold for cutaneous sensation, contraction of skeletal muscles occurs as a result of direct stimulation of nerve and muscle fibers. At about the same level of current, the phrenic and vagus nerves are also stimulated. Stimulation of the phrenic nerves produces tetanic contraction of the diaphragm. Stimulation of the vagus nerves produces the usual spectrum of parasympathetic activity, which includes slowing or arrest of the heart and increased gut motility. In addition, sympathetic nerve fibers are stimulated, yielding effects that oppose the parasympathetic activity; particularly evident is vasoconstriction in many vascular beds. To assign a magnitude for these phenomena, Geddes and Baker (1969) passed sinusoidal current through the thoraxes of dogs ranging in weight from 10 to 18 kg. The dogs were anesthesized with sodium pentobarbital and artificially respired while femoral artery blood pressure was recorded as an indicator of cardiac activity. Using first the metal-band neck–abdomen electrodes, then transthoracic plate electrodes, the current at each frequency was increased until vagal slowing of the heart was observed. The threshold currents at different frequencies required to produce vagal slowing of the heart are given in Fig. 17, which illustrates that in the 10–18-kg animal, vagal stimulation is easily achieved with low-frequency currents on the order of 50 mA applied with either neck–abdomen or transchest electrodes. Figure 17 also shows that the threshold current for vagal stimulation increases with increasing frequency. For example, the threshold current for vagal

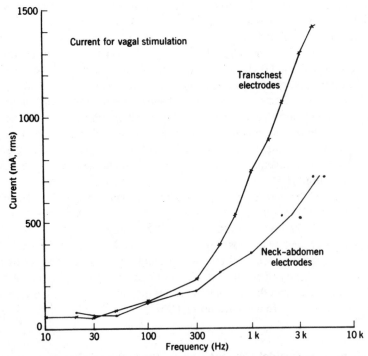

Figure 17 Average threshold sinusoidal current for vagal stimulation using transchest and neck-abdomen electrodes applied to dogs weighing 10–18 kg. Vagal stimulation was observed by slowing of the heart rate.

stimulation with neck–abdomen electrodes at 5 kHz is about 12 times that required at 60 Hz. With transchest electrodes, the current required to obtain cardiac slowing at 5 kHz is 16 times that required at 60 Hz. Proof that slowing of the heart was caused by stimulation of the vagus nerves was verified by the administration of atropine, which blocked the effect.

Ventricular Fibrillation. When thoracic current is further increased, ventricular fibrillation occurs; this is a condition of complete asynchronous contraction and relaxation of all the ventricular fibers, resulting in a loss of cardiac output. Figure 18 illustrates the precipitation of ventricular fibrillation by the direct application of current to the ventricles. Once started, ventricular fibrillation rarely, if ever, stops spontaneously in man and the larger domestic animals. If it continues for more than 3 min, irreversible damage may occur to the central nervous system, although the heart itself can be resuscitated.

In the normal subject, the passage of a relatively low-intensity current of low frequency through the thorax will produce ventricular fibrillation. In particular, ordinary lighting sources are more than sufficient to produce fibrillation; the critical factors are the current intensity, pathway, duration of exposure, and frequency of the current. Although it is not desirable to experiment on humans to determine the current threshold for fibrillation, studies have been carried out on experimental animals having body weights comparable to the human to identify the dangerous current levels at various frequencies (Ferris et al., 1936; Geddes and Baker, 1969).

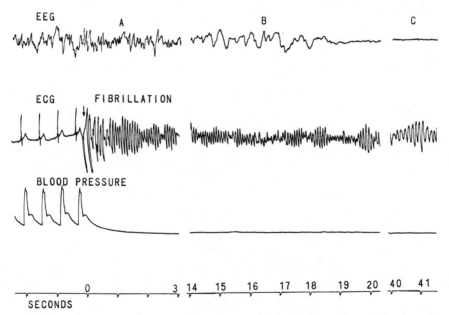

Figure 18 The EEG, ECG, and femoral artery blood pressure of a dog before (left) and after precipitation of ventricular fibrillation by the application of current to the heart. Observe that after about 20 sec of loss of blood pressure, the EEG became isoelectric.

In a series of experiments on dogs, Geddes and Baker determined the threshold current required to produce ventricular fibrillation, using sinusoidal current of various frequencies. Several electrode arrangements were used, and current was passed through the thoraxes of anesthetized animals in which breathing was assisted with a respirator. Blood pressure and the ECG were recorded as indicators of cardiac function. The procedure consisted of choosing a frequency and increasing the current slowly while watching the animal's blood pressure and electrocardiogram carefully. A consistent sequence of events occurred with each animal as the current was increased. The first event was strong contraction of skeletal muscles; this was followed by arrest of spontaneous respiratory movements, vagal slowing of the heart, and initially in most animals there was evacuation of the bladder and bowel. Finally, ventricular fibrillation occurred and blood pressure dropped to a near-zero value. After about 20 sec of fibrillation, the ventricles were defibrillated electrically using high-intensity 60-Hz current applied to transchest electrodes. The procedure was repeated over a frequency range extending from 20 to 3000 Hz. The results (Fig. 19) clearly illustrate that as frequency was increased, more current was required to produce ventricular fibrillation. It is particularly important that in the frequency range extending from 20 to 300 Hz, fibrillation was produced in the dog

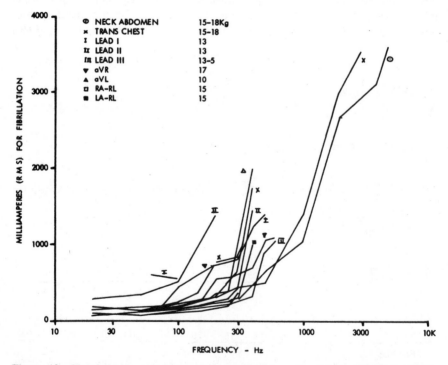

Figure 19   Threshold sinusoidal current for precipitation of ventricular fibrillation in the dog using various electrode locations. Ventricular fibrillation was precipitated by gradually increasing the current while monitoring the electrocardiogram and blood pressure.

with relatively low currents applied to the electrode arrays. Noteworthy is the fact that the threshold for fibrillation in the region between 20 and 100 Hz is almost independent of frequency. Above 100 Hz the current required to initiate fibrillation is markedly higher, and with all electrode systems the current required to produce ventricular fibrillation increases with increasing frequency. Essentially the same data were obtained by Kouwenhoven and Hooker (1936), who, using interrupted direct current, found that the threshold current for fibrillation at 1500 Hz was about 10 times that at 60 Hz. Much earlier, Prévost and Battelli (1900) discovered that the threshold voltage for fibrillation at 2000 Hz was 10 times that for 200 Hz.

The magnitude of thoracic current necessary for the precipitation of ventricular fibrillation at any frequency is related to the size of the subject and the current pathway. Since the low-frequency threshold current for fibrillation is adequately described by the current required at 60 Hz, the effect of body size in relation to fibrillation threshold can be studied at this frequency. Ferris et al. (1936) carried out the first quantitative studies of this type, using guinea pigs, rabbits, cats, dogs, pigs, sheep, and calves. Geddes et al. (1973) carried out similar studies. All these data are plotted in Fig. 20 for the various species and electrode locations; the duration of current flow for the studies was 5 sec.

Figure 20 shows that the threshold for 5 sec of 60-Hz current required for the precipitation of ventricular fibrillation is dependent on the weight of the subject and the location of the electrodes. The straight lines describing these relationships were calculated by the least squares method from the data. It is interesting to note the difference in threshold currents for the electrode positions employed. The values required for the precipitation of venticular fibrillation with electrodes on the forelimbs (lead I) are about three times those required when the current is applied between the fore and hind limbs (leads II and III). In general, the 60-Hz current required to initiate ventricular fibrillation varies approximately as the square root of body weight.

Particularly important in Fig. 20 is the value of 60-Hz current required to initiate ventricular fibrillation in the 70-kg animal (which approximates the weight of an adult man). From Fig. 20 it would appear that 215 mA rms of 60-Hz current flowing for 5 sec through the left arm–left leg circuit (lead III) will fibrillate the ventricles if species differences are disregarded. Only a slightly higher current (260 mA) is required between the right forelimb and left hind limb (lead II), but a much higher current (670 mA) is required when applied across the forelimbs (lead I). Dalziel (1956) estimated that a 60-Hz thoracic current of 100–275 mA would in all likelihood produce ventricular fibrillation in humans.

It was stated earlier that in addition to frequency, electrode location, and body weight, the duration of exposure to current affected the threshold value for the precipitation of ventricular fibrillation. A study of the significance of this factor was carried out by Geddes et al. (1973). Figure 21a illustrates the manner in which the threshold current for the precipitation of ventricular fibrillation increases with a decrease in the duration of exposure to 60-Hz current. The data for lead III (left forelimb to left hind limb) were chosen for presentation because the current required with lead III was the lowest of the three limb leads. The illustration also shows

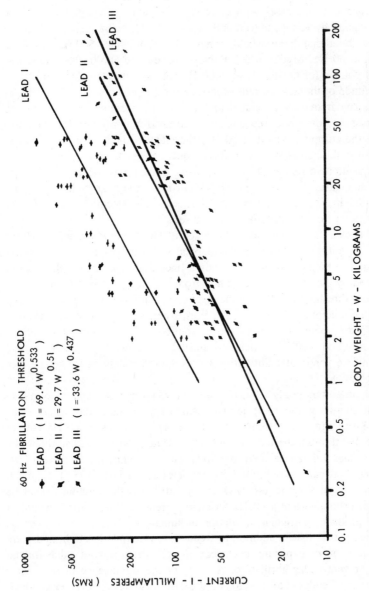

Figure 20 Threshold 60-Hz current (applied for 5 sec) required to precipitate ventricular fibrillation in animals of various body weights. (Lead I, right to left forelimb; lead II, right forelimb–left hind limb; lead III, left forelimb–left hind limb.) [Redrawn from L. A. Geddes et al., *IEEE Trans. Biomed. Eng.* **BME-20**:465–468 (1973).]

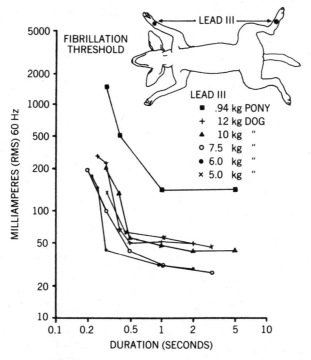

Figure 21a Threshold 60-Hz current required to precipitate ventricular fibrillation when the period of exposure is varied. [From L. A. Geddes et al., *IEEE Trans. Biomed. Eng.* **BME-20**:465–468 (1973). By permission.]

that for a given body weight the amount of current required to induce ventricular fibrillation increases with decreasing duration of exposure. For a duration of exposure in excess of about 1 sec, the threshold current for the precipitation of ventricular fibrillation decreases very little. Figure 21*b* presents data obtained by Roy et al. (1977) in which the 60-Hz current for precipitating ventricular fibrillation was measured as a function of current exposure time using catheter electrodes of different areas. It is evident that decreasing the exposure time below a few seconds increases the current required for precipitating fibrillation.

In summary, the important factors pertaining to the precipitation of ventricular fibrillation with body-surface electrodes are the electrode locations (current pathway), current frequency, and duration of exposure to the current. The current required increases when the duration of exposure becomes shorter than about 3 sec. An increase in frequency above about 100 Hz also increases the current required for fibrillation. The region on the body surface were current gains easiest access to the ventricles is the apex-beat area on the left anterior chest. At this site, the apex of the heart is closest to the rib cage, there being a notch in the lung. It is for this reason that in closed-chest cardiac pacing and ventricular defibrillation, one electrode is located at this site (Geddes et al., 1977, 1984).

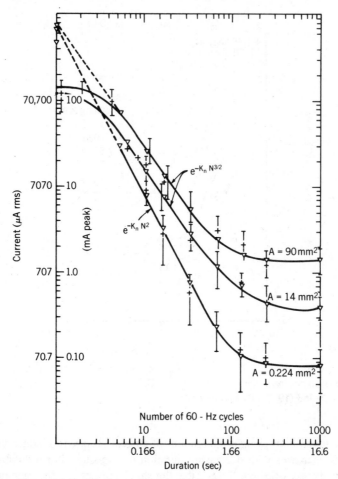

Figure 21b Threshold 60-Hz current required for ventricular fibrillation with direct-heart electrodes and for current applied for different durations. Vertical bars indicate standard deviation for (+) experimental average values and (▽)-calculated values. [Redrawn from O. Z. Roy et al., *IEEE Trans. Biomed. Eng.* **BME-24**(5):430–435 (1977).]

Leakage Current. Ventricular fibrillation is a hazard that can result from leakage currents associated with power-line apparatus connected to human subjects. This subject has been researched thoroughly by professional and standards-promulgating groups. A consensus is beginning to emerge that quantitates the current level and duration of exposure. In addition, there is a growing awareness of the importance of current entry and exit sites, as well as electrode area in relation to the hazard. The present thought on this important subject is contained in the ANSI/AAMI Proposed Standard, "Safe Current Limits for Electromedical Apparatus" (1982a).

Catheter-Borne Current. The most dangerous situation for the precipitation of ventricular fibrillation exists when a catheter or catheter electrode is placed in the right or left ventricle. Mechanical stimulation of the myocardium by the catheter tip as the heart beats can cause extrasystoles and tachycardia, which can lead to ventricular fibrillation. However, when the catheter is filled with an electrolyte (e.g., saline or blood), or when a catheter electrode (for temporary cardiac pacemaking) is in a ventricle, the opportunity arises for leakage current to gain access to the ventricular myocardium. In such a circumstance, a very small current can precipitate ventricular fibrillation. To provide quantitative data on this point, many investigators have carried out studies to determine the threshold current required to induce ventricular fibrillation. The important variables are frequency, duration of current flow, and electrode area. As shown in Fig. 21, with 60-Hz current, for body-surface and direct-heart electrodes the threshold is lowest when the current flow is longer than a few seconds. Most of the 60-Hz threshold current studies have used current exposure times in this range; Table 4 presents the data reported in the literature. Some investigators used catheter electrodes of various areas; others used electrolyte-filled catheters. Inspection of the threshold current data for fibrillation reveals that the current increases with increasing electrode area as shown by Starmer and Whalen (1973) and Roy et al. (1976, 1977). Thus, in specifying the

Table 4   60-Hz Ventricular Fibrillation Thresholds for Dogs

Exposure Time	Current (μA rms)		Electrode Type and Size	Reference
	RV	LV		
Increase to fibrillation	140–205 (min 60)	110–162 (min 75)	#7 catheter #7 Pt electrode	Weinberg and Artley (1962)
2 sec	258 (av) ($\pm$200 variability)		#7 catheter electrode	Whalen et al. (1964)
Not given	20		Bipolar catheter electrode	Staewen et al. (1969)
5 sec	60–430	300–430	#7F catheter	Geddes and Baker (1971)
10 sec	428[a]	485[a]	Catheter	Lee and Scott (1973)
			Catheter electrode	Starmer and Whalen (1973)
2 sec	2990 1290 340		5.06 (cm^2) 1.19 (cm^2) 0.85 (cm^2)	
15 sec	64–1190		Catheter	Roy et al. (1976)
>4 sec	1130 296 64		0.9 cm^2 0.14 cm^2 0.00224 cm^2	Roy et al. (1977)

[a]Assumed to be rms current.

lowest current required for ventricular fibrillation with 60 Hz, the electrode area must be specified; increasing the area increases the current required to precipitate fibrillation.

It was stated earlier that frequency is an important factor in precipitating ventricular fibrillation. To provide information on this point, Geddes and Baker (1971) applied sinusoidal current to saline-filled catheters in the left and right ventricles of dogs; the duration of current flow was 5 sec. An indifferent electrode was applied to the left leg. Blood pressure and lead III electrocardiogram were recorded, and the threshold current for fibrillation was determined in a frequency range extending from 30 to 350 Hz. The ventricular fibrillation threshold current levels appear in Fig. 22, which indicates that the lowest current for fibrillation occurs in the frequency range between 30 and 100 Hz. In this frequency region, current values ranging from 50 to 400 μA (rms), applied for 5 sec, produced ventricular fibrillation.

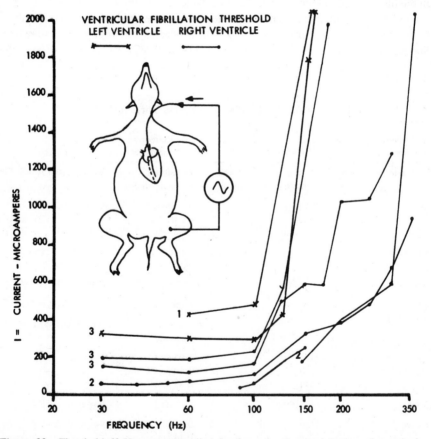

Figure 22 Threshold 60-Hz current applied for 5 sec for the precipitation of ventricular fibrillation with catheters in the right and left ventricles. [From L. A. Geddes and L. E. Baker, *J. Assoc. Adv. Med. Instrum.* **5**(1):13–18 (1971).]

It is important to recall that the current levels in Fig. 22 apply when the catheter tip is in contact with the endocardium. Even a slight displacement of the catheter tip raises the current requirements for ventricular fibrillation. Therefore the data in Fig. 22 represent the worst-case situation.

In practice, it is a voltage source that causes current to flow. To shed light on the implications of the data in Fig. 22, it is necessary to consider two distinct situations: in one a catheter electrode is placed in a ventricle, and in the other a saline-filled catheter. In the first case, the electrode impedance amounts to about 500 Ω at 60 Hz; a voltage of 25 mV (rms) would cause 50 μA (rms) of 60 Hz current to flow and precipitate ventricular fibrillation. With saline- and blood-filled catheters, the situation is entirely different, as was clearly pointed out by Monsees and McQuarrie (1971). Using resistivity values of 70 and 150 Ω-cm for physiological saline and blood, respectively, the resistance of a typical cardiac catheter can be calculated. For example an 8F catheter has an internal diameter of 1.42 mm; for a 100-cm length, its resistances when filled with saline and blood are 0.44 and 0.95 MΩ, respectively. The voltages necessary to cause 50 μA (rms) to flow in these catheters, to precipitate ventricular fibrillation when the tips are in contact with the endocardium, are 22 and 47.5 V (rms), respectively. The two cardiac catheter situations described indicate that special precautions must be taken to prevent cardiac catheters from carrying 60-Hz current.

Legal Electrocution

In view of the hazardous current thresholds just described, it is of interest to consider the currents that have been used for the legal execution of convicted criminals. Much has been written on this subject, and an excellent account of the circumstances surrounding the first legal executions, starting in 1890, was presented by MacDonald (1892), who also reported the pathological findings on the first seven electrocutions. More recently, Bernstein (1973) described the heated controversy between Edison and Westinghouse on the subject of death by electric current. It will be recalled that Edison strongly advocated the use of direct current because of its high safety and Tesla championed alternating current because it could be transmitted efficiently over large distances using high voltage which, with a transformer, could be reduced to any convenient voltage at the receiving end of the transmission line.

In the first legal executions, about 1500–1700 V was applied to wetted sponge electrodes in contact with the head and sacrum. About 2–7 A of 60-Hz current flowed, the current being applied initially for 20 sec and reapplied shortly thereafter. In some installations, direct current was used with equal success. The pathological findings associated with death from electric current have been reported by Spitzka and Radash (1912), Jex-Blake (1913), Jaffe (1928), Langworthy (1930), Hassin (1933), Pritchard (1934), and Alexander (1938). These reports indicate that there is virtually complete thermal destruction of the central nervous system in legal electrocution; brain temperatures as high as 140°F have been measured. Ventricular fibrillation has also been reported. There is general agreement that in legal execution consciousness is lost instantly and death is due to thermal destruction of the central nervous system.

Painful Stimulation

With a given electrode type, when the current is increased to a value above the perception threshold, a variety of sensations can be encountered depending on the electrode area, location, current level, frequency, and waveform. The variation in sensation probably results from the possibility of simultaneous stimulation of touch, pressure, temperature, and pain receptors and/or their afferent nerve fibers. Despite the many studies carried out in which a variety of current waveforms were applied to electrodes on the surface of human skin, it is difficult to specify the kind of sensation that will be perceived; nonetheless there appears to be some agreement. Using low-frequency sinusoidal current, the sensation under large-area electrodes is often described as buzzing, throbbing, or tingling. Under electrodes a few square millimeters or less in area, a stinging, burning, or painful sensation is frequently reported.

An interesting sensation, described as a pinprick, can be obtained under a small-area ($\sim$ 0.5 mm) electrode when the voltage is gradually increased; at a critical voltage the pricking sensation is encountered. Mueller et al. (1953) studied this phenomenon using 1200-Hz sinusoidal voltage, which was increased linearly while both voltage and current were recorded. At the point when the pricking sensation was observed, the current was seen to increase markedly, and the impedance under the small-area electrode decreased suddenly. The decrease in impedance was due to a highly localized breakdown of the skin dielectric.

Current levels above the perception threshold are applied to electrode arrays for sensory communication (Gilmer, 1961) and in psychophysiological studies for conditioning. In the latter case, the goal is to achieve a perceptible stimulus that can be controlled in its intensity but is still nonhazardous to the subject. Reviews of the studies in these fields were presented by Notermans (1966) and Pfeiffer (1968).

An early study aimed at differentiating between a perceptible (touch) and painful electrical stimulus was reported by Anderson and Munson (1951), who found that the pain threshold for sinusoidal current was about 25 dB above the perception threshold in the frequency range extending from 100 to 10,000 Hz. Gibson (1963), in a preliminary study, discovered that a rectangular pulse lasting 0.5 msec provided the highest ratio of a painful to a perceptible stimulus. Measurable differences in threshold were found between hairless and hairy skin, the former requiring less current for pain and perception. The polarity of the stimulus also affected the perception and pain thresholds. With cathodal stimuli the thresholds were lower, but anodal stimulation produced less reddening under the active (small-area) electrode. In these studies, 11-mm-diameter active electrodes were used.

Having selected the optimum pulse duration (0.5 msec), Gibson conducted two series of experiments in which the number of pulses, with a frequency of 100 Hz, was varied to determine the perception and pain thresholds. In the second series, the frequency of the 0.5-msec stimuli was varied, and the thresholds for pain and

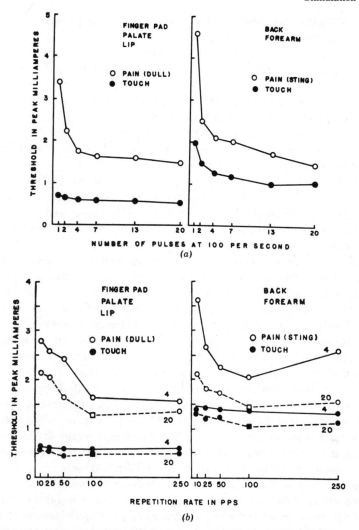

Figure 23 Threshold current for perception and pain using an active electrode (11 mm in diameter) applied to various areas of the body. (*a*) Values for pain and perception using rectangular pulses (0.5-msec duration; 100-Hz frequency) for different exposure times created by varying the number of stimuli applied. Values for 4 and 20 pulses, each 0.5 msec in duration, for different repetition rates. [From R. H. Gibson, *Proc. 2nd Int. Congr. Technol. Blindness* **2**:183–207 (1963). By permission.]

perception were determined for stimuli consisting of 4 and 20 pulses. Figure 23 presents the data obtained, which indicate that the current thresholds for perception and pain, determined with 1–20 stimuli (0.5 msec in duration with a frequency of 100 Hz), depend on the site stimulated, the hairless tissues requiring less current for both perception and pain. The current required for pain and perception decreased initially with an increasing number of pulses, but a further increase beyond about

4 for hairless tissue and about 10 for hairy tissue decreased the pain and perception thresholds insignificantly.

In the second study, in which 4 and 20 stimuli (each 0.5 msec in duration) were delivered at varying frequencies, it was clearly demonstrated that a frequency of about 100 Hz is generally optimum to evoke pain and perception with the least current. The threshold currents for both sensations were lower with 20 stimuli than with 4. These studies indicate that a stimulation period lasting 0.2 sec using 0.5-msec pulses having a frequency of 100 Hz appears to be optimum for evoking perception and pain. In general the pain perception threshold current ratio was found to range between 1.3 and 2.4 for the various body sites.

Numerous other studies have led to a description of the parameters for a painful stimulus. Table 5 is a representative compilation. Even though extensive studies such as those of Gibson (1963), Pfeiffer et al. (1971) Tursky and Watson (1964) have been conducted using a variety of waveforms, the readily available 60-Hz current seems to be preferred by many investigators.

There is no agreement on the parameters to be specified to provide a controlled and reproducible pain sensation. For various physical and psychophysiological reasons, a reproducible stimulus intensity is difficult to establish. There have been attempts to normalize a painful sensation by expressing the stimulus in terms of current density, that is, milliamperes per square millimeter of electrode area. Jackson and Riess (1934), Forbes and Bernstein (1935), and Nethken and Bulot (1967) have examined the validity of this technique and found that the current density decreased with increasing electrode area. This means that the threshold current decreases with decreasing area. This fact was put to practical use by Furman et al. (1975) to increase the longevity of batteries in cardiac pacemakers. However, caution must be exercised when estimating the current required with electrodes of different areas, because it is well known that the current-density distribution under an electrode is not uniform, being much higher under the perimeter than under the center. Stimulation occurs at the site of highest current density.

Most investigators have emphasized that a constant-current circuit should be used, regardless of the stimulus waveform. However, a few feel that current is not the quantity most associated with pain intensity; these investigators (Forbes and Bernstein, 1935; Gilmer, 1937) believe that power is the best descriptor for painful stimuli.

Since the application of electric current to the skin results in stimulation of a variety of receptors of different types, a pure pain sensation is difficult to establish, quantitate, and reproduce. For this reason, investigators have placed electrodes over regions where there are pain fibers only. Apparently the first to use this technique was Adrian (1919), who placed electrodes on the glans penis and produced a painful sensation using capacitor pulses of current. More recently, Goetzl et al. (1943) and Harris and Blockus (1952) applied stimuli to the tooth pulp to evoke pain. Although the sensation produced in each case was true pain, it has been difficult to standardize and quantitate the pain stimulus, which would be a highly desirable result for studies on the ability of drugs (analgesics) to raise the pain threshold. Nonetheless there are devices used to produce painful electrical

TABLE 5 Stimulus Parameters for Pain Sensation

Reference	Stimulus Waveform	Current[a] (mA)	Electrode Size and Location	Remarks
Notermans (1966)	Square wave, 100 Hz; 50% duty cycle, 40 pulses	0.39–0.65 p	Conical, 1-mm radius, dorsum of 2nd finger	Pinprick pain
Gibson (1963)	Rectangular, 0.5 msec, 100 Hz; 4–20 pulses	1.5 p	11-mm diameter active electrode is anode; various sites	Optimum number of stimuli
Gibson (1963)	Rectangular, 0.5 msec, 100 Hz; 20 pulses	1.5 p	11-mm diameter active electrode is anode; various sites	Optimum frequency for stimulus
Pfeiffer (1971)	Square wave, 50–150 Hz; 50% duty cycle	1–2 p	4 small points on skin of forearm	
Pfeiffer and Stevens (1971)	Rectangular 120 Hz, 3.2 msec	0.8–1.8 p	4 small points on skin of forearm	0.5 sec on, 0.5 sec off
Steinbach and Tursky (1965)	Sine wave, 60 Hz	1.82–10.23 pp	Annular electrode on dorsum of forearm	Applied for 1 sec
Sigel (1953–1954)	Square wave, 10 msec	—	1.5 × 2 in. saline pad on volar upper forearm	Pinprick sensation with 5 V
Plutchich and Bender (1966)	Square wave, 50 msec	0.7–0.85 p	1 cm diameter on tips of fingers	Applied for 5 sec
Hill et al. (1952)	Sine wave, 60 Hz	4.42–4.67 r	3 × 5 cm electrodes on palm and dorsum of hand	Applied for 0.1 sec
Hawkes and Warm (1960)	Sine wave, 100 Hz 500 1,000 5,000 10,000	1.0 r 1.9 r 2.0 r 5.5 r 10 r	Active electrode on fingertip	

489

TABLE 5 (*Continued*)

Reference	Stimulus Waveform	Current[a] (mA)	Electrode Size and Location	Remarks
Tursky and Watson (1964)	Sine wave, 60 Hz	1–3 pp 8.5 pp	Concentric electrode (Tursky, 1965) on forearm; inner electrode = 56.4 mm²; outer = 430 mm²	Untreated skin; treated skin applied for 0.5 sec
Higgins et al. (1971)	Sine wave, 60 Hz	3.5–4.2	Concentric electrode on left forearm (Tursky, 1965)	In conjunction with another test
Sternbach and Tursky (1965)	Sine wave, 60 Hz	6.12–10.23 pp	Concentric electrode (Tursky, 1965) on left forearm	Applied for 1 sec

[a] p = peak; pp = peak-to-peak, r = rms.

stimuli, and the name given to the measurement of pain threshold is algesimetry. A good account of the difficulties encountered is presented in Beecher's book (1959), which deals with the measurement of subjective responses.

When electrical stimuli are used to produce a painful sensation, it is of paramount importance to consider the safety of the subject. Although any site can be selected for application of the stimuli, it is important to examine all the current pathways to be sure that the heart is not included either directly or indirectly because of the presence of another electrode (e.g., ground) on the subject or a ground fault in the output circuit of the stimulator used to generate the painful stimulus. The safest method of applying painful electrical stimuli places both the active and indifferent electrodes on the same body segment and uses a stimulator with an isolated output circuit. The concentric electrode described by Tursky et al. (1965) offers a practical method of confining the current. The insertion of low-current fuses in series with the output terminals of the stimulator provides additional protection. Adoption of these two safeguards will do much to provide maximum safety for the subject and make it easier for the investigator to defend his or her technique to reviewers and critics.

Psychophysiologists who conduct studies on small animals in cages with electrodes on the floor face a particularly difficult problem in delivering a painful stimulation through the animals' feet unless the floor electrodes are kept clean. Fecal matter and urine can initially short-circuit the electrodes, and dry feces can cover the electrodes with a semi-insulating covering, making it difficult to deliver a controllable painful shock. Alternating current, direct current, and high-voltage pulses have all been used with varying degrees of success. A good review of the techniques was presented by Campbell and Teghtsoonian (1958).

PRACTICAL APPLICATIONS OF STIMULATION

There are many instances when stimuli are applied to produce a desired physiological response. Increasing in popularity are the many applications of skeletal muscle stimulation, either directly or via the motor nerve. Such techniques embrace the new field of functional electrical stimulation (FES). Cardiac pacing with direct-heart and transchest electrodes is now over 25 years old. The application of a relatively strong shock to transheart or transchest electrodes is the only safe and effective therapy for ventricular fibrillation. To diminish or abolish certain types of pain, bursts of short-duration stimuli are applied to skin-surface electrodes; this technique is called transcutaneous electrical nerve stimulation (TENS). These applications are described in the following pages.

Skeletal Muscle Stimulation

In physical therapy and in functional electrical stimulation, stimuli are delivered to motor nerves and muscles to elicit contraction. In the former case, the goal is to exercise the muscle, and in the latter case, the goal is to produce a desired limb movement, usually in patients with spinal cord paralysis. Recall that below the level of injury in the spinal cord, all voluntary control of muscles (and sensation) is lost, yet the motor nerves and muscles are intact and are capable of contracting in response to electrical stimuli.

Before discussing some of the applications of myoneural stimulation, it is of value to recognize the appropriate type of stimulus to evoke muscular contraction. It is the action potential of skeletal muscle fibers that triggers release of the contractile force. Whether initiated physiologically (by the motor nerve) or by direct electrical stimulation, the action potential is the same and is almost over before the contractile force is released. Figure 24 illustrates this point.

The consequence of the short duration of the action potential in relation to the duration of the twitch (the response to a single stimulus) is that another stimulus can be delivered during the twitch, causing an increase in the contractile force. This remarkable property of skeletal muscle can be demonstrated by delivering short bursts of stimuli of increasing frequency. Figure 25a illustrates the response when this method of stimulation is employed using repetitive electrical pulses. It is clear that as the frequency of stimulation is increased, the individual twitches fuse to provide a sustained force, which is called tetanic contraction. Not surprising, the tetanic force is several times greater than the twitch force. Figure 25b illustrates this phenomenon by demonstrating that during tetanic (sustained) contraction produced by repetitive nerve stimulation there are discrete muscle action potentials.

There is another important property that relates to the force developed by skeletal muscle—the response to initial stretch (loading) of the muscle fibers. It is a fundamental property of skeletal (and heart) muscle that (up to a point), an increased force of contraction occurs when the resting muscle is stretched. This point is illustrated in Fig. 26, for a situation in which the muscle was stretched between stimuli (delivered at 1/sec). Note that as the muscle was stretched, the resting tension increased and the force of contraction increased dramatically. Soon, however, the stretch was such that the muscle was no longer able to increase its force of contraction.

A practical point must be made regarding muscle contraction produced by electrical stimulation. When stimulating electrodes are placed on the skin over a muscle or inserted into it, the force developed depends on the number of muscle fibers

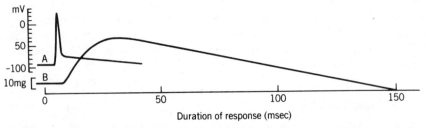

Figure 24   (A) Transmembrane potential and (B) contractile force generated by skeletal muscle in the frog in response to a single stimulus. [Redrawn from A. L. Hodgkin and P. Horowicz, *J. Physiol.* **136**:17P–18P (1957).]

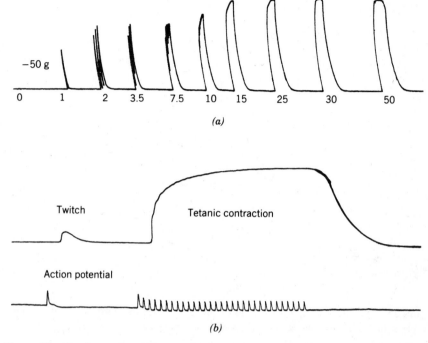

Figure 25   The force released by repetitive stimuli. (*a*) Force delivered by short bursts of increasing frequency results in the progression from a twitch to a tetanic contraction. (*b*) Action potentials accompanying a twitch and a tetanic contraction are shown in this myogram.

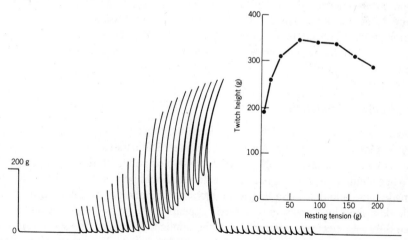

Figure 26   The increased force of contraction due to increasing stretch. This isolated frog gastrocnemius muscle was stimulated once per second, and between stimuli the muscle was stretched slightly. Note the increased force of contraction (up to a point) with increased stretch.

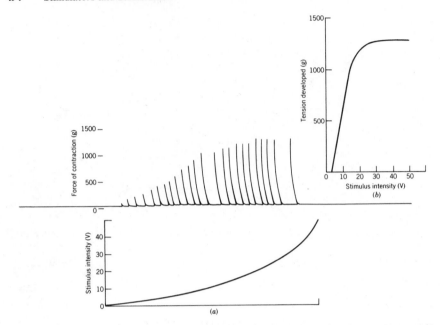

Figure 27   The effect of increasing stimulus strength applied to an isolated gastrocnemius muscle stimulated once per second. (*a*) Force of contraction corresponding to stimulus intensity; (*b*) a plot of force versus stimulus intensity.

stimulated. Increasing the intensity of the stimulating current will increase the number of muscle fibers stimulated until all of the muscle fibers (and axons) in the region are stimulated. Beyond this point, no additional force will be developed. Figure 27 demonstrates this point by illustrating the increase in the force of contraction produced by single stimuli of increasing intensity. Note that for this isolated frog gastrocnemius muscle, no additional force was produced when the stimulus was in excess of 30 V.

Motor-Point Stimulation

Regions on the surface of the body where the threshold for stimulating muscle groups is lowest are called motor points. Figure 28 illustrates motor points for the face and neck muscles; Fig. 29 identifies the motor points on the arm.

When stimulating a motor point, the cathode should be placed over it; the anode is made large and distant so that it produces no stimulation. The concentric electrode described by Tursky et al. (1965) appears to be of value in this situation, since only one electrode assembly need be applied. However, the successful use of a concentric electrode requires careful attention to details. For example, to obtain reasonable penetration of current, the inner diameter d_i of the outer ring electrode should be three or more times the diameter d of the central electrode. The area of

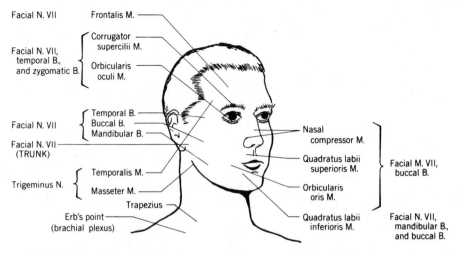

Facial N. VII — Frontalis M.

Facial N. VII, temporal B., and zygomatic B. — { Corrugator supercilii M. / Orbicularis oculi M. }

Facial N. VII — { Temporal B. / Buccal B. / Mandibular B. }

Facial N. VII (TRUNK)

Trigeminus N. — { Temporalis M. / Masseter M. }

Trapezius

Erb's point (brachial plexus)

Nasal compressor M.

Quadratus labii superioris M. } Facial M. VII, buccal B.

Orbicularis oris M.

Quadratus labii inferioris M. — Facial N. VII, mandibular B., and buccal B.

Figure 28 Motor-point chart showing the sites on the skin for the least current required to stimulate the muscles identified.

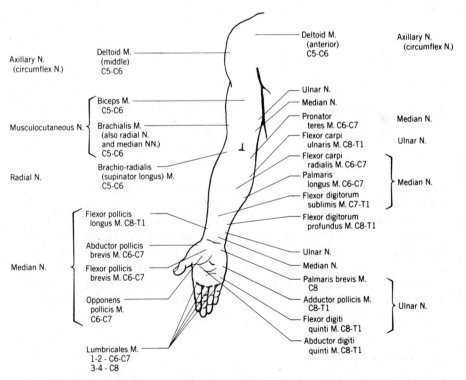

Axillary N. (circumflex N.)

Deltoid M. (middle) C5-C6

Deltoid M. (anterior) C5-C6 — Axillary N. (circumflex N.)

Musculocutaneous N. { Biceps M. C5-C6 / Brachialis M. (also radial N. and median NN.) C5-C6 }

Radial N. — Brachio-radialis (supinator longus) M. C5-C6

Median N. { Flexor pollicis longus M. C8-T1 / Abductor pollicis brevis M. C6-C7 / Flexor pollicis brevis M. C6-C7 / Opponens pollicis M. C6-C7 }

Lumbricales M. 1-2 - C6-C7 3-4 - C8

Ulnar N.
Median N.
Pronator teres M. C6-C7 — Median N.
Flexor carpi ulnaris M. C8-T1 — Ulnar N.
Flexor carpi radialis M. C6-C7
Palmaris longus M. C6-C7 } Median N.
Flexor digitorum sublimis M. C7-T1
Flexor digitorum profundus M. C8-T1

Ulnar N.
Median N.
Palmaris brevis M. C8
Adductor pollicis M. C8-T1 } Ulnar N.
Flexor digiti quinti M. C8-T1
Abductor digiti quinti M. C8-T1

Figure 29a Motor points of anterior aspect of upper extremity.

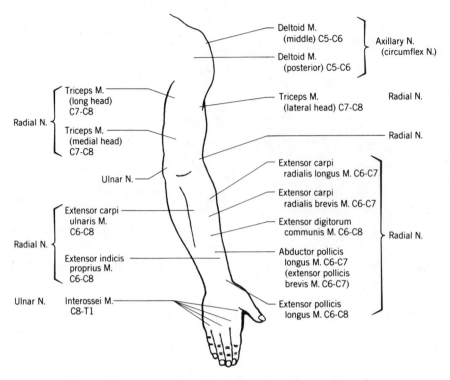

Figure 29b   Motor points of posterior aspect of upper extremity.

the ring electrode should be 10 or more times that of the central electrode. There-fore, $d_i = 3d$ and

$$10\pi d^2/4 = \pi(d_o - d_i)^2/4,$$

where d_o and d_i are the outer and inner diameters of the ring. Thus, once d is chosen, the values of d_i and d_o can be calculated.

There is an important precaution in using the concentric electrode when it is applied to the skin surface with conductive electrode paste. To avoid short-cir-cuiting between the ring and central electrode, the electrode paste must be placed only on the central and ring electrodes. The region between them, and the corre-sponding skin surface, must be kept dry. An easy method of accomplishing this goal is to use a conducting adhesive cut to match the dimensions of the central and ring electrodes (see Chap. 9).

Stimulus Parameters

When stimulating motor points the goal is to obtain the maximum contractile force with the least sensation. Because of the differences in chronaxies (and mem-brane time constants) between motor nerve and sensory and pain receptors, theory predicts that a short-duration stimulus should be used and that the stimulus repetition rate should be just high enough to obtain a tetanic contraction. For human skeletal muscle, stimuli with a repetition rate of 30–50/sec produce a smooth tetanic contraction. The use of lower frequencies will produce an incomplete tetanus; the use of higher frequencies will produce unnecessary fatigue of the myoneural junctions.

Several studies have been carried out to determine the best electrical parameters for stimulating skeletal muscle with skin-surface electrodes placed over the appropriate motor points. In all cases, the goal was to obtain the maximum contractile force with the least skin sensation. Vodovnik et al. (1965) compared sine and square waves used to raise the finger and concluded that frequencies in excess of 500 Hz were more comfortable. They also found that rectangular and trapezoidal waves 100–300 μsec in duration, with a repetition rate of 20–40/sec, were acceptable to the patients. Milner et al. (1970) investigated the stimulus parameters for contraction of the quadriceps, tibialis anterior, and gastrocnemius muscles with skin-surface electrodes. They found that stimuli having a duration of 200 μsec, repeated at the rate of 50/sec, were acceptable to the patients. Gracanin and Trnkoczy (1975) stimulated the peroneal nerve with skin-surface electrodes to obtain a constant torque of 5 N-m, measured at the ankle. They concluded that a rectangular pulse of 300-μsec duration was more comfortable than one of 1000-μsec duration. They also found that a 300-μsec rectangular pulse was preferable to a symmetrical biphasic wave consisting of two 150-μsec pulses. Some investigators used sine waves to produce contraction of the finger muscles and found that a 2-msec burst of 10-MHz sine waves repeated at a rate of 100/sec was acceptable to the patients. Finally, Bowman and Baker (1985) conducted a study to determine the preferred pulse duration, wave shape, and stimulator output circuit. The quadriceps muscle was stimulated, and a torque of 27 N-m was obtained at the knee joint. The pulse repetition rate was 35/sec, and the duration of stimulation was 1.5 sec. They found that the patients overwhelmingly preferred the 300-μsec pulse over the 50-μsec pulse, strongly preferred a symmetrical biphasic pulse (a 150-μsec pulse followed by a 150-μsec pulse in the opposite direction), and had an inconsistent preference for a constant-voltage versus a constant-current stimulator.

The foregoing studies have shown that short-duration stimuli should be used to minimize skin sensation when stimulating motor points. It is clear, however, that more studies are needed to determine the optimum stimulus duration. In our experience, stimuli less than 100 μsec in duration are far more comfortable than those of longer duration. In fact, stimuli of 5–10 μsec (which are difficult to generate with adequate current), produce excellent muscle contractions with little skin sensation. Whether such short-duration stimuli are applicable to patients is yet to be established. Moreover, the contradictory findings with the symmetrical biphasic wave must be resolved.

Functional Electrical Stimulation

Perhaps the most exciting uses for muscular stimulation are embraced by the field of functional electrical stimulation (FES), the name used to describe the use of electrical stimuli to achieve motion in the arms and legs in patients who are paralyzed, usually due to spinal cord injury. In such patients the motor nerves and muscles beyond the point of spinal injury are capable of responding to electrical stimuli. Schemes for deriving controlled trains of stimuli have been devised to achieve foot dorsiflexion in patients with drop foot and to provide hand and finger motion in patients with high spinal cord injury. Programmed stimuli have been delivered to the leg muscles to achieve leg bracing, bicycle pedaling, and walking.

Drop Foot. One of the frequent difficulties encountered by hemiplegic patients is drop foot—an inability to tilt the foot upward (dorsiflexion) that results in a shuffling gait. Until recently, a leg brace was used to assist walking. Liberson et al. (1961) showed that foot dorsiflexion could be produced by electrical stimulation of the peroneal nerve with skin-surface electrodes. Since then, others have reported successful application of this technique.

Liberson et al. (1961) used skin-surface electrodes and a special switch to activate a peroneal nerve stimulator. Using short-duration pulses (20–250 μsec) with a frequency of 30–100/sec, successful dorsiflexion was obtained in seven patients with peak currents of less than 90 mA. Closure of the heel switch prevented stimulation when the heel was on the ground; such a device is known as a heel-off switch. Vodovnik et al. (1966) described a similar but improved system in which the heel-off switch triggered a timing circuit that controlled the duration of the stimulation. Successful automatic dorsiflexion of the foot was achieved. However, Vodovnik stated that all patients desired a more compact system.

Waters (1977) reviewed his experience with drop foot patients in whom peroneal nerve stimulation was applied. He pointed out that it was often difficult to find the optimal location for skin-surface electrodes and that patients often complained of an unpleasant sensation due to the stimuli. To solve both problems in 13 patients, he used an implanted stimulus receiver with the output connected to electrodes placed around the peroneal nerve. The stimulus (33/sec, 20-μsec duration, and 0.4–0.8 V) was delivered by the implanted receiver via a coil taped to the skin over the implant. A switch in the heel caused the stimulator to be activated during the swing phase. Figure 30 illustrates the gait without and with foot dorsiflexion.

In commenting on the results, Waters stated that patient selection is important, not only from the viewpoint of the neurological deficit, but also for considerations of cognition and motivation. At surgery, careful selection of the branches of the peroneal nerve is necessary to achieve a balanced dorsiflexion.

Leg Bracing. Waters (1977) described stimulation of the motor branches of the femoral nerve in four patients, using an implanted stimulus receiver to contract the quadriceps muscle, thereby locking the knee joint. This goal was achieved by using a heel-off switch (with an adjustable time delay), that caused the leg to extend during the terminal swing, thereby permitting the patient to walk without a long leg brace.

Waters stated that patient selection is necessary for best results. Moreover, the femoral nerve branches must be selected carefully at surgery to minimize sensation

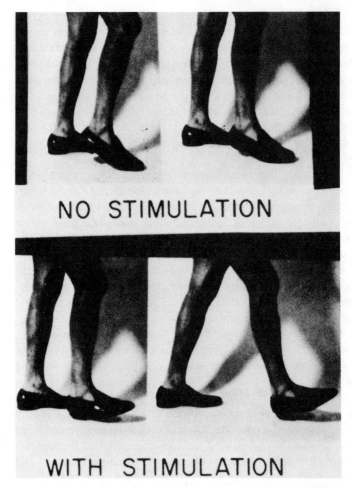

Figure 30   Gait of a paraplegic patient with drop foot without (above) and with (lower) an implanted peroneal nerve stimulator, which produces foot dorsiflexion. [From R. Waters, in *Functional Electrical Stimulation*. F. T. Hambrecht (ed.). Dekker, New York, 1977. By permission.]

and to obtain a uniform locking of the knee joint. He recommended exclusion of the fibers to the sartorius muscle and the saphenous sensory fibers; the latter can produce reflex withdrawal of the leg.

Hand and Finger Motion. Patients with cervical (neck) spinal-cord lesions exhibit a loss of muscle control and sensation beyond the level of the lesion. For example, in addition to suffering a total distal paralysis and sensory loss, patients with a C5 (cervical) lesion have lost control of the muscles of the forearm and hand; there is also a sensory loss below the mid-forearm. However, most retain shoulder, head, and neck control as well as arm rotation and elbow flexion. If the lesion is lower (C6), there is slightly less functional and sensory loss in the upper extremities. Some wrist control is retained, and sensation extends further down the arm, often to the fingers. With lower cervical lesions, the upper arm deficits are much less. Recall that since the distal spinal motor neurons are intact, the motor nerves and muscles persist; however, the lack of use of the muscles gives rise to disuse atrophy, which is reversible by active physical therapy (i.e., electrically induced exercise of the muscles). Because the muscles are capable of contracting, there is the opportunity to apply functional electrical stimulation to produce desired hand and finger movements.

One of the earliest uses of stimulation to produce finger motion in a quadriplegic patient was reported by Long and Masciarelli (1963). A 19-year-old boy was fitted with a spring-loaded hand splint that provided grasp. Electrodes were applied to the motor point of the extensor digitorum, which opened the grasp when stimulated. Stimuli of 200-μsec duration with a frequency of 55/sec were used to contract the finger extensor muscles. Output of the stimulator was controlled via a potentiometer actuated by the opposite forearm. At the time the paper was published (1963), the "electrophysiologic hand splint" had been in successful use for a year.

Peckham and Mortimer (1977) reported studies in which shoulder movement was used to control stimulation of the finger muscles. Elevation of the shoulder directed stimulation of the finger flexors; shoulder depression caused stimulation of the extensors. Percutaneous wire electrodes were inserted into the forearm for muscle stimulation. Muscle force was graded by controlling the frequency and width of the stimuli. In this study, five patients were equipped with the finger-control system, which performed successfully. Only a 2-hr training period was required. The patients used the system for eating, drinking, writing, typing (with a pencil), and holding a cigarette. Later, Peckham (1983) reported further use of the system to stimulate more hand muscles and identified the use of myoelectric signals from normal muscles as additional control information.

Programmed Neuromuscular Stimulation

For many paraplegics and some quadriplegics, there is the possibility that programmed neuromuscular stimulation can provide locomotion and walking. However, it must be recognized that even the simplest routine muscular acts involve the coordinated use of many muscles. For example, walking along a level surface involves about 40 muscles. Avoiding obstacles, stair climbing, and rising from the seated to the upright position are complex integrated muscular acts that require considerable muscular force and coordination. Nonetheless, the first steps have been taken to provide patterned movement in paralyzed patients through the use of programmed stimulation.

The first attempts to provide walking for hemiplegic patients appear to have started about 1970 in Yugoslavia. Vodovnik and co-workers summarized these early studies and their progress over 7 years (Vodovnik et al., 1977). Starting with quantitative data on bone and joint motion in normal subjects, they proceeded to create a six-channel programmed stimulating system to improve the walking capabilities of 10 hemiplegic patients. The following muscles were stimulated using skin-surface electrodes: triceps surae, quadriceps, hamstrings, gluteus maximus, gluteus medius, and sartorius. They reported very good results in enabling these subjects to walk but stated that patient selection is an important consideration.

Having built up muscle strength in two paraplegic patients using electrical stimulation, Petrofsky and Phillips (1983) and Petrofsky et al. (1983), developed a system first designed to permit bicycle pedaling, then walking along a level surface. The muscle groups receiving stimuli via skin-surface electrodes were the quadriceps, iliacus, gastrocnemius, tibialis anterior, and the hamstrings. Sensory input was provided by position indicators on the hip, knee, and ankle. Additional supervisory sensors were provided to limit the range of joint motion. Pressure sensors were used to report on the force under the foot. The system was activated by shoulder motion: a forward thrust of one shoulder caused the leg on that side to move forward.

The system developed by Petrofsky et al. has been able to produce primitive walking, but the investigators point out that much more research is needed to perfect it. Additional sensors (e.g., body position sensed by a gyroscope) will improve the gait. Much additional research will be needed to provide a means for moving sideways and climbing stairs—activities that are an important part of the everyday life of normal subjects. Particularly important is a means to regain the upright position after falling to the ground.

Cardiac Pacing

Direct Heart Pacing. Rhythmic stimulation of the ventricles (or atria), called cardiac pacing, is applied when the ventricles, the main pumping chambers of the heart, do not beat frequently enough owing to loss of their drive from the atrial pacemaker, the SA node. Typically, ventricular pacing is achieved with a catheter electrode in the right ventricle connected to an implanted pacemaker. Figure 31 illustrates a typical location for the pacemaker and its catheter electrode. Choice of the pacing pulse duration derives from the strength–duration curve for charge.

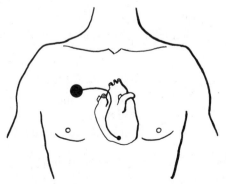

Figure 31 The site most frequently used for pacemaker implantation. The pacemaker is located in a subcutaneous pouch, and its catheter electrode is passed into the right ventricle via a small venous branch.

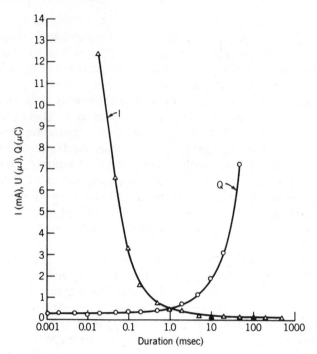

Figure 32   Strength–duration curves for stimulating cardiac muscle. *I*, current; *Q*, charge.

Figure 32 illustrates the strength–duration curves for current (*I*) and charge (*Q*) for stimulating mammalian ventricles with single rectangular pulses of current of different durations delivered during the diastolic interval. The general relationships are those predicted by theory and reveal that the membrane time constant is about 2 msec.

Since all of the charge *Q* comes from the battery in the implanted pacemaker, choice of stimulus duration is based on the minimum charge, which occurs with a duration of less than 1 msec. Typically 0.5 msec or less is used (Furman et al., 1975). The waveform is trapezoidal, and typical peak currents vary from 1 to 10 mA.

Figure 33 illustrates normal sinus rhythm (left) and sinus node arrest (center) with a slow ventricular rhythm; note the reduction in blood pressure. On the right the pacemaker was activated to stimulate the ventricles.

Closed-Chest Pacing.   In emergency situations of cardiac arrest, it is becoming popular to pace the ventricles with chest-surface electrodes; one (the cathode) placed over the apex-beat area and the other (the anode) on the right chest wall. This was the method used by Zoll (1952) when he introduced cardiac pacing in humans with 2-msec stimuli (Fig. 34*a*).

To illustrate the importance of locating the cathode on the apex beat area, Geddes et al. (1984) mapped the pacing thresholds at points 1 in. apart on the dog

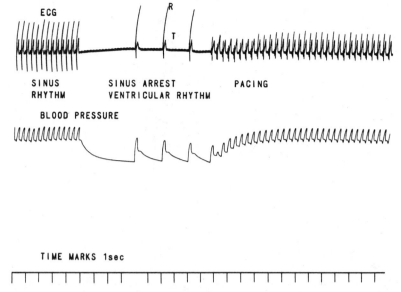

ECG

R

T

SINUS   SINUS ARREST   PACING
RHYTHM   VENTRICULAR RHYTHM

BLOOD PRESSURE

TIME MARKS 1sec

Figure 33   The ECG and blood pressure with normal sinus rhythm (left) and with sinus arrest (center), showing the slow ventricular rate. On the right, the pacemaker was activiated.

chest using single 10-msec rectangular pulses. Threshold isocurrent pacing contours that were constructed are shown in Fig. 34b and c. Note that the lowest pacing current was 30 mA (peak) and coincided with the apex-beat area, the point on the chest where the apex of the ventricles is closest to the left chest surface. In humans, pacing thresholds range from 50 to 150 mA (peak) for 10-msec rectangular pulses (Geddes et al., 1985a,b).

Due to the early appearance of implanted pacemakers and because of the muscle twitching and unpleasant skin sensation it caused in many patients, closed-chest pacing was abandoned. However, Zoll et al. (1981) pointed out quite correctly that in emergency situations in which a patient becomes unconscious due to sudden cardiac arrest, closed-chest pacing can be a life-saving procedure.

The use of closed-chest pacing brings up important considerations relative to stimulation of all of the tissues between the precordial electrodes and the heart. In the current path are sensory and pain receptors, motor nerves, and skeletal muscles, all of which have their own excitability characteristics defined by their membrane time constants (and chronaxies). The desideratum with closed-chest pacing is to pace the ventricles with the least stimulation of other tissues, because the patient is very likely to regain consciousness during precordial pacing, which may have to be continued until a permanent pacemaker is implanted.

Complicating the situation is the fact that some structures that should not be stimulated are nearer the electrodes; their rheobases and differing membrane time constants (and chronaxies) make closed-chest pacing a compromise in the choice of the optimum stimulus duration. Cutaneous receptors and motor nerves have

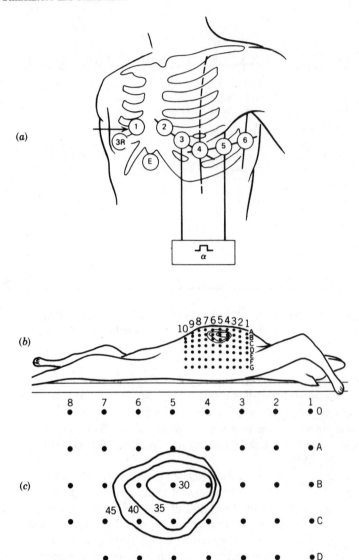

Figure 34 Placement of electrodes on the chest for closed-chest pacing. (*a*) The location used by Zoll (1952); (*b*, *c*) isocurrent pacing contours on the left chest of the dog.

relatively short membrane time constants (0.05–0.5 msec). Moreover, they are close to the skin-surface electrodes, so their rheobasic values will be less than those for deeper tissues. The membrane time constant of mammalian cardiac muscle is about 2 msec, and it is distant from the skin-surface electrodes, so its rheobase will be high.

Figure 35 clearly illustrates that as stimulus duration is decreased, the strength–duration curve for cardiac muscle ($\tau = 2$ msec) rises before those for tissues

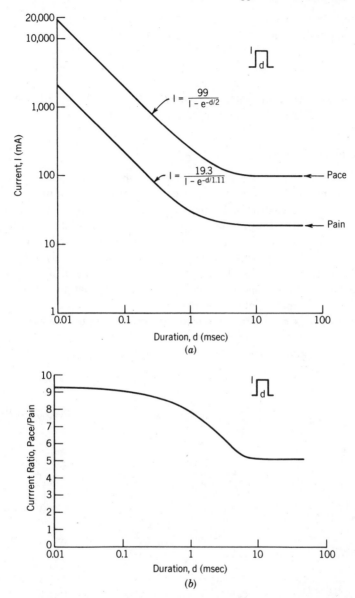

Figure 35 (*a*) Threshold for cardiac pacing and pain for stimuli of differing duration applied to chest electrodes. (*b*) Ratio of pacing to pain current versus stimulus duration. (From Geddes et al., 1985.)

having shorter membrane time constants, such as motor nerves ($\tau = 0.1$ msec) and cutaneous receptors ($\tau = 1.1$ msec). Therefore it is logical to choose a long-duration stimulus for pacing. Figure 35*a* presents strength–duration curves for pain and cardiac pacing and shows that the rheobase for cardiac stimulation with chest-surface electrodes is higher than that for pain receptors (because the latter are closer to the electrodes). Therefore, choice of the optimum duration is based on the least ratio of the current required for cardiac pacing to that for stimulating cutaneous pain receptors. Figure 35*b* demonstrates that the choice is in favor of a longer duration. This situation was discussed in the section dealing with stimulation of deep-lying tissue. Typically 10–20-msec stimuli are used for closed-chest pacing, and some motor nerve stimulation and pain occur. However, the strength–duration curves provide a basis for minimizing these side effects.

Ventricular Defibrillation

Ventricular fibrillation is a lethal cardiac arrhythmia that results in circulatory collapse due to a sudden loss of coordination of the contraction of the individual muscle fibers of the ventricles. Normal ventricular pumping and the precipitation of ventricular fibrillation were illustrated in Fig. 18. Defibrillation is achieved by massive stimulation of all the excitable ventricular fibers, rendering them inexcitable. After the pulse of stimulating current, the ventricles are ready to receive their rhythmic excitation. Figure 36 illustrates electrical ventricular defibrillation by passage of a short-duration pulse (~ 5 msec) of current through the ventricles. Note the immediate resumption of cardiac pumping.

A defibrillator is a powerful stimulator that delivers a pulse of current through the heart to terminate ventricular fibrillation (and several other types of arrhythmias). Direct-heart or thoracic electrodes can be used as shown in Fig. 37.

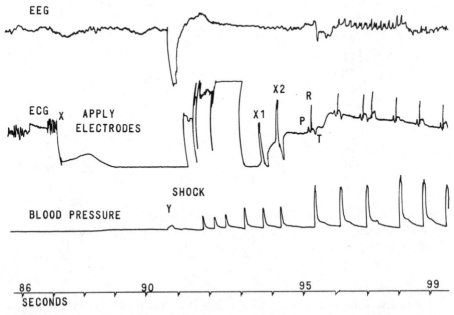

Figure 36 The EEG, ECG, and blood pressure prior to and after electrical ventricular defibrillation. Observe the prompt restoration of cardiac pumping and restoration of the EEG.

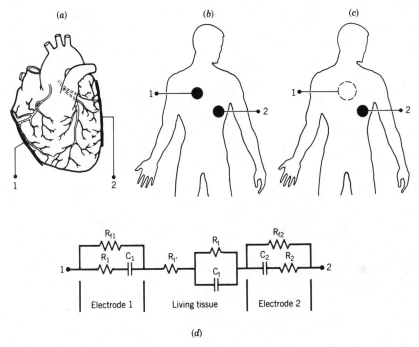

Figure 37 Defibrillating electrodes applied (*a*) directly to the heart, (*b*) to the precordium, and (*c*) to the chest and back. (*d*) The approximate equivalent circuit.

With either thoracic electrode placement (transchest or chest-to-back), it is important to locate one electrode over the apex-beat area so that current gains easy access to the heart. To illustrate this point, Geddes et al. (1977) mapped the threshold (damped sine wave) current for defibrillation in the dog using a small-area electrode (1 in. in diameter) paired with a large-area electrode on the right chest or on the back. The threshold current was expressed in amperes per kilogram, and isocurrent defibrillation contours were plotted. Figure 38 illustrates the results for both locations of the large-area electrode. Observe that the lowest current was required for defibrillation with the small-area electrode over the apex-beat area.

Line-operated and portable battery-operated defibrillators are available. In the latter category, the batteries are rechargeable. Many defibrillators contain an ECG monitor (oscilloscope or stripchart recorder) to first identify fibrillation and then verify successful defibrillation.

Defibrillating Current Waveforms. Two types of current pulses are used: (1) the damped sine wave and (2) the trapezoidal wave (Fig. 10). Damped sine waves can be either overdamped (Fig. 10*D*) or underdamped (Fig. 10*E*). There are also two types of trapezoidal waves—low-tilt (square or rectangular wave; Fig. 10*A*) and high-tilt (Fig. 10*C*). Tilt is the fractional decrease in current during the pulse. Typical durations *d* for the damped sine wave range from 4 to 12 msec, and for the trapezoidal wave from 5 to 30 msec. The majority of defibrillators are of the damped sine wave type.

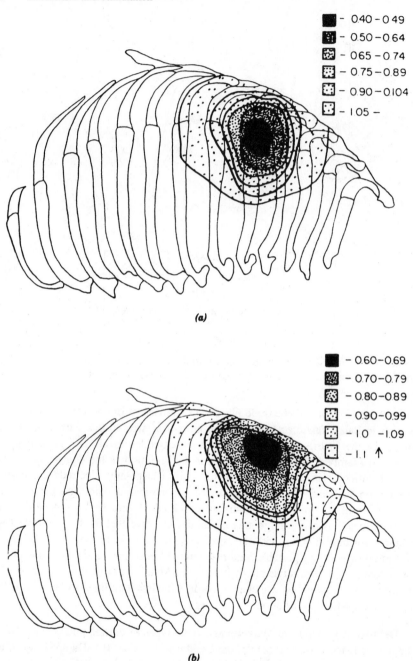

Figure 38   Threshold current dose (A/kg) lines for defibrillating the dog heart (a) with a large indifferent electrode on the right chest and a small exploring electrode on the left chest and (b) with a large indifferent electrode on the back and a small exploring electrode on the chest. [From L. A. Geddes et al., *Am. Heart J.* **94:**70, 71 (1977). With permission.]

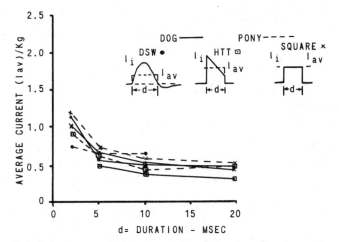

Figure 39   Threshold average current (I_{av}) per kilogram versus duration required for defibrillating dog and pony hearts with the damped sine wave (DSW), high-tilt trapezoid (HTT), and square wave pulses of current. (Redrawn from W. A. Tacker and L. A. Geddes, *Electrical Defibrillation.* CRC Press, Boca Raton, FL, 1980.)

Ventricular defibrillation obeys the strength–duration concept for tissue stimulation. Since the threshold current (for any pulse duration) is almost linear with heart and body weight, it is possible to plot the strength–duration curve in a normalized form. Because the average current law applies (Bourland et al., 1978; Geddes et al., 1985a, b), the normalized strength–duration curves for average current are almost superimposable for damped sine, rectangular, and high-tilt trapezoidal waves. Figure 39 illustrates this graphically.

Although it is current flow through the heart that arrests arrhythmias, the output of defibrillators is specified in terms of energy (watt-seconds or joules). A typical damped sine wave defibrillator stores 400 J. The low-tilt trapezoidal wave defibrillator stores 250 J, and the high-tilt defibrillator stores 400 J.

In a carefully controlled dog study, the efficacy of the damped sine and constant-tilt (60%) trapezoidal waves were compared by Hinds et al. (1987), who found that they were equal. Two measures of efficacy were compared, delivered energy and percent successful defibrillation. Both waveforms were applied to each animal in the series.

Stored versus Delivered Energy.   Standard test conditions have been established for determining the energy-delivery capabilities of defibrillators. Since the resistance of the average human thorax is about 50 Ω, defibrillators are rated on the basis of the energy delivered to a 50-Ω noninductive resistor. Due to the internal defibrillator resistance r, the delivered energy is less than the stored energy. When delivered energy is reported, it usually refers to the energy delivered to a 50-Ω noninductive resistor. The energy required to defibrillate the ventricles of an adult human subject with direct-heart electrodes is 5–10 J; a typical heart impedance is

25–35 Ω. With chest-surface electrodes, the energy required for adult human subjects is 200–400 J. Typically, the chest impedance is 50 Ω (25–125), and the peak current for a damped sine wave defibrillator is 50 A (Machin, 1978). Additional information on defibrillation thresholds can be found in Tacker and Geddes (1980).

Defibrillator Circuits

The heart of every defibrillator is a high-voltage energy-storage capacitor. Defibrillators differ only in the way this capacitor is discharged to deliver the desired current waveform. As stated previously, there are two basic types of defibrillators: damped sine wave and trapezoidal (truncated exponential).

Damped Sine Wave Defibrillator. The circuit for the damped sine wave defibrillator is shown in Fig. 40. The energy-storage capacitor C is charged to a voltage V from a power supply P. When the defibrillating pulse of current is delivered to the subject (R_L), the capacitor is discharged through an inductor L, the result being a damped sine wave of current; R_i is the internal resistance, mainly the resistance of the inductor (L).

In a typical damped sine wave defibrillator, C = 16 or 32 μF, with a voltage rating of 7000 or 5000. The inductor (L) is typically 10–50 mH, with a low internal resistance R_i. Whether the current waveform is under-, over-, or critically damped depends on the relationship between L, C, and R_i and R_L. The damping D is given by

$$D = \frac{R}{2}\sqrt{\frac{C}{L}},$$

where $R = R_L + R_i$. When $D < 1$ the circuit is underdamped; $D = 1$ represents critical damping, and $D > 1$ identifies the overdamped condition. The current equations and the delivered energy values for all three cases are shown in Table 6.

For all cases of damping, the delivered energy U_d is given by

$$U_d = \frac{U_s R_L}{R_i + R_L},$$

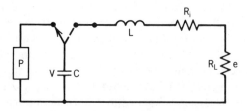

Figure 40   Circuit diagram of a typical damped sine wave defibrillator.

TABLE 6 Damped Sine Wave Defibrillator Equations

	Underdamped ($D < 1$) $a = \dfrac{R}{2L}$; $b = \sqrt{\dfrac{1}{LC} - \dfrac{R^2}{4L^2}}$	Critically Damped ($D = 1$) $a = \dfrac{R}{2L}$; $b = 0$	Overdamped ($D > 1$) $a = \dfrac{R}{2L}$; $b = \sqrt{\dfrac{R^2}{4L^2} - \dfrac{1}{LC}}$
Current i	$\dfrac{V}{bL} e^{-at} \sin bt$	$\dfrac{Vt}{L} e^{-at}$	$\dfrac{V}{2bL}\left[e^{-(a-b)t} - e^{-(a+b)t} \right]$
Peak current, I_p	$\dfrac{V}{L\sqrt{a^2+b^2}} \exp\left(-\dfrac{a}{b}\tan^{-1}\dfrac{b}{a} \right)$	$\dfrac{V}{aeL}$	$\dfrac{V}{2bL}\left[e^{-(a-b)t_p} - e^{-(a+b)t_p} \right]$
Time to peak, t_p	$\dfrac{1}{b}\tan^{-1}\dfrac{b}{a}$	$\dfrac{1}{a}$	$\dfrac{1}{2b}\ln\dfrac{a+b}{a-b}$
Stored energy	$\dfrac{CV^2}{2}$	$\dfrac{CV^2}{2}$	$\dfrac{CV^2}{2}$
Energy delivered to R	$\dfrac{V^2R}{4b^2L^2}\left[\dfrac{1}{a} - \dfrac{a}{a^2+b^2} \right]$	$\dfrac{V^2R}{4a^3L^2}$	$\dfrac{V^2R}{4L^2}\left[\dfrac{1}{a(a^2-b^2)} \right]$
Energy delivered to R_L	$CV^2R_L/2(R_i + R_L)$	$CV^2R_L/2(R_i + R_L)$	$CV^2R_L/2(R_i + R_L)$
			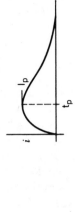

$R = R_i + R_L$, R_i = internal resistance of defibrillator, R_L = subject resistance (load), C = capacitance, L = inductance, D = damping = $R\sqrt{C}/2\sqrt{L}$.

where

$$U_s = \frac{CV^2}{2}.$$

A simple technique for determining R_i, C, and L was described by Babbs and Whistler (1978). It involves merely discharging the defibrillator into at least two load resistances R_L, which provide less than critical damping.

Trapezoidal Wave Defibrillator. The circuit for the trapezoidal (trancated exponential wave) defibrillator is shown in Fig. 41. The energy-storage capacitor (C) is charged from a power supply (P) and discharged through the subject R_L by triggering SCR1. The discharge is terminated by triggering SCR2, which short-circuits (crowbars) the capacitor. The resulting voltage and current waveform is a truncated exponential of duration d (Fig. 10C), which corresponds to the time between the triggering of SCR1 and SCR2. In addition to the SCRs, the defibrillator has an internal series resistance R_i and a parallel resistance R_p, the latter being required to assure operation of the SCRs over a wide range of R_L; R_p is usually much larger than R_L.

The decrease in voltage and current during the waveform is described in terms of tilt, which is the fractional decrease. Tilt is defined as follows:

$$T = \frac{E_i - E_f}{E_i} = \frac{I_i - I_f}{I_i},$$

where E and I are the voltage and current and the subscripts i and f denote initial and final values, respectively.

The tilt T is determined by the value of C in the defibrillator, the duration d of the current pulse, and the subject resistance R_L, as well as R_i, the internal resistance. There are two types of trapezoidal wave defibrillator; one is a low-tilt type in which C is large and d varies from about 5 to 30 msec. In this type, the delivered energy is selected by controlling the pulse duration d. In the other type the pulse duration is fixed at about 5 msec, the tilt is high ($\sim$ 60–80%), and the energy is selected

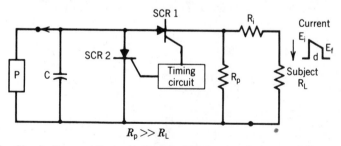

Figure 41   Circuit diagram of a typical trapezoidal (truncated exponential) wave defibrillator.

TABLE 7   Trapezoidal Wave Defibrillator

Item	Equation
Current waveform $(t = 0\text{-}d)$	$I_f = I_i\, e^{-t/(R_i + R_L)C}$
Tilt, T	$T = \dfrac{I_i - I_f}{I_i} = 1 - \dfrac{I_f}{I_i}$ $T = 1 - e^{-d/(R_i + R_L)C}$
Stored energy, U_s	$U_s = \dfrac{CV^2}{2}$
Delivered energy, U_d (to R_L)	$U_d = \dfrac{E_i I_i}{2}\left(\dfrac{d}{\ln\,(I_i/I_f)}\right)\left(1 - \dfrac{I_f^2}{I_i^2}\right)$ $U_d = \dfrac{I_i^2\, R_L d}{2\,\ln\left(\dfrac{1}{1-T}\right)}(2T - T^2)$
Average current, I_{av}	$I_{av} = \dfrac{TI_i}{\ln\,[1/(1 - T)]}$

by the voltage on the capacitor. The stored energy in the low-tilt defibrillator is typically 250 J; in the high-tilt unit, 400 J.

The total energy delivered by the capacitor to the resistive load R_L is shown in Table 7, which also presents expressions for average current and stored energy.

In all cases, the energy U_d delivered to the subject (load resistance R_L) is

$$U_d = \frac{E_i I_i}{2}\left(\frac{d}{\ln I_i/I_f}\right)\left(1 - \frac{I_f^2}{I_i^2}\right).$$

Babbs et al. (1980) described a simple method of determining the internal components (C, R_i, R_p) of the trapezoidal wave defibrillator. Briefly, this method involves measurement of the voltage and current waveforms when the defibrillator is discharged into several load resistors.

The American National Standards Institute (ANSI) has prepared a standard for defibrillators. Published by the American Association for the Advancement of Medical Instrumentation (AAMI) in 1981, the Standard covers delivered energy levels for damped sine and trapezoidal wave defibrillators and recommends testing procedures (AAMI, 1982, 1985). The appendix provides the rationale for adoption of this standard.

Transcutaneous Electrical Nerve Stimulation (TENS)

Transcutaneous electrical nerve stimulation (TENS) is a technique whereby electrical stimuli are applied to skin-surface electrodes to reduce or abolish pain. The electrodes are placed on specific skin sites, and short-duration stimuli are applied.

Wall and Sweet (1967) called attention to the fact that pain could be suppressed by electrical stimulation of large-diameter nerve fibers (A fibers). Accordingly, they carried out studies on eight patients using direct-nerve and transcutaneous electrical stimulation. They used 0.1-msec rectangular wave stimuli having a frequency of 100/sec. Superficial nerves were stimulated using needle or wire electrodes—a needle or wire paired with a skin-surface electrode or two skin-surface electrodes. In each case the stimulus intensity was increased until a tingling sensation was perceived by the patient. In general, 2 min of stimulation provided about $\frac{1}{2}$ hr of pain relief.

The use of TENS has expanded rapidly, being employed in a wide variety of situations to relieve the pain associated with athletic injuries, trauma, surgical procedures, cancer, and childbirth. Among the many conditions now treated with TENS are migraine, bursitis, tennis elbow, tendonitis, rheumatoid arthritis, tinnitus, diabetic neuropathy, radiculopathies, carpal tunnel syndrome, shoulder-hand syndrome, osteoarthritis, sciatica, sinus headache, and hemiplegic pain. Although pain from any cause is amenable to TENS treatment, only a small percentage of subjects experience complete relief. Nonetheless, adequate relief is obtained about 50% of the time.

Electrode Placement. At present, there is no standard technique to guide placement of the electrodes for TENS. Mannheimer (1978) and Mannheimer et al. (1978) recommended that the best sites were motor, acupuncture, and/or trigger points. A trigger point is a site where pressure evokes a specific sensation, usually pain. In general, one electrode is placed over, or just proximal to, the site of pain and over a superficial nerve. The other electrode is placed distally at a convenient site. Uniform contact with the skin is essential to prevent the development of localized regions of high current density. Usually a conducting paste is employed. The current intensity is increased until a tingling is perceived. Excess current will result in muscular contraction; inadequate current will not stimulate the underlying large-diameter sensory nerve fibers.

If, after several minutes of stimulation, the pain sensation is not reduced, the stimulus frequency is usually altered. If success is still not achieved, other electrode sites are investigated until a satisfactory response is obtained. Optimally, a half-hour or more of pain relief is obtained with a few minutes of stimulation; however, longer periods of stimulation are not at all uncommon. In practice, the physician or therapist will conduct preliminary trials with TENS. When the treatment procedure has been established, the patient takes the TENS unit home for treatments as prescribed or needed.

Stimulating Current. It is generally agreed that the large-diameter A (sensory) nerves are the targets for TENS current. This being so, it is useful to recall that the chronaxie for these fibers is much shorter than that for C (pain) fibers. Li and Bak (1976) measured the chronaxie values for A and C fibers in the cat saphenous nerve at 29.3°C; Fig. 42 was composed from their data and demonstrates that with decreasing duration the threshold for stimulating C fibers rises at a longer duration

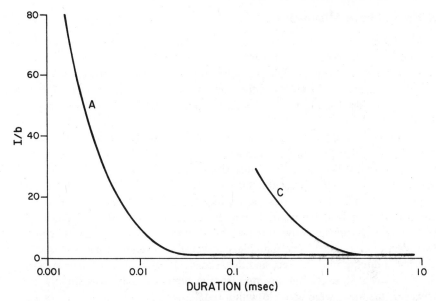

Figure 42   Strength–duration curves for sensory and motor fibers (A) and pain fibers (C) in the cat saphenous nerve at 29.3°C. [Redrawn from C.-L. Li and A. Bak, *Exp. Neurol.* **50:**67–79 (1976).]

than for A fibers. Therefore, the best pulse duration for stimulating A fibers selectively is less than 0.1 msec.

Although the electrophysiological characteristics of the large A fibers dictate that a short-duration stimulus should be used for TENS, there is not complete agreement on the optimal current pulse or on the frequency of the stimuli. The frequencies used vary between 10 and 100 per second. A waveform that is gaining popularity consists of bursts (3/sec) of seven 80-μsec biphasic pulses; the equivalent frequency of the burst is 85 Hz.

It is difficult to identify typical output current and voltage levels because different values are needed with the different waveforms, frequencies, and electrodes. Moreover, the optimum type of output circuit (e.g., constant-current or constant-voltage) has not been specified; many prefer the constant-current type. Standards are now being drafted by the American Association for the Advancement of Medical Instrumentation (AAMI).

The proposed standard (NS4-1983) specifies the output in several ways using a 100-Ω resistive load. Maximum charge and current are specified. The maximum charge per pulse is $20 + 1.8$ ($35t$) μC, where t is the pulse duration in milliseconds, with t being measured at 50% of the pulse amplitude. The maximum average current is 10 mA into a 100-Ω load. These recommendations are provisional, and modifications will likely be made. For a summary of the various waveforms, pulse durations, and frequencies, see Health Devices (1981).

Reciprocal-Pulse Stimulation

The term reciprocal pulse is used here to identify a stimulus consisting of an upward wave followed by a downward one, the two waves being time locked closely. Some use the term biphasic to identify this waveform; however, "biphasic wave" could mean two pulses in the same direction. The reciprocal pulse is beginning to be used in chronic TENS stimulation applications because it results in no net current flow.

It is customary to use a single unidirectional rectangular or trapezoidal (truncated exponential) pulse to stimulate excitable tissue. When the pulse rises from and returns to zero, it is essentially a pulse of direct current. Lilly et al. (1955) called attention to this fact and pointed out that when a train of such unidirectional pulses is used for stimulating nervous tissue, there is injury at the electrode sites. To eliminate this galvanic type of lesion, he devised and used a reciprocal pulse consisting of an upward wave followed by a downward wave, the areas under the two waves being equal. The individual waveforms resembled half-sinusoids; the first had a duration of 48 μsec, and the second, 35 μsec. The separation between the pulses was 38 μsec. The inverted (shorter duration) pulse was slightly larger; however, the areas were equal to within 0.4%.

Lilly et al. (1955) used their reciprocal pulse waveform for chronic stimulation of the sensorimotor cortex of the monkey. A 2-sec train of 60/sec reciprocal pulses was delivered every 30 sec for 4–5 hr/day for 5–6 weeks. It was found that the threshold for stimulation decreased slightly over a 6-week period and no neural damage was produced at the electrode sites.

It is useful to speculate on the mechanism of stimulation in Lilly's study. Because the second (downward) pulse was delivered 136 μsec after the onset of the first, it is likely that the first pulse initiated the response and the second fell in the refractory period. The second downward pulse probably served to provide zero net current flow for the duration of the reciprocal pulse.

Those who use transcutaneous electrical nerve stimulation (TENS) for the relief of pain are beginning to employ the reciprocal pulse because it has been found that skin reactions at the electrode sites are less. The waveforms produced by the various commercially available TENS stimulators are described in *Health Devices* (1981). Those who use skin-surface electrodes to stimulate motor nerves in functional electrical stimulation (FES) have also found less skin reaction under electrodes when the reciprocal pulse is used. In most cases, the downward pulse starts with the end of the upward pulse.

It is difficult to know how to characterize the duration and amplitude of the reciprocal pulse since the upward and downward waves have no time separation. There is no doubt that such a zero-net-current waveform can stimulate; a familiar example is sinusoidal alternating current. There has been no fundamental research directed toward analyzing the transmembrane movement of charge in response to the reciprocal-pulse stimulus. One study by Bourland et al. (1982) compared the threshold peak current for defibrillation using a unidirectional rectangular wave with that required by a reciprocal pulse having the same total duration. It was found that the threshold currents, measured from zero to the peak, were essentially the same for both waveforms. Whether this special case of massive tissue stimulation is representative of stimulating a simple strip of excitable tissue is not known, and research needs to be directed toward this area.

For long-term stimulation, the zero-net current—i.e., the zero charge transfer characteristic of the reciprocal pulse—minimizes the risk of electrolytic decomposition of electrodes and tissue fluids. It is for the future to establish the practical value of this waveform. However, Donaldson and Donaldson (1986) pointed out that capacitive coupling to the electrodes achieves, in part, the desired charge balance. With platinum electrodes, the electrode–electrolyte capacitance provides a degree of capacitance coupling. They advocated that in practice the balanced (Lilly) pulse is not needed with platinum electrodes.

Training Collar

An interesting telestimulator is used in animal obedience training (Tortora, 1981). The stimulator is mounted in a collar (Fig. 43) and receives its command by a radio signal. Connected to two rod electrodes that penetrate the fur of the animal,

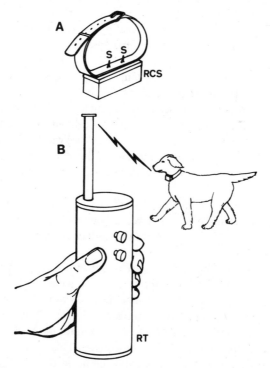

Figure 43 (A) Training collar, showing the radio-controlled stimulator (RCS) and stimulating electrodes S. (B) The trainer transmits a radio signal to the telestimulator by pressing a button on the transmitter. (Redrawn from D. E. Tortora, *Understanding Electronic Dog-Training.* Tri-Tronics Inc., Tucson, AZ, 1981.)

the stimulator has a high-voltage, constant-current output circuit and delivers a train of pulses, each 200–300 μsec in width and repeated with a frequency of 200–300/sec. The voltage is in the range of 1200–1500 V across a 100,000-Ω load. Some models produce short bursts of stimuli in response to the radio signal.

A shock is delivered to the animal when it barks or exhibits some other undesired behavior, and the animal quickly learns to stop the undesired behavior to avoid the shock. This technique is called avoidance training.

There is little danger to an animal wearing the training collar. Although the vagus and sympathetic nerves are in the neck, the combination of a short period of stimulation (a second or so) and short duration of each pulse minimizes the risk of stimulating these structures. However, the cutaneous receptors are strongly stimulated and provide the unpleasant sensation to the animal.

Stimulator Output Circuits

Although a variety of waveforms are used to stimulate excitable tissue, the output circuit that delivers such stimuli to the stimulating electrodes can be either of two types that have quite different operating characteristics. These are the constant-voltage and the constant-current circuits. Many stimulators are neither purely constant-voltage nor constant-current. Nonetheless, an understanding of the characteristics of each type is essential in evaluating the operation of a stimulator and in testing it to determine its stimulating capabilities.

Constant-Voltage Circuit. The constant-voltage stimulator provides an output that, for a given voltage setting, is capable of delivering a current that is inversely proportional to the impedance of the electrode–subject circuit connected to it. This means that the stimulator has a very low internal (output) impedance. Figure 44a illustrates the constant-voltage stimulator, with the waveform of the stimulus sketched in the circle representing the generator and the resistance r representing the internal impedance, which is low with respect to that of the electrode–subject circuit, Z_s.

Figure 44b illustrates the output characteristics with respect to varying the impedance Z_s of the electrode–subject circuit. Note that the output voltage remains constant for all values of Z_s; however, the delivered current increases as Z_s is decreased.

In Figure 44a, if the impedance Z_s of the electrode–subject circuit is purely resistive, the waveform of the current will be the same as that of the voltage. However, as shown in Chapter 9, the electrode–electrolyte interface (and living tissue) have capacitive and resistive components; the net result is that for all stimulus waveforms other than sine waves, the waveform for the current in the constant-voltage circuit is not the same as that of the voltage. This is illustrated in Fig. 44c, which was derived from stimulating a motor point on the arm with a small-area (0.31-cm^2) electrode and a large (4 cm $\times$ 5 cm) plate electrode on the same arm. Note that the presence of the capacitive component of the electrode–electrolyte interface and that of the tissues results in a peaking of the current pulse, which is not present in the voltage pulse.

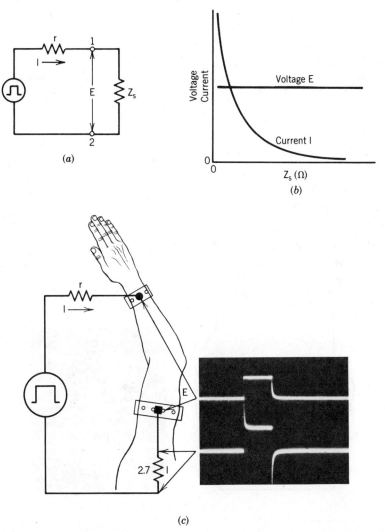

(a)

(b)

(c)

Figure 44 (a) The constant-voltage stimulator and (b) its output characteristics with different impedances Z connected to it. (c) Voltage E and current I waveforms for a constant-voltage stimulator having an internal impedance $r = 25 \ \Omega$. (The peak voltage is 20 V, and the duration is 2 msec.)

Constant-Current Circuit. The constant-current output circuit provides the same current, irrespective of the impedance Z_s of the electrode–subject circuit. This means that the internal impedance of the stimulator is very high. Figure 45a illustrates an idealized constant-current output circuit in which the waveform of the stimulus is sketched in the circle representing the generator and the resistance R represents the internal (output) impedance of the stimulator; Z_s is the impedance of the electrode–subject circuit. For the stimulator to function as a constant-current

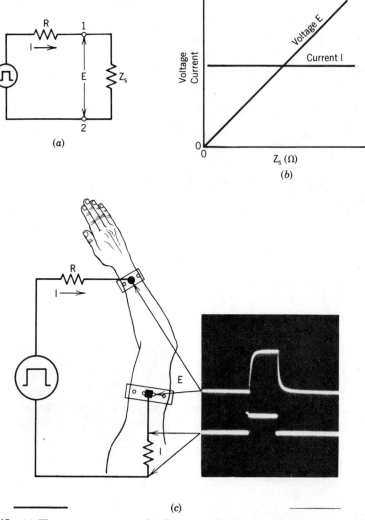

Figure 45 (a) The constant-current stimulator and (b) its output characteristics, with different impedances Z_s connected to it. (c) Voltage E and current I waveforms from a constant-current stimulator having an internal impedance $R = 100 \text{ k}\Omega$. (The peak current is 2 mA, and the duration is 2 msec.)

device, the internal impedance R is very high with respect to the impedance Z_s of the electrode–subject circuit.

Figure 45b illustrates the output characteristics of the constant-current circuit as the impedance of the electrode–subject circuit Z_s is varied. Note that the current remains constant for all values of Z_s; however, the voltage increases linearly with a linear increase in Z_s.

In Figure 45a, if the impedance Z_s is purely resistive, the waveforms of the current and voltage are the same. However, as shown in Chapter 9, the electrode-electrolyte interface (and living tissue) have capacitive and resistive components. The net result is that for all waveforms other than the sine wave the waveform for the voltage is not the same as that of the current. This point is illustrated in Fig. 45c, which was derived from stimulating a motor point on the arm with a small-area (0.31-cm^2) electrode and a large (4 cm $\times$ 5 cm) plate electrode on the same arm. It is clear that the presence of the capacitive component of the tissues and the electrode–electrolyte interface results in a rounded waveform for the voltage, which is not present in the rectangular current waveform.

Isolated Output Circuit. Many stimulators provide a negative-going (cathodal) output pulse that is referred to ground. While this is adequate for most stimulating applications, it causes great difficulty when recording an action potential evoked by the stimulus. This situation arises because the stimulus is many times larger than the action potential and is conductively coupled into the measuring apparatus by the common ground. Although a high common-mode rejection ratio in the measuring apparatus favors rejection of this ground-referred stimulus artifact, another technique, developed by Schmitt (1943), greatly reduces pickup of the stimulus during the recording of an evoked bioelectric response.

A technique of stimulus isolation is shown in Fig. 46 that consists of using the stimulus to modulate a radiofrequency oscillator that transmits a carrier signal across an air gap. The signal is then detected by a tuned circuit (L-C), to which is connected a diode (D) and an integrating capacitor (C_i) and resistor (R_i). This circuit recovers the stimulus waveform as shown. A capacitor C'' is used to block the dc component due to the unidirectional stimulus.

The radiofrequency (rf) isolation technique can provide a high degree of isolation (e.g., a few picofarads to ground) for the stimulus. The figure of merit of a stimulus-isolation circuit is the capacitance to ground from either output terminal.

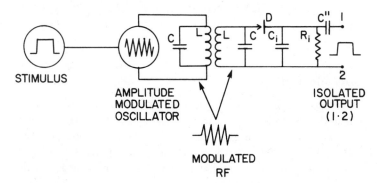

Figure 46 The radiofrequency (rf) isolated stimulator. The stimulus amplitude modulates a high-frequency oscillator, which delivers its output to the primary of a tuned circuit (L-C), the secondary of which feeds a diode (D) and integrating capacitor and resistor (C_i, R_i), which recovers the stimulus. A blocking capacitor (C'') removes any dc component from the stimulus.

The intensity of the stimulus is controlled by the amplitude of the stimulus used to modulate the rf oscillator. Special circuit arrangements can be provided to accommodate waveforms that have both negative- and positive-going phase. In addition, stimulus-isolation circuits can be made to approximate the characteristics of a constant-voltage or constant-current output circuit, the latter being the easier to provide.

It should be obvious that a transformer with a low primary-to-secondary capacitance can be used for stimulus isolation. However, if the stimulus pulse has a long duration, there will be considerable waveform distortion. This will also occur if the secondary of the transformer is highly resonant. This latter effect can be diminished by placing a resistor of the appropriate magnitude across the secondary terminals to provide damping.

Stimulus isolation can also be achieved by the use of an optical coupler, which consists of a light-emitting diode (LED) facing a photodiode. The stimulus is delivered to the LED, and the photodiode recovers it and usually triggers a battery-operated stimulator that is isolated from ground.

Manufacturers of stimulus-isolation units strive to provide the lowest output capacitance to ground and to the stimulator that drives it. To benefit maximally from this low capacitance, the stimulus isolator should be placed as close to the stimulating electrodes as possible to minimize the length of the wiring. Extension cables should never be connected to the output of a stimulus-isolation unit. If an extension cable is needed, it should be placed between the stimulator and the isolation unit.

To close this section on isolated stimulator output circuits, it is useful to recall that the isolation is capacitive. Typical isolation amounts to from a few to perhaps 10 picofarads (pF). While the reactance ($1/2\pi fC$) of such a capacitance (C) is high at 60 Hz, it is not high for electrosurgery or diathermy currents. For example, at 1 MHz, the reactance of 10 pF is 15,900 Ω. At 27 MHz diathermy frequency, it is $1/27$ of this value. Moreover, capacitive isolators have a finite breakdown voltage and can be destroyed by electrosurgical or diathermy voltages; therefore, precautions must be taken to avoid exposing the isolating circuit to excessive voltage.

Electrodeless Stimulation

Since the discovery of magnetic induction by Faraday and Henry in the early 1800s, there has been much speculation about the effect of magnetic fields on living organisms. Many inconclusive experiments have been performed; these are well summarized by Becker (1983). Both steady and changing fields have been applied to examine the effect on living tissue; however, it is the changing field that is important because of its ability to induce eddy currents of sufficient magnitude to cause stimulation of excitable tissue.

Since 1896 it has been known that the magnetic field surrounding a coil carrying a changing current can induce eddy currents in living tissue and cause stimulation of receptors and nerve fibers. The changing magnetic field has been produced by passing alternating current through a coil and by discharging a capacitor into it.

The flow of eddy current in the tissue gives rise to a voltage drop that causes stimulation. The more rapidly the magnetic field changes, the larger the induced voltage. Perhaps the most attractive feature of magnetically induced stimuli is the reduced skin sensation compared to stimulation with skin-surface electrodes. In the latter case the superficial current density is high, and consequently the stimulation is strongest under the skin-surface electrodes. A high stimulus intensity must be applied when deep-lying tissues are to be stimulated, which causes great discomfort when skin-surface electrodes are used.

It was d'Arsonval (1896) who first reported magnetically induced stimulation by passing 42-Hz current through a coil into which the head was placed. He wrote:

"There occurs, when one plunges the head [into the coil], phosphenes and vertigo, and in some persons, syncope. . . . The alternating magnetic field modifies the form of muscular contraction and produces, in living beings, other effects that are easy to demonstrate and of which I am pursuing the study at this time."

D'Arsonval clearly demonstrated the ability of an alternating magnetic field to stimulate retinal receptors and motor nerves. He gave little information on his coil other than stating that it was made of thin-walled brass tubing, that it was excited with 110 V, and that the current was 30 A. He devised a thermocouple ammeter to measure this current. Beer (1901), unaware of d'Arsonval's study, reported flickering light sensations due to a magnetic field. His paper contains no quantitative information on the coil or the field strength used.

Magnetically induced phosphenes, which are bright spots in the visual field, became the subject of considerable interest at this time when alternating current was being developed commercially. Thompson (1910), the pioneer of electrical engineering, Dunlap (1911), and Magnusson and Stevens (1911, 1914) all carried out studies on magnetophosphenes, as they were called. Thompson, unaware of d'Arsonval's paper, constructed a coil of 32 turns of stranded copper wire (cross-sectional area of 0.2 in.^{2}) with an internal diameter of 9 in. and 8 in. long. He applied 50-Hz current (up to 180 A), which produced a field of 5760 ampere-turns, with an rms field strength at the center of 1000 cgs units. At the mouth of the coil, the field strength was about two-thirds of this value. On inserting his head into this coil, with his eyes closed and in a darkened room, he reported "a faint flickering illumination, colorless, or of a slightly bluish tint," being brighter in the peripheral field. Even in daylight with eyes open, the visual sensation could be perceived. Some subjects reported a taste sensation.

Dunlap (1911) suspected that the phosphenes reported by Thompson's subjects might be due to suggestion produced by the loud hum of the transformer when the current was applied to the coil. To investigate this situation, Dunlap constructed a coil of 27 turns of stranded wire (37 strands, each 0.082 in. in diameter); the coil was 8 in. long and elliptical in cross section (9 in. × 10.5 in. minor and major axes). The coil was suspended from the ceiling and could be lowered over the subject's head. The current was 200 A at 60 Hz, producing a field of 5400 ampere-turns. Not all subjects perceived the flickering reported by Thompson. (Note that the field strength is slightly less than that reported by Thompson.)

To settle the matter of sound-induced suggestion, Dunlap plugged the subject's ears, and the loud transformer hum was produced with and without current in the coil. The transformer hum without current in the coil was produced by switching the transformer to a load resistor carrying the same current as was passed through the coil. Dunlap concluded that the flickering-light phenomenon was real. He also reported that the phenomenon could be perceived with the eyes either closed or open in a moderately lighted room. Additional tests were conducted with 440 A (60 Hz) applied to the coil; the flickering was more distinct and even perceived by the subjects who could not see it in the first tests. When the frequency was changed to 25 Hz and with 480 A flowing in the coil, the response was striking, the whole visual field appearing illuminated. Flickering could also be perceived with the head below the coil, and the sensation was described as disagreeable. However, none of the subjects reported any other sensation.

Magnusson and Stevens (1911, 1914) carried out studies with a large coil that could be placed over the subject's head. No phosphenes were perceived when direct current was flowing in the coil. However, they were seen when the current flow was initiated and interrupted (make and break). With the make shock, the phosphenes consisted of a horizontal luminous bar moving downward. On the break, the bar was dimmer and moved upward. Reversing the polarity of the field did not change the direction of movement of the light bars.

Magnusson and Stevens then carried out a series of studies on the importance of frequency and field strength in producing phosphenes in human subjects. Below 25 Hz, the phosphenes appeared to follow the magnetic field. For a given field strength, the phosphenes appeared brighter with 20–30-Hz current. The threshold for 60-Hz current was 3000–4000 ampere-turns. Above 90 Hz, the phosphenes became faint, even with severalfold higher field strength.

After more than three decades of disinterest in eddy-current stimulation, Walsh (1946) presented a paper on retinal stimulation in humans using ac fields having frequencies ranging from 5 to 90 Hz, with field strengths up to 900 G. The familiar colorless, peripheral-field flickering sensation was reported. When the coil was close to the eye, maximal flickering was perceived. When the coil was over the occiput, no flickering was reported. The flickering diminished with constant stimulation; prolongation could be achieved by moving the eyes. Recovery occurred within a few seconds of cessation of stimulation. They reported that the sensation was similar to that when 100-Hz current was passed through the head using directly applied electrodes.

Magnetophosphenes were also described by Barlow et al. (1947), using a coil of 397 turns of 16-gauge copper wire, and measuring 10.5 cm i.d., 20.7 cm o.d., and 7.3 cm long. Into the coil was placed a laminated core 5.3 cm × 2.9 cm in cross section and 37 cm long. The core was placed a few centimeters from the side of the head. With 20 A of 60-Hz sinusoidal current, phosphenes were perceived. The field strength was 7940 ampere-turns, which corresponded to an intensity of 900 G measured by a search coil.

To illustrate that the phosphenes were due to electrical stimulation of the retina, Barlow et al. placed an active electrode on the side of the forehead and a reference electrode on the back of the forearm. With 0.3 mA of 60-Hz current, phosphenes were perceived.

In their studies, Barlow et al. (1947) stated that the phosphenes were usually colorless, but occasionally they were bluish and sometimes slightly yellow. No phosphenes could be perceived when the core of the coil was placed over the occipital area, the site of the visual cortex.

Stimulation of an exposed motor nerve by a 60-Hz ac field was reported by Kolin et al. (1959). The magnetic field was produced in a laminated core of square cross section, with one end being tapered to a pyramidal shape. A frog nerve-muscle preparation was looped around the pyramidal part of the core. With a field of 6000 G (rms) at 60 Hz, a strong tetanic contraction was produced in the gastrocnemius muscle. No dimensions or data were given on the coil or the current.

Bickford and Fremming (1965) were able to produce a twitch in the frog and rabbit gastrocnemius muscle by stimulating the sciatic nerve with a pulsed magnetic field having a strength of 20–30 kG produced by discharging a 200-μF capacitor into an air-core inductor of about 250 μH having a resistance of less than 1 Ω. The resonant frequency of the circuit was 500 Hz, and the damping coefficient was about 0.10. The capacitor could be charged to 2000 V. Using the same technique, they stimulated the peroneal, sciatic, and ulnar nerves noninvasively in humans and obtained a twitch in the associated muscles. Surprisingly, with the field directed toward the eye, no phosphenes were perceived even in the presence of a twitch in the orbital muscles.

Some of the theoretical aspects of inducing current in living tissue were discussed by Rentsch (1965). He pointed out that the coupling efficiency between a coil and tissue is inherently small, being on the order of 10^{-5}. Therefore high energies must be delivered to the excitation coil to produce an adequate current in the tissue for stimulation. Using a coil of 30 turns and 20 cm in diameter (inductance 365 μH and resistance 10 Ω), placed against the chest, he was able to twitch the chest muscles by discharging a 10-μF capacitor, charged to 1500 V, into the coil. The energy stored in the capacitor was 11.25 J. He speculated that the technique might be of value in dentistry to identify viable nerve supply to a tooth.

Exposed dog and rabbit motor nerves were stimulated by Maass and Asa (1970) with a magnetic field produced by discharging a capacitor bank (18–22 μF) into a 100-turn coil wound on a toroidal core that was cut across its diameter to allow placing the nerve in the center of the toroid. The excitation coil was on one half of the toroid, and a sense coil was placed on the other to measure the field strength. The energy delivered by the capacitor bank was less than 2 J, and the duration of the pulse appearing across the ends of the sense coil was between 30 and 100 μsec. Compared to the parameters used by other investigators, this is remarkably low energy.

Bursts of high-frequency induced current were used by Oberg (1973) to stimulate exposed frog sciatic nerve. A ferrite toroid of 25 mm internal diameter and 31.5 mm^2 cross-sectional area was used to produce the magnetic field. An air gap of 1–2 mm was cut in the toroid for insertion of the motor nerve. Different shapes for the air gap were investigated. A coil made of 0.2-mm-diameter copper wire was wound on the toroid; the inductance was 25–30 mH, and the resistance was 4–4.5 Ω, depending on the model used. Great care was taken to provide shielding and very low leakage current. The coil was excited with bursts of sinusoidal current

1–100 kHz in frequency; the duration of the burst was selectable from 0.1 msec to 10 sec. A pickup coil in the air gap was used to measure the field strength. Typically, 20 V at 20 kHz was applied to the energizing coil on the toroidal core. Tetanic contractions were produced with a variety of stimulus burst durations and frequencies. Oberg found that the efficiency of stimulation was best when the nerve was at the edge of the air gap in the toroidal core, rather than in the center where the field is more uniform. He pointed out that the design of the air gap merits careful consideration.

Magnetically induced stimulation of the muscles of the hand, face, and shoulders in humans and stimulation of the phrenic, ulnar, and femoral nerves in the dog was reported by Hallgren (1973). A flat coil of 20 turns of 14-gauge copper wire with an iron core 1 in. in diameter (inductance 2–4 μH) was energized by discharging a 500-μF capacitor charged to 200 V. The charge–discharge circuitry permitted the delivery of stimuli having a frequency up to 45/sec. However, at this high rate, the coil became very hot after 1 min. A water-cooling jacket was added to solve this problem. Perhaps the most significant finding in this study is that none of the human subjects reported pain from the stimulation.

Polson et al. (1982) described the use of an eight-turn flat coil, 35 mm in diameter, to stimulate the median nerve in humans, causing the thumb muscles to twitch. The muscle action potential was recorded. The coil was made with 2-mm-diameter copper wire and had an inductance of 3 μH. A bank of twelve 500-μF capacitors charged to 500 V was discharged into the coil. The stored energy was 750 J, and the peak current was 6800 A, producing a peak field strength of 2.2 T.

Twitches in the muscles of the arm and leg of humans were produced by Barker et al. (1985), who placed a flat coil 10 cm in diameter on the scalp. The current pulse (4000 A) was derived from a capacitor bank. The electromyogram of the thumb muscles was recorded with skin-surface electrodes. The subjects reported that the muscle twitches were produced "without causing distress or pain." The maximum frequency of stimulation was once every 3 sec.

Magnetically induced stimulating current has advantages over stimulation with skin-surface electrodes. Recall that the sensory receptors are largely in the skin, which overlies a layer of fat. To stimulate tissue below the fat layer, the current must pass through all the invervening tissues, usually causing pain or discomfort. With magnetically induced stimulation, the current in the skin and fat is low because of their high resistivities. Magnetic fields pass freely through all living tissues and induce eddy currents, causing potential differences that produce stimulation. Although only a small amount of current flowing in a tissue is needed for excitation, the effective coupling between the coil and the tissues is very low. Therefore, rather large currents are needed in the excitation coil to produce rather small eddy currents in the excitable tissue.

Magnetically induced stimulation is usually achieved by discharging a capacitor into a low-resistance air-core inductor. The high flux densities required largely preclude the use of ferromagnetic materials because of their saturation characteristics. It is the changing current flow in the coil that produces the changing magnetic field that produces the eddy current that stimulates. Figure 47a illustrates a typical

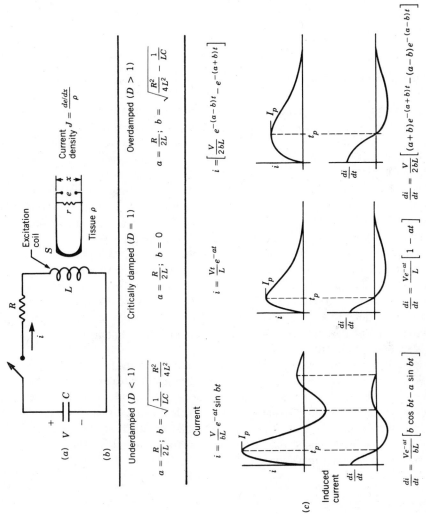

Figure 47 (a) Typical magnetic (eddy-current) stimulator and (b) excitation-coil current (*i*) and (c) induced current (*di/dt*) waveforms for the underdamped (*D* < 1.0), critically damped (*D* = 1.0), and overdamped (*D* > 1.0) conditions. Damping $D = R\sqrt{c}/2\sqrt{L}$.

527

stimulator. The excitable tissue is represented by a single-turn coil (S) connected to a resistor (r). The current i that flows in the excitation coil depends on the voltage V to which the capacitor (C) is charged and the damping coefficient D, which depends on the relationship between the inductance L, capacitance C, and resistance R. It is desirable to achieve low damping. Damping D is given by

$$D = \frac{R}{2}\sqrt{\frac{C}{L}}.$$

Figure 47*b* illustrates the current waveform i in the excitation coil L when the charged capacitor C is discharged. The magnetic field mirrors the current waveform. The voltage e induced in the one-turn coil S that represents the tissue depends on the rate of change of the current (di/dt). Because of this, it is highly desirable to employ a high current flowing through a coil of low inductance. Therefore, every effort is taken to use large-diameter wire to keep resistance R as low as possible and $D < 1.0$.

Because the eddy-current stimulus depends on the rate of change current in the excitation of coil, the waveform of the stimulus e will be quite different from that of the current in the excitation coil, as shown in Fig. 47*c*. Note that the duration of the induced stimulus (di/dt) measured from the onset to the first zero crossing is much less than that of the current i flowing in the excitation coil. Observe that the waveform of e consists of two phases, positive and negative, whereas that in the excitation coil is unidirectional (with critical damping or overdamping) and polyphasic with $D < 1.0$. In practice, the effective duration of the first stimulus wave is usually quite short, typically a fraction of a millisecond. Such pulses are best applied to stimulate tissues with short chronaxies and membrane time constants, such as nerve fibers.

Stimulation is achieved by exceeding a critical current density J in the excitable tissue. The current density is equal to the voltage gradient (de/dx) divided by the resistivity ρ of the medium carrying the current. The voltage gradient de/dx is the voltage e divided by the small distance x over which it exists. At present, there are no data that specify the current density (and pulse duration) needed to excite various tissues. It is estimated that a rheobasic average current density of 1–2 mA/cm^2 is required for stimulation.

Stimulation with Capacitive Electrodes

A capacitor consists of two conductors separated by an insulator (dielectric). A capacitive electrode consists of a conductor covered by an insulator, and the tissue constitutes the other conductor. Such an electrode is traditionally used as a dispersive electrode for electrosurgical (0.5–2 MHz) current or to deliver diathermy (13.56 or 27.12 MHz) current to warm tissue. Capacitive electrodes have infrequently been used to stimulate excitable tissue. However, because of their unique properties and the special requirements that they impose on the stimulator, they merit some discussion.

One unusual form of capacitive electrode used to stimulate motor nerves percutaneously by Batrow and Batrow (1963) is similar to the vacuum tube electrodes used with old diathermy units (see Geddes, 1984b). The Batrow electrode (Fig. 48) consisted of a glass chamber at the end of a bent glass tube in which there was argon at a low pressure. A metal electrode protruded from the glass tube within the handle. When the active surface of the glass chamber was placed on the skin over a motor point and a high-voltage, short-duration pulse was applied between the glass electrode and a dispersive electrode on the subject, the gas in the glow chamber glowed, forming a conductor within the chamber. The capacitive current caused stimulation of the motor nerve, producing a twitch in the associated muscle. The voltage pulse was typically 30–60 kV, and the duration of the pulse was in the range of tens of microseconds.

Interestingly, the Batrow capacitive electrode produced minimal skin sensation for neuromuscular stimulation. The combination of a short-duration pulse, which is inefficient for stimulating sensory receptors, and a capacitive electrode, with its relatively uniform current distribution thereunder (Pearce and Geddes, 1980), reduces the skin sensation dramatically. If a small moistened pad is placed between the glass electrode and the skin, there is virtually no skin sensation. Surprisingly, this technology has seen little use in neuromuscular stimulation. Such a capacitive electrode could be made easily without the glowing gaseous conductor.

Geddes et al. (1987) described a capacitor electrode suitable for motor-point stimulation (Fig. 49a) that was constructed from No. 7740 fused silica tubing (13 mm o.d., 11 mm i.d.). The dielectric constant is 5.1. The tubing was heated in a flame to close the end and blown to form the end chamber, 1 in. in diameter and

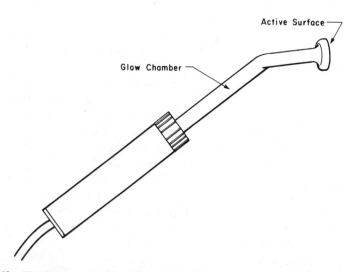

Figure 48 The Batrow capacitive electrode, which contains argon gas at a low pressure. When a high-voltage pulse is applied, the gas ionizes, becoming one conductor of the capacitive electrode. The glass is the dielectric, and the skin of the subject is the other conductor of the capacitive electrode.

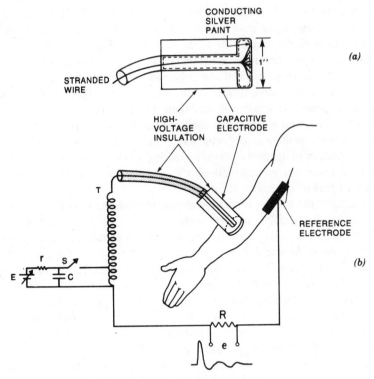

Figure 49 (*a*) The capacitive electrode and (*b*) the method of applying a high-voltage, short-duration pulse of current to it. S is a triggered thyratron or SCR.

slightly more than 1 mm thick. The electrode within the chamber was formed by passing a stranded wire down the tube so that the strands spread radially when the terminal portion of the wire entered the end chamber. The stranded wire was advanced further until the individual strands were all in contact with the surface of the end of the chamber. Then conducting silver paint (Silver Print, Cat. 21-22, General Cement Co.) was injected via a long thin-walled tube so that it covered all of the radial strands. In this way, the electrode consisted of the inner diameter of the chamber. When placed on the skin, the capacitance is on the order of 5 pF.

The stimulator consisted of an autotransformer of the ignition-coil type. Into the primary was discharged an 8-μF capacitor. The maximum open-circuit voltage was variable to 60 kV. Figure 49*b* illustrates the stimulator, the active capacitive electrode on the skin of the forearm, and the large-area reference conducting electrode on the back of the upper arm. This figure includes a sketch of the current waveform with the capacitive electrode applied to the skin.

Stimulation of the motor points of the forearm produced twitches and tetanic contractions with ease, causing little skin sensation. Even less sensation was perceived when a thin, 1-in.-diameter gauze pad, lightly moistened with tap water, was placed between the skin and the capacitive electrode.

Another type of capacitive stimulating electrode, described by Schaldach (1971), was designed for cardiac pacing. The electrode consisted of electrochemically deposited tantalum oxide on a pacemaker electrode. Schaldach pointed out that such an electrode behaves like a pure capacitor and that no electrolytic action can occur at the interface with tissue. Stimulation results from a change in the charge distribution at the interface. In animal trials it was found that only a thin fibrotic layer covered the dielectric and that the capacitance remained stable. Only one-third as much energy was needed to pace the heart as for a conventional electrode of the same area.

Capacitive stimulating electrodes have relatively high impedance and therefore require high voltages to achieve stimulation. They are well suited to short-duration pulses and for this reason will probably be best suited to skin-surface stimulation of large-diameter nerve fibers, which have short chronaxies and membrane time constants.

The design of a capacitive stimulating electrode merits special care because of the high voltages required and the small electrode–subject capacitance. The high voltage requires that the dielectric of the capacitive electrode be a material of low loss and high dielectric strength. The thickness of the dielectric must be able to withstand the applied voltage.

REFERENCES

Adrian, E. D. 1916. The electrical reactions of muscles before and after nerve injury. *Brain* **39**:1–33.

Adrian, E. D. 1919. The response to human sensory nerves to currents of short duration. *J. Physiol.* **53**:70–85.

Alexander, L. 1938. Electrical injuries to the central nervous system. *Med. Clin. North Am.* **22**:663–688.

Anderson, A. B., and W. A. Munson. 1951. Electrical excitation of nerves in the skin at audiofrequencies. *J. Acoust. Soc. Am.* **23**:155–159.

Association for the Advancement of Medical Instrumentation (AAMI). 1982. *American National Standard Cardiac Defibrillator Devices.* AAMI, Arlington, VA (plus errata ANSI/AAMI DF2 Err 1985).

Association for the Advancement of Medical Instrumentation (AAMI). 19 . *Standard for Transcutaneous Electrical Nerve Stimulation (Proposed).* AAMI, Arlington, VA.

Association for the Advancement of Medical Instrumentation (AAMI/ANSI). 1982a. *Safe Current Limits for Electromedical Apparatus.* AAMI, Arlington, VA.

Association for the Advancement of Medical Instrumentation (AAMI/ANSI). 1982b. *Standard Cardiac Defibrillator Devices.* AAMI, Arlington, VA.

Ayers, G. M., S. W. Aronson, and L. A. Geddes. 1986. Comparison of the ability of the Lapicque and exponential strength-duration curves to fit experimentally obtained perception threshold data. *Australas. Phys. Eng. Sci. Med.* **9**(3):111–116.

Babbs, C. F., and S. J. Whistler. 1978. Evaluation of the operating internal resistance, inductance and capacitance of intact damped sine wave defibrillators. *Med. Instrum.* **12**:34–37.

Babbs, C. F., S. J. Whistler, and L. A. Geddes. 1980. Evaluation of the operating internal resistance and capacitance of intact trapezoidal waveform defibrillator. *Med. Instrum.* **14**:67–69.

Barker, A. T., R. Jalinous, and I. L. Freeston. 1985. Noninvasive magnetic stimulation of human motor cortex. *Lancet* **2**:1106–1107.

Barlow, H. B., H. L. Kahn, and E. G. Walsh. 1947. Visual sensations aroused by magnetic fields. *Am. J. Physiol.* **48**:372.

Batrow, J., and P. Batrow. 1963. Electrophysiotherapy apparatus. U.S. Patent 3,077,884, February 1963.

Becker, R. O. 1983. Biological effects of magnetic fields. *Med. Electron. Biol. Eng.* **1**:293–302.

Beecher, H. 1959. *Measurement of Subjective Responses.* Oxford Univ. Press, London and New York.

Beer, B. 1901. Ueber das Auftraten einer objectiven Lichtempfindung in magnetischen Felde. *Wien. Klin. Wochenschr.* **15**:108–109.

Bernstein, T. 1973. A grand success. *IEEE Spectrum* **10**:54–58.

Bickford, R. G., and B. D. Fremming. 1965. Neural stimulation by pulsed magnetic fields in animals and man. *Dig. 6th Int. Conf. Med. Biol. Eng.* Paper 7.

Blair, H. A. 1932. On the intensity-time relations for stimulation by electric currents. *J. Gen. Physiol.* **15**:177–185, 709–729, 731–755.

Bourland, J. D., W. A. Tacker, and L. A. Geddes. 1978a. Strength- duration curves for trapezoidal waveforms of various tilts for transchest defibrillation in animals. *Med. Instrum.* **12**:38–41.

Bourland, J. D., W. A. Tacker, L. A. Geddes, and V. Chaffee. 1978b. Comparative efficacy of damped sine wave and square wave current for transchest ventricular defibrillation in animals. *Med. Instrum.* **12**:42–45.

Bourland, J. D., J. L. Wessale, M. J. Kallok, W. A. Tacker, and L. A. Geddes. 1982. Ventricular defibrillation threshold in dogs using reciprocal pulses. *Proc. 17th Annu. Meet. Assoc. Adv. Med. Instrum., 1982* p. 15.

Bowman, B. R. and L. L. Baker. 1985. Effects of waveform parameters on comfort during transcutaneous neuromuscular electrical stimulation. *Ann. Biomed. Eng.* **13**:59–74.

Brazier, M. A. B. Electrical Activity of the Nervous System. 1951. London, Sir Isaac Pitman 220 pp.

Campbell, B. A., and R. Teghtsoonian. 1958. Electrical and behavioral effects of different types of shock stimuli on the rat. *J. Comp. Physiol. Psychol.* **51**:185–192.

Dalziel, C. F. 1956. Effects of electric shock on man. *IRE Trans. Med. Electron.* **5**:44–62.

d'Arsonval, A. 1893a. Action physiologique des courants alternatifs à grande fréquence. *Arch. Physiol. Norm. Pathol.* **5**:401–408, 780–790.

d'Arsonval, A. 1893b. Influence de la fréquencies sur les effets physiologiques des courants alternatifs. *C. R. Hebd. Seances Acad. Sci.* **116**:630–633.

d'Arsonval, A. 1896. Dispositifs pour la mesure des courants alternatifs de toutes frequences. *C. R. Seances Soc. Biol. Ses Fil.* **2**:450–451.

d'Arsonval, A. 1897. Action physiologique des courants alternatifs a grande frequence. *Arch. Electr. Med.* **7**:133.

Dominguez, G., and A. Fozzard. 1970. Influence of extracellular K concentration on cable properties and excitability of sheep purkinje cardiacfibers. *Circ. Res.* **26**:565–574.

Donaldson, N. de N., and P. E. K. Donaldson. 1986. When are actively balanced biphasic (Lilly) stimulating pulses necessary in a neurological prosthesis. *Med. Biol. Eng. Comput.* **24**(1):41–49, 50–56.

Dunlap, K. 1911. Visual sensations from the alternating magnetic field. *Science* **33**:68–71.

Ferris, L. P., B. G. King, P. W. Spence, and H. B. Williams. 1936. Effect of electric shock on the heart. *Electron. Eng.* **85**:498–515.

Forbes, T. W., and A. L. Bernstein. 1935. The standardization of sixty-cycle electric shock for practical use in psychological experimentation. *J. Gen. Psychol.* **12**:436–442.

Fozzard, H. A. 1966. Membrane capacitance of the cardiac purkinje fiber. *J. Physiol.* **182**:255–267.

Fozzard, H. A., and M. Schoenberg. 1972. Strength–duration curves in cardiac purkinje fibers. *J. Physiol.* **236**:593–618.

Furman, S., J. Garvey, and P. Hurzeler. 1975. Pulse duration variation and electrode size as features in pacemaker longevity. *J. Thorac. Cardiovasc. Surg.* **60:**382–389.

Geddes, L. A. 1984a. The background of electromedicine. *IEEE Eng. Med. Biol.* **3**(4):8–23.

Geddes, L. A. 1984b. A short history of the electrical stimulation of excitable tissue. *Physiologist* **27**(1):S1–S47.

Geddes, L. A., and L. E. Baker. 1969. Hazards in the use of low frequencies for the measurement of physiological events by impedance. *Med. Biol. Eng.* **7:**289–296.

Geddes, L. A., and L. E. Baker. 1971. Response to the passage of electric current through the body. *J. Assoc. Adv. Med. Instrum.* **5:**13–18.

Geddes, L. A., and J. D. Bourland. 1985. Tissue stimulation: Theoretical considerations and practical applications. *Med. Biol. Eng. Comput.* **23**(2):131–137.

Geddes, L. A., P. Cabler, A. G. Moore, J. Rosborough, and W. A. Tacker. 1973. Threshold 60-Hz current required for ventricular fibrillation in subjects of various body weights. *IEEE Trans. Biomed. Eng.* **BME-20:**465–468.

Geddes, L. A., S. S. Grubbs, P. S. Wilcox, and W. A. Tacker. 1977. The thoracic windows for electrical ventricular defibrillation current. *Am. Heart J.* **94**(1):67–72.

Geddes, L. A., W. D. Voorhees, C. F. Babbs, R. Sisken, and J. DeFord. 1984. Precordial pacing windows. *Pace* **7:**806–812.

Geddes, L. A., C. F. Babbs, W. D. Voorhees, and A. Aronson. 1985a. Choice of the optimum duration for precordial cardiac pacing. *Pace* **8:**862–869.

Geddes, L. A., M. Niebauer, C. F. Babbs, and J. D. Bourland. 1985b. Fundamental criteria underlying the efficacy and safety of ventricular defibrillating current waveforms. *Med. Biol. Eng. Comput.* **23**(2):122–130.

Geddes, L. A., M. Hinds, and K. Foster. 1987. Stimulation with capacitive electrodes. *Med. Biol. Eng. Comput.* **25**(3):359–360.

Gibson, R. H. 1963. Requirements for the use of electrical stimulation of the skin. *Proc. Int. Congr. Technol. Blindness* **2:**183–207.

Gilmer, B. von H. 1937. The sensitivity of the finger to alternating electrical current. *Am. J. Psychol.* **49:**444–449.

Gilmer, B. von H. 1961. Toward cutaneous electropulse communication. *J. Physiol.* **52:**211–222.

Goetzl, F. R., D. Y. Burrill, and A. C. Ivy. 1943. A critical analysis of algesimetric methods with suggestions for a useful procedure. *Q. Bull. Northwestern Univ. Med. Sch.* **17:**280–291.

Gracanin, F., and A. Trnkcozy. 1975. Optimum stimulation parameters for minimum pain in the chronic stimulation of innervated muscle. *Arch. Phys. Med. Rehabil.* **56**(6):243–249.

Hallgren, R. 1973. Inductive nerve stimulation. *IEEE Trans. Biomed. Eng.* **BME-20**(6):470–472.

Harris, S. C., and L. E. Blockus. 1952. The reliability and validity of tooth-pulp algesimetry. *J. Pharmacol.* **104:**135–148.

Hassin, G. B. 1933. Changes in the brain in legal electrocution. *Arch. Neurol. Psychiatry* **30:**1046–1060.

Hawkes, G. R., and J. S. Warm. 1960. The sensory range of electrical stimulation of the skin. *Am. J. Psychol.* **73:**485–487.

Higgins, D. B., B. Tursky, and C. E. Schwartz. 1971. Shock elicited pain and its reduction by concurrent tactile stimulation. *Science* **172:**866–867.

Health Devices. 1981. Transcutaneous electrical nerve stimulator (TENS) units. *Health Devices* **10**(8):179–195.

Hill, H. E., H. G. Flanary, C. H. Konetsky, and A. Winkler. 1952. Relationship of electrically induced pain and the amperage and wattage of the shock. *J. Clin. Invest.* **31:**464–472.

Hill, A. V. 1935. Excitation and accommodation in nerve. *Proc. R. Soc. Med.* **B119:**305–354.

Hinds, M., G. M. Ayers, J. D. Bourland, L. A. Geddes, W. A. Tacker, and N. E. Fearnot. 1987. Comparison of the efficacy of defibrillation with the damped sine and constant tilt current waveforms in the intact animal. *Med. Instrum.* **21**(2):92–96.

Irnich, W. 1980. The chronaxie and its practical importance. *Pace* **3**:292–301.

Jackson, T. A., and B. F. Riess. 1934. Electric shock with different size electrodes. *J. Gen. Psychol.* **45**:262–266.

Jaffe, R. H. 1928. Electropathology. *Arch. Pathol.* **5**:837–870.

Jex-Blake, A. J. 1913. Death by electric currents and by lightning. *Brit. Med. J.* **1**:425–430, 492–498, 548–552, 601–603.

Kennelly, A. E., and E. F. W. Alexanderson. 1910. The physiological tolerance of alternating-current strengths up to frequencies of 100 kilocycles per second. *Electron. World* **50**:154–156.

Kolin, A., N. Q. Brill, and P. J. Broberg. 1959. Stimulation of irritable tissues by means of an alternating magnetic field. *Proc. Soc. Exp. Biol. Med.* **102**:251–253.

Koslow, M., A. Bak, and C. L. Li. 1973. C-fiber excitability in the cat. *J. Neurol.* **41**:745–753.

Kouwenhoven, N. B., and D. R. Hooker. 1936. Electric shock; effects of frequency. *Electron. Eng.* **55**:384–386.

Lacourse, J. B., W. T. Miller, M. Vogt, and S. M. Selkowitz. 1985. Effects of high frequency current on nerve and muscle. *IEEE Trans. Biomed. Eng.* **BME-32**(1):82–86.

Langworthy, O. R. 1930. Abnormalities in the central nervous system by electrical injuries. *J. Exp. Med.* **51**:943–968.

Lapicque, L. 1909. Definition experimental de l'excitation. *C. R. Hebd. Seances Acad. Sci.* **67**(2):280–283.

Lapicque, L. 1926. *L'excitabilité en function du temps.* Presses Univ. de France, Paris, 371 pp.

Lee, W. R., and J. R. Scott. 1973. Thresholds of fibrillating leakage currents along ventricular catheters. *Cardiovasc. Res.* **7**:495–500.

Li, C-L., and A. Bak. 1976. Excitability characteristics of the A and C fibers in the peroneal nerve. *Exp. Neurol.* **50**:67–79.

Liberson, W. T., H. J. Holmquist, D. Scot, and M. Dow. 1961. Functional electrotherapy. *Arch. Phys. Med. Rehabil.* **42**:101–105.

Lilly, J. C., J. R. Hughes, E. C. Alvord, and T. W. Gallin. 1955. Brief non-injurious electric waveform for stimulation of the brain. *Science* **121**:468–469.

Long, G., and V. D. Masciarelli. 1963. Electrophysiologic splint for the hand. *Arch. Phys. Med. Rehabil.* **44**:495–503.

Maass, J. A., and M. M. Asa. 1970. Contactiless nerve stimulation and signal detection by inductive transducer. *IEEE Trans. Magn.* **MAG-6**(2):322–326.

MacDonald, C. F. 1892. The infliction of the death penalty by means of electricity. *Trans. Med. Soc. State N. Y.* pp. 400–427.

Machin, J. W. 1978. Thoracic impedance of human subjects. *Med. Biol. Eng. Comput.* **16**:169.

Magnusson, C. E., and H. C. Stevens. 1911. Visual sensations caused by the changes in the strength of a magnetic field. *Am. J. Physiol.* **29**:124–136.

Magnusson, C. E., and H. C. Stevens. 1914. Visual sensations created by a magnetic field. *Philos. Mag.* [6] **28**:188–207.

Mannheimer, G. S. 1978. Electrode placement for transcutaneous electrical nerve stimulation. *Phys. Ther.* **58**(12):1455–1462.

Mannheimer, G. S. et al. 1978. *Clinical Transcutaneous Electrical Nerve Stimulation.* Davis, Philadelphia, PA.

Milner, M., A. O. Quanbury, and J. V. Basmajian. 1970. Surface electrical stimulation of the lower limb. *Arch. Phys. Med. Rehabil.* **51**:540–548.

Monsees, L. R., and D. G. McQuarrie. 1971. Is an intravascular catheter a conductor? *Med. Electron. Data* **12**:26–27.

Mueller, E. E., R. Loeffel, and S. Mead. 1953. Skin impedance in relation to pain threshold testing by electrical means. *J. Appl. Physiol.* **5**:746–752.

Nethken, R. P., and M. A. Bulot. 1967. Threshold of electrical sensation on the upper human arm. *Trans. Reg. 3rd IEEE Meet.*

Notermans, S. L. H. 1966. Measurement of the pain threshold determined by electrical stimulation and its clinical application. *Neurology* **16**:1071–1086.

Oberg, P. A. 1973. Magnetic stimulation of nerve tissue. *Med. Biol. Eng.* **11**(1):55–64.

Pearce, J. A., and L. A. Geddes. 1980. The characteristics of capacitive electro-surgical dispersive electrodes. *Proc. 15th Annu. Meet. Assoc. Adv. Med. Instrum., 1980.*

Pearce, J. A., J. D. Bourland, W. Neilsen, L. A. Geddes, and M. Voelz. 1982. Myocardial stimulation with ultrashort duration current pulses. *Pace* **5**:52–58.

Peckham, P. H. 1983. Restoration of upper extremity function. *IEEE Eng. Med. Biol.* **2**(3):30–32.

Peckham, P. H., and J. T. Mortimer. 1977. Restoration of hand function in the quadriplegic through electrical stimulation. In *Functional Electrical Stimulation.* F. T. Hambrecht (ed.). Dekker, New York, 547 pp.

Petrofsky, J. S., and C. A. Phillips. 1983. Computer controlled walking in paralyzed individuals. *J. Neurol. Orthop. Surg.* **4**:153.

Petrofsky, J. S., H. Heaton, and C. A. Phillips. 1983. Outdoor bicycle for exercise in paraplegics and quadriplegics. *J. Biomed. Eng.* **5**:292–298.

Pfeiffer, E. A. 1968. Electrical stimulation of sensory nerves with skin electrodes for research, diagnosis, communication and behavioral conditioning: A survey. *Med. Biol. Eng.* **6**:637–651.

Pfeiffer, E. A. and S. Stevens, D. S. Problems of electro-aversive shock in behavior therapy. Neuroelectric Research, D. V. Reynolds and Sjoberg, A. E., Eds. Springfield, IL. 1971.

Plonsey, R. 1969. *Bioelectric Phenomena.* McGraw-Hill, New York, 380 pp.

Polson, M. J. R., A. T. Barker, and I. L. Freeston. 1982. Stimulation of nerve trunks with time-varying magnetic fields. *Med. Biol. Eng. Comput.* **20**:243–244.

Prévost, J. L., and F. Battelli. 1900. Influence du nombre des périodes sur les effets mortels des courants alternatifs. *J. Physiol. Pathol. Gen.* **2**:755–766.

Pritchard, E. A. 1934. Changes in the nervous system due to electrocution. *Lancet* **1**:1163–1167.

Ranck, J. S. 1975. Which currents are excieted in extracellular stimulation of mammalian central nervous system. *Brain Res.* **98**:417–440.

Rentsch, W. 1965. The application of stimulating currents with magnetic inductive energy transmission. *Dig. 6th Int. Conf. Med. Biol. Eng., 1965* Paper 7-5.

Ritchie, A. 1944. The electrical diagnosis of peripheral nerve injury. *Brain* **67**:314–330.

Roy, O. Z., J. R. Scott, and G. C. Park. 1976. 60 Hz ventricular fibrillation and pump failure threshold versus electrode area. *IEEE Trans. Biomed. Eng.* **BME-23**(1):45–48.

Roy, O. Z., G. C. Park, and J. R. Scott. 1977. Intracardiac fibrillation threshold as a function of the duration of 60Hz current and electrode area. *IEEE Trans. Biomed. Eng.* **BME-24**(2):430–435.

Schaldach, M. 1971. New pacemaker electrodes. *Trans. Am. Soc. Artif. Intern. Organs* **17**:29–35.

Schmitt, O. H. 1943. A radiofrequency coupled tissue stimulator. *Science* **107**:432.

Sigel, H. 1953–1954. Prick threshold stimulation with square wave current. *Yale J. Biol. Med.* **26**:145–154.

Spitzka, E. A., and H. E. Radash. 1912. The brain lesions produced by electricity. *Am. J. Med. Sci.* **144**:341–347.

Staewen, W. S. 1964. Electric shock hazards. *Md. State Med. J.* **13**:70–73.

Staewen, W. S., M. Mower, and B. Tabatznik. 1969. The significance of leakage currents in hospital electrical devices. *J. Mt. Sinai Hosp.* (*N.Y.*) **15**:3–10.

Starmer, C. F., and R. E. Whalen. 1973. Current density and electrically induced ventricular fibrillation. *Med. Instrum.* **7**(2):158–161.

Starmer, C. F., H. McIntosh, and R. E. Whalen. 1971. Electrical hazards and cardiovascular function. *N. Engl. J. Med.* **284**:181–186.

Sternbach, R. A., and B. Tursky. 1965. Ethnic differences among housewives in psychophysiological and skin-potential responses to electric shock. *Psychophysiology* **2**:241–246.

Tacker, W. A., and L. A. Geddes. 1980. *Electrical Defibrillation.* CRC Press, Boca Raton, FL, 192 pp.

Thompson, S. P. 1910. A physiological effect of an alternating magnetic field. *Proc. R. Soc. London, Ser. B,* **82**:396–397.

Tortora, D. F. 1981. *Understanding Electronic Dog Training.* Tri-Tronics, Inc., Tucson, AZ, 119 pp.

Tursky, B., and P. D. Watson. 1964. Controlled physical and subjective intensity of electrical shock. *Psychophysiology* **1**:151–162.

Tursky, B., P. D. Watson, and D. N. O'Connor. 1965. A concentric shock electrode for pain stimulation. *Psychophysiology* **1**:296–298.

Vodovnik, L., C. Long, E. Regenos, and A. Lippay. 1965. Pain response to different tetanizing currents. *Arch. Phys. Med. Rehabil.* **46**:187–192.

Vodovnik, L., M. Dimitrijevic, T. Prevoc, and M. Logar. 1966. Electronic walking aids for patients with peroneal palsy. *World Med. Electron.* **4**(2):58–61.

Vodovnik, L., A. Stanic, and R. Kralj. 1977. Functional electrical stimulation in Ljubljana. In *Functional Electrical Stimulation.* F. T. Hambrecht (ed.). Dekker, New York, 547 pp.

Wall, P. D., and W. H. Sweet. 1967. Temporary abolition of pain in man. *Science* (Jan. 6):108–109.

Walsh, P. 1946. Magnetic stimulation of the human retina. *Fed. Proc.* **5**(1)(Part 2):109–110.

Waters, R. 1977. Electrical stimulation of peroneal nerves in man. In *Functional Electrical Stimulation.* F. T. Hambrecht (Ed.). Dekker, New York, 547 pp.

Weinberg, D. I., and J. C. Artley. 1962. Electric shock hazards in cardiac catheterization. *Circ. Res.* **1**:1004–1009.

Weiss, G. G. 1901. Sur la possibilité de rendre comparables entre eux les appareils: A l'excitation. *Arch. Ital. Biol.* **35**:413–446.

Whalen, R. E., C. F. Starner, and H. D. McIntosh. 1964. Electrical hazards associated with cardiac pacemaking. *Ann. N.Y. Acad. Sci.* **111**:922.

Zoll, P. M. 1952. Resuscitation of the heart in ventricular standstill by external cardiac stimulation. *N. Engl. J. Med.* **247**:768.

Zoll, P. M., R. M. Zoll, and A. H. Belgard. 1981. External noninvasive electrical stimulation of the heart. *CRC Crit. Care Med.* **9**:393.

11

Detection of Physiological Events by Impedance

INTRODUCTION

Often it is necessary to measure a physiological event for which there is no specialized transducer. In many circumstances transduction can be carried out by means of the impedance method if the event can be caused to exhibit a change in dimension, dielectric, or conductivity or a rearrangement of these components. The elegantly simple technique requires only the application of two or more electrodes, and it has been used successfully for many years to detect a remarkable variety of physiological events. It is extremely practical for phenomena that produce a large change in one or more of the quantities just mentioned. With the simplest "transducers"—that is, appropriately placed electrodes—the impedance between them may reflect seasonal variations, blood flow, cardiac activity, respired volume, bladder, blood, and kidney volumes, uterine contractions, nervous activity, the galvanic skin reflex, the volume of blood cells, clotting, blood pressure, and salivation. In some instances the impedance is dissected into its resistive and reactive components; in others, the total impedance is measured. Often only a change in impedance, with or without resolution into its components, contains information sufficient to describe the physiological event. Many of the techniques that have been employed are presented in this chapter.

The impedance method offers all the advantages of the indirect techniques used in the biomedical sciences, the most important being that in many applications the integument need not be penetrated to make the measurement. Since electrodes are very easy to apply, practicality is an attractive feature of the method. Because a specialized transducer is not required, the same electrodes and the same impedance apparatus often can be used to detect a variety of events in humans and animals. In the absence of a transducer, the response time is governed mainly by the event. If the electrodes are small enough, they offer little restraint to the subject and need not modify the phenomenon under study. Unlike many transducers, electrodes are affected little by temperature and barometric pressure changes. This property makes the impedance method practical for monitoring events under changing environmental conditions. In addition, because the usually bothersome galvanic potentials produced when metallic electrodes come into contact with electrolytes are not a part of the signal when the impedance method is employed, the problem of canceling these unwanted voltages is eliminated. A further advantage of the impedance method is obtained through employment of carrier-system techniques, which permit the use of narrow-band amplifiers with consequent enhancement of the signal-to-noise ratio.

The impedance method is subject to the limitations inherent in many indirect techniques. Since frequently the signal is obtained at a distance from the phenomenon, resolution is compromised, and the signal is often difficult to calibrate in true physiological terms. However, uncalibratible signals that directly reflect a physiological event can have considerable value for monitoring changes under a variety of experimentally controlled conditions. Uncalibrated tracking signals have value in time-domain studies.

SAFETY CONSIDERATIONS

When the impedance method is used to measure physiological events, the current used must not stimulate or heat the tissues. When current is passed through living tissue, special consideration (Geddes et al., 1964, 1969, 1971b) must be given to the structures between the electrodes. Muscle (skeletal, cardiac, and smooth), nerve fibers, sensory receptors, glands, and body fluids all form part of the current-carrying circuit. The parameters for electrical stimulation of the irritable tissues in the current path can be found in their strength–duration curves, which are plots of the threshold current required for excitation versus the duration of the single testing stimulus. This subject is discussed extensively in Chapter 10.

When sinusoidal alternating current is used to measure physiological events by impedance, it is necessary to use frequencies and intensities that do not stimulate excitable tissue. Sinusoidal alternating current can be roughly equated to a train of short-duration pulses, with a duration equal to the period, that is, $1/\text{frequency}$. Since the strength–duration curves for all excitable tissues rise with decreasing duration, it is obvious that the minimum risk of stimulation is achieved by using high-frequency alternating current. In practice, frequencies in excess of 1 kHz are used; typically frequencies from 10 to 100 kHz are used. It should be obvious that the risk of tissue stimulation decreases with increasing frequency. Conversely, with the higher frequencies, more current can be used safely to measure a physiological event, thereby providing a larger signal. However, there may be reasons for choosing the frequency on the basis of the nature of the electrical properties of the tissues between the impedance-measuring electrodes; this subject is discussed in the section dealing with the impedance of tissues.

With the low current intensities used to measure physiological events, tissue heating is not a problem. Currents in the range of 50 μA at frequencies above 1 kHz and up to a few milliamperes at 100 kHz are typical. Of course, the location of the electrodes with respect to excitable tissues constitutes an important factor in helping decide the safe current level and frequency. More information on these points can be found in Chapter 10.

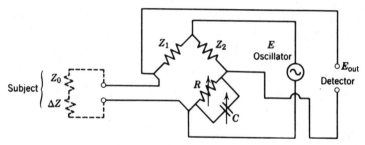

Figure 1 Impedance bridge.

IMPEDANCE-MEASURING CIRCUITS

There are two basic impedance-measuring circuits: the bridge and bipolar and tetrapolar circuits. With the bridge circuit (Fig. 1), the bridge is adjusted (balanced) so that the output voltage is zero when the impedance (and phase angle) of R and C are equivalent to those of Z_0. Then the output is proportional to ΔZ. The bridge circuit can be converted to a constant-current circuit by making Z_1 high with respect to $Z_0 + \Delta Z$. Thus, the current through the subject is independent of the subject impedance (Z_0).

With the bipolar symmetrical constant-current circuit (Fig. 2), the two resistances (R, R) are made high with respect to $Z_0 + \Delta Z$. Therefore, the output voltage (E_{out}) is linearly proportional to $Z_0 + \Delta Z$. This condition identifies constant-current operation, in which the current through the subject is independent of the subject impedance (Z_0).

With the tetrapolar constant-current circuit (Fig. 3), current is admitted to the subject by two electrodes (1, 4) connected to a voltage source via two resistors (R, R) that are high in value with respect to the impedance appearing between electrodes 1 and 4. Alternatively, an active constant-current source can be used. The output voltage (E_{out}) is obtained from two potential-measuring electrodes (2, 3) and is proportional to $Z_0 + \Delta Z$.

The properties of the bridge and constant-current bipolar and tetrapolar constant-current circuits will now be described.

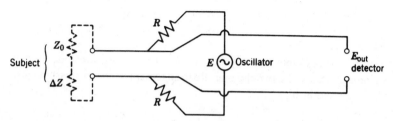

Figure 2 Symmetrical bipolar constant-current circuit. (For simplicity the constant-current circuit is illustrated by an oscillator and two resistances. R, R, which are much larger than $Z_0 + \Delta Z$.)

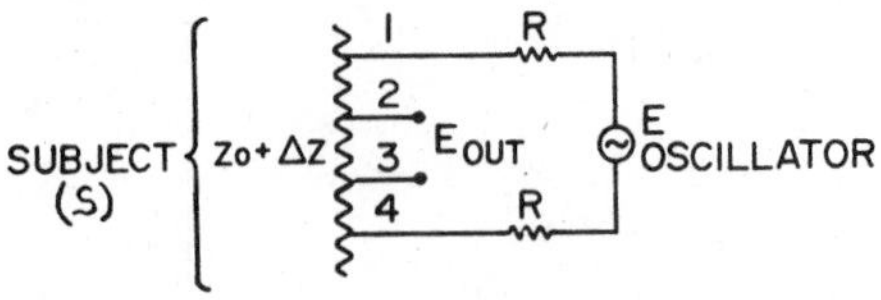

Figure 3   The tetrapolar constant-current circuit.

Bridge Circuit

When two electrodes are employed, the impedance bridge circuit diagramed in Fig. 1 can be used. In such an arrangement, the oscillator voltage E is applied to two opposite corners of the bridge and the detector is connected to the other two. When the ratio arms Z_1, Z_2 are resistors of equal value, the impedance bridge becomes a comparison bridge. The balancing arm RC may consist of parallel resistance and capacitance decade units that are adjusted to balance the bridge for the basal (Z_0) impedance between the electrode terminals. At balance, the value of the balance arm gives the equivalent parallel resistive and reactive components of the tissue–electrode circuit. If R and C are placed in series and the bridge is balanced, the new values for R and C give the equivalent series circuit between the electrode terminals. These equivalents are valid only for the frequency employed. With most bridges the impedance is measured in terms of a parallel or a series equivalent, but not both. Often it is desirable to transform one equivalent into the other; for example, if in a given case R_s and C_s are the series resistance and capacitance at a particular frequency f, the parallel equivalents R_p and C_p at the same frequency are given by

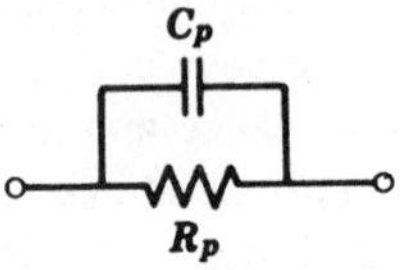

is equivalent to

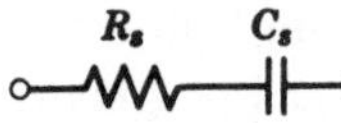

$$R_p = \frac{1 + (2\pi f C_s R_s)^2}{4\pi^2 f^2 C_s^2 R_s}, \qquad R_p = R_s + \frac{X_s^2}{R_s},$$

$$C_p = \frac{C_s}{1 + (2\pi f C_s R_s)^2}, \qquad X_p = X_s + \frac{R_s^2}{X_s}.$$

Frequently it is desirable to carry out the reverse process, that is, to express a series circuit in terms of a parallel one. Rearrangement of the expressions just given provides the relationships

$$R_s = \frac{R_p}{1 + (2\pi f C_p R_p)^2}, \qquad C_s = C_p\left[1 + \frac{1}{(2\pi f R_p C_p)^2}\right].$$

With the bridge circuit, the changes in impedance reflecting the physiological event produce a varying output voltage (E_{out}), which, after amplification and demodulation, is displayed to produce a record related to changes in the physiological event. It must be emphasized that an output is obtained if there is a change in either the resistive or the reactive component or in both. If it is desired to examine the magnitude of each component individually, a phase-sensitive detector is required.

If the bridge is operated at the balance point and without the use of a phase-sensitive detector, an output voltage is obtained if the impedance being measured increases or decreases. Under this operating condition, direction indication is lost. However, if after the bridge has been initially balanced, it is then unbalanced slightly by the addition of a small resistance in series with the impedance being measured, the output voltage from the bridge will increase and decrease with the impedance being measured. The amount of resistance added is dictated by the maximum change in impedance required to drive the bridge toward the balance point.

Precautions must be taken in using the bridge circuit to avoid having the size of the output voltage become dependent on the magnitude of Z_0, the basal impedance. For the same ΔZ, if Z_0 is small, more current will flow through Z_1 and Z_0, and the output (ΔE_{out}) will be large. This sensitivity dependence on Z_0 can be eliminated by making Z_1 much greater than $Z_0 + \Delta Z$, which allows the bridge to have the properties of the constant-current circuit, which is described next.

Bipolar Constant-Current Circuit

The constant-current bipolar electrode system is depicted in Fig. 2. Current from the oscillator is fed symmetrically to the electrodes through two resistances R, R, which are high in value with respect to the total impedance between the electrode terminals. With this circuit configuration the current through the subject is determined by these resistances and the oscillator voltage E and is independent of the electrode–subject impedance ($Z_0 + \Delta Z$). The detector is connected across the electrodes, and the voltage present is a function of the basal impedance between the electrodes (Z_0) and any change ΔZ due to the physiological event. It can easily be shown that the voltage across the electrodes is given by

$$E_{out} = \frac{E(Z_0 + \Delta Z)}{2R + Z_0 + \Delta Z}.$$

If R is made much greater than Z_0 and ΔZ is much less than Z_0, then

$$E_{out} \doteq \frac{E(Z_0 + \Delta Z)}{2R} \doteq \frac{EZ_0}{2R} + \frac{E\Delta Z}{2R}.$$

Demodulation of these signals after amplification yields a large constant signal ($EZ_0/2R$) plus a smaller one ($E\Delta Z/2R$) proportional to the impedance change due to the physiological event. The larger signal, reflecting the basal impedance of the electrode–subject circuit, is often eliminated from the output by blocking this dc component with a capacitance or by canceling it with an opposing voltage.

Tetrapolar Circuit

The tetrapolar circuit (Fig. 3) for measuring impedance (or its change) permits attainment of the highest accuracy because, when properly applied with a constant-current source, it eliminates all electrode–subject impedance errors. The tetrapolar circuit was introduced by Bouty in 1884 to measure the resistivity of electrolytes with high accuracy.

With the tetrapolar circuit (Fig. 3), current I is injected into the tissue by two current-injecting electrodes (1 and 4). The tissue impedance-dependent voltage (E_{out}) is obtained from two potential-measuring electrodes (2 and 3). When a constant-current source is used to inject the measuring current, its value is independent of the impedance of the two electrode–subject impedances (Z_{1S} and Z_{4S}) and that of the tissue between electrodes 1 and 4 (Z_{S1-4}). This requirement is met when the output impedance ($2R$) of the current source is large with respect to Z_{1S} + Z_{S1-4} + Z_{4S}.

When the current-injecting electrodes (1, 4) are widely spaced with respect to the potential-measuring electrodes (2, 3), there arises the best opportunity to achieve a uniform current distribution between the potential-measuring electrodes.

The voltage (E_{out}) appearing between the potential-measuring electrodes (2, 3) is proportional to the current injected (I), the impedance of the tissue between the potential-measuring electrodes (Z_{S2-3}), and their separation. Therefore, E_{out} = IZ_{S2-3}. Now, if a voltage-measuring instrument has an input impedance that is high with respect to the sum of the impedances of the two electrode–subject interfaces (Z_{2S}, Z_{3S}) and that of the tissue between the potential-measuring electrodes (Z_{S2-3}), the potential-measuring instrument indicates the true voltage E_{2-3}; therefore E_{2-3} = IZ_{S2-3}; Z_{S2-3} = Z_0 + ΔZ; and E_{2-3} = E_{out}.

The method of calibrating the tetrapolar system is simple and merely requires disconnecting all four electrodes from the subject and connecting the potential-measuring electrodes (2, 3) to a calibrated noninductive resistor. Electrode 1 is then connected to electrode 2, and electrode 4 is connected to electrode 3. Thus the tetrapolar system is converted to a bipolar system for calibration.

When the bipolar or tetrapolar methods are used to measure a physiological event by impedance, the desired signal usually rides on a large undesired (basal) signal (Z_0), which must be removed. If (after demodulation) only the change in impedance is desired, capacitive coupling with an adequately long time constant is satisfactory. However, if both the basal impedance Z_0 and its change ΔZ are of interest, it is necessary to subtract the large output signal that represents Z_0. Although easy to do with a bucking voltage applied after the impedance signal is demodulated, the baseline recording will reflect the value of Z_0 plus any instability in the amplitude of the constant-current source. This problem can be eliminated by deriving the bucking voltage from the constant-current source; use of this technique was described by Worley and Geddes (1982) and is applicable to the bipolar and tetrapolar methods.

Figure 4 illustrates block diagrams for bipolar and tetrapolar impedance-measuring circuits in which a constant-current source is created by using an oscillator connected to a step-up transformer delivering current to the subject via two resistors that are high in value with respect to the impedance of the subject. The oscillator is also connected to a buffer amplifier (A_b), which delivers its output to a rectifier/filter (demodulator) circuit with a long time constant. From this circuit is derived a direct voltage proportional to the basal impedance Z_0. This signal is amplified and fed into a summing amplifier (A_3) to subtract the basal-impedance signal from the $Z_0 + \Delta Z$ signal. The Z_0 balance (BAL) control adjusts the amount of canceling that is applied. Figure 5 illustrates a practical tetrapolar circuit embodying the principles just described (Worley et al., 1982).

Resistive and Reactive Components

Up to this point, the discussion has focused on use of the absolute value of impedance (or its change) to represent the physiological event. As will be pointed out subsequently, at the frequencies used for this purpose the impedance is largely resistive. However, because cells have capacitive membranes, there is a small

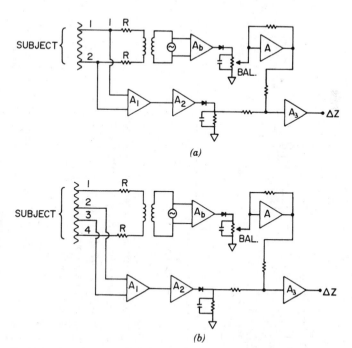

(a)

(b)

Figure 4 Technique for balancing to permit direct-coupled recording with (a) bipolar and (b) tetrapolar constant-current circuits.

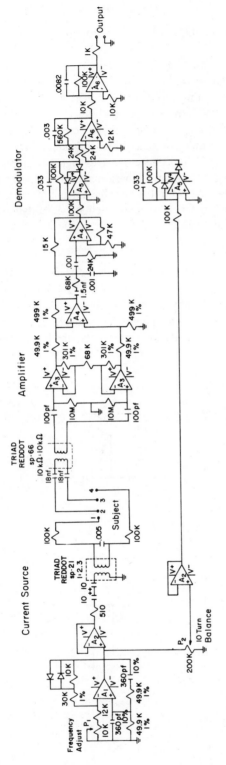

Figure 5 Circuit diagram of a tetrapolar constant-current isolated-input impedance recorder. For bipolar operation, terminals 1 and 2 are joined and 3 and 4 are joined. [Courtesy of N. E. Fearnot and redrawn from *Physiologist* 25(3):175–177 (1982).]

Output Current: 88 μA p-p
Oscillator Frequency: 9 KHz
Sensitivity: 100 mV/Ω
Dynamic Range 1300 Ohms
Operational to Zero Ohms

Notes:
1. Capacitors are in μF, unless otherwise stated.
2. Resistances are in ohms, 1/4 watt, 5%, " " "
3. A1: TL061; A2-4, A6: TL062; A5: TL072.
4. 1% Resistors are RN600 series.
5. Diodes are IN 4148's
6. [N]: Edge connector pin number

reactive component to the impedance signal. Occasionally it is desirable to separate the reactive and resistive components of the tissue between the electrodes and measure each as well as any changes that may occur in them. Ackmann and Seitz (1984) have described a tetrapolar circuit for this purpose and demonstrated its use to record the resistive and reactive changes in impedance that occur with respiration in the isolated perfused dog lung.

CURRENT-DENSITY DISTRIBUTION

When current is applied to living tissue, the spatial manner in which current is distributed is virtually unknown because of differing resistivities of tissues and fluids and because of their particular arrangement between the current-injecting electrodes. Except for a few simple cases, it is this situation that limits estimation or the calibratability of many physiological events detected by impedance. Moreover, there is no simple method for accurate measurement of current-density distribution in anisotropic tissue. The insertion of a voltage-measuring probe provides a voltage that is dependent on the current density and the resistivity of the material surrounding the probe. Knowledge of the resistivity allows calculation of the current density, provided introduction of the probe does not alter the current distribution. It must also be recognized that living tissue has different electrical properties in different directions; therefore accurate specification of the local current density requires knowledge of the resistivity and voltage gradient along three axes. The practical measurement of these quantities is by no means easy. Those who desire to explore this difficult but important problem are directed to the reviews presented by Baker and Geddes (1970a, 1971).

Although measurement of current-density distribution is a formidable task, an estimate of current distribution can be made by knowing the resistivity values of various body tissues and fluids. Reviews of the extensive literature on this subject have been presented by Schwan (1963) and Geddes and Baker (1967).

TISSUE RESISTIVITY

Although the resistivities of many biological specimens have been measured, some of the values appearing in the literature were determined without due regard to electrode impedance errors. Table 1 lists representative resistivity values. It is important to note that dead tissue exhibits a lower resistivity than living tissue.

With alternating current of the frequencies and intensities (nonstimulating and nonheating) used to measure physiological events, there appear to be no detectable alterations in cell function due to current flow. The effect of current density on body tissues and fluids has not been adequately investigated. Most body fluids are not simple electrolytes but are suspensions of cells and large molecules. The extent to which these fluid components are modified by current awaits investigation. One study by Poppindiek et al. (1964) pertinent to the techniques in which blood flow

TABLE 1   Resistivities of Biological Specimens

Specimen[a]	Resistivity (Ω-cm)	Species
Blood	150[b]	Human
Plasma	50–60	Mammal
Cerebrospinal fluid	65	Human
Bile	60	Cow, pig
Urine	30	Cow, pig
Cardiac muscle	400[c]	Dog
Skeletal muscle (T)	1600	Dog
Skeletal muscle (L)	300	Dog
Lung	1500	Mammal
Kidney	370	Mammal
Liver	820	Dog
Spleen	885	Dog
Brain (R)	580	Mammal
Fat	2500	Mammal
Skin (stratum corneum)	500 (at dc)[c]	Human
	200 (at 1 MHz)[c]	
Skin (keratin)	8×10^6 (dc)[c]	
	3000 (at 1 MHz)[c]	

[a] R = random orientation; T = transverse current; L = longitudinal current.

[b] Values for body temperature and the low-frequency region (<1 MHz). Magnitude depends on packed-cell volume.

[c] Yamamoto and Yamamoto (1976). Anisotropy ratio 2.0 (Van Oosterom et al., 1979).

Source: L. A. Geddes and L. E. Baker, *Med. Biol. Eng.* **5**:271–293 (1967).

was measured by impedance change, showed that no detectable change occurred in canine blood when it sustained a current density of 0.5 A/cm² for 3 hr. Studies on the nonthermal effects of current flow on other biological tissues and fluids will undoubtedly be carried out. There are only limited data on the impedance offered by living tissue to high current densities such as are used in ventricular defibrillation.

BLOOD RESISTIVITY

Blood is a suspension of red cells, white cells, and platelets in plasma, an electrolyte containing a myriad of other dissolved and suspended substances. The percentage of cells in a blood sample is called the packed-cell volume (H). Because the red cells are by far the most numerous, their percentage, which is called the hematocrit, is very nearly equal to the packed-cell volume except in certain disease states. Blood cells themselves contain electrolytes surrounded by an insulating membrane; therefore the resistivity of a blood sample is dependent on its packed-cell volume (H). Blood is an electrolyte, and its resistivity is dependent on temperature. Moreover, because of the capacitive nature of the cell membranes, the resistivity is dependent on the frequency of measurement.

Maxwell (1904) developed an expression for the resistivity of a suspension of spheres of known resistivity in an electrolyte of known resistivity. Fricke (1925), by including a form factor (f), extended the Maxwell expression to allow its application to suspensions of nonspherical particles. The Maxwell–Fricke expression for the resistivity ρ of a suspension of blood cells in plasma of resistivity ρ_p with a packed-cell volume of $H\%$ is

$$\rho = \rho_p \frac{1 + (f - 1)H/100}{1 - H/100}.$$

The form factor (f) for spheres is 1.5. It has been shown by Cole et al. (1969) that the Maxwell–Fricke expression is valid over a considerable range for a suspension of particles of various shapes, including rods. Figure 6 presents plots of the foregoing expression for various form factors (f). For convenience, the ratio of ρ/ρ_p is plotted versus packed-cell volume H. It will be of interest to compare the shapes of these curves and those obtained by measurement of blood samples.

Because a semilogarithmic plot of resistivity versus packed-cell volume is nearly linear, an exponential representation of the form $\rho = Ae^{\alpha H/100}$, where A and α have values for the type of blood and H is the packed-cell volume, can be employed. Note that the Maxwell–Fricke expression predicts an infinite value for the resistivity of a sample of packed cells ($H = 100\%$); the exponential representation

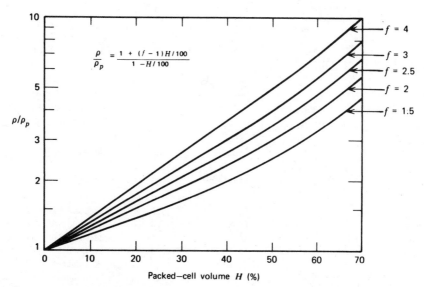

Figure 6 The Maxwell–Fricke expression for the resistivity (ρ) of a blood sample in terms of plasma resistivity (ρ_p), a form factor f, and packed-cell volume H.

predicts a finite value for packed cells. Since an H above 80 is usually incompatible with life, either expression can be used to represent the relationship between resistivity and H. Ease of calculation, of course, favors the Maxwell–Fricke expression; however, a form factor must be chosen for its use. The exponential representation is easier to derive from measured data using the least-squares method, and it does not require selection or determination of the form factor.

Values for the resistivities of blood samples have been presented in reviews by Schwan (1963) and Geddes and Baker (1967). However, resistivity data for body temperature are not common. At present, values for body temperature ($37°C$) are available for human blood at 1 kHz (Rosenthal and Tobias, 1948) and for dog blood at 100 kHz (Kinnen et al., 1964a,b) and at 25 kHz (Geddes and Sadler, 1973). The values obtained in these studies are presented in Table 2. Figure 7 shows the type of relationship for canine blood for 0–70% H using the exponential expression to represent the data.

Mention was made earlier of the importance of temperature control in resistivity measurement. Blood, like most electrolytes, exhibits a negative temperature coefficient of resistivity amounting to about $2\%/°C$.

Sedimentation Rate

Special precautions must be taken when measuring the resistivity of samples of blood. Apart from preventing clotting and eliminating electrode impedance errors,

TABLE 2   Resistivity of Blood at Body Temperature

Species	Maxwell–Fricke Expression	Exponential Expression	Frequency (kHz)	Reference
Human		$62.9e^{0.0195H}$	1	Rosenthal and Tobias (1948)
Human	$\dfrac{58.0(1 + 0.75H/100)}{1 - H/100}$	$53.2e^{0.022H}$	25	Geddes and Sadler (1973)
Human		$51.6e^{0.024H}$		
Dog		$56.6e^{0.022H}$	100	Kinnen et al. (1964)
Dog	$\dfrac{58.6(1 + 1.25H/100)}{1 - H/100}$	$53.7e^{0.025H}$	25	Geddes and Sadler (1973)
Dog		$55.5e^{0.024H}$		Geddes (1987)
Cow	$\dfrac{58.3(1 + 0.5H/100)}{1 - H/100}$	$54.2e^{0.020H}$	25	Geddes and Sadler (1973)
Horse	$\dfrac{61.5(1 + H/100)}{1 - H/100}$	$57.0e^{0.024H}$	25	Geddes and Sadler (1973)
Sheep		$55.6e^{0.020H}$	25	Geddes and Sadler (1973)
Sheep		$56.9e^{0.019H}$	25	Geddes and Sadler (1973)
Camel		$56.4e^{0.0162H}$	25	Geddes and Sadler (1973)
Camel		$56.4e^{0.016H}$	25	L. A. Geddes (unpublished)
Goat		$58.3e^{0.015H}$	25	L. A. Geddes (unpublished)
Cat		$53.9e^{0.023H}$	25	L. A. Geddes (unpublished)
Monkey		$53.7e^{0.019H}$	25	L. A. Geddes (unpublished)
Baboon		$57.5e^{0.019H}$	25	L. A. Geddes (unpublished)

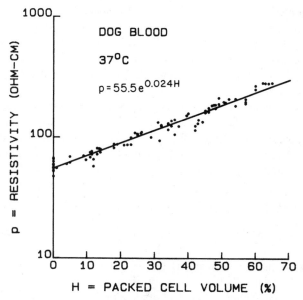

Figure 7   The relationship between blood resistivity ρ and packed-cell volume H.

attention must be given to controlling the temperature of the sample and maintaining the cells in a suspended state. If blood is allowed to stand undisturbed, the cells will fall to the bottom of the container, leaving plasma above. The rate of this process, called sedimentation, depends on the type of blood and whether inflammatory disease is present. Normal equine blood cells settle in a few minutes, whereas bovine blood cells settle very slowly and a month may be required for them to settle completely. The rate of sedimentation is increased in certain inflammatory diseases, and "sed rate" has been used as a diagnostic measurement.

Sedimentation rate has been measured by resistivity change by Nelson and Wilkinson (1972). The conductivity cell, which contained multiple platinum electrodes, measured 1×0.3 cm by 10.3 cm in height. The resistivity change showed a characteristic pattern with time as the cells settled. Attractive as this method appears, these authors pointed out that the optimum cell design had not been achieved.

Hematocrit Meter

Hematocrit is the volume percentage of red cells in the blood; packed-cell volume is the volume percentage of all cells in blood. Both are measured by placing a blood sample in a tube and centrifuging it to precipitate the cells. When this is done, the cellular components lie packed below the plasma, and the percentage of red cells can be measured by simple scaling. Above the red cells is a thin buffy coat that consists of the other cells. Because the red cells are the most numerous, the packed-cell volume is virtually equal to the hematocrit.

Because the resistivity of a blood sample depends on the percentage of cells, it is possible to measure resistivity to obtain a measure of packed-cell volume, that is, the approximate hematocrit. This technique was reported by Okada and Schwan (1960), who used a tiny (0.02 mL) conductivity cell. The resistivity was measured at 10 kHz using two platinum electrodes. The measuring bridge was temperature-compensated. A meter indicated the resistivity, and the scale was calibrated in terms of hematocrit.

The attractive feature of the resistivity method for measuring packed-cell volume is that it eliminates the need for centrifugation. The reading obtained is not quite hematocrit, although in normal subjects the difference is small. With disease, there can be a considerable increase in the population of other cells. As a screening tool, the hematocrit meter might be useful.

Resistivity of Flowing Blood

Blood is a suspension of cells that are distributed according to the velocity of flow and the geometry of the conduit that carries the stream. Suspended material migrates toward the axial stream as the flow velocity increases. In the case of blood, the suspended cells have a variety of shapes. The discoid red cells are the most numerous and exhibit a change in orientation as the flow velocity is increased from zero. At rest, their orientation is virtually random, although they will settle if flow is not restored.

When blood flows in an artery, the velocity is pulsatile and the diameter changes in a similar manner. Therefore, there will be a complex periodic redistribution of cells within the flowing stream. Moreover, since the red cells have about nine times the resistivity of plasma, their redistribution will result in a resistivity change. Thus if the impedance of a vessel carrying blood is measured, three components can contribute to a change with flow: (1) diameter change, (2) cell orientation, and (3) axial accumulation of cells. If the impedance of flowing blood is measured in a rigid tube, the latter two components will contribute.

The first to report a change in resistivity with blood flow velocity were Sigman et al. (1937), who used beef blood and measured the resistivity along the direction of flow. They found a resistivity decrease with increasing velocity. The decrease reached an asymptote that was about 5% below the stationary value. They also found that the percentage decrease depended on the hematocrit: plasma exhibited no resistivity decrease with increasing flow velocity. Other electrolytes behaved the same as plasma. They attributed the decrease in blood resistivity to red cells clumping together in the axial flow stream.

Velick and Gorin (1940) used ellipsoidal avian red cells to investigate the mechanism of resistivity change with flow velocity. They reported that red-cell orientation was an important contribution. Coulter and Pappenheimer (1949) measured the resistivity of bovine blood in the direction of flow and found that resistivity decreased with increasing velocity. The decrease was dependent on the hematocrit; Fig. 8 illustrates their results. They also showed that the reduced-resistivity asymptote was reached at a velocity well below that for turbulent flow for all values of hematocrit. In commenting on their study (which involved much more than resis-

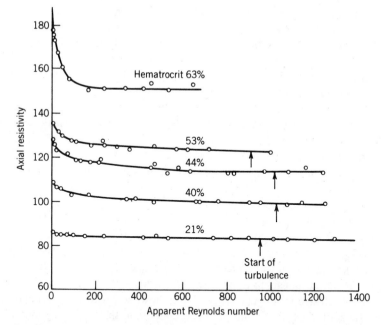

Figure 8   The decrease in axial resistivity with increasing flow velocity expressed in terms of Reynolds number. [Redrawn from N. Coulter and J. E. Pappenheimer, *Am. J. Physiol.* **159**:401–408 (1949).]

tivity measurement), they stated that blood is a two-compartment fluid (plasma and cells) and that flow consists of a peripheral plasma sheath with a central core of plasma and cells, which are nonconducting and become oriented, thereby resulting in an increased cross section for current flow.

Using a rigid circular flow tube, Moskalenko and Naumenko (1959) also reported the decrease in resistivity of cat, dog, and human blood with an increase in flow velocity. Like others, they reported that the effect was hematocrit-dependent. Baker and Mistry (1983) carried out a study using an aortic model in which the resistivity of dog blood was measured along the direction of flow. They found that in the range of laminar flow the resistivity decreased, the amount being hematocrit-dependent. The maximum decrease amounted to about 5% for a hematocrit of 40%.

Liebman et al. (1962–1963) measured the resistivity change of human blood in the direction of flow in rigid tubes of diameters ranging from 0.76 to 16 mm. In all cases, the resistivity decreased with increasing flow, the percentage being larger for the larger diameter tubes. The importance of conduit dimensions in determining the relationship between resistivity and blood flow was further reported by Kanai et al. (1976). Using a conduit with a rectangular cross section (3 mm × 30 mm) and 300 mm long, they measured the resistivity both in the direction of flow and transverse to it. They reported a maximum reduction in resistivity of 20% in the direction of flow and a maximum increase of 10% transverse to flow. From this study they concluded that the reduction in resistivity was due mainly to red-cell orientation. A similar study by Sakamoto and Kanai (1979) used a conduit with a rectangular cross section (2 mm × 20 mm) and 400 mm long. They reported a reduction in longitudinal resistivity and an increase in transverse resistivity with increasing flow velocity.

Kanai et al. (1976) studied the resistivity change due to pulsatile forward and backward flow with a frequency of 0.3–5 Hz. They reported that the resistivity change occurred with twice the frequency of the pulsatile flow. This is easily understood because both forward and backward flow will produce the same type of resistivity change. The magnitude of the change was inversely dependent on the frequency of the pulsatile flow, becoming very small above 3 Hz. The same result was reported by Sakamoto and Kanai (1979).

The foregoing studies indicate that there are four factors that contribute to the change in resistivity of blood flowing in a conduit: (1) geometry, (2) packed-cell volume, (3) axial migration of cells, and (4) reorientation of cells. The research to date appears to indicate that cell reorientation occurs with quite low flow velocity; axial accumulation appears to occur with higher flow velocities. The magnitude of the resistivity change is, in general, not large; however, whether it is important in a given situation depends on the principle underlying the measuring system. Because the resistivity change is nonlinearly related to blood flow and occurs over a small range of flow, it is unlikely to be of significant value in measuring blood flow (Dellimore and Gosling, 1975), although it can be used to detect the presence or absence of flow.

Noninvasive Measurement of Packed-Cell Volume

An ingenious noninvasive method of determining packed-cell volume was described by Yamakoshi et al. (1980). The method, which is illustrated in Fig. 9, employs four electrodes on a finger immersed in a temperature-controlled solution of selectable resistivity. Current is admitted to the finger in the solution by electrodes 1 and 4. The potential detected between electrodes 2 and 3 reflects the parallel impedance of the finger and the surrounding fluid. This impedance shows pulsatile changes.

To measure the packed-cell volume, the pulsatile impedance changes are recorded as the resistivity of the environmental solution is varied continuously. As the resistivity of the environmental solution approaches that of the blood in the finger, the amplitude of the pulsatile impedance decreases. When the resistivity of the environmental fluid equals that of the blood, the pulsatile impedance changes disappear. When the environmental fluid has a lower resistivity, the pulsatile impedance changes are inverted. Figure 10 illustrates this sequence of events.

By determining the resistivity (ρ) of fluid that eliminates the pulsatile impedance changes, the packed-cell volume (approximate hematocrit) can be calculated from $\rho = Ae^{\alpha H}$, where A and α are given in Table 2. Figure 11 illustrates the relationship

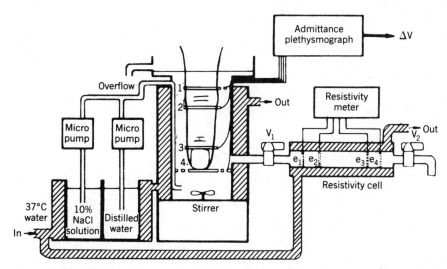

Figure 9 Equipment employed to determine hematocrit noninvasively. [Redrawn from K.-I. Yamakoshi et al., *IEEE Trans. Biomed. Eng.* **BME-27**:156–161 (1980).]

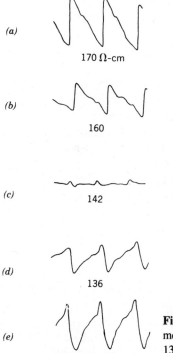

(a)

170 Ω-cm

(b)

160

(c)

142

(d)

136

(e)

130

Figure 10 Pulsatile impedance changes in the environmental fluid when the resistivity is changed from 170 to 130 Ω-cm. [Redrawn from K.-L. Yamakoshi et al., *IEEE Trans. Biomed. Eng.* **BME-27**:156–161 (1980).]

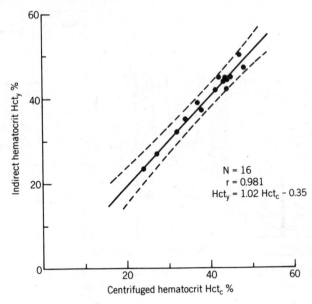

Figure 11   The relationship between indirectly and directly measured hematocrit values. [Redrawn from K. I. Yamakoshi et al., *IEEE Trans. Biomed. Eng.* **BME-27**:156–161 (1980).]

between indirectly and directly measured hematocrit values reported by Yamakoshi et al. (1980).

Shimazu et al. (1982) also used the resistivity-matching technique to determine the resistivity of blood in the human forearm. The method employed venous-occlusion plethysmography in which the impedance of the forearm is measured before and after inflation of a blood pressure cuff central to the four electrodes on the forearm. With this technique the forearm impedance decreases when the venous outflow is occluded, and the member swells. By measuring the impedance change with the arm in saline solutions of different, but known, resistivities, a solution could be found that produced no impedance change with venous occlusion. Under this condition, the resistivity of the solution is equal to that of the blood. The values so obtained were within $\pm 2\%$ of the measured blood resistivity.

Resistivity Matching

The technique of Yamakoshi et al. (1980) just described is an example of resistivity matching. Faced with the need to obtain a uniform current density distribution through an isolated heart for ventricular defibrillation studies, Niebauer et al. (1984) employed this technique. The method consisted of suspending an isolated beating dog heart in an isoresistive and isotonic volume conductor. The heart was first suspended in a solution of 5% dextrose in water (D5W), which has a very high resistivity and is isotonic. A pair of electrodes in the volume conductor, spaced widely enough to allow the heart to be lowered into the space between them, were used to measure the 20-kHz impedance. With the D5W solution there was a large change in impedance as the heart was introduced into the volume conductor between the electrodes. Resistivity matching was accomplished by withdrawing a volume of the D5W and adding an equal volume of 0.9% saline, which has a low resistivity (55 Ω-cm at 37°C) and is isotonic. When the heart was lowered into the volume conductor, the impedance change was less. By continuing to withdraw D5W add 0.9% saline, and introduce the heart, a point was reached when no impedance change occurred when the heart was introduced to the region between the electrodes. At this point the resistivity of the environmental fluid was equal to the average resistivity of the heart at 37°C.

ELECTRODE SYSTEMS

When the impedance technique is used to measure a physiological event, one of two methods is employed. With both, the physiological event is placed between the measuring electrodes in such a way that the event alters the current-density distribution between the electrodes, thus manifesting itself as a change in impedance. In one method, the electrodes are in ohmic contact with the preparation and a relatively low impedance circuit is formed; in the other, the electrodes are insulated from the subject and a relatively high impedance capacitive circuit results.

Although the circuits described earlier are those most frequently employed, in some cases in which movement has been converted into corresponding changes in capacitance the variation in capacitance has been employed to frequency modulate a carrier. On a few occasions a direct voltage was applied to the electrodes and the physiological event altered the conductivity and/or capacitance of the circuit, thereby modulating the direct current.

Guard-Electrode Technique

When the conducting property of a specimen is measured with electrodes that are small with respect to its size, the current spreads beyond the electrodes as in Fig. 12a. This situation, which often exists when physiological events are measured by impedance, plagued the early physicists seeking an accurate value for the resistivity of a material. Current spread also occurs when a small electrode is used in conjunction with a large electrode, as in Fig. 12b. To achieve a uniform current density distribution under an electrode, a guard-ring electrode is applied. Figure 12a and b shows that the current distribution with small and large electrodes applied to a conducting specimen extends well beyond both electrodes. To obtain a uniform current-density distribution under the smaller electrode, a concentric guard electrode is placed around the smaller electrode and the potential of the guard electrode is maintained at the potential of the smaller electrode used for current measurement (see Fig. 12c). Note that this technique prevents current spread from the smaller electrode connected to the current meter and achieves a more uniform current-

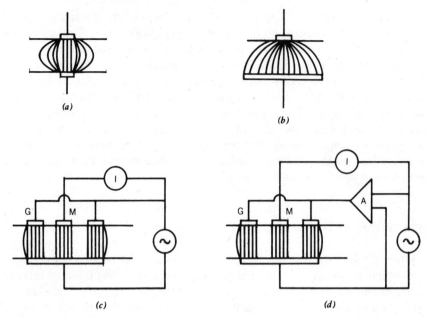

Figure 12 Current spread in a conductor and the use of a concentric guard electrode (*G*) to achieve uniform current density distribution. (*a*) Current spread in a conductor with similar electrodes. (*b*) Current spread with different sized electrodes. (*c*) Current spread with guard electrode maintained at same potential as measuring electrode (*M*). (*d*) Guard electrode driven by a unity-gain amplifier (*A*).

density distribution in the specimen. The current flowing in the guard electrode is not measured; it merely aids in providing a uniform current-density distribution around the main current path in the specimen. The modern method of applying a guard electrode employs an operational amplifier of unity gain to drive the guard electrode; this technique is illustrated in Fig. 12*d*.

The guard-electrode technique is sometimes applied when the constant-voltage system is used to measure impedance or impedance change. Graham (1965) reported its use in the measurement of respiration in the human with a chest-to-back electrode arrangement operated at 50 kHz. Without the guard applied, the basal impedance was 400 Ω, which increased to 404 Ω with inspiration. When the electrode on the back was guarded, the basal impedance was 8000 Ω, and the same inspiratory volume increased the impedance by 80 Ω. In this application, which measured the ventilation of one lung, a 20-fold respiratory impedance change was obtained by using the guard-electrode technique. In a similar study, Cooley and Longini (1968) chose the guard-electrode technique to detect respiration in humans and dogs. Application of the guard increased the measured basal transthoracic impedance. The ratio of the change in respiratory transthoracic resistance using the guard-electrode technique to that with simple bipolar electrodes varied with the size of the guarding electrode; ratios ranging from 39 to 67.5 were obtained.

Lifshitz and Klemm (1966) and Lifshitz (1970) applied guard electrodes to each of a bipolar pair of electrodes on the head to detect pulsatile cerebral blood flow by the method known as rheoencephalography. The basal impedance and the pulsatile changes were compared with and without the guard electrode, using the constant-voltage method with frequencies ranging from 25 kHz to 2 MHz. The average ratio of the basal impedance with guarded electrodes to that with unguarded electrodes was 3.39. When the amplitude of the pulsatile impedance with guarded electrodes was compared with the unguarded values, it was found that use of the guard electrodes more than doubled the size of the desired pulsatile impedance change.

Severinghaus (1971) reported the use of a single electrode carrying 100-kHz current guarded by four driven segments applied to the chest to detect pulmonary edema in humans. In the following year, Severinghaus et al. (1972) added four additional potential-sensing electrodes between the driven four-quadrant electrodes and the central measuring electrode. With this system, which mainly measured the impedance of the region below the guarded electrode, apparent lung resistivity was measured. Only a small decrease in resistivity was found to accompany a relatively large increase in intrathoracic fluid. However, the respiratory impedance change amounted to 63 Ω/L in an adult human. This high impedance coefficient is consistent with the values obtained by others who have used guarded electrodes to detect respiration.

Sahakian et al. (1985) compared the ability of the bipolar, tetrapolar, guarded bipolar, and guarded tetrapolar electrode systems to reject movement artifacts while recording respiration in humans by transthoracic impedance change. Of all of the electrode–circuit configurations, they found that the use of two concentric electrodes (each with a total area of 33.5 cm^2) connected in the bilateral guarded bipolar configuration (Fig. 13) was the optimum, reducing the artifacts by 66%.

It should be recognized that the guard-ring technique was designed for use with isotropic material; its application to living tissue is not strictly in accord with proper application, and the benefit may not be fully realized. Plonsey and Collin (1977) pointed out that without a priori knowledge of the distribution of the material that experiences a conductivity (or capacity) change, the method cannot be applied to its best advantage.

Electrodeless Impedance Measurement

By the use of electromagnetic induction, it is possible to measure the resistivity of a conducting substance without applying electrodes; this technique is used quite extensively in geophysical exploration. The first to apply this method to obtain signals reflecting respiration and pulsatile blood flow were Tarjan and McFee (1968, 1970), who employed three identical rigidly mounted coaxial coils separated by a distance approximately equal to their radii. The central coil was energized with 100-kHz current, and the two outer coils were connected in series opposition, as in Fig. 14. The arrangement therefore constitutes a differential transformer. With the three-coil assembly well removed from conducting materials, amplitude and

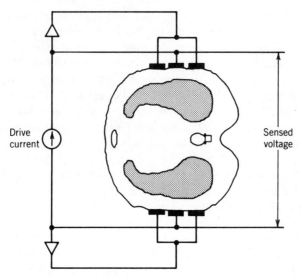

Figure 13 Symmetrically guarded concentric bipolar electrodes for measuring transthoracic impedance. [Redrawn from A. V. Sahakian et al., *IEEE Trans. Biomed. Eng.* **BME-32**(6):448–451 (1985).]

phase adjustments were made to obtain the smallest possible unbalance signal from the coils connected in series opposition.

When such a balanced three-coil assembly is brought near conducting material, a current is induced in it. The magnitude of the current is proportional to the conductivity. The induced current produces a magnetic field of its own, which alters the voltage induced in one or both of the two pickup coils. With fixed geometry, the unbalanced voltage can be detected and processed to provide a measure of the conductance of the material and any variations it experiences.

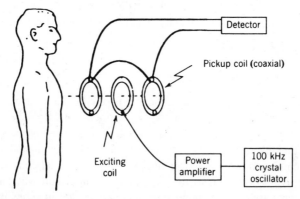

Figure 14 The electrodeless method of measuring impedance and impedance change using electromagnetic induction. [From P. P. Tarjan and R. McFee, *Ann. N.Y. Acad. Sci.* **170**:462–475 (1970). By permission.]

Tarjan and McFee (1968, 1970) detected respiration in the human by mounting the coil assembly a short distance from the thorax. By carefully placing the axis of the coil assembly over the heart and requesting that the subject hold his or her breath at full inspiration, recordings strikingly similar to ventricular volume changes were obtained. With the assembly placed near the head, the investigators recorded pulsatile changes reflecting cerebral blood flow. In this application, they were even able to detect metallic tooth fillings.

The electrodeless method for detecting impedance changes exhibits some interesting characteristics. For many reasons, the elimination of electrodes provides great practicality and allows nonstressful measurements to be made. Magnetic fields penetrate readily into biological tissue, and subintegumental events can be detected more easily than by the use of surface electrodes. However, with electromagnetic induction, the magnitudes of the signals provided by physiological events are small, and they decrease with increasing distance from the coil assembly; thus care must be exercised to obtain the optimum placement of the coil assembly that constitutes the transducer. If artifacts are to be avoided, the subject must not move with respect to the coil assembly. It is also important to prevent the induced currents from attaining a magnitude sufficient to stimulate irritable tissue or to cause heating. Finally, as with all other impedance-measuring techniques, it is difficult to calibrate the signal obtained in terms of the magnitude of the physiological event. Nonetheless, as pointed out earlier, if the signal tracks a physiological event faithfully, it can be used to obtain timing and relative-amplitude information.

IMPEDANCE OF LIVING TISSUE

The unit of living tissue is the single cell, which can be idealized as an electrolyte containing a variety of subcellular structures necessary for metabolism, repair, and reproduction (if the cell exhibits this latter property), enveloped completely by a membrane having a low electrical leakage in the resting state. The passive capacitance values for cell membranes range from 0.1 to 12 $\mu F/cm^2$, with a typical value of about 1.0 $\mu F/cm^2$ (Cole, 1933). The resistivity of cytoplasm ranges from 10 to 30,000 Ω-cm; 300–400 Ω-cm are typical values for mammalian cells (Cole, 1933). Biological tissue consists of an aggregation of cells of differing shapes bonded together and surrounded by tissue fluids that are electrolytes. Therefore, current passing through a specimen of living tissue can pass around the cells by way of the environmental fluid (Fig. 15a) if the current is dc or varies slowly (low frequency). If the frequency is high enough, the reactance of the capacitance of the cell membranes will be small, and current will flow through the cytoplasm as well as the environmental fluid (Fig. 15b). Therefore, the low-frequency impedance is high and the high-frequency impedance is low, as idealized in Fig. 15c. The transition from the high to the low value is characteristic for the type of tissue and reflects the capacitive nature of cell membranes. This characteristic feature of living tissue, recognized by Philippson (1920), led to the concept of equivalent circuits. The circuit at the right in Fig. 16 is frequently used to describe the passive electrical

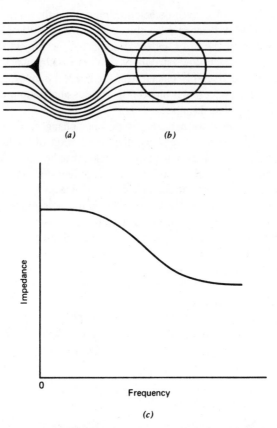

(a)   *(b)*

(c)

Figure 15 Pathways for (*a*) low-frequency current and (*b*) high-frequency current for a cell in an electrolyte; (*c*) the resulting idealized impedance–frequency characteristic.

behavior of biological specimens. In the measurement of the impedance–frequency characteristics of tissue, precautions must be taken to avoid stimulation of the tissue and to assure awareness of errors introduced by the impedance of the electrode-tissue interface, which increases with decreasing frequency. The latter phenomenon makes it difficult to obtain accurate low-frequency impedance and dc resistance measurements with a bipolar electrode system. In such cases, the tetrapolar method is required.

To display the electrical properties of tissue specimens in a more informative manner, Cole (1929, 1933) employed the impedance–locus method used earlier by Carter (1925) to describe the impedance and phase angle of two-terminal networks containing resistances and reactances. With this method the series-equivalent reactance is plotted against resistance. For the idealized circuit on the right in Fig. 16*a*, the impedance-locus plot consists of a semicircle of radius $R_m/2$ on the resistance axis with its center located at $R_s + R_m/2$ units from the origin (Fig. 16*b*). The line joining the origin to a point on the semicircle is the impedance (Z_f)

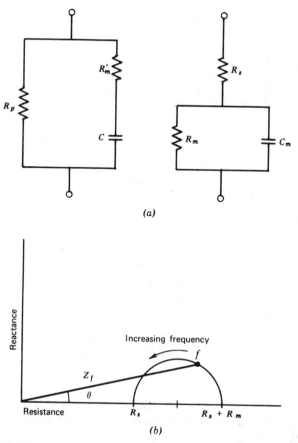

Figure 16   (a) Idealized equivalent circuits for living tissue; (b) the impedance–frequency characteristics for living tissue represented by the impedance locus (reactance versus resistance). Z_f is the impedance at frequency f, and θ is the phase angle.

at the frequency f. Increasing the frequency moves the point f in a counterclockwise direction on the semicircle. The angle θ made by the impedance vector with the resistance (horizontal) axis is the phase angle between the voltage and current measured at the terminals of the network. In the capacitive circuit shown, the current leads the voltage under steady-state sinusoidal conditions.

When the impedance-locus method is used to display the impedance–frequency characteristics of a biological specimen, the pattern obtained is slightly different from that in Fig. 16b. Typical impedance–frequency and phase–frequency characteristics for a single frog egg suspended in an electrolyte are shown in Fig. 17 (Cole and Guttman, 1942); Fig. 18 is the impedance-locus plot for the same specimen. Recalling that the resistivity of electrolytes is constant over a considerable frequency range, it is interesting to note that the circuit measured between the electrode terminals exhibits capacitive reactance (due to the cell membrane). The

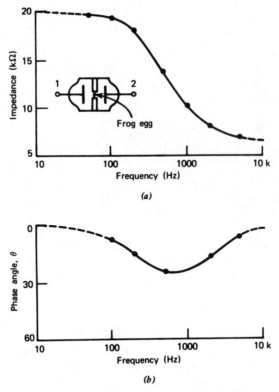

(a)

(b)

Figure 17 (a) Impedance–frequency characteristic of a single frog egg in an electrolyte; (b) phase–frequency characteristic. [Redrawn from K. S. Cole and R. M. Guttman, *J. Gen. Physiol.* **25:**765–775 (1942).]

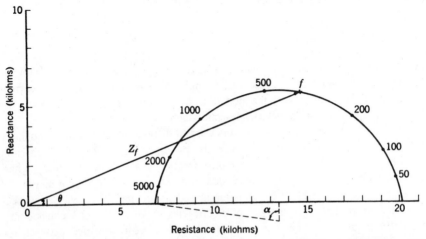

Figure 18 Impedance-locus plot for a single frog egg suspended in an electrolyte. [Redrawn from K. S. Cole and R. M. Guttman, *J. Gen. Physiol.* **25:**765–775 (1942).]

center of the semicircle in the impedance-locus plot lies slightly below the resistance axis because the cell membrane is not an ideal capacitor. A line between the point where the arc of the semicircle crosses the resistance axis and the center of the circle makes an angle α with a perpendicular line through the center of the circle. This angle is the membrane phase angle. If the cell membrane were a perfect insulator, α would be $90°$, the tangent of α would be infinity, and the center of the semicircle would be on the resistance axis. Additional information on the impedance locus of living tissue can be found in a paper by Ackmann and Seitz (1984) and a book by Schanne et al. (1978).

An alternative and quicker method of collecting data from which the impedance-locus plot can be obtained was described by Teorell (1947). With this method, a low-frequency square wave generator of known resistive output impedance applies current to the biological specimen. By careful measurement of the waveform of voltage across the specimen and of the current in the circuit, it is possible to obtain the necessary data to plot the impedance locus. Although the data require time to process, the method has the attractive feature of tracking a fairly rapid change in the components of tissue impedance. To date little use has been made of this technique, which is quite common in circuit analysis.

SEASONAL VARIATIONS IN IMPEDANCE

The conducting properties of the body have been found to vary throughout the year. For example, Crile et al. (1922) discovered that the resistivity of excised samples of biological material depended on the time of the year during which they were removed. Barnett (1940) noted that the 11.16-kHz impedance measured between electrodes on the upper arms of 20 normal subjects varied cyclically over the period of a year. During the winter months the impedance was stable in the vicinity of 100 Ω; it increased to 140–250 Ω during the summer, an increase of 40–150%. There also occurred a 1–4-degree increase in phase angle during the summer. Similar changes were exhibited by the majority of 50 patients institutionalized and undergoing psychiatric treatment. Barnett explained the impedance change on the basis of alterations in epidermal thickness.

ENDOCRINE ACTIVITY

Since the composition and proportions of the body are profoundly affected by the endocrine system, changes in the levels of various circulating hormones would be expected to be revealed in the impedance between electrodes on subjects in which there are alterations in endocrine function. For example, in diseases of the thyroid gland, gross somatic changes occur. In hypothyroidism there is a characteristic increase in body proportions. The skin is thick, dry, coarse, yellowish, and characterized by heavy deposits of subcutaneous material. The hyperthyroid subject is thin and has a warm, soft, moist skin. Such gross differences in body composition have been found to alter the impedance measured by electrodes placed on the surface of the body.

Brazier (1935) reported that in the intact human the phase angle (in radians) is directly related to thyroid function. In normal subjects, with both arms immersed up to the elbows in saline solutions serving as electrodes, she measured the impedance and phase angle at 20 kHZ and noted a difference in the phase angle between males and females. In 150 women with thyrotoxicosis she found that the phase angle was directly related to the metabolic rate and was independent of meals, muscular exercise, and the effect of autonomic drugs. Less correlation was found for hypothyroidism, but there was a measurable change when treatment of such subjects with thyroid-stimulating drugs or thyroid extract was begun.

Response to Brazier's paper was almost immediate. Horton and Van Ravenswaay (1935) reexamined the data. By strategically locating electrodes they were able to measure the impedance of the superficial and deep layers of the arms separately. However, they were unable to establish a distinct correlation with thyroid function.

Barnett (1937) thoroughly investigated the problem and was able to obtain impedance values for the skin and deep tissue layers. The phase angle for normal skin was 71.5 degrees, and for deep tissue layers 5–10 degrees. He found that the important quantity was not the phase angle, which was almost constant, but the impedance value. He plotted the skin impedance for normal, hyperthyroid, and hypothyroid individuals in a range of frequencies extending from below 100 Hz to above 40 kHz. The three curves were significantly different, the curve for the hypothyroid subjects lying above that for the normal, and the curve for the hyperthyroid lying below. Choosing 11.15 kHz, Barnett studied 458 cases and showed that a plot of basal metabolic rate (BMR) versus the reciprocal of the impedance correlated almost 80%. A BMR of -2% was equivalent to 109.7 Ω, and a range of 84–135 Ω represented a BMR spread of $+10$ to -13%.

Although the impedance method uncovers changes in the conducting properties of the body that are related to thyroid function, in comparison to other thyroid tests it is not an adequately sensitive indicator for clinical use.

In the studies of impedance associated with thyroid dysfunction, small changes in impedance in the human were observed to be related to age and sex (Brazier, 1935). The impedance changes reflecting estrogenic activity in the white rat were reinvestigated by Farzaneh (1953). Using approximately 100 animals and measuring the 15-kHz impedance between the limbs, at estrus he observed a decrease in impedance of 20% and an increase in phase angle of approximately 5 degrees. In ovariectomized animals, the phase angle remained constant but the impedance varied slightly. Farzaneh also observed that thyroid activity altered the impedance. Much more remains to be investigated to discover the cause of the impedance changes that accompany changes in the level of estrogenic hormones in the circulation. Certainly, the fluid shifts encountered in these circumstances must play an important role.

BLOOD VOLUME CHANGES

Underwood and Gowing (1965) reported that the impedance between widely spaced electrodes on experimental animals reflected blood volume. In their studies on dogs and cats, they used a bipolar electrode arrangement; one electrode was placed on the sternal notch and the other in the lumbar region. A 10-kHz square wave of current was employed, and the impedance change was measured as blood was withdrawn from the animals. A 10% change in blood volume was found to produce a 1.5-Ω change in impedance.

Geddes and Baker (1971) verified these observations, using a tetrapolar electrode arrangement applied to dogs. The current electrodes were placed on the right forelimb and left hind limb, and the potential electrodes on the left forelimb and right hind limb. A 50-kHz constant-current system was used. Withdrawal of blood increased the impedance; the addition of blood decreased it. A coefficient of 0.16% change in impedance for a 1% change in blood volume was obtained. A nearly linear relationship was observed for a +30% change in blood volume (calculated on the basis of blood constituting 7% of body weight). The addition of isotonic saline, which has a lower resistivity than blood, produced larger changes in impedance.

Berman et al. (1971) measured the 100-kHz tetrapolar impedance change in dogs in response to hemorrhage, shock, and the intravascular infusion of saline. Small changes in impedance accompanied hemorrhage and shock, and they obtained a decrease in impedance of 0.012 Ω/per milliliter of saline infused into the vascular system. Luepker et al. (1973) obtained similar results with dogs.

Attempting to identify the individual extracellular and intracellular fluid volume changes. Salansky and Utrata (1972), using rabbits and guinea pigs, characterized the impedance measured between the hind limbs by the circuit appearing in Fig. 16a. They represented the extracellular fluid compartment by R_p and the intracellular current pathway by the series circuit ($R'_M C$). The magnitudes of the components of each of these two current pathways were determined by making impedance measurements at 1 and 800 kHz. Using a variety of maneuvers, blood and body fluid volume changes were induced, and their effect on the intracellular and extracellular equivalent circuits was examined. The investigators found that changes in extracellular fluid volume primarily affected the value of R_p.

Despite the attractiveness of the method of using total body impedance to identify blood loss or infusion, the impedance change obtained is small. Underwood and Gowing used bipolar electrodes that required an extremely stable electrode-subject impedance. The tetrapolar electrode system is more appropriate for such measurements because it eliminates errors due to the impedance of the measuring electrodes.

INTRATHORACIC FLUID

Detection of the accumulation of fluid within the thoracic cavity is of considerable clinical importance. Since the fluid that accumulates is an electrolyte, attempts have been made to use changes in basal thoracic impedance to quantitate the accumulation or disappearance of such fluid.

Van DeWater et al. (1970a, 1971, 1972) and Dove et al. (1971b) employed the tetrapolar method used in thoracic impedance cardiography to measure changes in chest fluid volume in human subjects. Both groups found that aspiration of pleural fluid increased the basal 100-kHz thoracic impedance slightly. Typical values of impedance change were in the range of 1 mΩ/mL of fluid aspirated. Pomerantz et al. (1969, 1970) measured 100-kHz impedance changes in dogs and humans using the tetrapolar electrode technique. In the dog they obtained a decrease in impedance of about 6 mΩ/mL of saline infused into the thoracic cavity. In a human subject with pleural effusion, they obtained an increase in impedance of 5 mΩ/mL of fluid withdrawn. Luepker et al. (1973) obtained similar results using dogs. Severinghaus (1971) and Severinghaus et al. (1972) used a four-quadrant guarded electrode applied to the thoraxes of dogs to measure the 100-kHz change in lung impedance in response to saline infusion. A decrease in impedance amounting to 1% was produced by a 4% increase in lung water.

Although the impedance method can detect a change in thoracic fluid volume, a relatively large volume change is required to produce a reliable impedance change. In dogs and humans the magnitude of the impedance change is in the vicinity of 10 mΩ/mL of fluid volume change. With a stable tetrapolar constant-current instrument and mechanically stable potential-measuring electrodes, the method can be used to monitor changes in intrathoracic fluid volume; however, it cannot distinguish between the presence of intravascular and extravascular fluid. Moreover, the resting expiratory level must be stable to permit interpretation of the impedance change as a change in thoracic fluid. Within these constraints, the noninvasive nature of the tetrapolar impedance technique may be of clinical value for monitoring thoracic fluid shifts if the measuring electrodes can be retained in the same plane for prolonged periods (or replaced in exactly the same locations) and if respiratory impedance changes do not obscure measurement of the basal impedance.

To obtain a number that is related to pulmonary fluid, it is becoming popular to divide the basal impedance Z_0 by the separation of the potential-measuring electrodes on the chest. It is hoped that the quantity Z_0/L will allow comparison among patients and hence indicate the need for diuretics to reduce pulmonary fluid. It would seem that inclusion of body weight in the normalizing factor Z_0/L may improve its value.

RESPIRATION

Mention was made in Chapter 4 of the studies by Atzler and Lehmann and Fenning, who employed the capacitance change principle to detect respiration. Other investigations have been carried out in which the impedance changes between two or four electrodes in direct contact with the chest wall have been employed to detect respiration. A good review of the circuits used in these studies was presented by Pacella (1966).

While recording cardiac impedance pulses with electrodes on the thorax, Nyboer (1944) noted variations in the baseline impedance that correlated with a simultaneously recorded spirogram. Schaefer et al. (1949) developed an impedance system for recording respiration in animals and humans, using electrodes inserted subcutaneously in the chest wall. That such transthoracic impedance changes were related to the volume of air moved was demonstrated by Goldensohn and Zablow (1959), who passed a 10-kHz constant current between electrodes on the wrists and detected the respiratory signal from similar electrodes placed farther up on each arm. Geddes et al. (1962) described a two-electrode constant-current system in which respiration was detected by measuring the 50-kHz impedance changes appearing between electrodes placed on the surface of the chest of animals and humans. A high correlation between impedance change and volume of air breathed has been demonstrated by Goldensohn and Zablow (1959), Geddes et al. (1962), Robbins and Marko (1962), Hanish (1962), Allison (1962), Allison et al. (1964), McCally et al. (1963), Kubicek et al. (1963, 1964), Ax et al. (1964), Baker and Geddes (1965, 1966), Pallett and Scopes (1965), and Hamilton et al. (1965).

Figure 19 is a typical three-channel record of an electrocardiogram, an impedance pneumogram, and a spirogram in the human subject made with electrodes at the level of the xiphoid process and along the midaxillary lines. While the recording was being made, the subject was asked to vary his depth of respiration. The impedance and ECG recordings were made from the same pair of electrodes (Geddes et al., 1962). The excursions of the spirometer were detected by coupling a low-torque potentiometer to the pulley suspending the bell (Chap. 2). Using the same impedance pneumograph, Geddes and Baker have recorded respiration from horses, dogs, monkeys, cats, rabbits, rats, mice, alligators, frogs, and a camel. The magnitude of the impedance change encountered with respiration depends on body size and the location of the electrodes.

Choice of Frequency

Throughout the years there has been some discussion concerning the importance of frequency for measurement of the respiratory impedance change. Apart from safety considerations, which call for the use of a high-frequency current to avoid tissue stimulation, there appears to be no particular advantage to the choice of one frequency over another. This fact is illustrated by Fig. 20a, which shows the impedance change in a human subject produced by a vital capacity maneuver. It is noted that the change in transthoracic impedance from full inspiration to maximum expiration is practically the same in the frequency range of 50–600 kHz.

Figure 20b presents a continuous impedance–frequency plot obtained on a dog using a variable-frequency constant-current generator connected to transthoracic electrodes placed along the midaxillary lines at the level of the xiphoid process. The animal was connected to a constant-volume respirator to maintain a constant tidal volume. In the frequency range extending from 10 Hz to 100 kHz, the impedance change for a constant respiratory volume is essentially the same. The decrease is basal (resting expiratory level) impedance reflects both the decrease in electrode-subject impedance and the reactive nature of the cells that constitute the thorax of the animal.

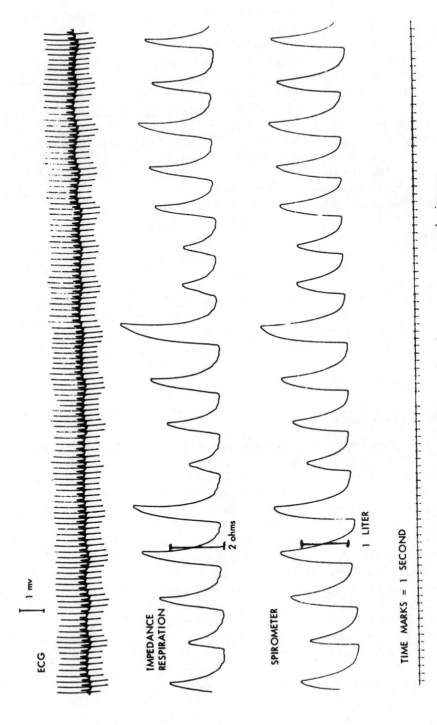

Figure 19 An electrocardiogram, impedance pneumogram, and spirogram.

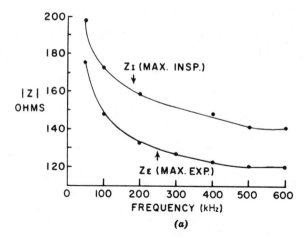

Figure 20   (*a*) The relationship between impedance change and volume of air at different frequencies. [Redrawn from Baker and Geddes, *Am. J. Med. Electron.* **4**:75 (1965). By permission.] (*b*) Impedance–frequency characteristic of a dog measured with a variable-frequency constant-current generator connected to transthoracic electrodes. During the measurement the animal was respired with a constant-volume respirator.

Impedance–Volume Relations

The relationship between impedance change ΔZ and volume of air moved (ΔV) is approximately linear under most circumstances. For the human, the coefficient $\Delta Z/\Delta V$ depends on the size of the subject and the location of the electrodes. In the studies carried out by Baker and Geddes (1965a,b), who used bipolar electrodes, a fairly good linearity was obtained for all electrode locations studied. In general they found coefficients ranging from 6.0 Ω/L for adults of slight build to 1.0 Ω/L for heavy subjects. Kubicek et al. (1964) reported a coefficient of 1.2 Ω/L air breathed. The studies reported by Allison (1962), in which a tetrapolar electrode system was used, indicated a coefficient of 0.3–0.4 Ω/L. Figure 21, taken from Baker's investigation (1966), indicates the degree of linearity obtained in human subjects of differing builds with bipolar electrodes placed on midaxillary lines at different levels on the chest. Inspection of this illustration shows that the coefficient $\Delta Z/\Delta V$ is largest for adults of slight build.

A variety of electrode locations have been studied. For example, Weltman and Ukkestad (1969), like Goldensohn and Zablow (1959), placed electrodes on the upper arms and measured the respiratory changes in impedance at 50 kHz and obtained values for $\Delta Z/\Delta V$ in the range of 0.6–2.5 Ω/L. They reported that the linearity between ΔZ and ΔV was superior to that obtained with other electrode locations. Khalafalla et al. (1970) carried out low-frequency (280-Hz) respiratory-impedance measurements on humans using 14 different lead configurations and obtained values for $\Delta Z/\Delta V$ ranging from 0.1 to 1.31 Ω/L.

Figure 22 summarizes the values for $\Delta Z/\Delta V$ obtained by the authors on dogs and humans using transthoracic electrodes. Clearly the values for $\Delta Z/\Delta V$ are

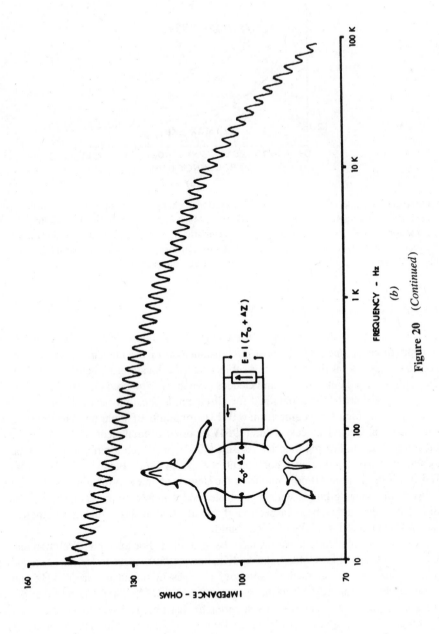

FREQUENCY - Hz

(b)

Figure 20 (Continued)

$E = I(Z_0 + \Delta Z)$

$Z_0 + \Delta Z$

IMPEDANCE - OHMS

160

130

100

70

10

100

1 K

10 K

100 K

dependent on electrode location and body size; however, the data in this illustration do not reveal the linearity of the $\Delta Z/\Delta V$ relationship. This point is demonstrated by Fig. 21 (Baker et al. 1966a), which shows the linearity of the impedance change with the volume of air inspired by subjects of differing somatotypes. With tall thin subjects (ectomorphs), the largest amplitude is obtained with transthoracic electrodes at the level of the xiphoid process. However, the best linearity is obtained with electrodes higher on the chest near the axilla, the price paid being a smaller value for $\Delta Z/\Delta V$. With endomorphs (corpulent subjects), all values for $\Delta Z/\Delta V$ are smaller, and the best linearity is obtained with electrodes near the axilla, as is the case with the mesomorph. Similar observations have been reported by Kubicek et al. (1964), Hamilton et al. (1965), and Logic et al. (1967).

Valentinuzzi et al. (1971) conducted a study of the impedance change per liter of air inspired in subjects of widely differing body weights, using transthoracic electrodes placed to obtain the maximum value for $\Delta Z/\Delta V$. Their data (Fig. 23)

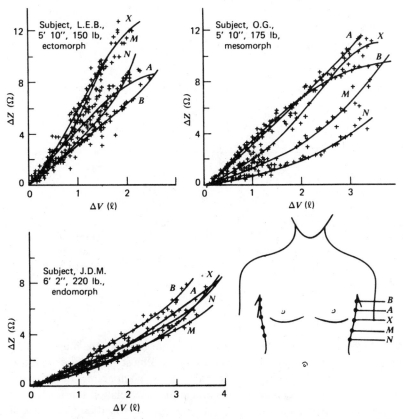

Figure 21 Transthoracic impedance changes (ΔZ) versus respired volume measured (ΔV) with bipolar electrodes applied to subjects of light, medium, and heavy builds. [From L. E. Baker et al. *Med. Biol. Eng.* **4**:374 (1966). By permission.]

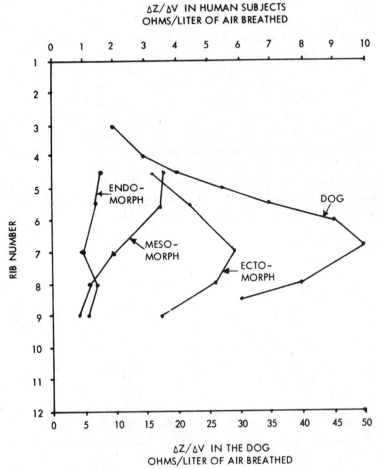

ΔZ/ΔV IN HUMAN SUBJECTS
OHMS/LITER OF AIR BREATHED

ΔZ/ΔV IN THE DOG
OHMS/LITER OF AIR BREATHED

Figure 22   The relationship between the maximum impedance coefficient [$\Delta Z/\Delta V$ (Ω/L)] and electrode location in subjects of differing body types. Note the general inverse relationship between impedance coefficient and body proportions and the influence of electrode location. [From L. E. Baker and L. A. Geddes. *Ann N.Y. Acad. Sci.* **170:**667–688 (1970b). By permission.]

reveal an inverse relationship between the maximum value for the impedance coefficient in ohms per liter and body weight. This almost hyperbolic relationship ($\Delta Z/\Delta V = 453/W^{1.08}$, where W is the body weight in kilograms) has been called the law of impedance pneumography. An approximate relationship for the maximum value of the impedance coefficient in ohms per liter is $1000/W$, where W is the body weight in pounds. Depending on somatotype and electrode location, an impedance change as small as one-fifth of this value can be encountered.

ΔZ/ΔV (Ω/l)

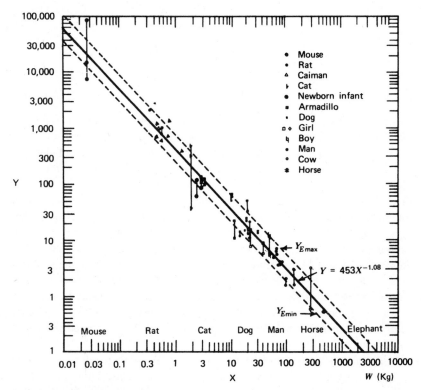

Figure 23 The inverse relationship between impedance change (ΔZ) in ohms per liter of air breathed (ΔV) and body weight (W), called the law of impedance pneumography, obtained with transthoracic electrodes located for maximum ΔZ/ΔV. [From M. E. Valentinuzzi et al., *Med. Biol. Eng.* **9:**157–163 (1971). By permission.]

Capacitive Component

Over the years there has arisen some discussion regarding the capacitive component of the transthoracic impedance change that accompanies respiration. Baker and Geddes (1965) showed that the capacitance change accompanying respiration is small. Hamilton et al. (1965) presented recordings showing volume change (ΔV) and the transthoracic resistance change (ΔR) and capacitance change (ΔC) during respiration in the human subject. The ΔR and ΔC recordings tracked volume change equally well. A penetrating quantitative study of the relative importance of ΔR and ΔC was carried out by Pasquali (1967), who employed transthoracic electrodes ranging in size from 1 to 64 cm² applied to the human thorax, measuring the components of the thoracic impedance and their change at 100 kHz. From an extensive series of measurements, Pasquali concluded that although the percentile changes in resistance and capacitance were approximately equal, the capacitance change contributed negligibly to the transthoracic impedance change because the reactance change was small compared with the resistance change accompanying respiration. In a similar study, Cooley and Longini (1968) concluded that the respiratory impedance change was mainly resistive.

Guard-Ring Technique

Use of the guarded-electrode technique has been applied to obtain signal enhancement in the detection of the respiratory impedance change. Graham (1965) reported a 20-fold increase in impedance change by using the guarded-electrode method. Similarly, Cooley and Longini (1968) reported ratios ranging from 39 to 67.5. In both cases, along with this signal enhancement, guarding produced an increase in basal (resting expiratory level) impedance. In a study directed toward detecting intrathoracic fluid accumulation by measurement of lung resistivity, Severinghaus et al. (1972) used a guarded electrode paired with an unguarded one applied to the human thorax. The measuring electrode was guarded by four driven segments arranged around the central measuring electrode. The potentials used to drive each of the four segments were obtained from four small electrodes located between the measuring and guard electrodes. Although only a small impedance change was accompanied by an alteration in intrathoracic fluid volume, the respiratory impedance change was large, amounting to 63 Ω/L. No comparisons were made using unguarded electrodes.

Sahakian et al. (1985) investigated the efficacy of several unguarded and guarded electrode systems with a view to reducing movement artifacts. They found that a bilaterally guarded bipolar electrode system was slightly superior to other electrode–circuit configurations.

It is clear that guarding produces an enhancement in respiratory impedance change. However, more studies must be carried out to determine the optimum size and location for guarded electrodes.

Origin of the Impedance Pneumogram

Ever since it was found that an increase in transthoracic impedance accompanied inspiration, there has been speculation regarding the factors that contribute to the respiratory impedance change. The matter is unsettled because measurements of current-density distribution have not been carried out to determine the pathways of the current injected by thoracic electrodes. Some investigators believe that a respiratory redistribution of blood in the pulmonary vascular circuit contributes importantly to the inspiratory impedance increase; this theory has been countered on many occasions. Others believe that despite the small fraction of injected current traversing the lungs, the increase in lung resistivity with inspiration is the major contributor to the impedance change. Baker et al. (1966), using dogs, found that approximately 80% of the injected current traversed the posterior thoracic path and 5% passed through the anterior path. Approximately 10% of the current flowed through the liver and diaphragm, and 5% flowed through lung tissue. Many investigators believe that dimensional changes of the thorax and/or redistribution of its contents underlie the impedance change. At this time, it is difficult to assign the degree of contribution made by each factor associated with the respiratory impedance signal.

Esophageal Impedance Pneumogram

Respiration, cardiac impulses, and the electrocardiogram can be obtained from electrodes on a catheter in the esophagus. Geddes (1984) investigated the importance of electrode location and separation for esophageal electrodes for recording respiration and the ECG. Figure 24 is a typical canine record of respiratory and cardiac impedance changes and the volume change measured with a spirometer; the ECG was obtained from the same electrodes.

In the typical 15-kg dog, the largest respiratory impedance change was obtained with an electrode separation of 11.5 cm. The largest ECG signal was obtained with a spacing of 5.5 cm.

Other events such as body temperature and heart sounds can be obtained from within the esophagus. The application of a thermistor to the catheter permits measurement of core body temperature. The heart sounds are very loud and clear when detected by a tiny piezoelectric crystal mounted on the esophageal catheter (Geddes et al., 1974a). It is easy to build a multipurpose catheter (which need not be small in diameter) to acquire many useful vital signs from within the esophagus.

Characteristics of Impedance Pneumography

Practicality is probably the most attractive feature of the impedance method for measurement of respiration. Nothing is simpler than affixing electrodes to a subject

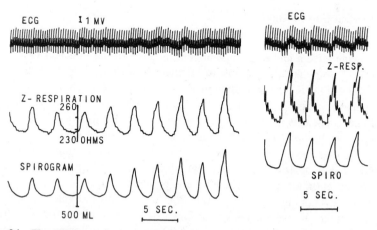

Figure 24 The ECG and impedance pneumogram obtained from esophageal electrodes (7.5-cm spacing) and the spirogram obtained from a dog. The section on the right was made with the electrodes placed to favor detection of the cardiac impedance changes. [From L. A. Geddes, *Med. Biol. Eng. Comput.* **22**(1):90–91 (1984).]

and connecting them to the recording equipment. Since the impedance change is related to the volume of air moved, the method can be calibrated. Although calibration requires the use of a spirometer or other volume-measuring instrument, the calibrating device can be removed and respiratory volumes measured without obstructing the airstream. Another attractive feature of the method is availability of the electrocardiogram and cardiac impedance signals from the same electrodes.

Perhaps the most unattractive feature of the measurement of respiration by impedance is the need to calibrate each subject with a volume-measuring device. No single calibration factor can be specified for each species or subject. However, once a calibration value has been obtained on a subject for electrodes in a given location, this factor remains fairly constant.

As with any physiological event that is measured with electrodes, movement causes a variation in impedance and produces unwanted signals. Therefore precautions must be taken to avoid this complication.

BLOOD FLOW

When the impedance-change technique is applied to the determination of blood flow, three methods are available. With the first, cardiac output (liters per minute) is determined by applying the dilution technique. Stroke volume, that is, the systolic discharge from the ventricles is determined by measurement of the impedance change between electrodes placed on or in the heart. With the third method, which employs electrodes that encompass a segment of the body, attempts are made to calibrate the pulsatile impedance signal in terms of blood flow in the field between the electrodes. A variant of this method employs measurement of venous drainage.

Indicator-Dilution Method

Stewart (1921) showed that if a known concentration of indicator is introduced into a flowing stream and the temporal concentration of the indicator is measured at a downstream point, it is possible to calculate the volume flow. To illustrate the salient points of the indicator-dilution method, consider a fluid flowing at a constant rate in a tube of cross-sectional area a, as shown in Fig. 25a. Assume that m grams of a soluble and detectable indicator is rapidly introduced to form a uniform cylinder of indicator in the fluid. If a concentration detector is placed slightly downstream and its output is recorded, an idealized rectangular concentration–time curve of amplitude c will be recorded as the cylinder passes. The practical use of this idealized concentration–time curve will now be illustrated.

In a tube containing a flowing fluid, flow is equal to the velocity of flow v multiplied by the cross-sectional area a; flow $\phi = va$. Velocity is distance divided by time ($v = L/t$), and in the model the cylinder of indicator moves L units of distance in t sec, the value for t being identified on the concentration–time curve. Substituting L/t for velocity, $\phi = La/t$. It is not possible to measure La, the

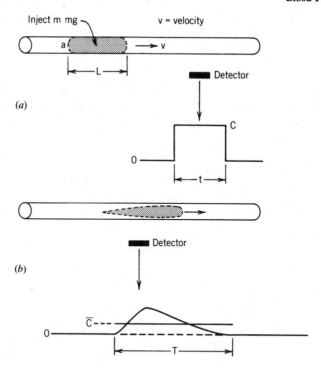

Figure 25 Genesis of the dilution curve.

volume V of the cylinder, but it is possible to measure concentration c, which is equal to m/V. Substituting this quantity gives

$$\text{Flow } \phi = \frac{m}{ct} = \frac{\text{mass of indicator injected}}{\text{concentration} \times \text{time}}.$$

The expression just derived illustrates that in the idealized case, if m g of indicator is injected and the downstream concentration–time curve is recorded, it is possible to calculate flow. In a practical situation, the cylinder of indicator would be spread out into a teardrop shape due to the velocity profile in the tube. Therefore, the concentration–time curve will rise rapidly and fall slowly as shown in Fig. 25b. However, a rectangular concentration–time curve can be obtained from this typical dilution curve by measuring the area under it and dividing by the base. Performing this operation provides a mean concentration $\bar{c}$ for the time T. Thus,

$$\text{flow} = m/\bar{c}T.$$

In this expression, m is the amount (in grams) of indicator injected, $\bar{c}$ is the mean height of the dilution curve that lasts T seconds. Note that $\bar{c}T$ is the area under the dilution curve.

There is an extremely important subtlety about the indicator-dilution flow expression. Note that it is only necessary to know the amount m of indicator injected and the downstream concentration–time curve. The concentration–time curve can be recorded from any downstream branch. The important requirement is that the injected indicator mixes with all of the flow. In the measurement of cardiac output, the indicator is injected into the right atrium, right ventricle, or pulmonary artery, and the dilution curve can be obtained by withdrawing arterial blood (from any large artery) into the detector at a constant rate. Alternatively, the injection can be made into the right atrium and the dilution curve obtained from the pulmonary artery.

Before describing practical application of the indicator-dilution method, several facts should be recognized, the most important of which is that cardiac output must remain constant for the duration of measurement. The characteristics of the indicator are also very important. Obviously, it must be detectable and not be a stimulant or depressant to the circulatory system. It must be negligibly lost between the injection and measuring sites. Indicators that are lost between the injection and measuring sites provide falsely high values for cardiac output because $\bar{c}$ is too small and is in the denominator of the flow expression. Indicators that are rapidly cleared from the circulation allow repeated determinations without indicator buildup. Indicators that are retained in the circulation can build up to excessively high concentrations if repeated determinations are made.

Saline Indicator Method

One of the earliest studies to determine cardiac output employed the impedance method. By measuring transarterial impedance in dogs and intravenously injecting 1.5% saline, Stewart (1897–1898, 1921) was able to identify the time of arrival and the passage of the blood containing the injected saline. He accomplished this by using a simple impedance bridge, one arm of which was the transarterial impedance. The alternating current for the bridge was derived from an inductorium. The detector was a telephone receiver. Passage of the hyperconducting blood unbalanced the bridge and directed the investigators to collect blood at the moment for future determination of its salinity. Cardiac output was determined by use of the dilution formula. Continuous recording of the change in conductivity of the blood as it passed an arterial detector was accomplished by Romm (1924) and by Gross and Mittermaier (1926). In both studies the conductivity curve was not calibrated because the information sought was circulation time. These two studies paved the way for investigations by Wiggers (1944), who employed a flow-through conductivity cell inserted in a femoral artery. Using the original Stewart constant-injection method, Wiggers obtained, in anesthetized dogs, cardiac output values that were in good agreement with those measured by other observers. White (1947) refined the method by devising two types of hypodermic needle electrodes that were inserted directly into an artery. As the injected saline passed the electrodes, the intraarterial impedance at 70 kHz was continuously recorded on an oscilloscope. Despite certain practical difficulties, he obtained cardiac outputs differing between -12 and $+22\%$ from the values obtained by the Fick method.

When saline is injected into the venous system and the dilution curve is detected in the arterial system, some of the saline is lost in the pulmonary vascular circuit. Since this affects the limit of accuracy attainable, the exact amount lost has been the subject of much debate, which has caused the accuracy of the saline method to be questioned. Chinard et al. (1962) stated that 5% of intravenously injected saline is lost in passing through the lungs. More recently, Grubbs et al. (1985), measured this loss in the dog and found it to be 15%.

An important point arises here: When there is no capillary bed between the injection and measuring sites, there is no saline loss. Thus, cardiac output measured by venous injection and pulmonary-artery detection of the dilution curve will not be in error, as will be shown subsequently. To eliminate the pulmonary circuit loss of saline, Goodwin and Saperstein (1957) used autogenous plasma instead of saline. Blood from an artery was withdrawn at a constant rate through a conductivity cell operated at 2500 Hz for conductivity measurements. In a series of 24 dogs, Goodwin and Saperstein compared the conductivity method and the Evans blue technique and obtained remarkably similar results. The difference in the mean values was 0.3%.

When saline is used as the indicator, the transducer is a downstream electrode assembly and the amplitude of the dilution curve is in ohms and represents the transient change in blood resistivity due to the indicator mixing with the blood. The dilution curve can be calibrated in terms of concentration of sodium chloride in blood if the manner in which blood resistivity decreases with the addition of sodium chloride is known. In other words, resistivity change can be converted to concentration change. At the frequencies used to obtain dilution curves (above 10 kHz), the impedance is mainly resistive; therefore the reactive component can be ignored with negligible error. With any electrode system used to measure the resistivity ρ of the solution, the measured resistance R is

$$R = k\rho,$$

where k is the conductivity cell constant (cm^{-1}).

When hypertonic sodium chloride is added to blood, the blood concentration c increases and the resistivity ρ decreases. Therefore,

$$\frac{dR}{dc} = k\frac{d\rho}{dc}.$$

Now it is necessary to measure how blood resistivity changes with the addition of sodium chloride. Measurements were made at 37°C on blood samples from several species to reveal the nature of the dependence of the resistivity on the amount of added sodium chloride and packed-cell volume H. Samples of the desired H in the range 0–70% were prepared by centrifuging the blood and adding the desired volume of cells to the plasma. To each of these samples, known amounts of sodium chloride were added and the concentration was calculated by dividing the weight of the added sodium chloride in grams by the volume of the blood sample in liters. Resistivity measurements were made with a variable-length conductivity cell (Geddes, 1973), which was surrounded by a temperature-controlled water jacket (37°C); the assembly was mounted on an agitator to prevent the blood cells from settling while measurements were being made. The conductivity cell was connected to a constant-current 25-kHz impedance-measuring instrument. A typical resistivity–saline concentration curve obtained for a canine blood sample appears in Fig. 26. This figure shows that the reduction in resistivity depends on packed-cell volume H, the value for $d\rho/dC$ being large for the high packed-cell volumes.

The values for $d\rho/dc$ were plotted versus packed-cell volume H, as shown in Figure 27 and reveal that the relationship is of the form

$$\frac{d\rho}{dc} = Be^{\beta H}.$$

Now it is undesirable to have to draw a blood sample to determine the packed-cell volume H to calculate the calibration factor $d\rho/dc$. It has been shown by Baker and Geddes (see earlier in this chapter), that the resistivity of blood depends on its packed-cell volume according to

$$\rho = Ae^{\alpha H}.$$

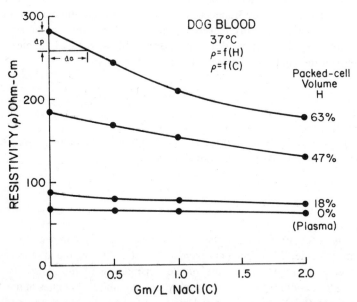

Figure 26 The manner in which blood resistivity decreases with the addition of sodium chloride to samples having different packed-cell volumes. [Redrawn from L. E. Geddes et al., *Cardiovasc. Res. Cent. Bull.* **10**:91–106 (1972).]

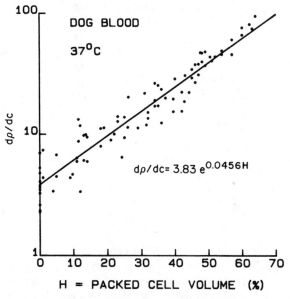

Figure 27   The manner in which $d\rho/dc$ depends on packed-cell volume H. [From L. A. Geddes, *IEEE-EMBS* **8**(1):22–27 1989.]

The baseline of the dilution curve reflects the blood resistivity ρ. Therefore the calibration factor $d\rho/dc$ can be determined by eliminating H from these two equations. This gives

$$H = \frac{1}{\beta} \ln \frac{1}{B} \frac{d\rho}{dc} \quad \text{and} \quad H = \frac{1}{\alpha} \ln \frac{\rho}{A}.$$

Equating these two expressions and solving provides

$$\frac{d\rho}{dc} = B \left(\frac{\rho}{A} \right)^{\beta/\alpha}.$$

Since the measured resistance R of the baseline of the dilution curve is equal to $k\rho$, the calibration factor becomes

$$\frac{d\rho}{dc} = B \left(\frac{R}{kA} \right)^{\beta/\alpha},$$

where B and β and A and α are species-dependent blood constants. Table 3 contains values for B and β, and Table 2, values for A and α.

It is now necessary to derive the cardiac output equation for the sodium chloride

TABLE 3   Values for $d\rho/dc$ at 37°C

Species	$d\rho/dc$
Dog	$3.83e^{0.0456H}$
Sheep	$4.15e^{0.041H}$
Camel	$3.975e^{0.354H}$
Human	$3.73e^{0.044H}$

indicator using these fundamental expressions. The equation for cardiac output (CO) in liters per minute is

$$CO = \frac{60m}{\overline{\Delta C} t},$$

where m is the amount of indicator injected (in grams), $\overline{\Delta C}$ is the mean concentration change of the dilution curve (grams per liter), and t is the duration of the dilution curve (seconds). Using the incremental (Δ) notation and recognizing that the dilution curve has a mean height of ΔR riding on a baseline of R, ΔC becomes

$$\Delta C = \frac{\Delta\rho}{B(R/kA)^{\beta/\alpha}}.$$

Substitution of this expression into the cardiac output equation yields

$$CO = \frac{60mB}{t\,\Delta\rho}\left(\frac{R}{kA}\right)^{\beta/\alpha}.$$

Now,

$$\Delta R = k\,\Delta\rho.$$

Substituting for $\Delta\rho$ yields the expression for cardiac output (in liters per minute):

$$CO = \frac{60mBk}{t\,\Delta R}\left(\frac{R}{kA}\right)^{\beta/\alpha},$$

where
m = the grams of indicator injected,
t = the duration of the dilution curve (seconds),
ΔR = the mean height of the dilution curve (ohms),
$t\,\Delta R$ = the area of the dilution curve (ohm-seconds),
k = the resistivity cell constant (cm^{-1}),
$A, B, \alpha,$ and β = species-dependent blood quantities (see Tables 2 and 3), and
CO = the cardiac output (liters/minute).

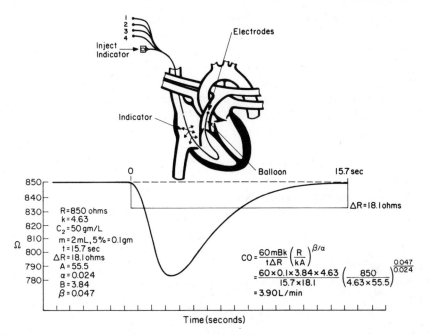

Figure 28 Placement of catheter-tip conductivity cell in the pulmonary artery to record a dilution curve (lower) resulting from injecting 2 mL of 5% saline indicator into the right atrium.

Figure 28 illustrates application of the saline method to determine cardiac output in the dog by injecting 2 mL of 5% saline ($m = 0.1$ g) into the right atrium and detecting the dilution curve in the pulmonary artery using a tetrapolar catheter-tip electrode having a cell constant k of 4.63, determined by measuring the resistance of a solution of known resistivity. The values for A, α, B, and β (for this animal) were entered into the equation along with R and ΔR to calculate cardiac output as shown in the figure.

The Forbidden Indicator. Worley et al. (1982) pointed out that when the concentration of the saline indicator is decreased below about 3% the cardiac output values are overestimated. In fact, if the indicator has a resistivity equal to that of the blood, no dilution curve will be produced. This indicator is known as the "forbidden indicator." To permit the use of saline having a concentration that approaches that of the forbidden indicator, while retaining accuracy, Voorhees et al. (1986) derived a mass-balance-based correction factor for application to the standard cardiac output equation. This factor (F) is

$$F = 1 - C_1/C_2,$$

where C_1 is the concentration of the indicator already in the blood and C_2 is the concentration of the indicator in the injectate. Note that as C_2 becomes much larger than C_1, the situation when the blood already contains no indicator or when the indicator has a high concentration with respect to its concentration in the blood, the correction factor becomes 1.0.

Since it is difficult to determine the concentration (C_1) of sodium chloride already in blood, another strategy, the use of resistivity, is used to evaluate it. The resistivity ρ of saline of concentration C at 37°C is

$$\rho = \frac{379.1}{C^{0.9149}}.$$

Now equating ρ to the blood resistivity, the equivalent concentration C_1 becomes

$$C_1 = \left(\frac{379.1}{\rho}\right)^{1.093}$$

Therefore the corrected cardiac output equation becomes

$$CO = \frac{60mBk}{t\,\Delta R}\left(\frac{R}{kA}\right)^{\beta/\alpha}\left(1 - \frac{C_1}{C_2}\right).$$

Substituting for C_1,

$$CO = \frac{60mBK}{t\,\Delta R}\left(\frac{R}{kA}\right)^{\beta/\alpha}\left[1 - \frac{1}{C_2}\left(\frac{379.1}{\rho}\right)^{1.093}\right].$$

From $R = k\rho$,

$$CO = \frac{60mBk}{t\,\Delta R}\left(\frac{R}{kA}\right)^{\beta/\alpha}\left[1 - \frac{1}{C_2}\left(\frac{379.1k}{R}\right)^{1.093}\right].$$

Verification Studies. The accuracy of the method illustrated in Fig. 28 was evaluated with 5% saline in 10 dogs by Grubbs et al. (1984) using the direct Fick (oxygen uptake) method as the reference. Over a range of cardiac output of 2–6 L/min, the average saline values were within 3.3% of the values obtained by the Fick method. Using the correction factor F and 3% saline as the indicator ($C_2 = 30$ g/L), Voorhees and Geddes (1984) compared cardiac outputs with the saline-indicator method with those obtained from a carefully calibrated pulmonary artery flowmeter. The 3% saline was injected into the right atrium, and the dilution curve was recorded from the pulmonary artery. In 455 comparisons in 10 dogs, the relationship between saline cardiac output (CO_s) and cardiac output with the electromagnetic flowmeter (CO_{em}), in liters per minute was

$$CO_s = 0.973CO_{em} - 0.0047,$$

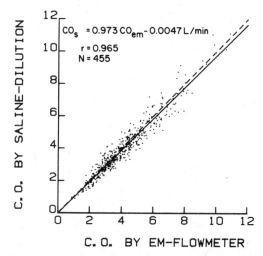

Figure 29 The relationship between saline cardiac output (CO_s) and cardiac output measured by a pulmonary artery electromagnetic flowmeter on the pulmonary artery (CO_{em}) in 10 dogs. [Redrawn from W. D. Voorhees et al., *Med. Instrum.* **19**(1):34–37 (1985).]

with a correlation coefficient of 0.965. The slope of the regression line (0.973) and the intercept (0.0047) were not significantly different from 1.0 and zero, respectively, at the $p = .01$ level. Figure 29 presents the results.

These studies by Grubbs et al. (1984) and Voorhees et al. (1986) clearly indicate that high accuracy is attainable with saline, a diffusible indicator, when it is used to measure cardiac output by right-atrial injection and pulmonary artery detection. In this situation there is no intervening capillary bed and therefore no indicator loss.

Flow-through Cell Technique. For studies in the experimental animal, it is often desirable to make repeated measurements of cardiac output using inexpensive equipment. Such a technique was described by Geddes et al. (1972); Fig. 30 illustrates the method in which a flow-through resistivity-measuring (conductivity) cell is placed in an arteriovenous shunt to record the dilution curve. In this application, the saline indicator is injected into the right external jugular vein. Since the injection is venous, the measurement is arterial, and the indicator is diffusable, it is expected that the cardiac output so obtained will be about 15% too high due to indicator loss in the pulmonary capillaries.

The flow-through resistivity-measuring cell is shown in Fig. 31. It consists of a plastic housing with screw caps that hold the stainless steel electrodes. Blood enters tangentially, swirls around the cell, and exits tangentially. The blood chamber is a cylinder 1 cm long and 1.129 cm in diameter (d). Thus the cross-sectional area is $0.785d^2$; therefore the cell constant $k = L/A = 1.00$. Thus, if the frequency used to measure the impedance between the electrode terminals is high enough (above 25 kHz), the electrode–blood interface impedance is low and the impedance

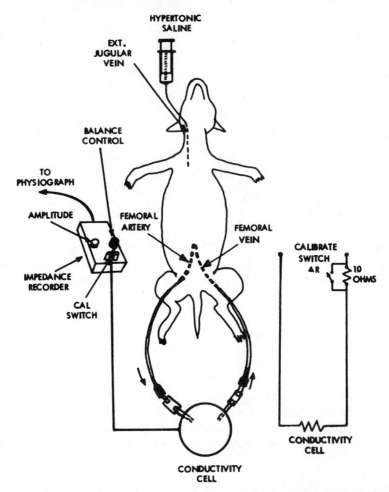

Figure 30 Arrangement employed to obtain multiple dilution curves without blood loss. The conductivity cell is placed in an arteriovenous shunt, and the indicator (sodium chloride solution) is injected into a large central vein (or the right atrium or ventricle). The dilution curve is obtained by continuously recording the impedance appearing between the terminals of the conductivity cell. Electrical calibration of the conductivity cell is achieved by short-circuiting a calibrating resistor (ΔR) in series with the conductivity cell.

so measured is close to the resistivity of the blood. Therefore, the baseline of the dilution curve is the blood resistivity. Electrical calibration of the dilution curve can be established by momentarily short-circuiting a 10-Ω resistor in series with the conductivity cell as shown in Fig. 30.

Because blood is caused to flow through the conductivity cell, it is necessary to use an anticoagulant (heparin, 1 mg/kg), which is usually satisfactory for a several-hour experiment. Figure 32 illustrates a typical record of impedance (resistiv-

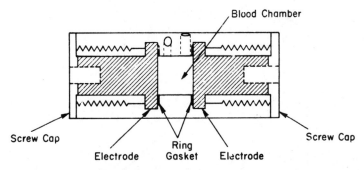

Figure 31 Flow-through blood-resistivity (conductivity) cell suitable for placing in an arteriovenous shunt to obtain dilution curves. Blood enters tangentially, swirls around, and exits tangentially. [Redrawn from D. S. Worley et al., *Physiologist* **25**(3):173–177 (1982).]

ity) decrease following the injection of 2 mL of 5% saline into the jugular vein. Note that the dilution curve exhibits recirculation, which must be removed.

Removal of Recirculation Error. Since the falling phase of the dilution curve is a good approximation to an exponential, semilogarithmic plotting of this portion of the curve will produce a straight line as shown in Fig. 33. Extrapolation of the linear portion to 1% of maximum concentration ($C_{max}/100$) will provide values that can be used to complete the dilution curve (dashed portion) shown in Fig. 32. The semilogarithmic extrapolation technique is frequently applied to dilution curves that exhibit recirculation. The method was introduced by Kinsman et al. (1929).

Referring to Fig. 32, the baseline resistance is 190 Ω, and the mean height and duration of the dilution curve are 4.35 Ω and 32 sec, respectively. The cell constant k is 1.0, and 2 mL of 5% saline ($m = 0.1$ g) was injected. The cardiac output is calculated from the equation

$$CO = \frac{60mBk}{t\,\Delta R}\left(\frac{R}{kA}\right)^{\beta/\alpha}$$

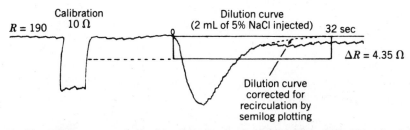

Figure 32 Dilution curve obtained by injecting 2 mL of 5% NaCl solution into the right atrium. The conductivity cell was placed in an arteriovenous shunt as shown in Fig. 30. The conductivity cell had an area A-to-length (A/L) ratio of $k = 1.0$.

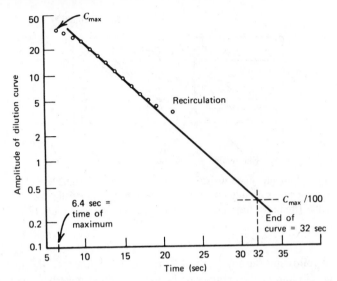

Figure 33 Semilog plot of the downslope of the dilution curve in Fig. 32. Note that the portion of the downslope of the dilution curve that is exponential is linear in the semilog plot. Extrapolation of the line joining the points forming the straight line allows the acquisition of values for the dilution curve during recirculation. In practice, extrapolation is carried out to find a time corresponding to 1% of the maximum height of the dilution curve. In this example the end of the dilution curve was found to occur at 32 sec, and the amplitudes between 15 sec (when recirculation became apparent) and 32 sec (the end of the curve) were used to complete the dilution curve in Fig. 32.

To illustrate, suppose the data are as follows:

$$m = 2 \text{ mL } 5\% = 0.1 \text{ g} \qquad A = 55.5$$
$$k = 1.0 \qquad \alpha = 0.024$$
$$t = 32 \text{ sec} \qquad B = 3.84$$
$$\Delta R = 4.35 \ \Omega \qquad \beta = 0.047$$
$$R = 190 \ \Omega$$

Then,

$$CO = \frac{60 \times 0.1 \times 3.84 \times 1.0}{32 \times 4.35} \left(\frac{190}{1.0 \times 55.5}\right)^{0.047/0.024}$$

$$= 1.84 \text{ L/min.}$$

The accuracy of the method just described was evaluated in dogs by Geddes et al. (1974a), using Evans blue in the reference method and bottled 5% saline and

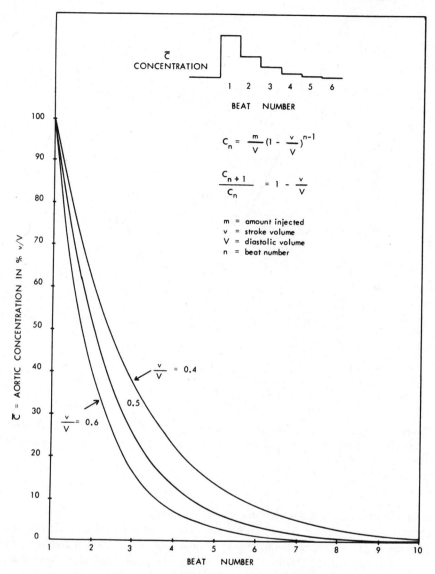

Figure 34   Fractional emptying of the left ventricle.

prepared saline as the indicators. With both saline indicators, the cardiac output was overestimated by 10–25%. The correlation coefficients with the two indicators were 0.91 and 0.98, respectively.

Ventricular Emptying. It is possible to measure stroke volume, end-diastolic volume, and ejection fraction by injecting a small amount of saline into a ventricle during diastole and measuring the stepwise change in impedance as the saline is washed out. Figure 34 illustrates the aortic concentration as the injected material

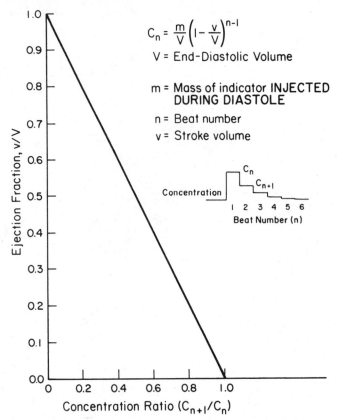

Figure 35 Ejection fraction versus concentration ratio for an indicator injected into a ventricle (during diastole), and concentration measured on a beat-by-beat basis in the outflow tract.

is cleared from the left ventricle for ejection fractions equal to 40, 50, and 60% of the diastolic volume V. The ejection fraction can be determined from the stepwise decrease in aortic concentration. Figure 35 is a plot of the ejection fraction v/V versus the concentration ratio C_{n+1}/C_n. Thus from calibrated records of these data, ventricular diastolic volume V and stroke volume v can be calculated. Cardiac output can also be determined by multiplying the stroke volume v by heart rate.

The fractional emptying of the left ventricle in the dog was determined by Holt (1957, 1962) and Holt and Allensworth (1957) using a modification of the sodium chloride indicator-dilution technique. By injecting a known amount of hypertonic sodium chloride into the left ventricle and continuously recording conductivity in the aorta, it was possible to calculate the volume of the left ventricle and the amount discharged per beat (stroke volume). Elegant as this technique is, it depends on the assumption that perfect mixing occurs in the left ventricle. That this is not always the case was shown by Irisawa et al. (1960).

The mathematical expression for the aortic concentration of a material injected into the left ventricle can be derived if two assumptions are made. The first is that the weight m (grams) of the material injected into the left ventricle is contained in a volume that is small with respect to the diastolic volume of the ventricle (V mL); the second is that uniform mixing takes place in the ventricle. The injection is made as quickly as possible just before systolic ejection. Then, if uniform mixing has occurred, and the stroke volume (v mL) remains constant for each beat, the aortic concentration (C mg/mL) will decrease in a stepwise fashion. For the first beat the aortic concentration will be (m/V) g/mL. The number of grams ejected is mv/V, and the number remaining in the ventricle is $m - mv/V$ or $m(1 - v/V)$ g. The ventricle then fills, and the diastolic volume is again V mL, into which this weight of material is diluted. The aortic concentration for the second beat is then $(1 - v/V)m/V$. The process continues to be repeated, and the general expression for the aortic concentration for the nth beat becomes

$$C_n = \frac{m}{V}\left(1 - \frac{v}{V}\right)^{n-1}$$

Stroke Volume by Direct Impedance Cardiography

Rappoport and Ray (1927) recorded the impedance changes in a tortoise heart as it was kept beating in vitro. The heart, suspended in a beaker of saline, constituted one electrode; the other was placed nearby in the solution. The investigators noted a change in impedance of 10% with each heart beat. Rushmer et al. (1953) affixed electrodes to the interior walls of the right and left ventricles of dogs. In one animal they placed electrodes at the apex and the base of the right and left ventricles. They recorded a decrease in impedance during diastole and an increase during systole. Although the recordings resembled those made with cardiometers, their studies on models and animals led them to believe that the method contained variables that were difficult to quantitate, and they abandoned the technique in favor of others that appeared more promising at that time. Mello-Sobrinho (1963) and Geddes et al. (1965, 1966) reinvestigated the value of the method, using electrodes (insulated except at the tip) inserted into the left ventricle at the base and the apex of canine hearts. Accordingly, the cardiac chambers functioned as conductivity cells of varying dimensions; the impedance decreased with filling and increased with emptying. Since the resistivity of cardiac muscle is several times that of blood, the current is largely confined to the ventricle. Figure 36 is a typical record of the 80-kHz impedance changes recorded with this technique. By making ventricular casts and measuring them, Mello-Sobrinho found that a 5-Ω change was equivalent to a 1-mL change in volume. Palmer (1970) obtained calibration factors of 0.5–1.7 Ω/mL by measuring cardiac output.

The ventricular stroke volume changes in atrial fibrillation and the increased stroke volume after restoration of normal sinus rhythm are dramatically illustrated by the impedance-stroke-volume method. On the left of Fig. 37, the atria are fibrillating and the ventricular stroke volume is irregular and small. Atrial fibril-

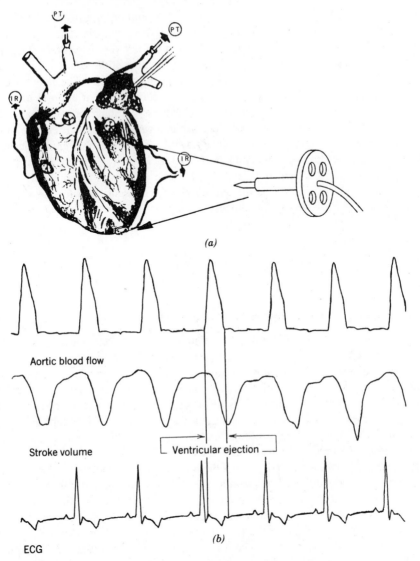

(a)

Aortic blood flow

Stroke volume   Ventricular ejection

(b)

ECG

Figure 36 (*a*) Method of recording stroke volume by measuring the impedance between a pair of electrodes inserted into a ventricle. (*b*) Aortic flow, impedance change, and ECG.

lation suddenly ceased at the center of the record, and the stroke volume became much larger, as shown. Note also the appearance of the atrial filling wave (ASV) when normal sinus rhythm returned.

It is possible to record the stroke-volume impedance changes with a catheter electrode in the left or right ventricle. However, the impedance-change curve is not exactly the same as that obtained with electrodes inserted through the ventricular

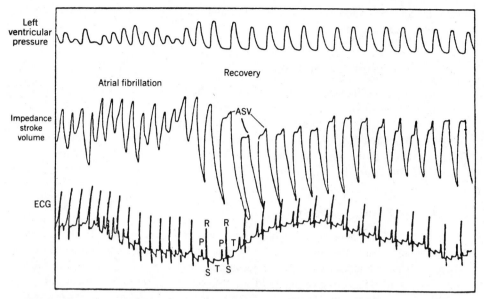

Figure 37 Ventricular volume changes during and after recovery from atrial fibrillation obtained using the method shown in Fig. 36.

walls at the base and apex. Palmer (1970) described the use of a bipolar catheter electrode in the left ventricle; using the Fick method to determine cardiac output, she found that the impedance change per milliliter of blood ejected was between 0.5 and 1.9 Ω/mL among the dogs studied.

Bourland et al. (1978) and Geddes et al. (1981) employed a bipolar right-ventricular catheter electrode to detect the absence of pulsatile impedance changes to identify ventricular fibrillation. This signal, along with the ECG change, directed the discharge of a capacitor to achieve ventricular defibrillation.

Investigators are beginning to use catheter electrodes to detect the pulsatile impedance changes in the ventricles to monitor stroke volume. Among these are Baan et al. (1981), McKay et al. (1984), Clavin et al. (1983), Salo and Walmer (1984), and Spinelli and Valentinuzzi (1986). From the data in the latter's paper, a coefficient of 0.86 Ω/mL was calculated.

There are several important considerations when using catheter electrodes in the ventricles. Of paramount importance is the spacing between the electrodes, which should be such that the electrodes are wholly within the chamber. Although a large pulsatile impedance change can be recorded, it may be contaminated by the proximity of the chordae and/or papillary muscles close to the electrodes.

Although it is possible to model the left and right ventricles geometrically to derive an estimate for the expected change in impedance for a given stroke volume, such models usually ignore the chordae and papillary muscles; consequently, the models, although useful, have limited value. Traditionally, the pulsatile impedance change has been calibrated by determining stroke volume by dividing cardiac output by heart rate. Thermodilution, dye dilution, and the Fick methods have been used to measure cardiac output.

The Pressure–Volume (*PV*) Loop

The ventricular impedance changes can be used along with ventricular pressure to create pressure–volume (impedance-change) loops; Fig. 38 is an example. The area inside such a loop represents the work done. The power can be calculated from the loop area divided by the time to complete the loop. The oxygen consumed is proportional to the power expended. The various phases of the ventricular cycle are nicely illustrated by such loops.

Impedance Plethysmography

The use of the impedance change technique for recording peripheral volume pulses was first described by Mann (1937). In a few years there appeared numerous papers on the subject, and the technique soon became known as impedance ple-thysmography. Pioneering in this field were Nyboer et al. (1943), Nyboer (1944, 1950, 1959). Brook and Cooper (1957), Polzer et al. (1960), and Polzer and Schuhfried (1961). Nyboer became the advocate of the tetrapolar electrode method, whereas most of the other investigators cited employed two-electrode systems. Although the literature shows that the impedance change is mainly resistive at the frequencies presently employed (20–100 kHz), Mann (1953) demonstrated the existence of a reactive component at 10 kHz when the impedance was measured between electrodes on each forearm.

With either the two- or the four-electrode system it is easy to obtain impedance

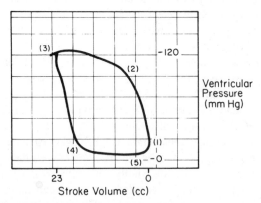

Figure 38 Pressure–volume loop from the canine left ventricle. Pressure was recorded from a catheter in the left ventricle; the impedance (volume) change was recorded from a bipolar electrode on the catheter. Ventricular contraction begins between 5 and 1; at 2, the aortic valve opens, and ejection continues to 3, at which time the aortic valve closes. From 3 to 4, the ventricle relaxes without filling, and at 4 the mitral valve opens and the ventricle starts to fill. (Redrawn from Palmer, 1970.)

changes strikingly similar to those recorded with capsule plethysmographs. The real difficulty lies in the lack of accurate methods to relate the impedance change to a volume change.

The basis for impedance plethysmography as applied to body segments is the decrease in impedance when a volume of blood is introduced between the measuring electrodes. The expression most frequently employed to relate the measured impedance change to the volume change can be derived by assuming that there is a homogeneous conducting material and a uniform current-density distribution between the measuring electrodes. Obviously these requirements are never satisfied in practical situations, and to minimize some of the resulting errors, current is introduced to the specimen by widely spaced electrodes. The current distribution between metal-band electrodes placed on homogeneous conducting cylinders of differing lengths can be seen in Figs. 39a and b. Note that in both cases there is the same distortion of the lines of equal current at each electrode, but in the central region a–a' (Fig. 39b) the current distribution is more uniform.

To illustrate how a volume change can be identified by a resistance change, we remove the conducting cylinder a–a' and place electrodes over its ends. For a length L, area A_0, and resistivity ρ, the resistance is $R_0 = \rho L / A_0$. Consider now the addition of a volume ΔV of conducting material to the segment without producing a change in length. The cross-sectional area will increase uniformly to A_1,

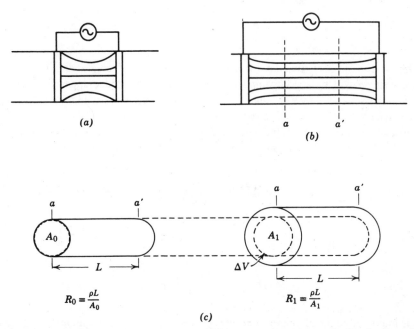

Figure 39 Simplified basis for impedance plethysmography: (a) current distribution with closely spaced and electrodes; (b) current distribution with widely spaced electrodes; (c) the result of adding a volume ΔV to the conducting cylinder a–a. $R_1 - R_0 = \Delta R = -(\Delta V / \rho)$ $(R_0 / L)^2$.

and the resistance measured between the electrode covering the ends will be $R_1 = \rho L / A_1$. The difference in resistance reflects the volume change; therefore,

$$\Delta R = R_1 - R_0 = \frac{\rho L}{A_1} - \frac{\rho L}{A_0} = \rho L \left(\frac{1}{A_1} - \frac{1}{A_0} \right),$$

but

$$V_0 = LA_0 \quad \text{and} \quad V_1 = LA_1.$$

Substituting,

$$\Delta R = \rho L \left(\frac{L}{V_1} - \frac{L}{V_0} \right)$$

$$= \rho L^2 \left(\frac{V_0 - V_1}{V_1 V_0} \right) = -\frac{\rho L^2 (V_1 - V_0)}{V_1 V_0}.$$

If V_1 is not appreciably larger than V_0 (i.e., the volume added, $\Delta V = V_1 - V_0$, is small), then,

$$\Delta R = - \left(\frac{\rho L^2}{V_0^2} \right) \Delta V.$$

Thus it can be seen that an increase in the volume of conducting material of resistivity ρ will be accompanied by a decrease in resistance appearing between electrodes separated by a distance L. Sometimes, instead of calculating the volume V_0 between the electrodes, the basal impedance value is used. This can be inserted into the formula by multiplying the expression $R_0 = \rho L / A_0$ by L/L to obtain $R_0 = \rho L^2 / V_0$. Substitution of this relationship in the foregoing equation gives

$$\Delta R = - \left(\frac{R_0^2}{\rho L^2} \right) \Delta V,$$

or by rearranging,

$$\Delta V = - \left(\frac{\rho L^2}{R_0^2} \right) \Delta R.$$

It is important to recall that this expression was derived assuming a uniform current-density distribution through a homogeneous conductor of uniform cross-sectional area. In the physiological application, this situation is almost never attained because when pulsatile blood flow measurements are made with the impedance method, the applied current is carried by at least two parallel conducting paths, tissue and blood. Although the resistivity of the latter is easy to measure, that of the former is not, because it consists of a variety of tissues, each having a characteristic value of resistivity. For this reason it is useful to perform an analysis of a two-compartment model to derive an expression for the change in blood volume that is reflected by a change in the impedance appearing between the potential-measuring electrodes (a–a' in Fig. 39*b*). It will be shown that when one makes fairly reasonable assumptions, the two-compartment model reduces to the one-compartment model just described.

Consider the two-compartment model illustrated in Fig. 40 in which A_t and A_b are the cross-sectional areas of the tissues and blood, respectively, and L is the spacing between the potential-measuring electrodes a, b. The resistivities of tissue and blood are ρ_t and ρ_b. Now the resistance R_{ab} appearing between electrodes a, b is given by

$$\frac{1}{R_{ab}} = \frac{1}{R_t} + \frac{1}{R_b},$$

where R_t and R_b are the resistivities of the tissue and blood paths, respectively. Accordingly,

$$R_t = \frac{\rho_t L}{A_t} \quad \text{and} \quad R_b = \frac{\rho_b L}{A_b}.$$

Substitution of these relationships and manipulation gives

$$R_{ab} = \frac{\rho_t \rho_b L}{\rho_b A_t + \rho_t A_b}.$$

Now it is assumed that when an increment of blood ΔV_b enters the region between the potential-measuring electrodes, the tissue area A_t remains essentially the same, or, stated another way, the change in area of the segment results from a small increase in the area of the blood conductor (A_b). Accepting this fairly

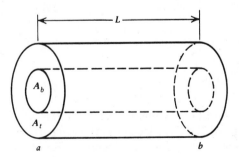

Figure 40 Two-compartment model for a body segment in which A_t represents its area occupied by tissue and A_b represents the area occupied by blood; $R_t = \rho_t L / A_t$ and $R_b = \rho_b L / A_b$ when R_t and R_b are the resistances of the tissue and blood paths, ρ_t and ρ_b are the tissue and blood resistivities, respectively, and L is the spacing of the potential-measuring electrodes.

reasonable physiological assumption permits derivation of an expression for the change in resistance appearing between the potential-measuring electrodes when blood enters the region between them.

Recalling that length multiplied by area is equal to volume, it is possible to multiply the right-hand side of the preceding expression by L/L and substitute for the volume of tissue $V_t = A_t L$ and the volume of blood $V_b = A_b L$ to obtain

$$R_{ab} = \frac{\rho_t \rho_b L^2}{\rho_b V_t + \rho_t V_b}.$$

To obtain a value for the change in resistance due to the entry of blood into the segment, it is merely necessary to differentiate R_{ab} with respect to V_b. Performing this operation, and recalling that V_t is assumed to be constant gives

$$dR_{ab} = -\left(\frac{\rho_b \rho_t^2 L^2}{(\rho_t V_b + \rho_b V_t)^2}\right) dV_b.$$

By remembering that $V_t = L A_t$ and $V_b = L A_b$, it is possible to make these substitutions and rearrange the expression to obtain a relationship that links the change in blood volume dV_b with the change in resistance dR_{ab}; carrying out this manipulation gives

$$dV_b = -\frac{(\rho_b A_t + \rho_t A_b)^2}{\rho_t^2 \rho_b} dR_{ab}.$$

Although this expression permits calculaton using a two-compartment model, it is practically impossible to determine the areas occupied by tissue (A_t) and blood (A_b). It is, however, convenient to use the basal resistance R_{ab} as a measure of their magnitudes. Therefore, as shown previously,

$$\rho_b A_t + \rho_t A_b = \frac{\rho_t \rho_b L}{R_{ab}}.$$

When this relationship is substituted into the expression for dV_b, the following is obtained:

$$dV_b = -\rho_b \left(\frac{L}{R_{ab}}\right)^2 dR_{ab}.$$

Note that this expression is the same as that derived for the change in resistance in a single blood cylinder when a volume of blood is added to it. In its application it is important to recall the basic assumptions: (1) The cross-sectional area of the tissue mass remained constant, (2) the area of the blood conductor increased with entry of a volume of blood into the region between the potential-measuring electrodes, and (3) the length L was constant.

If it is assumed that impedance Z may be substituted for resistance R, the expression for the blood volume change (ΔV) can be rewritten as

$$\Delta V = -\left(\frac{\rho L^2}{Z_0^2}\right) \Delta Z,$$

where ρ = resistivity of the blood,
L = distance (cm) between the potential-measuring electrodes,
Z_0 = basal impedance measured at end diastole, and
ΔZ = change in impedance attributable to the stroke volume in the absence of arterial runoff.

The negative sign merely signifies that the entry of blood produces a decrease in impedance between the potential-measuring electrodes.

When this simple expression is put to practical use to calculate the volume of blood (ΔV) entering the body segment between the potential-measuring electrodes, both physiological and physical factors come into play, making it difficult to determine ΔV accurately. It is important to note that the peak-to-peak amplitude of the pulsatile impedance change ($\Delta Z'$ in Fig. 41) is a measure of the difference

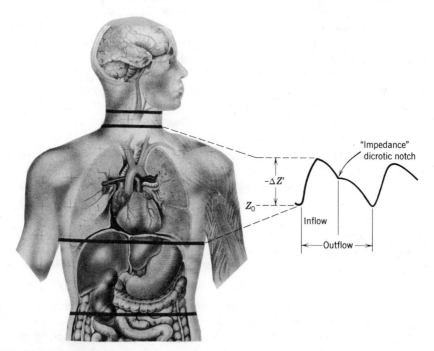

Figure 41 Location for the neck and chest electrodes for impedance cardiography. The outer two electrodes are for current injection; from the inner electrodes is derived a voltage that is proportional to the cardiac-induced impedance change $\Delta Z'$.

between blood flow into and out of the body segment between the potential-measuring electrodes. Since $\Delta Z'$ is supposed to measure the volume change produced only by the inflow of blood into the body segment, some means is required to estimate what this change would be in the absence of arterial runoff. Development of a suitable method is difficult in the case of thoracic impedance cardiography. Despite differences between the ideal and practical situations, the impedance method is useful and very convenient in estimating the change in blood volume of a body segment during each beat of the heart.

Impedance Cardiography

If electrodes are placed to encompass the thorax, impedance changes reflecting cardiac activity are recordable with ease. Bipolar and tetrapolar electrode arrangements have been placed on the arms, on either side of the thorax, on the back, and around the neck and chest at the level of the diaphragm. Clear cardiac impedance pulses can be recorded with any of these electrode configurations. When two electrodes are placed on the neck, as shown in Figs. 41 and 42a, they should be separated as widely as possible (by at least 3 cm) to ensure the most uniform current-density distribution. Some investigators use the forehead for the headward current-injecting electrode. Figure 42a illustrates the type of recording obtained from a human subject during breath holding. The electrocardiogram, recorded from the same pair of electrodes, is shown to identify the temporal location of the impedance change in the cardiac cycle.

A number of investigators have studied the thoracic impedance cardiogram, hoping to calibrate it in terms of the systolic discharge from the heart. Probably the earliest were Atzler and Lehmann (1932) and Atzler (1933, 1935), who placed metal-plate electrodes in front of and behind the thorax and detected ultrahigh-frequency impedance changes synchronous with cardiac activity. Because their circuit was mainly capacitive, they called the method ''Dielektrographie.'' Later Nyboer et al. (1940) described precordial impedance changes that also reflected cardiac activity. Probably in an attempt to standardize electrode placement, Holzer et al. (1945) measured the 14-kHz cardiac impedance pulses appearing between electrodes placed on the arms and legs. Their study examined the impedance pulses in human subjects in health and disease, measuring impedance changes by means of the standard electrocardiographic lead configurations. They called their method ''Rheokardiographie.''

Improving the capacitive method of Atzler and Lehmann, Whitehorn and Pearl (1949) employed a 10.7-MHz current and were able to record impedance pulses with high fidelity, stating:

''Values for stroke volumes, cardiac output and cardiac indices calculated from such records, on the basis of preliminary calibration of the instrument by introduction of known volumes of saline between the plates, fall within the range of accepted normal values, but conclusions as to the validity of the method are not yet possible.''

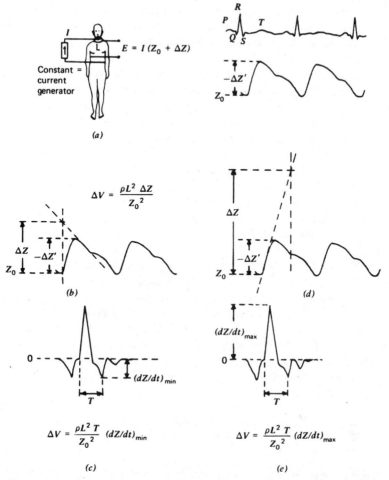

Figure 42 (*a*) A typical thoracic impedance cardiogram; to the left is the conventional electrode arrangement. A decrease in impedance ($-\Delta Z'$) is shown by an upward deflection in the recording. (*b*) The backslope extrapolation technique used to obtain the impedance change ΔZ, which reflects the total volume of blood entering the region between the potential measuring electrodes. Electronic differentiation of the impedance pulse $\Delta Z'$ provides a means of recording continuously the slope of the impedance pulse (*c*), and its use to obtain ΔZ, which is equal to $T(dz/dt)_{min}$. (*d*) The forward extrapolation technique for obtaining ΔZ. The steepest slope $(dZ/dt)_{max}$ is obtained by electrical differentiation (*e*), and ΔZ is equal to $T(dZ/dt)_{max}$.

Mann (1953), using his 10-kHz capacigraph, which recorded only the capacitance changes between single electrodes placed on each forearm, believed that these changes were due mainly to blood volume changes within the thorax, although he admitted the presence of smaller changes in the arms. Zajic et al. (1954), using 270 kHz applied to one electrode on the neck and another either in the pelvic area or on the thighs, observed changes in the impedance pulse with manuevers that were known to change stroke volume. In one study Nyboer (1959) presented records called radiocardiograms, taken at several levels on the precordium with his tetrapolar electrode system.

Thoracic impedance cardiography continues to be actively investigated because it is virtually the only noninvasive method available to estimate stroke volume (the volume of blood ejected with each heart beat). Figure 42 illustrates the methods used to obtain human thoracic impedance cardiograms from a tetrapolar electrode system employing a constant-current sinusoidal generator; at present a frequency in the range of 20–100 kHz is employed.

Nyboer, one of the pioneers in the use of electrical impedance to measure blood volume changes, developed what is now called the backslope or end-systolic extrapolation technique (1959) to obtain a value for the impedance change ΔZ that reflects the entry of blood between the potential-measuring electrodes when no outflow occurs. Allison and Nyboer (1965) verified the accuracy of the method using a hydraulic model.

Referring to Fig. 42b, just beyond the peak of the impedance pulse $\Delta Z'$ the physiological conditions are such that inflow to the thoracic segment between the potential-measuring electrodes (L cm apart) is minimum and outflow is maximum. It is fairly reasonable to assume that backward extrapolation of the steepest part of the postpeak impedance curve to a vertical line erected at the beginning of the pulse (which signals the beginning of ventricular ejection) would provide an impedance change ΔZ that corresponds to the inflow if no outflow existed. Therefore the stroke volume ΔV entering the segment can be calculated by using the expression given previously:

$$\Delta V = \frac{\rho L^2}{Z_0^2}(\Delta Z).$$

In this expression, ρ is the resistivity of the blood (in ohm-centimeters) for the packed-cell volume that exists, and Z_0 is the basal thoracic impedance between the potential-measuring electrodes, which are L cm apart. ΔZ is shown in Fig. 42b.

Because graphical extrapolation involves visual estimation of the steepest part of the immediate postpeak impedance curve, it is often more convenient to employ electronic differentiation to identify this slope and use a simple mathematical expression to derive the impedance change ΔZ that reflects volume inflow without outflow. Figure 42c illustrates application of the derivative to the impedance pulse (dZ/dt) to obtain the approximate ejection time T. Thus the slope $(dZ/dt)_{min}$, multiplied by the ejection time T, gives a corrected value for the impedance change ΔZ without outflow:

$$\Delta Z = T(dZ/dt)_{min}.$$

Entering the value for ΔZ into the expression just given allows calculation of the approximate stroke volume. Cardiac output is equal to stroke volume multiplied by heart rate.

The correction method developed by Kubicek et al. (1966) assumes that at the beginning of inflow to the interelectrode segment, outflow is minimal and inflow is maximal. Therefore forward extrapolation of the steepest part of the impedance pulse, if continued to the end of the ejection period T, which is often taken as the dicrotic notch in the impedance record (see Fig. 42d), would provide an impedance change ΔZ that is corrected for outflow. Entry of this value into the expression presented previously provides an approximate value for stroke volume ΔV. Often the impedance dicrotic notch is not prominent, and the onset of the second heart sound is used to identify the end of the ejection period. However, use of the electrical differentiation technique permits determination of the approximate ejection period T without the aid of the phonocardiogram.

Baker and Mistry (1981) evaluated blood flow values obtained by using the three extrapolation techniques shown in Fig. 42. Their preparation consisted of an isolated aorta in a fluid-filled chamber. Tetrapolar recording was used, and the blood flow in the aorta was made pulsatile by using a pump. They found that the maximum derivative method (Fig. 42c) produced the largest overestimate of flow. The forward projection method (Fig. 42d) overestimated less, and the backward projection method (Fig. 42b) overestimated flow the least.

Of all the methods for obtaining ΔZ, the maximum-derivative method (Fig. 42e) appears to be the most popular. With this concept, it is assumed that if the maximum rate of ventricular ejection continued throughout the ejection period T, the impedance change ΔZ would be $T(dZ/dt)_{max}$. This is a reasonable assumption because $(dZ/dt)_{max}$ occurs just after the beginning of ejection, and at this time the outflow from the arterial tree is minimum. Therefore the stroke-volume (SV) equation is

$$ \text{SV} = \rho \left(\frac{L}{Z_0} \right)^2 T \left(\frac{dZ}{dt} \right)_{max}, $$

where ρ = the resistivity of blood (Ω-cm),
L = the separation (cm) between the two inner (2, 3) potential-measuring electrodes,
Z_0 = the basal impedance between the potential-measuring electrodes (2, 3),
$(dZ/dt)_{max}$ = the maximum rate of change in impedance (Ω/sec), and
T = the ventricular ejection time (see Fig. 43).

The ventricular ejection time T can be obtained in several ways. Sometimes it is obtained from the derivative recording (Fig. 42e). At other times it is obtained from an arterial pulse recording, being the time from the start of the upstroke to the dicrotic notch. The time between the first and second heart sounds has also been used as a measure of T; however, it must be recalled that this time is slightly longer, because it includes the isovolumic period of ventricular contraction.

Calibration signals from the impedance cardiograph allow quantification of the record to obtain Z_0 and $(dZ/dt)_{max}$. Figure 43 illustrates a typical record.

The value for the resistivity ρ of blood depends on the percent packed-cell

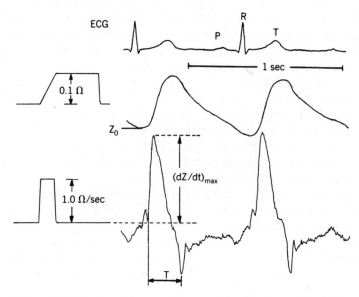

Figure 43   The impedance cardiogram and its time derivative dZ/dt.

volume H. For humans, the resistivity in ohm-centimeters was given by Geddes and Sadler (1973) as

$$\rho = 53.2e^{0.022H}.$$

Often it is undesirable to draw a blood sample to measure the packed-cell volume or resistivity. In these cases it is often assumed that a normal packed-cell volume of 40% exists and that therefore the resistivity at 37°C is 130 Ω-cm. Quail et al. (1981) advocated a value of 135 Ω-cm for general use. An alternative is to use the noninvasive method reported by Yamakoshi et al. (1980), which is described earlier in this chapter.

To illustrate a calculation of stroke volume SV, suppose the data are as follows: $\rho = 130$ Ω-cm, $L = 30$ cm, $Z_0 = 25$ Ω, $T = 0.22$ sec, $(dZ/dt)_{max} = 2.0$ Ω/sec. Using the equation presented earlier, the value for SV is obtained as follows:

$$SV = \rho \left(\frac{L}{Z_0}\right)^2 T \left(\frac{dZ}{dt}\right)_{max}$$

$$= 130 \left(\frac{30}{25}\right)^2 (0.22)(2.0)$$

$$= 82 \text{ mL}.$$

Verification Studies

Of particular importance is the relationship between cardiac output measured by impedance cardiography and values measured by conventional techniques such as the use of blood flowmeters and the indicator-dilution and Fick methods. Such comparisons have been made by Kinnen et al. (1964/), Allison (1966a,b), Kubicek et al. (1966), Harley and Greenfield (1968), Bache et al. (1969), Judy et al. (1969), Smith et al. (1969), Pomerantz et al. (1970), Kinnen (1970), Kubicek et al. (1970), Baker et al. (1971), Van de Water et al. (1971, 1973), Lababidi et al. (1971), Milleret and Barbe (1972), Naggar et al. (1975), Pate et al. (1975), Keim et al. (1976), Yamakoshi et al. (1976), Haffty et al. (1977), Denniston et al. (1976), Yu-Tang and Wen-Ti (1979), Boer et al. (1979), Miles et al. (1981), Edmunds et al. (1982), Judy et al. (1984, 1985), and Zhang et al. (1986). In some of these studies the correct value for blood resistivity was used; in others an assumed value or a room-temperature value was entered into the equation. Nonetheless, it would appear that, in general, impedance cardiography provides a value for cardiac output that agrees with the value obtained by an accepted method or overestimates cardiac output by as much as 25%.

A large number of studies have shown that impedance cardiography tracks changes in cardiac output very well. This point was made by Denniston et al. (1976) in a study of normal subjects exercising on a bicycle ergometer. Figure 44 illustrates the relationship between impedance cardiac output and true cardiac output. By correcting the data points (using the slope of the regression line in Fig. 44), Denniston replotted the data to show how well the impedance cardiac output tracks cardiac output, as measured with Cardio-green dye. Figure 45 presents the result.

Mohapatra et al. (1977) pointed out that the degree of overestimation of cardiac output by the impedance method is dependent on the packed-cell volume. From a study on infants they developed a logarithmic correction factor that when multiplied by the impedance cardiac output provided values in agreement with those obtained by a standard method. Edmunds et al. (1982) found this correction factor to be inadequate and proposed a linear correction based on packed-cell volume. At present there is no agreement on the equation for the correction factor that includes the packed-cell volume.

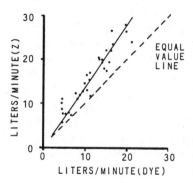

Figure 44 The relationship between impedance cardiac output Z and dye cardiac output in exercising subjects. [Redrawn from Denniston et al. (1976).]

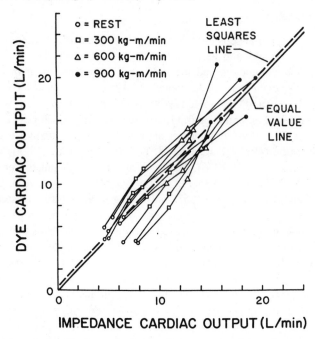

Figure 45 The relationship between dye cardiac output and impedance cardiac output (corrected) in subjects exercising on a bicycle ergometer. [Redrawn from J. C. Denniston et al., *J. Appl. Physiol.* **40**:91–95 (1976).]

A practical consideration worthy of note is the value for L, the separation between the two (inner) potential-measuring electrodes. Usually when this dimension is measured along the sternum, it differs from the magnitude measured along midaxillary lines and on the back. In this situation, the mean separation is sometimes taken. Denniston et al. (1976) were the first to report that use of L measured along the sternum provided values of cardiac output closest to those measured simultaneously, by dye dilution, in exercising subjections. Judy et al. (1984, 1985) found a much better agreement between impedance cardiac output and thermal-dilution output when the minimum separation was used for L.

In considering the accuracy of impedance cardiography it is useful to recognize that many oversimplifications were made in deriving the fundamental expression for stroke volume. It was assumed that current distribution was uniform and that the average resistivity of the thoracic contents was similar to that of blood; of course, the actual situation is far different. Whether a correction factor should be applied to Z_0 has not been considered. It may be that chest circumference or some other factor can be used to correct Z_0 so that impedance stroke volume comes closer to measured stroke volume. However, heroic efforts along these lines may not be rewarded. Perhaps it is best to recognize that impedance cardiography tracks stroke volume quite well in humans and animals and is perhaps the best noninvasive method available for this purpose.

Computer Averaging of the dZ/dt Waveform

Because the impedance cardiogram is obscured by body movement, it is often necessary to obtain and measure the recording during periods between breaths. This requirement is inconvenient and has somewhat limited the practical application of impedance cardiography. This problem is being partly solved by the use of signal averaging, which is ideally applicable because a timing signal (the R wave of the ECG) is already available from the thoracic electrodes.

Signal (ensemble) averaging is easily applied to remove non-R-wave locked artifacts from the dZ/dt signal, which bears an almost constant temporal relationship to the R wave of the ECG, which precedes it. Interfering signals do not share this relationship. Therefore, the R wave of the ECG can initiate repetitive sampling of the dZ/dt signal throughout its duration. Since the dZ/dt wave is time-locked to the R wave, each amplitude at the same time instant after the onset of sampling will be the same (or very nearly so). However, this is not true for the non-time-locked signals. Therefore an average amplitude at each instant after the onset of sampling will result in an enhanced dZ/dt signal, the artifact being effectively removed.

The use of R-wave-triggered averaging to enhance the dZ/dt signal was reported by Gollan et al. (1978) and Sheps et al. (1982). The interest of these investigators was to obtain a representative dZ/dt signal for measurement of the systolic timing intervals (see below). Muzi et al. (1985, 1986) described the use of ensemble averaging of the dZ/dt signal for the automatic calculation of stroke volume. They presented an excellent record (Fig. 46) that illustrates the signal-averaging process. In Fig. 46a is shown a dZ/dt record in which the baseline is moving due to respiration. The individual sampled signals are shown in Fig. 46b, and the averaged dZ/dt for five signals is shown in Fig. 46c. In their comparison of stroke volume obtained from computer (ensemble)-averaged dZ/dt signals and the same manually measured signal, the relationship between the ensembled average (EA) values versus manually measured (M) values was EA $= 0.91M + 4.31$, with a correlation coefficient of 0.972.

As stated previously, signal-averaging techniques applied to the dZ/dt signal will permit easier determination of stroke volume and cardiac output. Of course, values for ρ (blood resistivity) and L (electrode separation) must be entered for such automatic computation.

Systolic Time Intervals

Because the ΔZ and dZ/dt signals represent mechanical events, there is considerable interest in using these waveforms to extract information about the onset of systole and the beginning and end of ventricular ejection. The phonocardiogram and an arterial pulse pickup are traditionally used for this purpose. Since the timing of systolic events with respect to the R wave of the ECG reflects ventricular dynamics, extraction of timing information from the impedance cardiogram is of value to the clinician.

Figure 47 illustrates ECG, ΔZ, and dZ/dt recordings obtained by Peterson

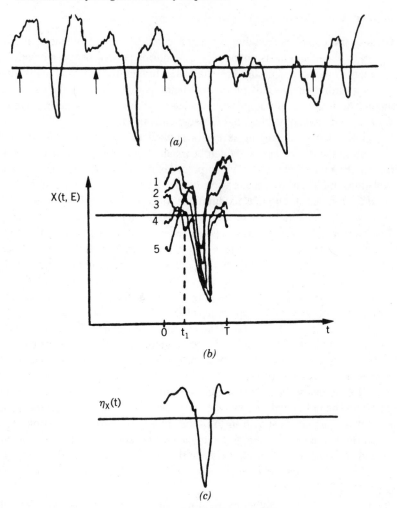

Figure 46 Record of (a) dZ/dt, (b) individual waves, and (c) average of four waves, using the R wave of the ECG as a time marker. [Redrawn from M. Muzi et al., *J. Appl. Physiol.* **58**(1):200–205 (1985).]

(1978) with dZ/dt labeled according to Lababidi et al. (1970). The A wave co-incides with the fourth heart sound and is atrial in timing. Takada et al. (1977) stated that the A wave reflects atrial contractility. Ventricular ejection commences with the B wave and continues to the X wave, when the aortic valve closes. The pulmonic valve closes at Y; O identifies opening of the mitral valve. The third heart sound (rapid ventricular filling) is associated with the Z wave. Most dZ/dt recordings allow identification of these components; however, in cardiovascular disease the identification is sometimes difficult.

The ability of the B-X interval to identify the left ventricular ejection time T has been documented by Labibidi et al. (1970, 1971), Hill et al. (1976), and Colin

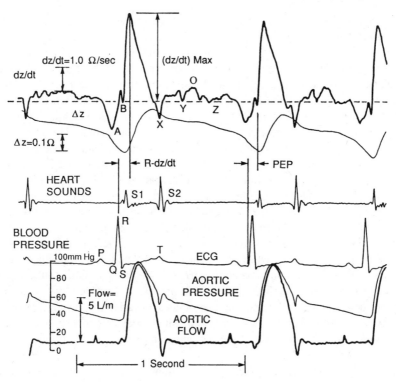

Figure 47 The dZ/dt and ΔZ impedance signals along with heart sounds, the ECG, arterial pressure, and aortic blood flow.

(1982). The preejection period (PEP), which is the time from electrical ventricular excitation to the onset of left ventricular ejection, reflects the metabolic status of the myocardium. This time is usually measured from the onset of the Q wave (or R wave if no Q wave is present) to the beginning of left ventricular ejection. When the ECG and dZ/dt recordings are used, the period is usually measured from the apex of the Q wave of the ECG to the B wave of the dZ/dt record.

Heather (1969) proposed that the ratio of $(dZ/dt)_{(max)}$ to the time from the Q wave to the peak of the dZ/dt recording would be a useful indicator of myocardial contractility. Because the Q wave is sometimes very small in amplitude, Hill and Merrifield (1976) advocated using the R wave for timing. Thus the Heather index, as it has come to be known, is the ratio of $(dZ/dt)_{(max)}$ to R-peak dZ/dt; this time is identified in Fig. 47. At present, clinical data are being accumulated on the value of the Heather index as a measure of contractility.

Genesis of the Impedance Cardiogram

As described earlier, the various waves in the thoracic impedance cardiogram (ΔZ) and its derivative (dZ/dt) have been correlated with systole and diastole of the atria and ventricles (Lababidi et al., 1970). However, the factors that underlie the genesis of the impedance cardiogram are not agreed upon, partly because the current pathway between the current-injecting electrodes is virtually unknown. The injected current flows through the extrathoracic and intrathoracic circulations. The former is smaller in extent but closer to the current-injecting electrodes. Both circulations have pulsatile components; those of the intrathoracic circulation consist of the pulmonary artery and the vascular bed of the lungs, the aorta, the atria, the ventricles, and the great veins. The pulmonary vascular bed, which is immediately below the rib cage, is large and carries the entire cardiac output. The aorta, which is deeper in the thorax, does not carry the entire cardiac output because of its many branches. A typical systolic change in aortic diameter is about 5%. The short pulmonary artery is deep within the thorax and pulsates with stroke volume. The four pulsating, blood-filled chambers of the heart all produce pulsatile impedance changes. The great veins expand and recoil when the heart beats. A considerable volume of blood is contained within the large deep thoracic veins.

In summary, the injected current passes through large vessels and vascular beds and heart chambers, all of which can contribute to a pulsatile impedance change. Moreover, these vessels and chambers carry blood with a variable (pulsating) velocity. As stated earlier in this chapter, the resistivity of blood is slightly dependent on its velocity. Thus, vessel and chamber dimension variations as well as resistivity change can contribute to the measured change in thoracic impedance. Many studies have been carried out to identify the participation of each factor in the genesis of the impedance cardiogram.

Bonjer et al. (1952), in a series of ingenious experiments that consisted of wrapping first the heart and then the lungs in rubber sheeting and perfusing each with a stroke pump, concluded that the thoracic impedance changes were due mainly to perfusion of the pulmonary vascular circuit by the output from the right ventricle and that only a small component was due to direct volume changes of the heart. Injecting 2 mL of 2% saline into the left and then the right ventricles of dogs during diastole, Geddes and Baker (1972) showed that when the saline was confined to the ventricles the thoracic impedance change due to the injection was small. However, with the first postinjection beat, the decrease in impedance was always larger for left ventricular injection. With right ventricular injection, the decrease in basal impedance Z_0 for postinjection beats appeared sooner, was larger in amplitude, and lasted longer. Injection into the aorta and pulmonary artery produced impedance changes larger than those produced by injection into the ventricles. Inferior vena cava injections produced small biphasic changes in thoracic impedance. Finally, the creation of atrioventricular block revealed a clear atrial component that occurs normally in the beating heart just before the upstroke of the ΔZ wave. The findings of these authors indicate that the impedance cardiogram contains both left and right ventricular components. Venous and atrial components, although present, are small.

Namon and Gollan (1970) used four 2.5 cm $\times$ 2.5 cm electrodes applied to the midline of the canine thorax and studied the 37-kHz resistive and reactive components of the pulsatile impedance change. Over a wide range of stroke volumes, they found that the magnitude of the reactive component varied between 25 and

100% of the amplitude of the resistive component. It was discovered that the amplitude of the reactance pulse correlated better with stroke volume (as measured by the indicator-dilution method) than did the amplitude of the pulsatile change in resistance. No data were given on values for stroke volume obtained from the reactive or resistive impedance pulses.

Namon and Gollan also recorded resistive and reactive thoracic impedance pulses from humans. The best results were obtained when the two current-injecting electrodes were placed on the back over the spine. No correlation data were presented in their initial study. Work in this direction has not continued. The use of spot (and strip) electrodes (Judy et al., 1984) has appeared from time to time; however, there has been no study to indicate the optional size and location in relation to anatomical landmarks.

Goto et al. (1981) conducted a series of ingenious experiments in dogs in which the flow in the pulmonary vascular circuit and the aorta could be made either pulsatile or nonpulsatile. While carrying out these maneuvers, they recorded impedance cardiograms and reported that both the right and left heart contribute to the impedance cardiogram. In another series of experiments in which only the pulmonary vascular circuit was made pulsatile or nonpulsatile, Saito et al. (1983) showed that the amplitude of the thoracic impedance cardiogram was reduced when the pulmonary circuit flow was made nonpulsatile, thereby adding confirmation to the studies by Goto et al. (1981). Baker and Mistry (1981), in a series of dog studies in which the pulmonary artery was occluded, showed that left ventricular ejection contributed 60% and right ventricular ejection contributed 40% to the thoracic impedance change.

Baker and Mistry (1981) conducted a series of model experiments to identify the contributions due to vascular volume and blood resistivity change. They concluded that both contributed to the impedance cardiogram. In a series of model experiments, Visser et al. (1981) concluded that the thoracic impedance cardiogram contained equal components due to vascular volume change and due to blood resistivity decrease with flow.

From the foregoing, it is quite clear that the thoracic impedance cardiogram contains components that are associated with vascular volume change and blood resistivity change with flow. An increase in the size of a vessel and the increase in blood flow that occurs in the vessel result in a decrease in impedance. Moreover, it is also clear that both left and right ventricular ejection contribute to the pulsatile decrease in thoracic impedance. However, there is no agreement on the extent to which these factors contribute to the impedance cardiogram.

Precordial Dilution Curve

When the direct-coupled method is used to record the arterial pulse, as in impedance cardiography, peripheral impedance plethysmography, and rheoencephalography, it is possible to record a dilution curve by injecting hyperconducting saline intravenously. Figure 48 illustrates such a dilution curve recorded from the thorax employing the tetrapolar electrode system used for impedance cardiography. Also

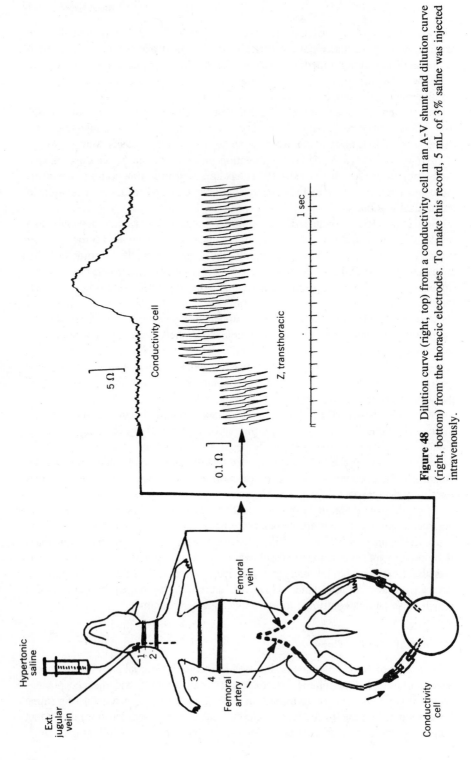

Figure 48 Dilution curve (right, top) from a conductivity cell in an A-V shunt and dilution curve (right, bottom) from the thoracic electrodes. To make this record, 5 mL of 3% saline was injected intravenously.

Hypertonic saline

Ext. jugular vein

Femoral vein

Femoral artery

Conductivity cell

Conductivity cell

Z, transthoracic

5 Ω

0.1 Ω

1 sec

shown is a dilution curve obtained from a flow-through conductivity cell placed in an arteriovenous shunt. To obtain these curves, 5 mL of 3% saline were injected into the right external jugular vein.

As yet, this technique for obtaining dilution curves, which only requires the use of body-surface electrodes, has not been put to practical use. It can provide information on circulation time.

Impedance Plethysmography of the Extremities

A reduction in blood flow to the extremities occurs in many types of cardiovascular disease. Accordingly, to assist in the diagnosis of peripheral vascular diseases and in evaluating the effect of therapeutic measures, considerable effort has been directed toward the development of quantitative methods to measure peripheral blood flow. The standard method available (venous-occlusion plethysysmography) is cumbersome to apply. The impedance method, however, is much easier to use and therefore offers attractive clinical possibilities. It has not seen extensive use because of difficulties in relating the impedance change, which is measured in ohms, to blood flow in units of milliliters per minute per gram of tissue (perfusion). Excellent accounts of the history and development of the impedance method are to be found in Nyboer's two monographs (1959, 1970).

Venous-Occlusion Plethysmography. Before describing impedance plethysmography of the extremities, the method that it may ultimately replace—namely, venous-occlusion plethysmography—must be understood because it provides a reasonably accurate measure of blood flow into an extremity. Most important, this technique will undoubtedly be used to verify the accuracy of the data obtained by impedance plethysmography.

The principle of the venous-occlusion plethysmographic technique was described by Brodie and Russell (1905). Figure 49 shows application of the pneumatic method to the finger and arm. (Water-filled systems have also been employed.) When applied to the finger (Fig. 49a), a hollow capsule is placed around a digit and sealed to it with any convenient thick paste (a disposable syringe barrel makes a convenient plethysmograph). The air in the chamber is connected to a sensitive pressure transducer, which in turn is connected to a graphic recorder. Also connected to the pneumatic system is a small syringe, which is used to inject a known volume of air for calibration purposes. Just central to the capsule, an inflatable cuff is wrapped around the finger. The cuff is employed to occlude venous outflow from the digit.

To measure digital blood flow, the apparatus is set up as in Fig. 49a. Because of the pulsatile expansion of the digit, small oscillations in pressure are recordable from the air surrounding the finger. When a determination of blood flow is to be made, the venous-occlusion cuff is suddenly inflated to about 50 mmHg, a pressure above venous and below arterial diastolic pressure. When this is done, arterial inflow starts to swell the digit, and the pressure in the capsule increases—at first, linearly with each heart beat, as in Fig. 49a. While the capsule pressure continues

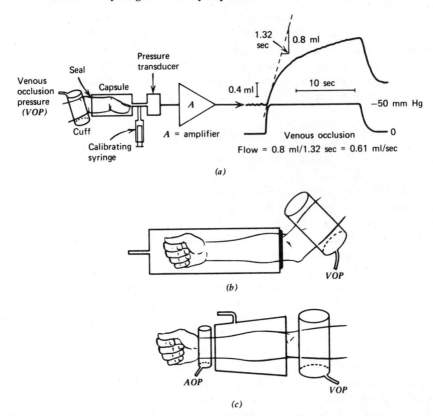

Figure 49 Application of venous-occlusion plethysmography to measure blood flow in (a) the digit, (b) forearm and hand, (c) and forearm only. The method consists of measuring the rate of swelling of the member when venous outflow is arrested by quickly inflating a cuff to venous occluding pressure (VOP), usually about 50 mm Hg. To measure flow in the forearm only, inflow and outflow to the hand are arrested by inflating the cuff to above arterial occluding pressure (AOP).

to increase, the linear rise gives way to an exponential rise because venous blood pressure increases and the net pressure driving the blood (arteriovenous) becomes less with each heart beat. A second reason for the exponential nature of the pressure rise relates to the nonlinear pressure–volume characteristic of the vascular bed. Continued application of the occluding pressure will result in venous pressure overcoming the pressure in the occluding cuff, and venous outflow will be reestablished. However, the measurement is not continued until this point is reached; the occluding pressure is reduced long before the plateau in capsule pressure is attained.

The blood flow per unit time into the digit is calculated by drawing a tangent to the capsule pressure curve where it departs from the baseline at the onset of venous occlusion. The slope of this tangent is converted to volume by recording capsule pressure while injecting a known volume of air while the finger is still inside the capsule. A time calibration is also placed on the record. Sample calculations for digital volume flow appear in Fig. 49a.

Figure 49 also shows how venous-occlusion plethysmography is applied to the hand and forearm (Fig. 49b) and to the forearm only (Fig. 49c). In the latter case, blood flow into the hand is arrested by inflating a cuff to well above arterial systolic pressure (arterial occluding pressure, AOP). The same technique is applied to measure blood flow in the lower extremities. Excellent descriptions of the pneumatic and hydraulic techniques have been presented by Burch (1944), Wise (1944), Abramson (1944), and Wolstenholme and Freeman (1954).

Impedance Plethysmography. When electrodes are applied to the finger within a closed chamber, as in Fig. 50, the pulsatile impedance change is strikingly similar to the pulsatile pressure change in the air within the chamber. This fact has been well documented with bipolar and tetrapolar electrode systems; an example of the latter from Nyboer's studies (1970) is illustrated in Fig. 50. It would seem that the two recordings reflect the same event, and it ought to be a straightforward task to verify the volume flow obtained by use of the impedance method with that determined by venous-occlusion plethysmography. However, such an investigation is very difficult to carry out using the finger because of the considerable artifact that the venous-occlusion technique imposes on the impedance method, as pointed out by Van der Berg and Alberts (1954). One such study was performed successfully by Young et al. (1967), who modeled a dog hind limb as a truncated cone (between the potential-measuring electrodes) and used a slightly different impedance expression: $\Delta Z / Z_0 = 1.6 \, \Delta V / V$, where ΔZ is the decrease in impedance when a volume ΔV entered the hind limb with a basal impedance Z_0 and volume V. An electromagnetic blood flowmeter probe was applied centrally to the femoral artery to examine the correlation of the flow calculated by the impedance method with that actually entering the member. Collateral circulation was virtually eliminated by ligating the middle sacral artery.

The results obtained by Young et al., who made measurements on five dogs, showed that the venous-occlusion impedance plethysmographic data obtained (using their formula) were 1.2% above the values for blood flow (in milliliters per minute as measured with the electromagnetic flowmeter). A plot of the impedance flow Z_f versus electromagnetic flowmeter E_f measurements provided the relationship $Z_f = 0.98E_f + 3.9$ mL with a correlation coefficient of 0.98, thereby indicating that venous-occlusion impedance plethysmography can provide quantitative blood flow data in an extremity.

When impedance plethysmography is applied to determine peripheral blood flow, there is no agreement on the best technique for converting the recorded impedance change to the volume of blood that flows through the body segment between the potential-measuring electrodes. At present, the extrapolation techniques shown in Fig. 42 offer the most promise. To the best of our knowledge, there have been no studies that compare segmental blood flow determined by nonocclusive impedance plethysmography with values obtained using a member-encircling capsule in con-

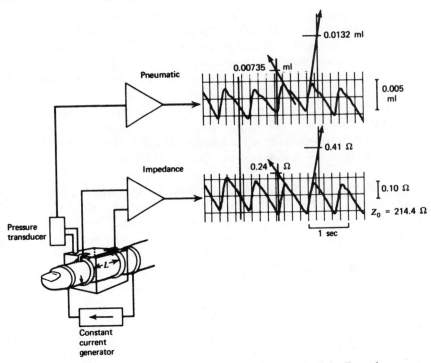

Figure 50 Pneumatic and impedance plethysmography of the digit. For a heart rate of 75/min; volume of digit = 14.5 mL; and length, L = 3.1 cm, the blood flow values are as tabulated below:

	Extrapolation Technique	
	Pneumatic	Impedance
Flow in mL/heart beat		
Backward	0.00735	0.00753
Forward	0.0132	0.0128
Flow in mL/(min) (100 mL of digit)		
Backward	3.80	3.89
Forward	6.83	6.62

junction with the venous-occlusion technique. Certainly the results of such a study would provide extremely valuable information. While anticipating the results of such work, it is of some interest to apply the graphical extrapolation techniques to both the pneumatic (pressure) and impedance recordings (Fig. 50) to examine the relation between the blood flows predicted by the two nonocclusive techniques.

The end-systolic (backslope) graphical construction has been applied to both the pneumatic and impedance recordings illustrated in Fig. 50. The volume of blood entering the region within the finger-surrounding capsule amounts to 0.00735 mL per heart beat for the pneumatic recording. For the impedance recording, the basal impedance Z_0 between the potential-measuring electrodes 3.1 cm apart and at the edges of the capsule is 214.4 Ω, and the extrapolated value for the impedance change ΔZ is 0.24 Ω. Using a typical value of 150 Ω-cm for the resistivity of blood, the predicted volume entering the body segment is

$$\Delta V = \frac{\rho L^2}{Z_0^2} \Delta Z = \frac{150 \times 3.1^2}{214.4^2} \times 0.24 = 0.00753 \text{ mL.}$$

The forward extrapolation technique has been applied to both the pneumatic and impedance recordings appearing in Fig. 50. The pneumatic recording indicates a flow of 0.0132 mL per heart beat. The extrapolated impedance change ΔZ amounts to 0.41 Ω, and, using the same values for L and Z_0, the volume obtained by the impedance method is

$$\Delta V = \frac{\rho L^2}{Z_0^2} \Delta Z = \frac{150 \times 3.1^2}{214.4^2} \times 0.41 = 0.0128 \text{ mL.}$$

It is customary to normalize the values for blood flow in terms of perfusion, namely flow in milliliters per minute per 100 (or grams) of tissue; therefore, the four values for digital flow have been calculated for a heart rate of 75 beats/min and a digital volume of 14.5 mL and are shown in Fig. 50. Table 4 indicates that these values compare reasonably well with digital blood flow obtained by venous-occlusion plethysmography using a member-encircling capsule. The agreement may be purely fortuitous, however, because the extrapolation techniques for the impedance pulse, as applied to the digit, have not been verified by flow determinations obtained by other methods.

Since the amplitude of the impedance pulse is lowered dramatically by any reduction in the lumen of the arterial supply, the impedance method offers an excellent noninvasive method for estimating the patency of the large arteries sup-

TABLE 4   Segmental Blood Flow in Humans

Body Segment	Perfusion n[mL/min (100 mL of segment)]		
	Normal	Maximum	Minimum
Finger	15–40	90	0.2
Hand	6 (0.5–16.5)	22	2.5 (0.3–4.7)
Forearm	2.9 (0.4–7.3)	12.6 (3.7–25.4)	0.7 (0.5–1.0)
Leg	1.4 (0.8–2.6)	3.6	1.2 (0.4–1.5)
Calf	1.4 (0.4–2.4)	—	—
Foot	2.7 (0.5–7.8)	18.1 (11–34)	—

Source: Data from D. S. Dittmer (ed.), *Handbook of Circulation.* Aerospace medical Laboratory; Wright Air Development Center, USAF Wright-Patterson AFB, OH, 1959.

plying the arm and leg. Applications of the impedance method to the arm and leg are illustrated in Fig. 51. Comparisons between the right and left sides often provide qualitative information on the symmetry of blood supply to the members. In addition, with the increase in vessel replacement surgery, impedance plethysmography of the members offers a convenient means of estimating the patency of a vascular prosthesis. Figure 51 presents typical recordings obtained from the arms and legs of human subjects.

It is obvious that there is a decrease in impedance due to an increase in segmental blood volume. However, when pulsatile impedance changes are recorded, there is interest in the role of resistivity change in the genesis of the impedance change.

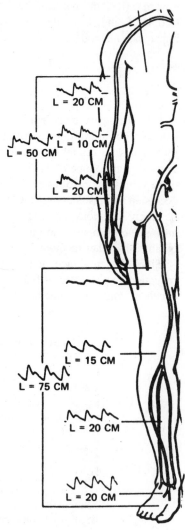

Figure 51   Impedance pulses obtained with different separations of electrodes applied to the extremities. [Redrawn from R. Allison, *J. Am. Geriatr. Soc.* **17**:685–693 (1969).]

Puera et al. (1978) addressed this issue by measuring the impedance of blood (26% hematocrit) flowing in a rigid tube and in a bovine carotid artery. The impedance was measured in the direction of flow and flow measured with an electromagnetic flowmeter. They concluded that only about 10% of the impedance change was associated with flow; the remainder was attributed to a volume change in the artery.

Impedance Phlebography. Venous occlusion by a blood clot in the limbs is difficult to detect, and there is a real danger of the clot becoming dislodged and passing through the right heart into the pulmonary vascular circuit, occluding blood flow to a region of lung where oxygen is taken up and carbon dioxide is released. Accordingly, any technique that offers promise of identifying venous clots is of considerable interest to the clinician. Wheeler et al. (1972), Gazzaniga et al. (1972, 1973), Dmochowski et al. (1972), Deuvaert et al. (1973), and Steer (1973) employed the impedance method to assess the venous drainage rate. Wheeler et al. (1972) designated the method "impedance phlebography." With this technique, the basal impedance of a segment of an extremity (arm or leg) is measured, and then venous outflow is occluded. A decrease in impedance occurs due to swelling of the member. On release of the venous occlusion, the segmental impedance increases, and its rate identifies the ability of the venous system to drain the engorged segment. If the major veins are obstructed by a blood clot, the initial volume increase (indicated by a decrease in impedance) is smaller than in the normal subject. On release of the venous occlusion, the rate of volume decrease (indicated by an increase in impedance) is smaller.

The method used by Wheeler (1973) and Wheeler et al. (1974), appears to be the most practical clinically. This method has become known as venous-occlusion impedance plethysmography or venous-occlusion phlebography (VOP), and the technique is illustrated in Fig. 52. Four metal-ribbon electrodes are placed around the member (arm or leg) in which venous drainage is to be evaluated. A blood-pressure cuff that is used to arrest venous outflow, but not arterial flow into the segment, is placed central to the four electrodes (toward the heart). This is accomplished by suddenly inflating the cuff, typically to between 30 and 60 mmHg. Prior to cuff inflation, the impedance recorder is connected to the four electrodes on the member. The two outer electrodes (1, 4) provide a constant, low-level (100–4000 μA) alternating current (25–100 kHz). The two inner electrodes (2, 3) detect the voltage, which is dependent on the applied current, the spacing between the electrodes, and the impedance of the intervening tissue. The impedance is inversely related to the volume of the tissue between the two inner electrodes. The voltage detected by the two inner electrodes is processed to provide a recordable signal, which identifies the limb segment volume and any changes that it experiences.

Prior to cuff inflation, the impedance record shows a steady baseline because arterial inflow and venous outflow are equal. Venous occlusion is accomplished by suddenly inflating the cuff to about 40 mmHg. Blood then starts to accumulate in the body segment, and the impedance decreases slowly, as indicated by a gradual rise in the recording (phlebogram) (Fig. 52). As venous pressure increases, the rate of rise in the recording decreases and typically reaches a plateau in about 45

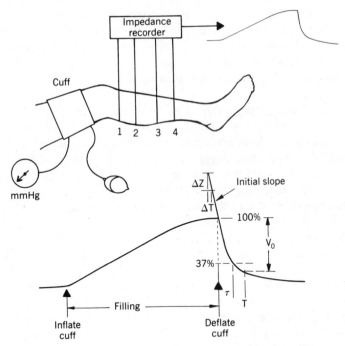

Figure 52 Principle employed in venous-occlusion plethysmography using electrical impedance to indicate segmented volume changes.

sec in normal subjects. Sometimes the occlusion period is shorter, i.e., 30–45 sec. The cuff is then deflated quickly (by 90% in 0.2 sec or less), and the venous system drains the engorged member. The normal impedance phlebogram displays a rapid exponential-like fall as shown in Fig. 52.

Several different measurements are made on the release portion of the impedance phlebogram. Since the outflow after cuff deflation approximates an exponential curve, the time constant τ (time to 37% amplitude after initiating deflation) is measured. Another measurement is the initial slope ($\Delta Z/\Delta T$) at the instant of cuff deflation. The fall V_0 (Fig. 52) at a specified time T is also a descriptor of the rapidity of venous drainage. Impaired venous drainage increases the time constant, decreases the initial slope and produces less fall to V_0 for the T-second value.

In a subject with impaired venous outflow, the post-cuff-deflation outflow time is increased as shown in Fig. 53, which illustrates how the time constant τ, initial slope $\Delta Z/\Delta T$ and fall to V_0 in time T are altered in venous-occlusive disease.

Anderson and Wheeler (1979) reported on the relative merits of each of these factors to identify venous occlusion; their data are shown in Table 5.

At present, venous-occlusion phlebography is one of the simplest methods for identifying deep venous occlusion. The technique is nonhazardous and requires minimal cooperation from the patient. Its place in clinical medicine is, however, yet to be established.

**TABLE 5   Evaluation of Methods for Analyzing
Impedance Phlebograms**

Method	% Accuracy
Time constant	88
Outflow slope	91
3-second amplitude	95

Source: F. A. Anderson and B. Wheeler, *Med Instrum.* **13**:350–354 (1979).

Cardiorespiratory Monitoring. The attractive features of the tetrapolar electrode system were employed to obtain cardiac and respiratory signals by Farag et al. (1985) and Wagner et al. (1987). In the former study, the electrodes were on a wrist band; in the latter they were on a neck band. In both cases, because the current (10 kHz) from a constant-current source was delivered to the outer electrodes, no electrode paste was required. Because the potential, reflecting the impedance change across the two inner electrodes, was applied to an amplifier with a high input impedance, no electrode paste was required for these electrodes either. Thus, the tetrapolar electrode system was applied to skin without preparation. Although the electrode–skin impedance is initially very high, it soon decreases because a small amount of perspiration accumulates under the electrodes, which prevents evaporation of perspiration. Figure 54 is a record made with the tetrapolar electrode system in the wrist band applied to a quiescent subject. The pulsatile

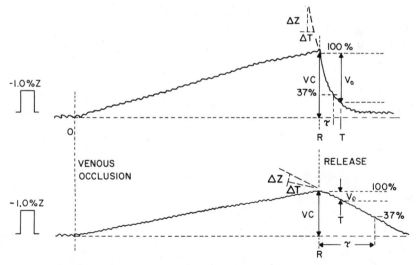

Figure 53 Venous-occlusion phlebogram for a normal subject (upper) and a subject with venous-occlusion disease (lower). Note the differences in postocclusion slope $\Delta Z/\Delta T$, time constant τ, and time T impedance change V_0. [Redrawn from F. A. Anderson and B. Wheeler, *Med. Instrum.* **13**:350–354 (1979).]

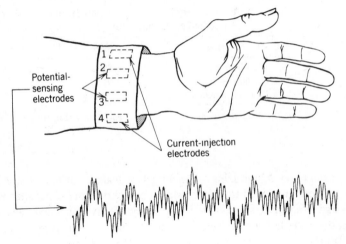

Figure 54   Dry tetrapolar electrodes in a wrist band used to detect cardiac and respiration-induced impedance changes.

cardiac impulses ride on a baseline that varies with respiration. The respiratory and cardiac signals can be separated by filtering.

Figure 55 illustrates cardiac and respiratory signals obtained from the neck band. The largest amplitude cardiac and respiratory signals do not occur with the same separation of the potential (inner) electrodes. A good compromise is to separate these electrodes by two-thirds of the hemicircumference of the neck and symmetrically locate them between the current electrodes.

The signals obtained with the tetrapolar wrist- and neck-band systems are small.

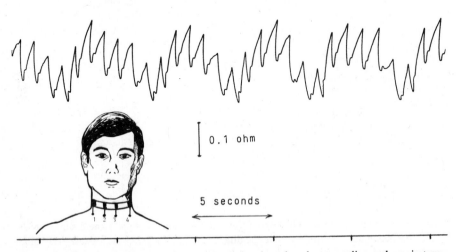

Figure 55   Dry tetrapolar electrodes in a neck band used to detect cardiac and respiratory-induced impedance changes.

For optimum results it is best to apply the bands to quiescent subjects. Movement produces artifacts that can be quite large. However, the attractive feature of these electrode systems is their quick application and the ease of monitoring unconscious subjects.

RHEOENCEPHALOGRAPHY

Jenkner (1957) introduced the term rheoencephalography to designate techniques that employ electrical impedance to assess cerebral blood flow. Measurement of cerebral circulation is difficult because the conventional pneumatic and hydraulic plethysmographic techniques, which employ a member-encircling chamber, cannot be employed. The only reliable method of determining the amount of blood that flows through the brain per minute was described by Kety and Schmidt (1945, 1948). With this technique, the subject inhales nitrous oxide (N_2O, 15%) and exhales to the atmosphere for a period of 10 min, the time necessary for cerebral venous blood to reach equilibration with the tension of N_2O in brain tissue. During the 10-min period, five paired samples of arterial and jugular vein blood are drawn and graphs are plotted of the arterial and venous blood concentrations of N_2O. From these data and using the dilution formula, cerebral blood flow per 100 gm of brain tissue can be calculated. Typically in humans the flow amounts to about 55 mL/min per 100 g of brain tissue.

Clearly measurement of cerebral blood flow is difficult, and any noninvasive, nonhazardous method for obtaining information on cerebral circulation is extremely attractive to the neurologist, the neurosurgeon, and the vascular surgeon. Probably for this reason Polzer and Schuhfried (1950) investigated the value of the impedance method to estimate cerebral blood flow. They placed a pair of electrodes on the head of a patient having an occlusion of one carotid artery and measured the 20-kHz pulsatile impedance changes, first on one side of the head and then on the other. On the affected side, the height of the pulsatile impedance change was diminished, indicating a possible relationship with cerebral blood flow. Since that time, numerous studies have been carried out; one book has been published (Jenkner, 1962), and three international symposia have been held on the subject (Martin and Lechner, 1965; Lechner et al., 1969; Markovich and Namon, 1965). Review papers have been presented by Lifshitz (1963a,b), Geddes et al. (1964), McHenry (1965), Perez-Borja and Meyer (1964), and Hadijev (1972). Although not all these reviews are laudatory of the method, there is considerable interest in the potential of rheoencephalography, and several instruments are available commercially. There is undeniable evidence that useful qualitative information regarding cerebral perfusion can be obtained by rheoencephalography, but there is no agreement on the optimum electrode placement or instrumentation technique. Therefore the results obtained must be evaluated in view of the type of recording technique employed.

A typical bipolar recording of the REG from a normal subject appears in Fig. 56. The electrodes were arrayed as shown, forehead to mastoid, and the impedance changes were measured at 70 kHz using about 1 mA (rms). The first and fifth

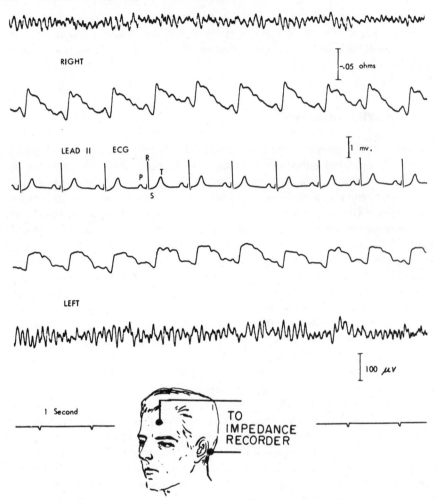

Figure 56 Rheoencephalogram (channels 2 and 4) and the electroencephalogram (channels 1 and 5) obtained from the same pairs of electrodes. The ECG (lead II) is included to illustrate the temporal locations of the REG in the cardiac cycle. A decrease in impedance is shown upward.

channels show the EEG; the second and fourth display the REG. The EEG and REG recordings were made from the same pair of electrodes. Lead II ECG was included as a temporal reference.

In this record, it is observed that the REGs from the right and the left sides are slightly different in waveform; this is a fairly common finding in normal subjects. Markovich and Namon (1965) reported that a 17% difference in area under pulses recorded from the right and left sides of the head is within normal limits. The pulse transmission time from the heart to the head is evident from the relationship between the R wave of the ECG and the onset of the impedance pulse. This interval is often described as the appearance time. It is cutomary to measure the peak amplitude (usually 20–200 mΩ) and the rate of rise of the impedance pulse (ohms per second). Often the time from the onset to the peak is also measured. It is hoped that alterations in these quantities will be found to accompany cerebrovascular disease.

As previously stated, the type of rheoencephalographic recording obtained is not unrelated to the type of circuit and the size and location of the electrodes applied to the subject's head. Since it has not been possible to quantitate recordings in terms of blood flow, recourse is made to comparison of the waveforms obtained from homologous areas of the head; an asymmetry usually indicates a difference in vascular supply. Therefore, two or more channels of data are usually recorded simultaneously, although serial single-channel recordings were made from homologous areas in the first studies by Polzer et al. (1960).

Figure 57a illustrates the method employed when two separate instruments, each with its own constant-current source, are used to compare the pulsatile impedance changes on two sides of the head. This technique has been designated REG I by Martin and Lechner (1965). The early studies employed impedance-bridge circuits (which often had the characteristics of a constant-voltage conductance-measuring system). To guarantee that cranial current of the same intensity flows on each side of the head, the constant-current circuit should be used; however, the frequencies of the current in the two channels must differ, and the amplifier demodulator (AD) for one channel must be sensitive only to current of its own frequency. Thus each channel must incorporate a constant source of alternating current and a narrow-band filter to select its own frequency of alternating current. Since the pulsatile impedance signal is very small, only the impedance change ΔZ is recorded; the basal impedance of the head (Z_0) is rejected by the use of capacitive coupling after demodulation. Usually a time constant in excess of 2 sec is employed. However, if it is desired to display the pulsatile impedance on a baseline that represents the basal impedance (Z_0) of the head, a biasing signal derived from the current source is applied to the amplifier demodulator. Lechner et al. (1966a,b) advocated recording the basal and pulsatile impedance, calling the record the "total rheoencephalogram."

With the method known as REG I, the same electrodes are used for current injection and potential measurement. Near the electrodes, the current density is highest; consequently impedance changes in these regions are more easily detected than are changes deep within the brain. This defect is attenuated by the two methods designated REG II and monopolar REG.

Probably because clinicians desire to obtain information about the circulation in many areas of the brain, Lechner and Rodler (1961) and Lechner et. (1966a,b) advocated the use of a single current source for multichannel rheoencephalography; their method is illustrated in Fig. 57b. The technique of recording was designated REG II by Martin and Lechner (1965). With this system, a sine wave generator applies a constant current to the head through electrodes placed on the forehead and occiput. The pulsatile impedance changes are detected by pairs of potential-

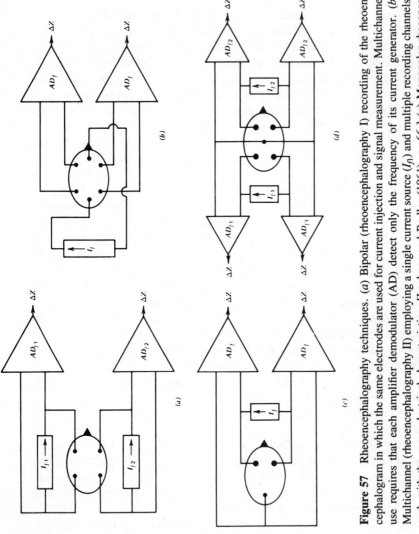

Figure 57 Rheoencephalography techniques. (a) Bipolar (rheoencephalogram in which the same electrodes are used for current injection and signal measurement. Multichannel use requires that each amplifier demodulator (AD) detect only the frequency of its current generator. (b) Multichannel (rheoencephalography II) employing a single current source (I_{fl}) and multiple recording channels, each with the same electrical characteristics. [Lechner and Rodler (1961), p. 66.] (c) Monopolar rheoencephalography employing large-area current-injecting electrodes (to obtain a low current density), which allows use of one current electrode and a single potential-measuring electrode. [Markovich and Namon (1965).] (d) Monopolar rheoencephalography employing large-area, current-injecting electrodes and two current sources to permit recording impedance pulses from four regions of the head. [Namon and Markovich (1970).]

measuring electrodes placed on the head as in Fig. 57*b*. As many pairs of potential-measuring electrodes as desired can be applied; therefore their size (and impedance) is unimportant when an amplifier/demodulator with a high input impedance is employed. An important practical attribute is that all the amplifier/demodulators are identical and sensitive only to the frequency of the applied alternating current. Separation of the current and potential electrodes ensures a more symmetrical and uniform current distribution; therefore, differences in circulation between cerebral hemispheres should be optimally displayed.

Markovich and Namon (1965) and Namon and Markovich (1966, 1970) pointed out that in the measurement of impedance the area of the electrodes used to apply current dramatically affects the amplitude of the measured impedance pulse. After documenting this fact, they recommended that the current electrodes should be no less than 6 cm in diameter (to obtain a low current density under them). These investigators detected pulsatile impedance changes using one current electrode paired with another potential-sensing electrode placed at any convenient location. Figure 57*c* illustrates the monopolar recording technique applied to detect the frontal-to-occipital impedance changes on the left and right sides of the head. Figure 57*d* illustrates the monopolar technique used to compare the vertex frontal and vertex occipital impedance pulses. With this arrangement, four different circulatory regions can be examined.

Lifshitz and Klemm (1966) and Lifshitz (1970) applied the guard-electrode technique to obtain a deeper and more uniform penetration of the current into brain tissue. They compared the basal and pulsatile impedance changes measured over a frequency range extending from 25 kHz to 2 MHz using unguarded and guarded electrodes applied to the heads of human subjects. They found that guarding more than trebled the basal impedance and more than doubled the pulsatile impedance change.

There is no agreement regarding the frequency of choice for any of the rheoencephalographic techniques just described. The first consideration, of course, is safety for the subject; this dictates that a frequency above 20 kHz be used to minimize the risk of stimulating cutaneous receptors. A second consideration relates to the peculiar arrangement of conducting tissues between scalp electrodes and the brain. For current to gain access to the brain by means of scalp electrodes, it must traverse the scalp and the skull, entering the brain through the cerebrospinal fluid. The resistivity of the scalp is much lower than that of the bony cranium, and the cerebrospinal fluid has a resistivity even lower than that of blood (Radvan-Ziemnowicz et al., 1964). Thus low-frequency current can easily pass between the electrodes through scalp tissue, and only a small fraction will pass through the high-resistivity calvarium to enter the brain. If the frequency is high enough, the reactance of the path constituted by the scalp, calvarium, and brain substance will be low, and current will gain easier access to the brain. Hence it ought to be possible to identify an empirically determined frequency that is high enough to secure current penetration into the brain to detect its pulsatile changes accompanying blood flow.

Two investigations have concerned themselves with the importance of the frequency of the current used for rheoencephalography. In a study by Gougerot and Marstal (1965), REG recordings were made in the frequency range extending from 400 to 8000 Hz. They concluded that there was no optimum frequency within this range. In a study that encompassed a much wider frequency range, Lifshitz and Klemm (1966) and Lifshitz (1970) found that increasing the frequency from 25 kHz to 2 MHz decreased the basal impedance and increased pulsatile impedance changes for both unguarded and guarded electrodes. Practical difficulties attributed to stray capacitance made it impractical to use frequencies above 500 kHz. Lifshitz therefore recommended a frequency of 120 kHz as a practical compromise, since the increase in size of the pulsatile impedance change above this frequency was small.

Although it is well known that the pulsatile impedance change detected by scalp electrodes is a reflection of pulsatile blood flow, there is no agreement on the relative contributions of the extracranial and intracranial circulations. However, the relative contributions of each can be demonstrated by the simple technique of placing a tight band caudal to the electrodes to cut off the extracranial blood flow. When this is done, there is a significant reduction in pulsatile amplitude with some electrode arrays and circuits; with others, in particular the REG II system, the reduction in amplitude is less, indicating deeper penetration of the current and better detection of intracranial circulation.

In evaluating the etiology of the cardiac-synchronous pulsatile impedance change, it must be remembered that the cerebral circulation is contained within a rigid container, the skull, and the simple plethysmographic model, which assumes that the pulsatile amplitude reflects member swelling and a temporal difference between inflow and outflow, may not be applicable. Nonetheless, an increase in blood volume between the measuring electrodes reduces the impedance. Lechner et al. (1965) proposed that the well-known reduction in blood resistivity with increasing blood flow velocity (see earlier in this chapter) contributes to the pulsatile impedance change. Certain maneuvers, known to alter cerebral blood flow, can be applied to reveal the types of relationships between the REG and blood flow. The first and foremost of these is occlusion of a carotid artery (by manual compression). This maneuver reduces the amplitude of the pulsatile impedance change on the side of the occlusion. However, the cerebral circulation is derived from four main vessels that eventually join at the circle of Willis at the base of the brain. Occlusion of one of these vessels does not totally deprive that side of the brain of circulation. Nonetheless, the result of transient occlusion of a carotid (or vertebral) artery may provide useful information regarding the possible contribution of the vessel that was occluded.

Other maneuvers that decrease brain perfusion also reveal themselves in the REG, although not always in a desirable manner. For example, venous compression or the performance of a Valsalva maneuver occludes venous outflow (and reduces brain perfusion) and usually increases the amplitude of the REG. Most important, body position, which also affects the resistance to venous outflow, influences the REG amplitude. In the head-up position the REG is smaller than it is when the body is horizontal. With the head-down position, the REG amplitude is increased.

In describing an REG, therefore, it is important to specify the position of the subject. It may be that useful clinical information can be derived from the REG changes that occur in response to body-position changes using a tilt table.

Another maneuver that reduces brain perfusion is hyperventilation, which reduces arterial pCO_2, thereby producing cerebral vasoconstriction. The expected reduction in the amplitude and decrease in steepness of the ascending limb of the REG are not always manifest with all recording methods. On the other hand, the inhalation of 5–7% CO_2 for 5–10 min increases the amplitude and slope of the REG (Hadijev, 1972).

An important factor determining the amplitude of the REG is heart rate. An increase in heart rate decreases the amplitude; a decrease in rate increases the amplitude. Therefore, heart rate should be known when measuring the components of the REG. The REG changes in response to an increase in heart rate have not been investigated extensively.

There are clearly identifiable changes in the REG following the administration of drugs; an excellent account of these has been presented by Hadijev (1972), who stated that nicotinic acid increases the rising phase of the REG pulse. Nitroglycerin increases the amplitude of the REG.

The clinical value of the various rheoencephalographic methods has not been established. Progress is slow because there are so many different techniques in use. Hadijev's review (1972) describes the clinical evaluations. The really attractive feature of the REG is that it is noninvasive and painless. A second attribute is its continuous recording aspect and its ability to indicate immediate changes in response to stimuli (carotid and jugular occlusion, hyperventilation, etc.). Although no method is available for converting the pulsatile impedance change to pulsatile flow, the potential for correlating REG changes with cerebrovascular disease exists and, with the passage of time, the useful correlations will be established. Its use as a safe screening technique may well be its most valuable contribution.

Bladder Volume

Bipolar and tetrapolar electrode systems have been used to measure the volume changes accompanying filling and emptying of the urinary bladder. Talibi et al. (1970) employed the tetrapolar electrode system to measure the impedance of the canine bladder containing different volumes of saline. In this study the impedance appearing between the potential electrodes applied to the bladder was represented by a parallel resistance (R_2)–capacitance (C_1) circuit in series with a resistance R_1 as identified in Fig. 58, which shows the method they employed and the data obtained. Their results indicate that the values for R_2 or C_1 could be used as quantities reflecting bladder volume.

A different method of measuring the volume of the canine urinary bladder was described by Waltz et al. (1971). The bladder was surgically exposed and two ring electrodes were applied to the bladder wall; then the incision was closed. Current from the ring electrodes flowed through the bladder contents and the surrounding tissues and body fluids. As the bladder filled, the ring electrodes moved farther

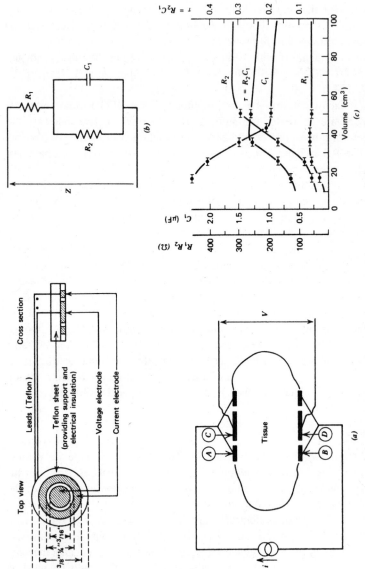

Figure 58 The measurement of urinary bladder volume using concentric (tetrapolar) electrodes. (a) The electrode system and its application to the bladder; (b) the equivalent circuit between the potential-measuring electrodes; (c) the manner in which the components of the equivalent circuit vary with bladder volume when saline is injected and withdrawn. [From M. A. Talibi et al., *Br. J. Urol.* **42**:56–65 (1970). By permission.]

apart in the conducting medium of the body, and the resistance measured between the electrode terminals increased. The interelectrode resistance change controlled the frequency of a resistance–capacity oscillator, which in turn was used to indicate bladder volume. Figures 59a and b illustrate the method employed and the relationship between bladder volume, interelectrode resistance, and frequency as a dog bladder was filled with saline and emptied.

Denniston and Baker (1975) developed a novel method of recording bladder emptying with body-surface electrodes applied to the dog. A constant-current (100-kHz) tetrapolar system was employed with one of the current-injecting band electrodes placed just above the xiphoid process and the other wrapped around both hind limbs (see Fig. 60). Two disk electrodes were used to measure the potential; one was placed midline on the abdomen over the umbilicus, and the other over the pubis. The bladder was catherized, and urine that was collected earlier was infused while impedance was recorded. The relationship between impedance change and urine volume indicated by Fig. 60 is 0.017 Ω/mL urine.

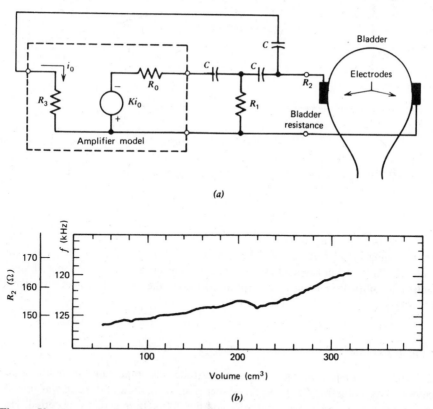

(a)

(b)

Figure 59 The measurement of urinary bladder volume by impedance. Electrodes were applied to the outer surface of the bladder of a 50-kg dog, and the interelectrode impedance was used to control the frequency of a resistance–capacity oscillator. [Redrawn from F. M. Waltz et al., *IEEE Trans. Biomed. Eng.* **BME-18**:42–46 (1971).]

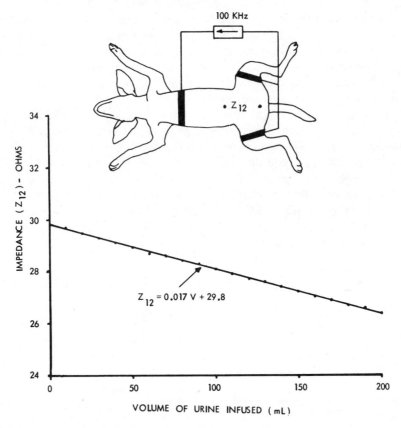

Figure 60   Bladder emptying in the dog. (Courtesy of J. C. Denniston and L. E. Baker.)

The method is elegantly simple and appears to be the only noninvasive method for recording bladder emptying. There is no reason to believe that the technique will not work in human applications, and it may be attractive in some clinical situations. With low-intensity current at 100 kHz, the method is obviously non-hazardous.

Kidney Volume

Variations in the impedance between electrodes encompassing the kidney were described by Lofgren (1951). He found that when a solution of dextran was forced into the rat kidney a decrease in the 2- and the 200-kHz impedance occurred. He then proceeded to employ the method to study the change in kidney volume in response to injections of drugs.

Uterine Contractions

Kornmesser and Nyboer (1962) developed an interesting noninvasive method of recording uterine contractions during labor in the pregnant human female. The method employed is sketched in Fig. 61. Four silver electrodes (10-cent coins) were mounted in a band that maintained the electrodes against the abdomen in the position shown in Fig. 61a. A low-intensity current (100 kHz) was admitted by the two outer electrodes (I_1, I_2), and the voltage, which is proportional to the impedance between the potential-measuring electrodes (E_1, E_2), was continuously recorded after amplification and demodulation.

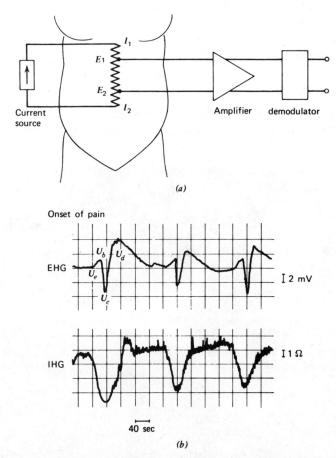

Figure 61 Arrangement of equipment for recording uterine contractions by impedance change, a record of which is called the impedance hysterogram (IHG). Also shown is the electrohysterogram (EHG), the voltage change that accompanies uterine contractions, detectable with electrodes placed on the abdomen. [From J. Nyboer and J. G. Kornmesser, *Harper Hosp., Bull.* **20**:248–261 (1962). By permission.]

The record of the impedance change between the two potential-measuring electrodes was called an impedance hysterogram (IHG). A typical example of uterine contractions from a pregnant human female appears in Fig. 61*b*, along with the electrohysterogram (EHG), which is a recording of the slow changes in potential detected by electrodes on the abdomen (Larks, 1960).

On the basis of clinical observations, Kornmesser and Nyboer suggested that the recorded impedance changes were related to mechanical displacement of the uterus during contraction. Such a suggestion is not without good foundation, because during contraction the uterine contents (fetus and amniotic fluid) were displaced in a direction away from the potential-measuring electrodes. Amniotic fluid and urine have the lowest resistives of all biological fluids (Geddes and Baker, 1967), and it is not surprising that displacement of this highly conducting mass is detectable with abdominal electrodes. Impedance hysterography would appear to be a safe practical method for recording the frequency of uterine contractions with properly placed electrodes, but little use has been made of this technique.

Nervous Activity

Certainly the most famous of all the impedance-change recordings is that presented by Cole and Curtis (1939), who showed (Fig. 62) that accompanying the

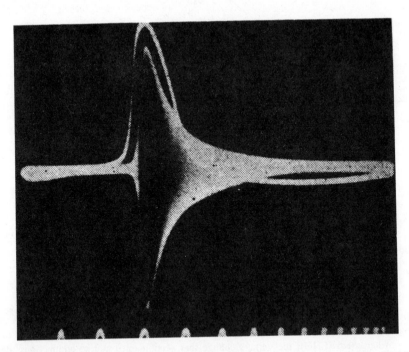

Figure 62 Action potential of the squid giant axon and the impedance change (10 kHz) that accompanies it, as signaled by an unbalance of the impedance bridge. Time marks 1.0 msec. [From Cole and Curtis, *J. Gen. Physiol.* **22**:649–670 (1939). By permission.]

action potential of nerve there is a transient decrease in transmembrane impedance. This impedance change led directly to investigations of the ion fluxes that underlie genesis of the action potential. Impedance changes associated with the activity of cerebral neurons have been recorded with extracellular electrodes. For example, Adey et al. (1962) recorded impedance changes in dendritic layers deep within the brain using 30 μV applied to coaxial electrodes, which measured the impedance change at 1000 Hz. They found that with the electrodes in the hippocampal area of cats, arousal decreased the resistive component of the impedance by 1–2%. On the other hand, sleep, and anesthesia produced by pentobarbital, increased the impedance by as much as 6%. In addition to these baseline shifts, rhythmic oscillations in impedance occurred in a frequency range extending from 0 to 20 Hz. Kado and Adey (1965) reported dissection of the impedance changes into resistive and reactive components. While recording impedance in the amygdala, hippocampus, and midbrain reticular formation in the cat, they observed that brief alerting stimuli decreased the resistance and increased the capacitance measured between electrodes in these regions. These interesting impedance changes await correlation with other parameters of nervous activity.

The impedance changes accompanying anoxia of the brain and spinal cord of cats have been demonstrated by Van Harreveld and Biersteker (1963). By clamping blood vessels and causing cats to breathe nitrogen, they produced tissue hypoxia that in both cases resulted in an increase of impedance amounting to 16–25%. Such changes were completely reproducible and reversible. Their significance at the cellular level awaits explanation.

An early study by Grant (1923) appeared to indicate some promise of applying the impedance method for locating brain tumors. Using a thin bipolar probe electrode connected to an impedance bridge, he found that as the probe was advanced into the brain, the impedance was constant until the tumor was encountered. When glioma tissue surrounded the electrodes, the impedance decreased by one-half to one-third.

Galvanic Skin Reflex

The terms galvanic skin response (GSR) [for psychogalvanic response (PGR)] and electrodermal response (EDR) designate two phenomena: the change in resistance and the appearance of a voltage measurable between one electrode in an area richly supplied by sweat glands and another in a region devoid of them. The change in resistance (the Féré effect) is now called the exosomatic response. The appearance of a voltage (the Tarchanoff phenomenon) is now termed the endosomatic response. Both events appear in response to an emotional stimulus and reflect a change in the activity of the autonomic nervous system. Frequently, only the resistance-change component is recorded.

Although direct current is usually employed to measure the resistance change, it is possible to observe the phenomenon by using the impedance method. The limiting frequency for its detection by impedance has not been established. McLendon and Hemingway (1930) observed that the GSR measured by dc resistance change was 45 times larger than the impedance change measured at 1.5 MHz. The two measurements were carried out simultaneously on human subjects. Using frequencies as high as 10 kHz, Forbes and Landis (1935) were able to detect the GSR in a few subjects. They pointed out, however, that there were gross individual differences. In some subjects the upper frequency was 1 kHz. Both Forbes (1936) and Montagu (1958) found a good correspondence between the potential change (endosomatic signal) and the impedance change in the low-frequency region below 100 Hz. Nichols and Daroge (1955), Tolles and Carberry (1959), and Taylor (1962) called attention to the advantages of using alternating current in minimizing electrode polarization problems in detecting the GSR. Nichols and Daroge employed 60 Hz, Tolles and Carberry used 5 Hz, and Taylor used 65 Hz. Nichols and Daroge stated that the amplitude of the GSR decreased with increasing frequency and that there is little response with frequencies above 1 kHz. At 60 Hz they found the response to be half that measured when using direct current. A similar decrease in the amplitude of the impedance change with increasing frequency was reported by Yokota and Fujimori (1962). More research must be carried out to correlate the effect of frequency on the impedance change with the resistive and voltaic components of the GSR. Because of the low frequency of the GSR signal, high-gain direct-coupled amplifiers are traditionally used, and drift has frequently been a problem. If the exosomatic component of the GSR can be adequately measured with alternating current, narrow band carrier amplifiers can be used to provide high stability and a high signal-to-noise ratio.

Blood Clotting

Impedance changes have been shown to accompany the clotting of blood. Rosenthal and Tobias (1948) measured such changes at 1 kHz in a thermostatistically controlled chamber in which a blood sample was placed. They noted an increase in resistivity after 5 min as the blood clot was forming. Blood samples treated with anticoagulants exhibited no such changes within a 1-hr period. The investigators noted the absence, with this technique, of the changes in clotting time that occur with motion of the blood. Henstell (1949) continued these studies using 60 Hz, with particular interest in the configuration of the electrodes. He found a circular loop with a horizontal crossbar to be the optimum shape. Using these electrodes he plotted impedance–time curves over a 48-hr period. He reported that with his electrodes the normal clot resistance for adult white males is $311 \pm 44.4\ \Omega$ and for adult white females $179 \pm 33.5\ \Omega$. The impedance clotting time was found to be 10.3 ± 1.0 min for normal males and 9.5 ± 0.94 min for normal females. He also noted changes in the impedance–clotting relationship in diseases of the blood.

An interesting conductivity cell for measuring coagulation time and clot retraction was described by Haley and Stolarsky (1951). Their conductivity cell contained a needle-and-plate electrode and accommodated 0.8 mL of blood. Impedance–time measurements were made at 10 kHz and at room temperature. The typical recording showed four transition points, and the second coincided with the occurrence of fibrin formation (verified by visual observation). The third transition correlated with clot formation, and the fourth with clot retraction. The largest change in impedance accompanied clot retraction; only a small change was associated with fibrin and clot formation.

A different approach to determine clotting time was taken by Richardson and Bishop (1957). The blood was contained in a tube fitted with two rod electrodes, and the assembly was placed on a platform that oscillated ±45 degrees from the horizontal, six times per minute. A record of the 60-Hz impedance change showed a sharp transition at the time the clot was formed.

Mungall et al. (1961) continued studies of the impedance changes in clotting blood. Using 100 kHz and a thermostatically controlled conductivity cell, they recorded resistive and reactive changes in blood over a 100-min period. Their records, made on normal subjects and patients with blood disorders, revealed several transitional points that await clarification.

In using impedance to detect blood clotting, attention must be directed to other factors that produce impedance change. Paramount among these are temperature and sedimentation rate. The design of a blood-containing cell must be such that no impedance change is produced by these two factors. Although temperature control is easily achieved, special care must be devoted to proper design of the electrodes to eliminate errors due to sedimentation. An interesting solution to both problems was presented by Ur (1970), who designed a differential system employing two conductivity cells; in one a sample of untreated blood was placed, and in the other was placed a sample of the same blood to which an anticoagulant had been added. The two cells formed two arms of an impedance bridge. With the passage of time, a characteristic difference in impedance was obtained that allowed determination of clotting time.

Salivation

An increase in the impedance of the canine submaxillary salivary gland accompanying secretion was noted by Bronk and Gesell (1926). Nervous stimulation and drug-induced salivation produced an impedance change of slightly more than 10% just before the appearance of saliva.

Blood Pressure in Microvessels

A very interesting application of the impedance method to measure blood pressure in tiny vessels is due to Wiederhelm and Rushmer (1964), who employed a micropipet (0.5–5 μm in diameter) as the sensor. It was filled with 2 M saline and connected to an electrical actuator that could apply pressure to the saline. The saline in the pipet and the blood in a tiny blood vessel of frog mesentery constituted an electrical resistance, the value of which depended on the position of the saline–blood interface in the microtip. The micropipet–animal resistance constituted one arm of a 1000-Hz impedance bridge. The detector consisted of an amplifier connected to the actuator. The bridge was then balanced and set to hunt for a fixed position of the meniscus. The current driving the actuator, which constantly rebalanced the bridge, was proportional to the blood pressure. The system exhibited a response time of 35 msec to a step function of pressure. The remarkably clean and faithful records revealed a blood pressure of 20/15 mmHg in the microcirculation of the frog mesentry.

Noninvasive Measurement of Blood Pressure. Swanson and Webster (1975) used the impedance method to determine blood pressure noninvasively. The current-injecting electrodes were applied to the member ahead of and beyond the blood pressure cuff, below which were five potential-measuring electrodes. Impedance changes were detected during cuff deflation. When cuff pressure fell below systolic pressure, the impedance pulse appeared between the distal pair of electrodes. Near mean pressure, the largest amplitude oscillations appeared between the electrode pair under the center of the cuff. These investigators chose a point where the oscillation amplitude fell to two-thirds of its maximum to identify diastolic pressure.

The method described by Swanson and Webster permits obtaining mean and systolic pressure unambiguously. The diastolic criterion is similar to that used in oscillometric methods of measuring blood pressure noninvasively (Geddes et al., 1983).

CONCLUSION

The flexibility of the impedance method to detect a wide variety of physiological events is its chief attribute. Its chief drawback is the difficulty encountered in calibrating the impedance in true physiological terms. Many studies are under way to establish the relationship between impedance values and physiological events. In many, the signals are being dissected into their resistive and reactive components, with a view to determining which component contains the more meaningful information. It is too soon, however, to draw conclusions regarding the true value of the impedance method for the measurement of physiological events.

A valuable asset to the impedance method is that a bioelectric event can often be obtained simultaneously from the same electrodes. Apart from its use in impedance cardiography and pneumography, this feature has been little exploited. Moreover, the event detected by the impedance-sensing electrodes is often mechanical in nature; in virtually all other situations where electrodes are used, the event recorded is bioelectric and contains no information on the mechanical event that it triggers.

A word of caution is addressed to those who will investigate the use of impedance or impedance change as a means of transduction. In every study adequate care must be exercised to guarantee that the change in impedance measured between the electrodes is due to the physiological event investigated and is not an artifact caused by changes in impedance at the electrode–electrolyte–tissue interfaces. In addition, the safety of the subject must always be borne in mind.

REFERENCES

Abramson, D. L. 1944. *Vascular Responses in the Extremities of Man in Health and Disease.* Univ. of Chicago Press, Chicago, IL.

Ackmann, J. J., and M. A. Seitz. 1984. Methods of complex impedance measurements in biologic tissue. *CRC Crit. Rev. Bioeng.* **11**(4):281–311.

Adey, W. R., R. T. Kado, and J. Didio. 1962. Impedance measurements in brain tissue using microvolt signals. *Exp. Neurol.* **5**:47–60.

Allison, R. D. 1962. Volumetric dynamics of respiration as measured by electrical impedance. Ph.D. thesis, Wayne University, Detroit, MI.

Allison, R. D. 1966a. Arterial-venous volume gradients as predictive indices of vascular dynamics. In *Instrumentation Methods for Predictive Medicine.* T. B. Weber and J. Poyer (eds.). Instrumentation Society of America, 215 pp.

Allison, R. D. 1966b. Stroke volume, cardiac output and impedance measurements. *Proc. Annu. Conf. Eng. Med. Biol.* Paper 8.5.

Allison, R. D., and J. Nyboer. 1965. The electrical plethysmography determination of pulse volume and flow in ionic circulatory systems. *New Istanbul. Contrib. Clin. Sci.* **7**:281–306.

Allison, R. D., E. L. Holmes, and J. Nyboer. 1964. Volumetric dynamics of respiration as measured by electrical impedance plethysmography. *J. Appl. Physiol.* **19**:166–173.

Anderson, F. A., and H. B. Wheeler. 1979. Venous occlusion plethysmography for the detection of venous thrombosis. *Med. Instrum.* **13**:350–354.

Atzler, E. 1933. Neues Verfahren zur Funktionsbeurteilung des Herzens. *Dtsch. Med. Wochenschr.* **59**:1347–1349.

Atzler, E. 1935. Dielektrographie. *Handb. Biol. Arbeitsmethoden* **5**:1073–1084.

Atzler, E., and G. Lehmann. 1932. Über ein neues Verfahren zur Darstellung der Herztätigkeit (Dielektrographie). *Arbeitsphysiologie* **5**:636–680.

Ax, A. F., R. Andreski, R. Courter, C. DiGiovanni, S. Herman, D. Lucas, and W. Orrick. 1964. Measurement of respiration by telemeter impedance strain gauge and spirometer. *Proc. ISA 2nd Natl. Biomed. Sci. Instrum. Symp.* pp. 1–12.

Baan, J., T. Jong, P. Kerkhof et al. 1981. Continuous stroke volume and cardiac output from intraventricular dimensions obtained with impedance catheter. *Cardiovasc. Res.* **15**:328–334.

Bache, R. J., A. Harley, and J. C. Greenfield. 1969. Evaluation of thoracic impedance plethysmography as an indicator of stroke volume in man. *Am. J. Med. Sci.* **258**:100–113.

Bagno, S. 1959. Impedance measurements of living tissue. *Electronics* **32**:62–63.

Baker, L. E. 1962. Impedance spirometry. *SWIRECO Conf. 1962.*

Baker, L. E., and L. A. Geddes. 1965. Quantitative evaluation of impedance spirometry in man. *Am. J. Med. Electron.* **4**:73–77.

Baker, L. E., and L. A. Geddes. 1966. Transthoracic current paths in impedance spirometry. *Proc. Symp. Biomed. Eng.*, Marquette University, Milwaukee **1**:181–186.

Baker, L. E., and L. A. Geddes. 1970a. The measurement of current density distribution in biological materials. *Proc. 2nd Int. Symp. Electrother. Sleep Electroanesth., Graz, Austria* **11**:3–11.

Baker, L. E., and L. A. Geddes, 1970b. The measurement of respiratory volumes in animals and man with use of electrical impedance. *N.Y. Acad. Sci.* **170**:667–688.

Baker, L. E., and L. A. Geddes. 1971. Factors affecting the measurement of current density distribution in living tissue. In *Neuroelectric Research.* D. V. Reynolds and A. E. Sjöberg (eds.). Thomas, Springfield, IL.

Baker, L. E., and G. D. Mistry. 1981. Assesment of cardiac function by electrical impedance. *Proc. 7th ICEBI 1981,* Tokyo, pp. 7–10.

Baker, L. E., L. A. Geddes, and H. E. Hoff. 1966a. A comparison of linear and non-linear characterizations of impedance spirometry. *Med. Biol. Eng.* **4**:371-379.

Baker, L. E., L. A. Geddes, H. E. Hoff, and C. J. Chaput. 1966b. Physiological factors underlying transthoracic impedance variations in respiration. *J. Appl. Physiol.* **21**:1491-1499.

Baker, L. E., W. V. Judy, L. E. Geddes, F. M. Langley, and D. W. Hill. 1971. The measurement of cardiac output by means of electrical impedance. *Cardiovasc. Res. Cent. Bull.* **9**:135-145.

Barnett, A. 1937. The basic factors involved in proposed electrical methods for measuring thyroid function (parts I-IV). *West. J. Surg., Obstet. Gynecol.* **45**:322-326, 380-387, 540-554, 612-623.

Barnett, A. 1938. The phase angle of the normal human skin. *J. Physiol.* **93**:349-366.

Barnett, A. 1940. Seasonal variations in the epidermal impedance of human skin. *Am. J. Physiol.* **129**:306-307.

Berman, J. R., W. L. Schertz, E. B. Jenkens, and H. V. Hufnagel. 1971. Transthoracic electrical impedance as a guide to intravenous overload. *Arch. Surg.* **102**:61-64.

Boer, P., J. C. Roos, G. G. Geyskes, and E. J. D. Mees. 1979. Measurement of cardiac output by impedance cardiography under various conditions. *Am. J. Physiol.* **237**(4):H491-H496.

Bonjer, F. H., J. van der Berg, and M. N. J. Dirken. 1952. The origin of the variations of body impedance occurring during the cardiac cycle. *Circulation* **1**:415-420.

Bourland, J. D., L. A. Geddes, R. S. Terry, M. H. Hinds, and J. T. Jones. 1978. Automatic detection of ventricular fibrillation for an implantable defibrillator. *Med. Instrum.* **12**(1):1-5.

Bourland, J. D., W. A. Tacker, L. A. Geddes, and W. Engle. 1979. A reliable detection system for an automatic implantable defibrillator. *Pace* **2**:A79.

Bouty, E. 1884. Sur la conductibilité électrique de dissolutions salines très étendues. *J. Physiol. (France)* **2**:325-355.

Brazier, M. A. B. 1935. The impedance angle test for thyrotoxicosis. *West. J. Surg., Obstet. Gynecol.* **43**:429-441, 514-527.

Brodie, T. G., and A. E. Russell. 1905. On the determination of the rate of blood flow through an organ. *J. Physiol.* **33**:XLVII-XLVIII.

Bronk, D. W., and G. Gesell. 1926. Electrical conductivity, electrical potential and hydrogen ion concentration measurements on the submaxillary gland of the dog recorded with continuous photographic methods. *Am. J. Physiol.* **77**:570-589.

Brook, D. L., and P. Cooper. 1957. The impedance plethysmograph—Its clinical application. *Surgery* **42**:1061-1070.

Burch, G. E. 1944. Sensitive portable plethysmograph. In *Methods in Medical Research*, Vol. 1. V. R. Potter (ed.). Year Book Publishers, Chicago, IL.

Carter, C. W. 1925. Graphic representation of the impedance of networks containing resistances and two reactances. *Bell Syst. Tech. J.* **4**:387-400.

Chinard, F. P., T. Enns, and M. F. Nolan. 1962. Indicator-dilution studies with "diffusible" indicators. *Circ. Res.* **10**:473-490.

Clavin, O. F., J. S. Spinelli, H. Alonso, and M. Valentinuzzi. 1983. *Diagramma presion-impedancia (DPZ) para el estudio de la function cardiaca*. Soc. Argent. Bioeng., Tucuman, Argentina.

Cole, K. S. 1929. Electric impedance of suspensions of spheres. *J. Gen. Physiol.* **12**:29-36.

Cole, K. S. 1933. Electrical conductance of biological systems. *Cold Spring Harbor Symp. Quant. Biol.* **1**:107-116.

Cole, K. S. 1968. *Membranes, Ions and Impulses.* Univ. of California Press, Berkeley and Los Angeles.

Cole, K. S., and H. J. Curtis. 1939. Electric impedance of the squid giant axon during activity. *J. Gen. Physiol.* **22**:649-670.

Cole, K. S., and R. M. Guttman. 1942. Electric impedance of the frog egg. *J. Gen. Physiol.* **25**:765-775.

Cole, K. S., C. L. Li, and A. E. Bak. 1969. Electrical analogues for tissues. *Exp. Neurol.* **24**:459-473.

Colin, J. 1982. Measurement of systolic time intervals by electrical plethysmography. *Aviat. Space Environ. Med.* **53**:62–68.

Cooley, W. L., and R. C. Longini. 1968. A new design for an impedance pneumograph. *J. Appl. Physiol.* **25**:429–432.

Coulter, N., and J. R. Pappenheimer. 1949. Development of turbulence in flowing blood. *Am. J. Physiol.* **159**:401–408.

Crile, G. W., H. R. Hosmer, and A. F. Rowland. 1922. The electrical conductivity of animal tissues under normal and pathological conditions. *Am. J. Physiol.* **60**:59–106.

Dellimore, J. W., and R. G. Gosling. 1975. Changes in blood conductivity with flow rate. *Med. Biol. Eng.* **13**(8):904–913.

Denniston, J. C., and L. E. Baker. 1975. Measurement of urinary bladder emptying using electrical impedance. *Med. Biol. Eng.* **13**:305–306.

Denniston, J. C., J. T. Maher, F. T. Reeves, J. C. Cruz, A. Gymerman, and R. F. Grover. 1976. Measurement of cardiac output by electrical impedance at rest and during exercise. *J. Appl. Physiol.* **40**:91–95.

Deuvaert, F. E., J. R. Dmochowsky, and N. P. Couch. 1973. Positional factors in venous impedance plethysmography. *Arch. Surg.* **106**:43–55.

Dmochowski, J. R., D. F. Adams, and N. P. Couch. 1972. Impedance measurements in the diagnosis of deep venous thrombosis. *Arch. Surg.* **104**:170–173.

Dove, G. B., B. E. Mount, and J. M. Van De Water. 1971a. Bioelectric impedance-clinical applications. *J. Am. Assoc. Adv. Med. Instrum.* **5**:111.

Dove, G. B., J. M. Van De Water, and R. W. Horst, 1971b. The application of impedance to the intensive care patient. *Proc. San Diego Symp. Biomed. Eng.* **10**:161–166.

Edmunds, A. T., S. Godfrey, and M. Tooley. 1982. Cardiac output measured by transthoracic impedance cardiography at rest, during exercise and various lung volumes. *Clin. Sci.* **63**:107–113.

Farag, A. A., W. A. Tacker, K. Foster, L. A. Geddes, and J. D. Bourland. 1985. Optimal detection of pulse and respiration signals from the wrist. *IEEE-EMBS Conf., 1985* Paper Session D-1.

Farzaneh, T. 1953. Endocrine factors influencing impedance and impedance angle. Ph.D. thesis, Ohio State University, Columbus. 124 pp.

Fenning, C. 1936–1937. A new method for recording physiological activities. I. *J. Lab. Clin. Med.* **22**:1279–1280.

Fenning, C., and B. E. Bonnar. 1936–1937. A new method for recording physiological activities. II *J. Lab. Clin. Med.* **22**:1280–1284.

Fenning, C., and B. E. Bonnar. 1939. Additional recordings with the oscillato-capacitograph. *J. Lab. Clin. Med.* **25**:175–179.

Forbes, T. W. 1936. Skin potential and impedance response. *Am. J. Physiol.* **117**:189–199.

Forbes, T. W., and C. Landis. 1935. The limiting AC frequency for the exhibition of the galvanic skin (psychogalvanic) response. *J. Gen. Psychol.* **13**:188–193.

Fricke, H. 1924. A mathematical treatment of the electrical conductivity of colloids and cell suspensions. *J. Gen. Physiol.* **6**:375–384.

Fricke, H. 1925. A mathematical treatment of the electric conductivity and capacity of disperse systems. *Phys. Rev.* (Ser. 2) **24**:575–587.

Gazzaniga, A. B., A. F. Pacela, R. H. Bartlett, and T. R. Geraghty. 1972. Bilateral impedance rheography in the diagnosis of deep vein thrombosis of the legs. *Arch. Surg.* **104**:515–519.

Gazzaniga, A. B., R. H. Bartlett, and J. B. Shobe. 1973. Bilateral impedance rheography in deep venous thrombosis. *Arch. Surg.* **106**: 835–837.

Geddes, L. A. 1962. Recording respiration and the EKG with common electrodes. *Aerosp. Med.* **33**:791–793.

Geddes, L. A. 1973. Measurement of electrolytic resistivity and electrode-electrolyte impedance with a variable-length conductivity cell. *Chem. Instrum.* **4**:157–168.

Geddes, L. A. 1984. Intraesophageal monitoring of the ECG and respiration in anesthetized animals. *Med. Biol. Eng. Comput.* **2**(1):90–91.

Geddes, L. A. 1989. Cardiac output using the saline-dilution impedance technique. *IEEE-EMBS* **8**(1):22–27.

Geddes, L. A., and L. E. Baker. 1967. The specific resistance of biological material—A compendium of data for the biomedical engineer and physiologist. *Med. Biol. Eng.* **5**:271–293.

Geddes, L. A., and L. E. Baker. 1971. Response to passage of current through the body. *Med. Instrum.* **5**(1):13–18.

Geddes, L. E., and L. E. Baker. 1972. Thoracic impedance changes following saline ejection into right and left ventricles. *J. Appl. Physiol.* **33**:278–281.

Geddes, L. A., and C. P. DaCosta. 1973. The specific resistance of canine blood at body temperature. *IEEE Trans. Biomed. Eng.* **BME-20**(1):51–53.

Geddes, L. A., and H. E. Hoff. 1963. The measurement of physiological events by impedance change. *Proc. San Diego Symp. Biomed. Eng.* **3**:115–122.

Geddes, L. A., and H. E. Hoff. 1964. Baylor Medical College, Houston, TX.

Geddes, L. A., and H. E. Hoff. 1965. Continuous measurement of stroke volume of the left and right ventricles by impedance. International Conference on Medical Electronics and Biological Engineering, Tokyo, 1965. *Jpn. Heart J.* **7**:556–565.

Geddes, L. A., and C. Sadler. 1973. The specific resistance of blood at body temperature. *Med. Biol. Eng.* **11**(3):336–339.

Geddes, L. A., H. E. Hoff, D. M. Hickman, and A. G. Moore. 1962. The impedance pneumograph. *Aerosp. Med.* **33**:28–33.

Geddes, L. A., H. E. Hoff, C. W. Hall, and H. D. Millar. 1964. Rheoencephalography. *Cardiovasc. Res. Cent. Bull.* **2**:112–121.

Geddes, L. A., H. E. Hoff, A. Mello, and C. Palmer. 1966. Continuous measurement of ventricular stroke volume by electrical impedance. *Cardiovasc. Res. Cent. Bull.* **4**:118–130.

Geddes, L. A., L. E. Baker, A. G. Moore, and T. W. Coulter. 1969. Hazards in the use of low frequencies for the measurement of physiological events by impedance. *Med. Biol. Eng.* **7**:289–296.

Geddes, L. A., C. P. DaCosta, and G. Wise. 1971a. The impedance of stainless-steel electrodes. *Med. Biol. Eng.* **9**:511–521.

Geddes, L. A., L. E. Baker, J. D. Bourland, and P. Cabler. 1971b. Response to the passage of sinusoidal current through the body. *Dig. 9th Int. Conf. Med. Biol. Eng., 1971* pp. 213–217.

Geddes, L. A., J. D. Bourland, and E. Arriaga. 1974a. Recording esophageal heart sounds with a catheter-tip contact microphone. *Cardiovasc. Res. Cent. Bull.* **13**(1):3–7.

Geddes, L. A., E. Peery, and R. Steinberg. 1974b. Cardiac output using an electrically calibrated flow-through conductivity cell. *J. Appl. Physiol.* **37**:972–977.

Geddes, L. A., J. D. Bourland, and R. S. Terry. 1981. Method of and apparatus for automatically detecting and treating ventricular fibrillation: U. S. Patent 4,291,699, September 29.

Geddes, L. A., M. Voelz, C. Combs, and D. Reiner. 1983. Characterization of the oscillometric method for measuring indirect blood pressure. *Ann. Biomed. Eng.* **10**(6):271–280.

Goldensohn, E. S., and L. Zablow. 1959. And electrical impedance spirometer. *J. Appl. Physiol.* **14**:463–464.

Gollan, F., P. N. Kirzakevich, and J. McDermott. 1978. Continuous electrode monitoring of systolic intervals during exercise. *Br. Heart J.* **40**:1340–1346.

Goodwin, R. S., and L. A. Saperstein. 1957. Measurement of the cardiac output in dogs by a conductivity method after a single intravenous injection of autogenous plasma. *Circ. Res.* **5**:531–538.

Goto, Y., H. Terasaki, Y. Saito, and T. Morioka. 1981. Effects of nonpulsatile flow in systemic and pulmonary circulation on impedance cardiography. *Proc. 5th ICEBI, 1981* Paper 1.2.1.

Gougerot, L., and N. Marstal. 1965. Quelques remarques sur la fréquence utilizée en rheoencephalographie. In *First Symposium on New Developments in the Field of Rheoencephalography*. F. Martin and H. Lechner (eds.). Verlag Wiener Medizinischen Akademie, Vienna, 298 pp.

Graham, M. 1965. Guard ring use in physiological measurements. *IEEE Trans. Biomed. Eng.* **BME-12**:197–198.

Grant, F. C. 1923. Localization of brain tumors. *JAMA* **8**:2168–2169.

Gross, R. E., and R. Mittermaier. 1926. Untersuchungen über das Minutenvolumen des Herzen *Pfluegers Arch. Gesamte Physiol.* **212**:136–149.

Grubbs, D. S., L. A. Geddes, and W. D. Voorhees. 1984. Right-side cardiac output determined with a newly developed catheter-tip resistivity probe using saline indicator. *Jpn. Heart J.* **25**(1):105–111.

Grubbs, D. S., L. A. Geddes, and J. Kusmic. 1985. Loss of indicator in the pulmonary circuit when measuring cardiac output. *Jpn. Heart J.* **25**(6):1047–1050.

Hadijev, D. 1972. Impedance methods for investigation of cerebral circulation. *Prog. Brain Res.* **35**:25–85.

Haffty, B. G., J. B. Singh, and R. A. Peura. 1977. A clinical evaluation of thoracic electrical impedance. *J. Clin. Eng.* **2**(2):107–116.

Haley, T. J., and F. Stolarsky. 1951. Changes in electrolytic resistance of blood following coagulation and clot retraction. *J. Appl. Physiol.* **4**:46–52.

Hamilton, L. H., J. D. Beard, and R. C. Kory. 1965. Impedance measurement of tidal volume and ventilation. *J. Appl. Physiol.* **20**:565–568.

Hanish, H. 1962. Telemetry of respiration and the electrocardiogram from the same pair of electrodes. *Proc. 15th Annu. Conf. Eng. Med. Biol.* pp. 1–66.

Harley, A., and J. C. Greenfield. 1968. Determination of cardiac output in man by means of impedance plethysmography. *Aerosp. Med.* **39**:248–252.

Heather, L. W. 1969. A comparison of cardiac output values by the cardiograph and dye dilution. NASA Prog. Rep. Contract 9-4500. NASA Manned Spacecraft Center, Houston, TX, p. 247.

Henstell, H. H. 1949. Electrolytic resistance of the blood clot. *Am. J. Physiol.* **158**:367–387.

Hill, D. W., and A. J. Merrifield. 1976. Left ventricular ejection and the Heather index. *Acta Anaesthesiol. Scand.* **20**:313–320.

Holt, J. P. 1957. Estimation of the residual volume of the ventricle of the dog's heart by two indicator dilution techniques. *Circ. Res.* **4**:187–195.

Holt, J. P. 1962. Left ventricular function in mammals of greatly different size. *Circ. Res.* **10**:798–806.

Holt, J. P., and J. Allensworth. 1957. Estimation of the residual volume of the right ventricle of the dog's heart. *Circ. Res.* **5**:323–326.

Holzer, W., K. Polzer, and A. Marko. 1945. *RKG, Rheokardiographie*. Wilhelm Maudrich, Vienna, 46 pp.

Horton, J. W., and A. C. Van Ravenswaay. 1935. Electrical impedance of the human body. *J. Franklin Inst.* **20**:557–572.

Irisawa, H., M. F. Wilson, and R. F. Rushmer. 1960. Left ventricle as a mixing chamber. *Circ. Res.* **8**:183–187.

Jenkner, F. L. 1957. Uber das Wert des Schadelrheogrammes fur die Diagnose cerebraler Gefasseto-rungen. *Wien. Klin. Wochenschr.* **69**:619–620.

Jenkner, F. L. 1959. Rheoencephalography. *Confinia Neurol.* **19**:1–20.

Jenkner, F. L. 1962. *Rheoencephalography*. Thomas, Springfield, IL, 81 pp.

Judy, W. V. 1969. Comparative evaluation of the thoracic impedance and isotope dilution methods for measuring cardiac output. *Aerosp. Med.* **40**:532–536.

Judy, W. V., F. M. Langley, K. D. McCowen, D. M. Stennett, L. E. Baker, and P. C. Johnson. 1969. Comparative evaluation of the thoracic impedance and isotope dilution methods for measuring cardiac output. *Aerosp. Med.* **40**:532–536.

Judy, W. V., H. Hall, and P. D. Toth. 1984. Evaluation of impedance cardiography in critical care medicine. *CRC Crit. Care Med.* **12**:270.

Judy, W. V., D. J. Powner, K. Parr, R. Demeter, C. Bates, and S. Marshall. 1985. Comparison of electrical impedance and thermal dilution measured cardiac output in the critical care setting. *CRC Crit. Care Med.* (June):13.

Kado, R., and W. R. Adey. 1965. Method for the measurement of impedance changes in brain tissue. *Dig. 6th Int. Conf. Med. Biol. Eng.* 638 pp.

Kado, R., W. R. Adey, and D. O. Walter. 1966. Regional specificity of impedance characteristics of cortical and subcortical structures evaluated in hyperapnea and hypothermia. *Abstr. Pap. 23rd Int. Congr. Physiol. Sci.* 549 pp.

Kanai, H., K. Sakamoto, and M. Miki. 1976. Impedance of blood; the effects of red cell orientation. *Dig. 11th Int. Conf. Med. Biol. Eng.* pp. 238–239.

Keim, H. J., J. M. Wallace, H. Thurston, D. R. Case, J. I. M. Drayer, and J. H. Labargh. 1976. Impedance cardiography for determination of stroke index. *J. Appl. Physiol.* **41**(5):791–799.

Kety, S. S., and C. F. Schmidt. 1945. The determination of cerebral blood flow in man by the use of nitrous oxide in low concentrations. *Am. J. Physiol.* **143**:53–66.

Kety, S. S., and C. F. Schmidt. 1948. The nitrous oxide method for the quantitative determination of cerebral blood flow in man: Theory, procedure and normal values. *J. Clin. Invest.* **27**:476–483.

Khalafalla, A. S., S. P. Stackhouse, and O. H. Schmitt. 1970. Thoracic impedance gradient with respect to breathing. *IEEE Trans. Biomed. Eng.* **BME-17**:191–198.

Kinnen, E. 1965. Estimation of pulmonary blood flow with an electrical impedance plethysmograph. Tech. Rept. SAM-TR-65-81. USAF School of Aerospace Medicine.

Kinnen, E. 1970. Cardiac output from transthoracic impedance variations. *Ann. N.Y. Acad. Sci.* **170**:747–756.

Kinnen, E., and C. Duff. 1970. Cardiac output from transthoracic impedance records using discriminant analysis. *J. Am. Assoc. Adv. Med. Instrum.* **4**:73–78.

Kinnen, E., and Kubicek, W. 1963. Thoracic cage impedance measurements. Impedance product system. Tech. Rept. SAM-TDR-63-69. USAF School of Aerospace Medicine.

Kinnen, E., W. Kubicek, P. Hill, and G. Turton. 1964a. Thoracic cage independance measurements. Tech. Doc. Rept. SAM-TDR-64-5. USAF School of Aerospace Medicine, 14 pp.

Kinnen, E., W. Kubicek, and R. Patterson. 1964b. Thoracic cage measurements. Impedance plethysmographic determination of cardiac output. Tech. Rept. SAM-TDR-64-15. USAF School of Aerospace Medicine.

Kinnen, E., W. Kubicek, and D. Witsoe. 1964c. Thoracic cage impedance measurements. Impedance plethysmographic determination of cardiac output. Tech. Rept. SAM-TDR-64-23. USAF School of Aerospace Medicine.

Kinsman, J. M., J. W. Moore, and W. F. Hamilton. 1929. Studies on the circulation I. Injection method: Physical and mathematical considerations. *Am. J. Physiol.* **89**:322–330.

Kirk, S., Y. Hukushima, S. Kitamura, and A. Ito. 1971. Transthoracic electrical impedance variations associated with respiration. *J. Appl. Physiol.* **30**:820–826.

Kornmesser, J. G., and J. Nyboer. 1962. Electrical and dynamic changes in uterine activity during labor. *Harper Hosp., Bull.* **20**:248–261.

Kubicek, W., E. Kinnen, and A. Edin. 1963. Thoracic cage impedance measurements. Tech. Rept. SAM-TDR-63-41. USAF School of Aerospace Medicine.

Kubicek, W. G., E. Kinnen, and A. Edin. 1964. Calibration of an impedance pneumograph. *J. Appl. Physiol.* **19**:557–560.

Kubicek, W. G., J. N. Kamegis, R. P. Patterson, D. A. Witsoe, and R. H. Mattson. 1966. Development and evaluation of an impedance cardiac output system. *Aerosp. Med.* **37**:1208–1212.

Kubicek, W. G., D. A. Witsoe, and R. P. Patterson. 1967–1968. Development and evaluation of an impedance cardiographic system to measure cardiac output and other cardiac parameters. NASA Rep. NAS 9-4500. NASA Manned Spacecraft Center, Houston, TX.

Kubicek, W. G., A. H. L. From, R. P. Patterson. D. A. Witsoe, A. Castenda, R. C. Lilleki, and R. Ersek. 1970. Impedance cardiography as a noninvasive means to monitor cardiac function. *J. Assoc. Adv. Med. Instr.* **4**:79–84.

Lababidi, Z., D. Ehmke, E. Durnin, F. Leaverton, and R. Lauer. 1970. The first derivative impedance scardiogram. *Circulation* **41**:651.

Lababidi, Z., D. A. Ehmke, R. E. Durnin, P. E. Leaveston, and R. M. Lauer. 1971. Evaluation of impedance cardiac output in children. *Pediatrics* **47**:870–879.

Lechner, H., and H. Rodler. 1961. Ein neue Method zur Registrierung intracranelier Kreislauf Veränderungen. *Elektromedizin* **6**:75.

Lechner, H., H. Rodler, and N. Geyer. 1965. Theoretical aspects of the nature of the rheoencephalogram. In *First Symposium on New Developments in the Field of Rheoencephalography.* F. Martin and H. Lechner (eds.). Verlag Wiener Medizinischen Akademie, Vienna, 298 pp.

Lechner, H., N. Geyer, and H. Rodler. 1966a. Die Funktion-rheographie. *Wien. Med. Wochenschr.* **116**:391–400.

Lechner, H., H. Rodler, and N. Geyer. 1966b. The technical development of field rheography. *Proc. Eur. Symp. Med. Electron., World Med. Electr.* pp. 150–153.

Lechner, H., N. Geyer, E. Lugarese, F. Martin, K. Lifshitz, and S. Mardovich. 1969. *Rheoencephalography and Plethysomographic Methods.* Excerpta Medica Foundation, Amsterdam, 239 pp.

Liebman, R. M., and F. Cozenza. 1962–1963. Study of blood flow in the dental pulp by an electrical impedance technique. *Phys. Biol. Med.* **7**:167–176.

Liebman, R. M., J. Pearl, and J. Bagno. 1962–1963. Electrical conductance properties of blood in motion. *Phys. Biol. Med.* **7**:177–194.

Lifshitz, K. 1963a. Rheoencephalography: I. Review of the technique. *J. Nerv. Ment. Dis.* **136**:288.

Lifshitz, K. 1963b. Rheoencephalography: II. Survey of clinical applications. *J. Nerv. Ment. Dis.* **137**:285.

Lifshitz, K. 1970. Electrical impedance cephalography; electrode guarding and analog study. *Ann. N.Y. Acad. Sci.* **170**:532–549.

Lifshitz, K., and K. Klemm. 1966. The use of electrode guarding in rheoencephalography. *Proc. 19th Annu. Conf. Eng. Med. Biol.* **8**:39.

Lofgren, B. 1951. The electrical impedance of a complex tissue and its relation to changes in volume and fluid distribution. *Acta Physiol. Scand.* **23**(Suppl. 81):1–51.

Logic, J. L., M. G. Maksud, and L. H. Hamilton. 1967. Factors affecting transthoracic impedance signals used to measure breathing. *J. Appl. Physiol.* **22**:362–364.

Luepker, R. V., J. R. Michael, and J. R. Warbasse. 1973. Transthoracic electrical impedance: Quantitative evaluation of non-invasive measure of fluid volume. *Am. Heart J.* **85**:83–93.

Mann, H. 1937. Study of the peripheral circulation by means of an alternating current bridge. *Proc. Soc. Exp. Biol. Med.* **36**:670–673.

Mann, H. 1953. The capacigraph. *Trans. Am. Coll. Cardiol.* **3**:162–175.

Markovich, S. E., and R. Namon. 1965. *Theory and Facts Concerning Rheoencephalography.* Grune & Stratton, New York, pp. 68–86.

Martin, F., and H. Lechner (eds.). 1963. *Rheoencephalographia.* Verlag Wiener Medizenschen Akademie, Vienna.

Martin, F., and H. Lechner (eds.). 1965. *First Symposium on New Developments in the Field of Rheoencephalography.* Verlag Wiener Medizinschen Akademie, Vienna, 298 pp.

Maxwell, J. C. 1904. *A Treatise on Electricity and Magnetism,* 3rd ed. Oxford Univ. Press (Clarendon), London and New York, 506 pp. (1st ed. 1873).

McCally, M., G. W. Barnard, K. E. Robins, and A. Marko. 1963. Observations with an electrical impedance respirometer. *Am. J. Med. Electron.* **2**:322–327.

McHenry, L. C. 1965. Rheoencephalography. *Neurology* **15**:507–517.

McKay, R. G., J. R. Shears, J. M. Aroesty et al. 1984. Instantaneous measurement of left and right ventricular stroke volume and pressure-volume relationships with an impedance catheter. *Circulation* **69**(4):703–710.

McLendon, J. F., and A. Hemingway. 1930. The psychogalvanic reflex as related to the polarization-capacity of the skin. *Am. J. Physiol.* **94**:77–83.

Mello-Sobrinho, A. 1963. Impedance plethysmography of the canine ventricles. M. S. thesis, Baylor College of Medicine, Houston, TX, 85 pp.

Miles, D. S., M. N. Sawka, S. W. Wilde, B. M. Doerr, M. A. B. Frey, and R. M. Glasser. 1981. Estimation of cardiac output by electrical impedance during arm exercise in women. *J. Appl. Physiol.: Respir., Environ. Exercise Physiol.* **51**(6):1488–1492.

Milleret, R., and R. Barbe. 1972. Note préliminaire sur une methode d'estimation du debit systoloque par voie extrème. *Ann. Anesthesiol. Fr.* **13**:307.

Mohapatra, S. N., K. L. Costeloe, and D. W. Hill. 1977. Blood resistivity and its implications for calculation of cardiac output by the thoracic electrical impedance technique. *Intensive Care Med.* **3**:1–5.

Molnar, G. W., J. Nyboer, and R. L. Levine. 1953. The effects of temperature and flow on the specific resistance of human venous blood. Rept. 127. U.S. Army Med. Res. Lab., Fort Knox, KY.

Montagu, J. D. 1958. The psychogalvanic reflex. *J. Neurol., Neurosurg. Psychiatry* **21**:119–128.

Moskalenko, Y. E., and A. I. Naumenko. 1959. Movement of the blood and changes in its electrical conductivity. *Bull. Exp. Biol. Med.* **47**:211–215.

Mungall, A. G., D. Morris, and W. S. Martin. 1961. Measurement of the dielectric properties of blood. *IRE Trans. Bio-Med. Electron.* **BME-8**:109–111.

Muzi, M., T. J. Ebert, F. E. Tristani, D. C. Jeutter, J. A. Barney, and J. J. Smith. 1985. Determination of cardiac output using ensemble-averaged cardiograms. *J. Appl. Physiol.* **58**:200–205.

Muzi, M., D. C. Jeutter, and J. J. Smith. 1986. Computer-automated impedance-derragdi cardiac indices. *IEEE Trans. Biomed. Eng.* **BME-33**:42–47.

Naggar, C. Z., D. B. Dobnick, A. P. Flessas, B. J. Kripke, and T. J. Ryan. 1975. Accuracy of the stroke index as determined by the transthoracic electrical impedance method. *Anesthesiology* **47**:201–205.

Namon, R., and F. Gollan. 1970. The cardiac electrical impedance pulse. *Ann. N.Y. Acad. Sci.* **170**:733–746.

Namon, R., and S. Markovich. 1966. Monopolar rheoencephalography. *EEG Clin. Neurophysiol.* **22**:272–273.

Namon, R., and S. Markovich. 1970. Monopolar rheoencephalography. *Ann. N.Y. Acad. Sci.* **170**:652–660.

Nelson, C. V., and A. F. Wilkinson. 1972. Electronic measurement of sedimentation rate. *J. Maine Med. Assoc.* **63**:160.

Nichols, R. L., and I. Darogue. 1955. An electric circuit for the galvanic skin response. *Am. J. Psychol.* **68**:455–461.

Niebauer, M. J., C. F. Babbs, L. A. Geddes, J. E. Carter, and J. D. Bourland. 1984. Functional cardiac depression by defibrillator shocks: Quantification of the safety factor for electrical defibrillation. *Jpn. Heart J.* **25**(5):773–781.

Nyboer, J. 1944. Electrical impedance plethysmography. In *Medical Physics*, Vol. 1. O. Glasser (ed.). Year Book Publishers, Chicago, IL, 744 pp.

Nyboer, J. 1950. Electrical impedance plethysmography. *Circulation* **2**:811–887.

Nyboer, J. 1959. *Electrical Impedance Plethysmography.* Thomas, Springfield, IL, 243 pp.

Nyboer, J. 1965. Tetrapolar electrical resistive impedance measurements as indices of vascular, cardiac and respiratory volume changes. *Proc. Eur. Symp. Med. Electron* Part 2.

Nyboer, J. 1970. *Electrical Impedance Plethysmography,* 2nd ed. Thomas, Springfield, IL.

Nyboer, J., S. Bagno, A. Barnett, and R. H. Halsey. 1940. Radiocardiograms. *J. Clin. Invest.* **19**:773.

Nyboer, J., S. Bagno, and L. F. Nims. 1943. The impedance plethysmograph, an electrical volume recorder. *Off. Sci. Res. Dev. Comm. Aviat. Med. Rep.* **149**:1-12.

Okada, R. H., and H. P. Schwan. 1960. An electrical method to determine hematocrits. *IRE Trans. Med. Electron.* **ME-7**:188-192.

Pacella, A. F. 1966. Impedance pneumography—A survey of instrumentation techniques. *Med. Biol. Eng.* **4**:1-15.

Pallett, J. E., and J. W. Scopes. 1965. Recording respirations in newborn babies by measuring impedance of the chest. *Med. Electron. Biol. Eng.* **3**:161-168.

Palmer, C. L. 1970. Continuous measurement of stroke volume by electrical impedance in the unanesthetized animal. Ph.D. thesis, Baylor College of Medicine, Houston, TX.

Pasquali, E. 1967. Problems in impedance pneumography. Electrical characteristics of skin and lung tissue. *Med. Biol. Eng.* **5**:249-258.

Pate, T. D., L. E. Baker, and J. P. Rosborough. 1975. The simultaneous comparison of the electrical impedance method for measuring stroke volume and cardiac output with four other methods. *Cardiovasc. Res. Cent. Bull.* **14**(2):39-52.

Patterson, R., W. G. Kubicek, E. Kinnen, G. Noren, and D. Witsoe. 1964. Development of an electrical impedance plethysmograph system to monitor cardiac output. *Proc. 1st Annu. Rocky Mt. Conf. Biomed. Eng.*, Colorado Springs, CO, pp. 56-71.

Perez-Borja, C., and J. S. Meyer. 1964. A critical evaluation of rheoencephalography in control subjects and in proven cases of cerebrovascular disease. *J. Neurol., Neurosurg. Psychiatry* **27**:66-72.

Peterson, J. W. 1978. A comparative study of extrapolation techniques used in impedance plethysmography, M.S. Thesis, University of Texas at Austin.

Petrovick, M. S., and J. Brumlik. 1961-1962. Clinical measurements of biological vibrations in normal and disease states. Symposium on Recent Developments in Research Methods and Instrumentation, National Institutes of Health, October 9-12, 1961. *Proc. 15th Ann. Conf. Eng. Med. Biol.* pp. 1-66.

Philippson, M. 1920. Sur la résistance électrique des cellules et des tissus. *Soc. Biol. (Belg.)* (Dec.):1399-1402.

Plonsey, R., and R. Collin. 1977. Electrode guarding in electrical impedance measurements of physiological systems. *Med. Biol. Eng. Comput.* **15**:519-527.

Plutchick, R., and H. R. Hirsch. 1963. Skin impedance and phase angle as a function of frequency and current. *Science* **141**:927-928.

Polzer, K., and F. Schuhfried. 1950. Rheographische Untersuchungen am Schädel. *Z. Nervenheilkd.* **3**:295-298.

Polzer, K., and F. Schuhfried. 1961. Application of rheography in vascular disease. *Spec. Issue, Z. Oesterr. Krank-Ztg.* **8-9**:5.

Polzer, K., F. Schuhfried, and H. Heeger. 1960. Rheography. *Br. Heart J.* **22**:140-148.

Pomerantz, M., R. Baumgartner, J. Lauridson, and B. Eiseman. 1969. Transthoracic electrical impedance for the early detection of pulmonary edema. *Surgery* **66**:260-268.

Pomerantz, M., F. Delgado, and B. E. Eiseman. 1970. Clinical evaluation of transthoracic electrical impedance as a guide to intrathoracic fluid volumes. *Ann. Surg.* **171**:686-694.

Poppendiek, H. E., G. L. Hody, N. D. Greene, J. L. Glass, and J. E. Hayes. 1964. *In vivo* study of the effects of alternating currents on some properties of blood in dogs. *Phys. Med. Biol.* **9**:215-217.

Powers, S. R., C. Schaffer, A. Boba, and Y. Nakamura. 1958. Physical and biologic factors in impedance plethysmography. *Surgery* **44**:53-61.

Puera, R. A., B. C. Penney, J. Arcuri, F. A. Anderson, and H. A. Wheeler. 1978. Influence of erotherocyte velocity on impedance plethysmographic measurements. *Med. Biol. Eng. Comput.* **16**:147-154.

Quail, A. W., F. M. Traugott, W. L. Porges, and S. W. White. 1981. Thoracic resistivity for stroke volume calculations in impedance cardiography. *J. Appl. Physiol.* **50**(1):191–195.

Radvan-Ziemnowicz, S. A., J. C. McWilliams, and W. E. Kucharski. 1964. Conductivity versus frequency in human and feline cerebrospinal fluid. *Proc. 17th Annu. Conf. Eng. Med. Biol.* 108 pp.

Rappoport, D., and G. B. Ray. 1927. Changes of electrical conductivity in the beating tortoise ventricle. *Am. J. Physiol.* **80**:126–139.

Richardson, A. W., and J. C. Bishop. 1957. A new accurate and reliable method to record blood coagulation times using an AC bridge principle. *J. Am. Pharm. Assoc.* **46**:553–555.

Robbins, K. C., and A. Marko. 1962. An improved method of measuring respiration rate. *Proc. 15th Annu. Conf. Eng. Med. Biol.* 66 pp.

Romm, S. O. 1924. Zur Bestimmungsmethode der Umlaufzeit des Blutes im Kreislauf. *Pfluegers Arch. Gesamte Physiol.* **202**:14–24.

Rosenbleuth, A., and E. G. del Pozo. 1943. The changes of impedance of the turtle ventricular muscle during contraction. *Am. J. Physiol.* **139**:514–519.

Rosenthal, R. L., and C. W. Tobias. 1948. Measurement of the electric resistance of human blood use in coagulation studies and cell volume determination. *J. Lab. Clin. Med.* **33**:1110–1122.

Rushmer, R. F., T. K. Crystal, C. Wagner, and R. Ellis. 1953. Intracardiac plethysmography. *Am. J. Physiol.* **174**:171–174.

Sahakian, A. V., W. J. Tompkins, and J. G. Webster. 1985. Electrode motion artifacts in electrical impedance pneumography. *IEEE Trans. Biomed. Eng.* **BME-32**:448–451.

Saito, Y., T. Goto, H. Terasaki, Y. Hayashida, and T. Morioka. 1983. The effects of pulmonary circulation pulsatility on the impedance cardiogram. *Arch. Int. Physiol. Biochim.* **91**:339–344.

Sakamoto, K., and H. Kanai. 1979. Electrical characteristics of flowing blood. *IEEE Trans. Biomed. Eng.* **BME-20**:687–695.

Salansky, I., and F. Utrata. 1972. Electrical tissue impedance of the organism and its relation to body fluid. *Physiol. Bohemoslov.* **21**:295–304.

Salo, R., and T. G. Walmer. 1984. Computer modeling of intracardiac impedance plethysmography. *IEEE-Symp. Biosensors, 1984* pp. 29–31.

Salo, R. W., B. D. Pederson, R. L. Olive, W. C. Lincoln, and T. G. Wallner. 1984. Continuous ventricular volume assessment for diagnosis and pacemaker control. *Pace* Part 11:1267–1272.

Schaefer, H., E. Bleicher, and F. Eckervogt. 1949. Weitere Beitrage zur elektrischen Reizung und zur Registrierung von elektrischen Vorgangen und der Atmung. *Pfluegers Arch. Gesamte Physiol.* **251**:491–503.

Schanne, O., E. Ruiz and P. Ceretti. 1978. *Impedance Measurements in Biological Cells.* Wiley, New York, 430 pp.

Schwan, H. P. 1955. Electrical properties of body tissues and impedance plethysmography. *IRE Trans. Bio-Med. Electron.* **BME-3**:32–46.

Schwan, H. P. 1963. Determination of biological impedances. In *Physical Techniques in Biological Research,* Vol. 6, Part B. G. Oster and A. W. Pollister (eds.). Academic Press, New York and London, 425 pp.

Schwan, H. P., and C. F. Kay. 1957. Capacitative properties of body tissues. *Circ. Res.* **5**:439–443.

Schwan, H. P., and K. Li. 1953. Capacitance and conductivity of body tissues at ultra high frequencies. *Proc. IRE* **41**:1735–1740.

Severinghaus, J. W. 1971. Electrical measurement of pulmonary edema with a focusing conductivity bridge. *J. Physiol.* **215**:53–55.

Severinghaus, J. W., C. Catron, and W. Noble. 1972. A focusing bridge for unilateral lung resistance. *J. Appl. Physiol.* **32**:526–530.

Sheps, D. S., M. L. Petrovich, P. N. Kirzakevich, C. Wolfe, and E. Craig. 1982. Continuous non-invasive monitoring during exercise. *Am. Heart J.* Apr:519–524.

Shimazu, I., K.-I. Yamakoshi, T. Togawa, and M. Fukoka. 1982. Evaluation of the parallel conductor theory for measuring human limb blood flow by electrical admittance plethysmography. *IEEE Trans. Biomed Eng.* **BME-29**(1):1-7.

Sigman, E., A. Kolin, L. N. Katz, and K. Jochim. 1937. Effect of motion on the electrical conductivity of the blood. *Am. J. Physiol.* **118**:708-719.

Smith, J. J., V. T. Wiedmeier, F. E. Tristani, and K. E. Cooper. 1969. Measurement of cardiac output during body tilt using impedance cardiography. *Fed. Proc.* **28**:643.

Smith, J. J., J. E. Bush, V. T. Wiedmeier, and F. E. Tristani. 1970. Application of impedance cardiography to study of postural stress. *J. Appl. Physiol.* **29**:133-137.

Smith, McK., L. A. Geddes, and H. E. Hoff. 1967. Cardiac output determined by the saline conductivity method using an extra-arterial conductivity cell. *Cardiovasc. Res. Cent. Bull.* **5**:123-134.

Spinelli, J. C., and M. E. Valentinuzzi. 1986. Conductivity and geometrical factors affecting volume assessment with an impedance catheter. *Med. Biol. Eng. Comput.* (Sept):460-464.

Steer, M. L. 1973. Limitations of impedance phlebography for diagnosis of venous thrombosis. *Arch. Surg.* **106**:44-48.

Stewart, G. N. 1897-1898. Researches on the circulation time and on the influences which affect it. *J. Physiol.* **22**:158-183.

Stewart, G. N. 1921. The output of the heart in dogs. *Am. J. Physiol.* **57**:27-50.

Sugano, H., and M. Oda. 1960. A new method for blood flow measurement. *Jpn. J. Pharmacol.* **10**:30-37.

Swanson, D. K., and J. G. Webster. 1975. Detecting systolic and diastolic blood pressure under a cuff using impedance plethysmography. *Proc. 28th Annu. Conf. Eng. Med. Biol.*, *1975* p. 118.

Takada, K., T. Fujinami, K. Senda et al. 1977. Clinical study of A waves. *Amer. Heart J.* **94**:710-717.

Talibi, M. A., R. Drolet, H. Kunov, and C. J. Robson. 1970. A model for studying the electrical stimulation of the urinary bladder of dogs. *Br. J. Urol.* **42**:56-65.

Tarjan, P. P., and R. McFee. 1968. Electrodless measurements of the effective resistivity of the human torso and head by magnetic induction. *IEEE Trans. Biomed. Eng.* **BME-15**:275-278.

Tarjan, P. P., and R. McFee. 1970. Electrodeless measurements of resistivity fluctuations in the human torso and head. *Ann. N.Y. Acad. Sci.* **170**:462-475.

Taylor, D. H. 1962. The measurement of galvanic skin response. *Electron. Eng.* **34**:312-315.

Teorell, T. 1947. Applications of square wave analysis to bioelectric studies. *Acta Physiol. Scand.* **12**:235-254.

Tolles, W. E., and W. J. Carberry. 1959. The measurement of tissue resistance in psychophysiological problems *Proc. Int. Conf. Electron. Biol. Eng.* pp. 43-49.

Tomberg, V. T. 1963. The high frequency spirometer. *Proc. Int. Cong. Med. Electron*, Liege, Belgium.

Tomberg, V. T. 1964. Device and a new method of measuring pulmonary respiration. *Proc. 17th Annu. Conf. Eng. Med. Biol.* 129 pp.

Underwood, R. J., and D. Gowing. 1965. An electronic method of detecting blood volume changes. *Anesthesiology* **26**:199-203.

Ur, A. 1970. Determination of blood coagulation using impedance measurements. *Biomed. Eng.* **5**:342-345.

Valentinuzzi, M. E., L. A. Geddes, and L. E. Baker. 1971. The law of impedance pneumography. *Med. Biol. Eng.* **9**:157-163.

Van der Berg, J., and A. J. Alberts. 1954. Limitation of electrical impedance plethysmography. *Circ. Res.* **2**:333-339.

Van De Water, J. M., K. S. Kagey, and G. B. Dove. 1970a. Clinical monitoring of thoracic fluid with electrical impedance. *Proc. 23rd Annu. Conf. Eng. Med. Biol.* Paper 25-4, p. 331.

Van De Water, J. M., I. T. Miller, E. N. C. Milne, G. F. Sheldon, and K. S. Kagey. 1970b. Impedance plethysmography. *J. Thorac. Cardiovasc. Surg.* **60**:641-647.

Van De Water, J. M., P. A. Philips, L. G. Thouin, L. S. Watanabe, and R. S. Lappen. 1971. Bioelectric impedance. *Arch. Surg.* **102**:541–547.

Van De Water, J. M., W. C. Watring, L. A. Linton, M. Murphy, and R. L. Byron. 1972. Prevention of postoperative pulmonary complications. *Surgery* **138**:229–233.

Van de Water, J. M., G. B. Dove, B. E. Mount, and L. A. Linton. 1973. Application of bioelectric impedance to the measurement of arterial flow. *J. Surg. Res.* **15**:22–29.

Van Oosterom, R. W., A. Van Oosterom, R. W. De Boer, and R. Th. Van Dam. 1979. Intramural resistivity of cardiac tissue. *Med. Biol. Eng. Comput.* **17**(3):337–343.

Van Harreveld, A., and P. A. Biersteker. 1963. Acute asphyxiation of the spinal cord and other sections of the nervous system. *Am. J. Physiol.* **206**:8–14.

Velick, S., and M. Gorin. 1940. The electrical conductance of suspensions of ellipsoids and its relation to the study of avian erythrocytes. *J. Gen. Physiol.* **23**:753–771.

Visser, K. R., R. Lamberts, and W. G. Zijlstra. 1981. Impedance cardiography and electrical properties of blood. *Proc. 5th ICEBI, 1981* Paper 1.1.3.

Voorhees, W. D., and L. A. Geddes. 1984. Right heart output using sodium chloride indicator. *Proc. Symp. Biosensors, IEEE-EMBS Meet., 1984* pp. 20–23.

Voorhees, W. D., J. D. Bourland, M. Lamp, J. C. Mullikin, and L. A. Geddes. 1985. Comparison of cardiac output techniques: right-side output by saline dilution and by perivascular electromagnetic flowprobe. *Med. Instrum.* **19**(1):34–37.

Voorhees, W. D., L. A. Geddes, J. D. Bourland, N. E. Fearnot, and J. T. Jones. 1986. The effective mass concept; an expression for the forbidden indicator phenomenon. *Med. Instrum.* **20**(3):130–134.

Wagner, J., L. A. Geddes, K. Foster, and A. Farag. 1987. Monitoring heart and respiratory activity by impedance change. *Med. Biol. Eng. Comput.* **25**(1):100–102.

Waltz, F. M., G. W. Timm, and W. E. Bradley. 1971. Bladder volume sensing by resistance measurement. *IEEE Trans. Biomed. Eng.* **BME-18**:42–46.

Weltman, G., and D. C. Ukkestad. 1969. Impedance pneumograph recording across the arms. *J. Appl. Physiol.* **27**:907–909.

Wheeler, H. B. 1973. Impedance testing for venous thrombosis. *Arch. Surg.* **106**:762–763.

Wheeler, H. B., D. Pearson, and S. C. Mullick. 1972. Impedance phlebography: Technique, interpretation and results. *Arch. Surg.* **104**:164–169.

Wheeler, H. B., J. A. O'Donnell, F. A. Anderson, and K. Benedict. 1974. Occlusive venous phlebography. *Prog. Cardiovasc. Dis.* **17**:199–203.

White, H. L. 1947. Measurement of cardiac output by a continuously recording conductivity method. *Am. J. Physiol.* **151**:45–57.

Whitehorn, W. V., and E. R. Pearl. 1949. The use of change in capacity to record cardiac volume in human subjects. *Science* **109**:262–263.

Wiederhelm, C. A., and R. F. Rushmer. 1964. Pre and post-ateriolar resistance changes in the blood vessels of the frog's mesentery. *Bibl. Anat.* **4**:234–243.

Wiggers, H. C. 1944. Cardiac output and total peripheral resistance measurements in experimental dogs. *Am. J. Physiol.* **140**:519–534.

Wise, C. S. 1944. Fluid-displacement and pressure plethysmography. In *Methods in Medical Research*, Vol. 1. V. R. Potter (ed.). Year Book Publishers, Chicago, IL.

Wolstenholme, G. E. W., and J. S. Freeman. 1954. *Peripheral Circulation in Man*. Little, Brown, Boston, MA.

Worley, D. S., and L. A. Geddes. 1982. Forbidden indicators in flow measurement using the saline dilution method. *Med. Biol. Eng. Comput.* **20**(4):745–748.

Worley, D. S., D. S. Grubbs, and L. A. Geddes. 1982. Repeated cardiac output determinations in the experimental animal. *Physiologist* **25**(3):175–177.

K. Yamakoshi, H. Ito, A. Yamada, S. Miura, and T. Tomino. 1976. Physiologic and fluid-dynamic investigations of the transthoracic impedance plethysmography method for measuring cardiac output. *Med. Biol. Eng. Comput.* (June):365–372.

Yamakoshi, K. I., H. Shimamazi, T. Togawa, M. Fukuoka, and H. Ito. 1980. Noninvasive measurement of hematocrit by electrical admittance plethysmography technique. *IEEE. Trans. Biomed. Eng.* **BME-27**(3):156–161.

Yamamoto, T., and Y. Yamamoto. 1976. Electrical properties of the epidermal stratum corneum. *Med. Biol. Eng. Comput.* **14**:151–154.

Yokota, T., and B. Fujimori. 1962. Impedance change of the skin during the galvanic skin reflex. *Jpn. J. Physiol.* **12**:210–224.

Young, D. G., R. H. Cox, E. K. Stones, and W. J. Edman. 1967. Evaluation of quantitative impedance plethysmography for continuous flow measurement. III. Blood flow determinations *in vivo. Am. J. Phys. Med.* **46**:1450–1457.

Yu-Tang, G., and S. Wen-Ti. 1979. Comparative study on measurement of stroke volume by impedance method and electromagnetic flow method. *Chin. Med. J.* **92**:79–94.

Zajic, F., Z. Fejfar, L. Franc, and J. Brod. 1954. Impedance plethysmography. *Physiol. Bohemoslov.* **3**:355–361.

Zhang, Y., M. Qu, J. G. Webster, W. I. Tompkins, B. A. Ward, and D. R. Bassett. 1986. Cardiac output monitoring by impedance cardiography during treadmill exercise. *IEEE Trans. Bio-Med. Eng.* **BME-33**(11):1037–1042.

12

The Bioelectric Events

ORIGIN OF BIOELECTRIC EVENTS

Electrical potentials exist across the enveloping membranes of living cells, and many cells have the ability to propagate a change in these potentials. Nerve, muscle, and gland cells, as well as many plant cells, exhibit this phenomenon, which is related to the functioning of the cell. When such a cell responds to a stimulus, the membrane potential exhibits a series of reversible changes, called the action potential. Action potentials, unlike many other physiological events, call for no specialized transducers for their detection. Suitable electrodes, amplification, and appropriate display are the only requirements for their presentation.

Because each type of cell exhibits a characteristic electrical activity, measurement of this activity yields important information relating to cellular function. From this fact has developed the clinical study of bioelectric signals, which deals with the measurement of the electrical activity of large numbers of cells. Because dysfunction frequently reveals itself in the bioelectric signal, much diagnostic information can be obtained from such recordings. In this chapter simplified explanations are presented of the manner in which living cells develop action potentials and present them to electrodes.

Although the bioelectric signals recorded from different cells vary considerably in amplitude and form, they all have a common origin in the membrane potential, which is the potential difference that exists between the interior and exterior surfaces of the cell. The enveloping membrane serves as a semipermeable barrier to the passage of certain substances and ions. The resulting ionic gradient is maintained by metabolic energy expended by the cell. In mammalian nerve cells, for example, the concentration of potassium ion is approximately 30 times higher inside the cell than in the extracellular fluid. On the other hand, sodium ion is approximately 10 times more concentrated in the fluid bathing the outside of the cell than in the intracellular fluid; similar conditions obtain for other ions. The net result is a potential difference across the membrane with the inside negative with respect to the outside. Membrane potentials vary within wide limits, ranging from a few tens of millivolts to about 100 mV. Table 1 presents the resting membrane potentials of a variety of cells measured under the circumstances indicated.

In response to a stimulus of adequate intensity to cause local depolarization, many types of cells propagate this disturbance over their membranes. The process

TABLE 1 Resting Membrane Potentials

Type of Tissue	Type of Environment	Membrane Potential[a] (mV)	Reference
Frog, myelinated axon	Excised—Ringer's	67.6 ± 1.4	Huxley and Stampfli (1951)
Rabbit, superior cervical ganglion cell	Excised—physiological solutions	65–80	Eccles (1955)
Cat, spinal motoneuron soma	In vivo	70	Coombs et al. (1955)
Cat, cortical pyramidal cell	In vivo	55	Phillips (1955)
Rat, skeletal muscle fiber	In vivo	99.8 ± 0.19	Bennett et al. (1953)
Dog, papillary muscle	Excised	85	Hoffmann and Suckling (1953)
Dog, auricle	Excised	85	Hoffmann and Suckling (1953)
Dog, Purkinje fiber	Excised—Tyrode's	90	Draper and Weidmann (1951)
Guinea pig, intestinal smooth muscle fiber	Excised—physiological solutions	51.5–70	Holman (1958)
Kid, Purkinje fiber	Excised	94	Draper and Weidmann (1951)
Frog, ventricle	In vivo—Ringer's	62	Woodbury et al. (1950)
Squid, giant axon	Excised—seawater	45	Hodgkin and Huxley (1939)
Frog, skeletal muscle	Excised—Ringer's	92.2	Adrian (1956)
Frog, myoneural junction	Excised—Ringer's	90	Nastuk (1953)

[a]Interior of the cell is negative with respect to the exterior.

of depolarization, reverse polarization, and repolarization constitutes the action potential. In nerve, the propagated disturbance travels at a rate governed by the nerve fiber diameter and the temperature. The speed of propagation in the fastest nerves is approximately 150 m/sec, which represents the highest rate of propagation in any tissue. In muscle, propagation is much slower and contraction follows development of the action potential.

ACTION POTENTIAL

The genesis of the action potential can be understood by considering a single strip of irritable tissue (as in Fig. 1) forming the whole or part of a cell in which the membrane is intact and an ionic gradient exists to produce a membrane potential of 70 mV. This potential is measured by placing an electrode A on the intact surface of the cell and inserting a microelectrode B into the cell. A microelectrode must be small with respect to the size of the cell so that its insertion will not produce cellular damage. In Fig. 1(2), at the arrow, the microelectrode has penetrated the cell membrane, revealing the resting membrane potential at electrode A.

Assume now that a stimulus intense enough to depolarize the membrane is applied elsewhere to the same cell. An ionic current will flow from the surrounding polarized region to the depolarized area. This current is adequate to depolarize the adjacent regions, and a wave of depolarization will travel in all directions over the membrane. In most cells the process does not consist merely of depolarization; a slight reverse polarization also is found to occur, causing the outside of the portion

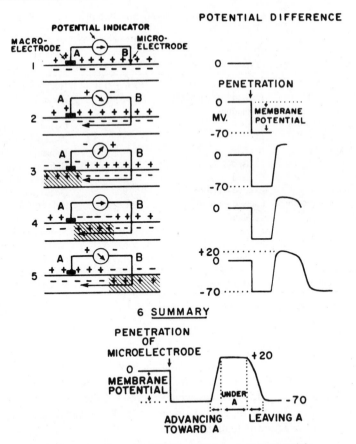

Figure 1   Genesis of the monophasic action potential.

of the cell which is active to be negative with respect to the inside. When this wave of depolarization–reverse polarization advances under electrode A [Fig. 1(3)], the potential indicator, which was previously indicating the membrane potential, shows a potential that drops to zero (depolarization of the membrane) and then a potential that is in the opposite direction to the membrane potential, indicating that the region of reverse polarization is under A. This sequence of events appears on the right of Fig. 1(3).

As the wave of depolarization–reverse polarization advances, in its wake the metabolic activity of the cell causes recovery (reestablishment of the membrane potential) to occur. Thus as the wave passes electrode A [Fig. 1(4)], the membrane potential is becoming restored, and when full repolarization has occurred, the potential indicator reads the membrane potential again [Fig. 1(5)]. When the wave passes point B, the potential indicator shows no change because the electrode is inside the cell.

This sequence of events is summarized in Fig. 1(6), in which it is seen that the fundamental bioelectric event consists of a traveling wave of changing membrane polarity; first depolarization, then reverse polarization, followed by reestablishment of the membrane potential. Most cells exhibit a rapid depolarization and slower repolarization. Action potentials of short duration are called spikes. In many cells during recovery the rate of repolarization slows, and another component appears called the negative afterpotential. Some cells overshoot their repolarization to produce what is called a positive afterpotential. Some even produce a second negative afterpotential before stabilization of the membrane potential occurs (Fig. 2). In pacemaker cells, before the propagated action potential, a spontaneous decay in membrane potential called the prepotential occurs. The prepotential is representative of an unstable membrane potential which upon reaching a critical value causes the cell to depolarize, resulting in a propagated action potential. In summary, a bioelectric event derives its form from the manner in which a cell membrane depolarizes and repolarizes to produce a simple or complex action potential. Compilations of the various forms of action potentials have been presented by Grundfest (1947, 1966a, b), Hodgkin (1951), and Durnstock et al. (1963).

Figure 2 diagrams the sequence of events that a hypothetical cell may display. Depolarization is rapid; repolarization is slower and follows a time course characteristic of the type of cell, resulting not in a flat-topped action potential, as sketched in Fig. 1, but in a smooth curve, as in Fig. 2, where there are four of the types of potential change that may be exhibited by an irritable cell: (1) the prepotential, (2) the spike, (3) the negative afterpotential, and (4) the positive afterpotential.

During passage of the wave of depolarization, a small quantity of heat is liberated, the membrane impedance drops, and there is movement of ions across the cell membrane. In mammalian cells, at the onset of depolarization there is a rapid inrush of sodium ions, followed by a slower outflow of potassium ions associated with recovery. In muscle cells there is an inflow of calcium ions. Metabolic energy is expended to restore the resting ionic gradients. Study of the transmembrane flux of ions constitutes an important part of basic electrophysiology and is important in understanding the action of many drugs.

Because the movement of ions represents moving charge, a magnetic field is

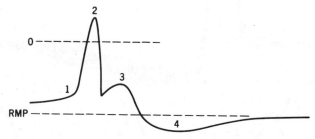

Figure 2 Changes in membrane potential for a hypothetical cell, showing the prepotential (1), spike (2), negative (3), and positive (4) afterpotentials: RMP is the resting membrane potential.

produced during depolarization and repolarization. Although small, it is detectable and elsewhere in this chapter the magnetograms of cardiac activity and neural activity are discussed.

The part of the cell that is occupied by the propagated wave of depolarization is unable to respond to a stimulus, and for this reason it is said to be refractory. However, during repolarization there is a cyclic variation in excitability, for a strong stimulus delivered early in the recovery phase will produce another response. Later, during the phase of the negative afterpotential (if it occurs), when the membrane is almost fully repolarized, a weaker stimulus will often produce a response. During a positive afterpotential (if it occurs), the effective stimulus would need to be stronger. Thus the action potential, in addition to indicating the time course of cellular activity, reveals the approximate time when it can be reactivated.

Figures 3–6 illustrate typical monophasic action potentials of various cells measured with microelectrodes. The monophasic action potential of a single nerve fiber of the squid is shown in Fig. 3. This fiber is so large ($> 100 \ \mu m$) that it is relatively easy to make a microelectrode to study the membrane and action potentials. In addition, the large size permits cannulation and replacement of the axoplasm with solutions of known ionic content. As illustrated, the membrane potential measured in seawater at 20°C was 45 mV, and during the spike the membrane potential became nearly +40 mV. Thus the total amplitude of the action potential was 85 mV. During the recovery phase a positive afterpotential was recorded.

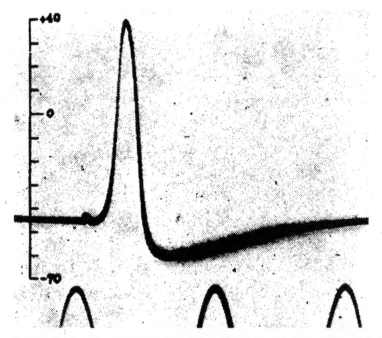

Figure 3   Membrane and action potential of giant axon of squid. Time pulses = 2 msec. [From A. L. Hodgkin and A. F. Huxley, *Nature* **144:**711 (1939). By permission.]

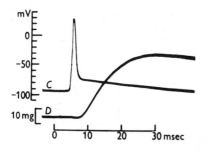

Figure 4 Action potential of a single skeletal muscle fiber in the frog (C) and the tension developed (D). [From A. L. Hodgkin and P. Horowicz, *J. Physiol.* **136**:18P (1957). By permission.]

The action potential for a single frog skeletal muscle fiber and its relationship to the twitch appears in Fig. 4 (Hodgkin and Horowicz, 1957). In this experiment the resting membrane potential was −92 mV, and at the peak of the spike the potential difference was +30 mV. During recovery a negative afterpotential is clearly visible.

The membrane potential changes in frog cardiac muscle are shown in Fig. 5. Starting from a resting value of about −55 mV, during peak activity the membrane potential became about +25 mV. Because recovery is prolonged in cardiac muscle, a relatively flat-topped monophasic action potential is produced. Clearly evident in this illustration is a positive afterpotential.

The electrical activity of smooth muscle of the guinea pig gut is presented in Fig. 6. During activity the membrane potential is seen to change from −46 to +10 mV. During recovery the afterpotentials previously mentioned can be seen.

ACTION POTENTIALS WITH EXTRACELLULAR ELECTRODES

Since body tissues and fluids are electrically conducting, there will be current flow in the environment of an active (depolarizing) and recovering (repolarizing) cell or cells. Therefore, suitably placed electrodes can be used to detect a voltage that reflects such a bioelectric event. The type of waveform detected depends on

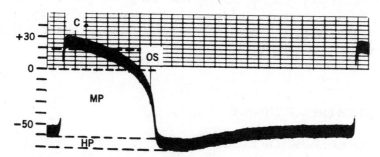

Figure 5 Membrane and action potential in a single cardiac muscle fiber in the frog. [From L. A. Woodbury et al., *Circulation* **1**:264–266 (1950). By permission of the American Heart Association.]

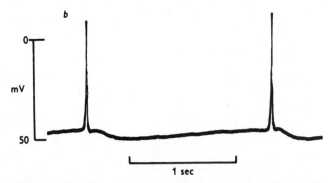

Figure 6   Membrane and action potential of single smooth muscle fiber of guinea pig gut. [From M. E. Holman, *J. Physiol.* **141**:466 (1958). By permission.]

the size and location of the electrodes and the temporal nature of the depolarization–repolarization process exhibited by the cell or cells, often designated the "bioelectric generator."

There is no doubt that the potential appearing between the terminals of electrodes that are strategically placed to record a bioelectric event represents a difference in the potentials existing under each electrode. However, relating this extracellularly recorded action potential to the excursion in transmembrane potential is by no means simple or straightforward. Nonetheless, two useful theories have been created that provide reasonable explanations for the potentials detected by extracellular electrodes. The older "interference" theory postulates that the extracellular electrodes detect a voltage that is the difference in potential occurring under each electrode and that the potential under each resembles an attenuated version of the excursion in transmembrane potential. Thus these two potentials, which are separated temporally by the propagation time, "interfere" with each other.

The newer "dipole" theory postulates that excitation and recovery can be equated to the movement of sets of dipoles that exist in the boundary between active (depolarized) and recovered (polarized) tissue. The propagation of excitation is signaled by an array of dipoles traveling with their positive poles facing the direction of propagation; recovery is signaled by the movement of dipoles with their negative poles facing the direction of propagation. As will be seen, each theory is more applicable in some recording situations than in others. Several examples will be presented to illustrate the application of each theory.

THE INTERFERENCE THEORY

Electrode Axis Parallel to Excitation

The interference theory can be illustrated by considering a situation in which both electrodes are "active"; that is, they are both located on the surface of a strip of irritable tissue, as in Fig. 7. In this idealized situation, it is assumed that the

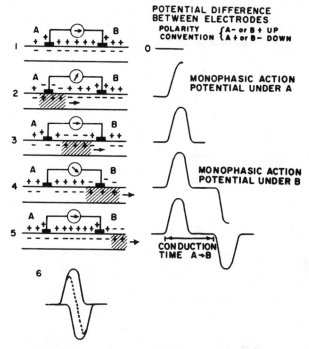

Figure 7   Genesis of the biphasic action potential.

electrodes are small and widely separated. The dimensions were chosen so that the traveling wave of excitation and recovery in the tissue occupies a small fraction of the electrode spacing. In addition, the bioelectric event is considered as a simple monophasic action potential without prepotentials or afterpotentials.

In Fig. 7(1), when the tissue is inactive, both electrodes are in regions of equal positivity, and the potential difference seen by the indicator is zero. When the region under electrode A is excited, this electrode becomes negative with respect to electrode B and the indicator rises [Fig. 7(2)]. As the wave of excitation passes onward toward electrode B and occupies the region between the two electrodes, the region under A is recovered and that under B is not yet excited. Under these conditions no voltage is registered by the potential indicator [Fig. 7(3)], and the first (upward) phase of the monophasic action potential has been completed. As the wave of excitation occupies the region under electrode B, this electrode becomes negative with respect to A; hence the potential indicator falls [Fig. 7(4)]. As the wave of excitation passes B, recovery occurs; the membrane potential is reestablished, the potential indicator reads zero, and the downward phase of the action potential is completed [Fig. 7(5)]. Under these circumstances the time between the two phases of the action potential is determined by the speed of propagation in the tissue and the spacing of the electrodes. If the electrodes are closely spaced, the two monophasic action potentials will fuse to form a continuous and symmetrical

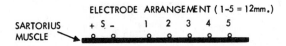

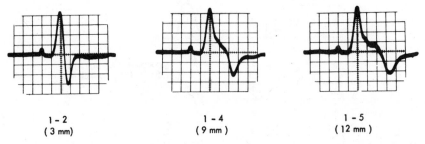

Figure 8   The effect of electrode spacing on the action potential of isolated frog sartorius muscle at room temperature: S = stimulus 0.5 msec; propagation velocity (calculated from record 1–5) = $12 \times 10^{-3}/6 \times 10^{-3}$ = 2 m/sec; time scale 2 msec. [From L. A. Geddes, *Electrodes and the Measurement of Bioelectric Events*. Wiley, New York, 1972.]

biphasic action potential. If the temporal relations are such that the monophasic action potentials overlap, a small action potential will result [see Fig. 7(6)].

Genesis of the biphasic action potential as just described is easy to demonstrate. For example, if two electrodes are placed on a strip of irritable tissue, as in Fig. 8, and the tissue is stimulated at one end, the traveling wave of depolarization and repolarization (action potential) will pass under electrode 1, then under electrode 2, describing a biphasic action potential. If now the distal electrode is moved further away, to positions 4 and 5, the two "interfering" phases of the biphasic action potential will be revealed. Moreover, knowing the polarity indication of the recorder, it is possible to identify the direction of propagation of excitation because propagated excitation is, in reality, a traveling region of negativity.

The Injury Potential

Between two points on the surface of intact, inactive, irritable tissue, there is no measurable potential difference. If the tissue under one electrode is depolarized, as by crushing or the application of potassium chloride ($\sim 2\%$) solution, this region becomes negative with respect to the intact surface, and the potential difference measured between these areas is called the injury potential. Since this region is largely depolarized, it cannot be excited or recover. If the tissue becomes active elsewhere, there will be detected an excursion in potential that occurs under the electrode over uninjured tissue. Interestingly enough, the type of waveform obtained with this situation strongly resembles the excursion in transmembrane potential and arises from and returns to a baseline representing the magnitude of the injury potential.

The injury potential is particularly easy to demonstrate and is frequently encountered when a needle electrode is advanced into irritable tissue to record a bioelectric event. To demonstrate the development of an injury potential, it is expedient to use irritable tissue that is spontaneously active—for example, cardiac muscle. In Fig. 9 the electrical activity of a turtle ventricle was recorded with two 0.6% saline-filled wick electrodes connected to a direct-coupled amplifier. The polarity was arranged so that negativity of the basal electrode (1), and consequently, positivity of the apical electrode (2), caused the recording pen to rise. In the upper record, for the first few beats, both electrodes were over uninjured tissue. Then a drop of 2% potassium chloride solution was placed on the apical wick electrode, causing injury (depolarization) to develop. Note that there occurred a diastolic depression of the baseline as the region under electrode 2 became progressively negative, and the electrogram altered characteristically. Because the myocardium under electrode 2 had been rendered inactive by chemical injury, the activity recorded came mainly from the tissue under electrode 1, which shows that when this tissue became active (negative), the indicator rose, revealing the characteristic action potential of cardiac muscle, rising from and returning to a baseline that represents the injury potential.

For the first few beats in Fig. 9b (lower) both electrodes were over uninjured tissue and the familiar R-T complex was seen. Then a drop of 2% potassium chloride solution was placed on the wick of electrode 1, causing injury (depolarization) to develop. Note that the diastolic baseline started to rise and the electro-

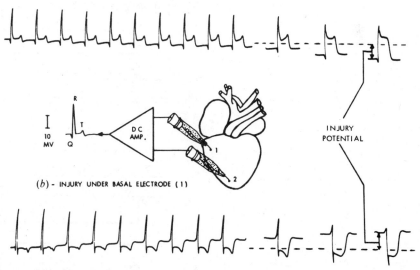

(a) - INJURY UNDER APICAL ELECTRODE (2)

(b) - INJURY UNDER BASAL ELECTRODE (1)

INJURY POTENTIAL

Figure 9 The injury potential. (a) Injury produced by placing a few drops of KCl under electrode 2, thereby depolarizing the tissue at this site; depression of the baseline indicates the development of injury under electrode 2. (b) Injury created under electrode 1 in a similar manner after injury was removed from under electrode 2.

gram developed its characteristic change as the tissue under electrode 1 became depolarized. When depolarization began, electrical activity was recorded from the uninjured tissue under electrode 2, which, when it detects activity, causes the indicator to be deflected downward to exhibit the characteristic electrical waveform of cardiac activity falling from and returning to a baseline that has been elevated by an amount representing the injury potential.

It is interesting to note the similarity between the form of the cardiac monophasic action potential produced by injury under a single electrode and the excursion in transmembrane potential obtained (Fig. 5) when transmembrane electrodes are employed. Indeed, long before the action potential of cardiac muscle had been recorded with transmembrane electrodes, Burdon-Sanderson (1879), hypothesized that the ECG was created by the algebraic sum of two such oppositely directed monophasic action potentials displaced in time, as diagramed in Fig. 14.

Electrode Axis Perpendicular to Excitation

In the situations analyzed thus far, the electrodes were placed along the direction of depolarization and repolarization. If they are placed opposite each other on either side of the uniform strip of irritable tissue, as in Fig. 10(1), the indicator will show no potential difference. When the wave of excitation arrives at the electrodes [Fig.

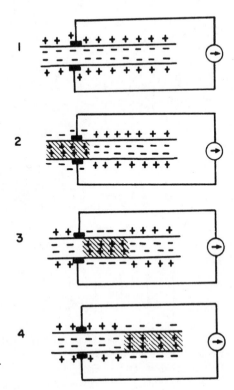

Figure 10   Electrodes at right angles to direction of propagation.

10(2)], depolarization and reverse polarization will occur simultaneously under both electrodes, and the indicator will show no potential difference. As the wave of excitation passes onward and repolarization occurs [Fig. 10(3, 4)], the indicator will continue to show no potential difference.

Consider excitation starting midway between electrodes 1 and 2 in Fig. 11. Excitation (or recovery) waves will arrive under electrodes 1 and 2 at the same instant. Therefore no potential will be recorded. It is to be noted that in this special case, excitation (or recovery) waves travel in the direction of the electrode axis.

The foregoing examples considered a uniform strip of irritable tissue in which the wave of excitation occupied a small portion of the tissue and was followed by recovery in a relatively short time. Although this situation is valid for nerve and skeletal muscle, it does not apply to cardiac muscle, in which the refractory period

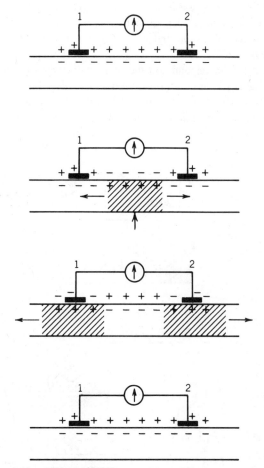

Figure 11 Simultaneous excitation and recovery in uniform tissue under electrodes 1 and 2 due to delivery of a stimulus midway between the electrodes, resulting in no recorded action potential.

is long and the wave of excitation advances and occupies the whole of the tissue before recovery occurs. Moreover, in many circumstances recovery does not necessarily travel in the same direction as excitation. Therefore, the action potentials developed under these conditions are expected to be different from those previously discussed.

Tissues with a Long Refractory Period

Figure 12(1) diagrams a strip of irritable tissue in which the refractory period is long. Assume that the tissue has been stimulated and that a wave of excitation advances and occupies the region under electrode A [Fig. 12(2)]. Thus A is negative with respect to electrode B, and the potential indicator rises. The wave of excitation continues to advance and ultimately occupies the region under electrode B. Because the refractory period is so long, recovery will not have occurred under electrode A; hence both electrodes are over active tissue, and the indicator shows no potential difference. Thus the first upward phase of the action potential will be described as in Fig. 12(3).

The events that follow depends on the manner in which recovery takes place. If the strip of irritable tissue is uniform, recovery follows in the same direction as excitation. If this situation obtains [Fig. 12(4)], recovery will occur first under electrode A. Under this condition electrode B is negative, A is positive, and the

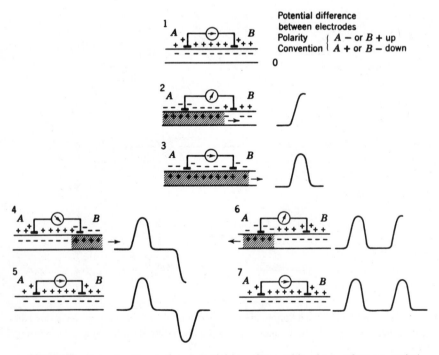

Figure 12   Genesis of an action potential in a tissue with a long refractory period.

potential indicator falls. When recovery occurs under electrode B, the potential indicator reads zero, and the second (downward) phase of the action potential is completed, as in Fig. 12(5).

In the sequence of events just described, the two phases of the action potential have a special meaning. The peak of the first upward monophasic action potential indicates excitation under electrode A. The end of this action potential shows that the whole tissue is active. The beginning of the downward wave indicates that recovery is starting under electrode A, and recovery under this electrode becomes complete when the peak of the downward action potential is reached. Completion of the downward action potential indicates full recovery of the tissue.

If the strip of irritable tissue is not uniform or if a metabolic gradient exists, the foregoing sequence of events will not occur. If, when all the tissue is active [Fig. 12(3)], recovery proceeds in the direction opposite to that of excitation, the second phase of the action potential will be different. In Fig. 12(6) recovery is shown to proceed from right to left, resulting in electrode B becoming positive with respect to A. Thus the potential indicator will rise, and the second phase of the monophasic action potential will be upward, that is, in the same direction as the first. As the tissue fully recovers, the second (upward) phase of the action potential is completed [Fig. 12(7)].

In the case just analyzed, the peak of the first upward phase described excitation under electrode A. At the end of the first monophasic action potential, when the indicator read zero, all the tissue was active. The beginning of the second upward phase indicated the start of recovery under electrode B, which was complete when the second upward monophasic action potential was completed.

Thus in irritable tissue, in which the refractory period is long, if the two phases of the action potential are in opposite directions, excitation and recovery travel in the same direction. If the two phases are in the same direction, excitation and recovery travel in opposite directions.

Figure 13 reveals how these fundamental circumstances underlie the genesis of the ECG when it is recorded with two electrodes on the heart. In Fig. 13a the ECG was obtained with a macroelectrode and a microelectrode which, in the first part of the record rested on the outside of a cardiac muscle cell. On the left of the illustration can be seen the familiar QRS-T complex of the ECG. In the middle of the record the microelectrode was pushed into a single cardiac muscle cell and the ECG was replaced by a monophasic action potential. Figure 13b shows the relationship between the ECG and the simultaneously recorded monophasic action potential.

In Fig. 14 are monophasic action potentials recorded from a frog ventricle. Applying the interference theory, the recorder sees the algebraic temporal sum of the monophasic action potentials; the voltage recorded is the familiar R-T complex of the ECG. This situation is diagramed in Fig. 14c. The solid line represents the summated ECG developed when excitation and recovery travel in the same direction; that is, the monophasic action potentials are alike but displaced in time. The dashed waveform in Fig. 14b illustrates the situation when recovery occurs earlier at the last electrode to become active. The effect is to make the T wave upward (dashed curve in Fig. 14c.)

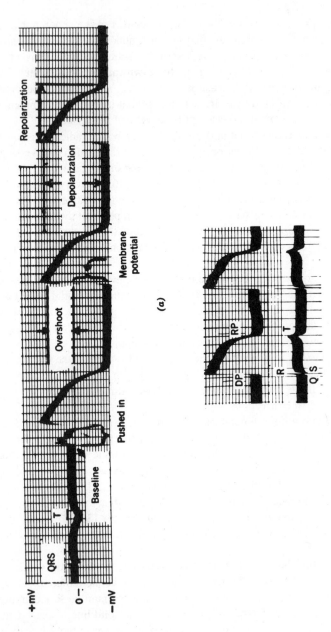

Figure 13 (*a*) Relationship of the electrocardiogram to the monophasic action potential. (*b*) Simultaneously recorded monophasic action potentials and the ECG. [From H. H. Hecht, *Ann. N.Y. Acad. Sci.* **65:**700–740 (1956–1957). By permission.]

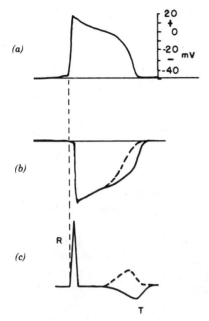

(a)

(b)

(c)

Figure 14 Summation of the monophasic action potentials to produce the ECG. (From H. E. Hoff and L. A. Geddes, *Experimental Physiology*, Baylor Medical College, Houston, TX, 1966. By permission.)

The ECG, as conventionally recorded, reflects the potential difference between a pair of electrodes on the surface of the body. The origin of this time-dependent potential difference resides in the muscle fibers that make up the two masses of the heart—the atria and the ventricles—each fiber producing its own action potential. Thus the ECG is the result of the temporal and spatial summation of the activities of all the myocardial fibers. Notwithstanding the obvious complexity of the resultant potential difference, it is interesting to see how the nature of the fundamental bioelectric generator, the monophasic action potential, reveals itself in recordings made with appropriately placed surface electrodes.

The manner in which initial polarity indicates direction of propagation of the wave of excitation can be demonstrated easily. For example, in the normal mammalian heart, because excitation of the ventricles advances generally from base to apex and the polarity for recording the ECG is chosen so that in lead II negativity of the right arm electrode (hence, positivity of the left leg) causes the indicator to deflect upward, the monophasic action potentials summate to cause the R wave of the ECG to be upward, as in Fig. 14c. If excitation travels in the opposite direction (apex to base), the downward monophasic action potential will occur first and the R wave will be inverted.

In the experimental animal, if excitation is forced to travel in the normal direction from the base to the apex, by application of a stimulus to the base of the heart, the R wave is upward, as shown by R′ in Fig. 15. If excitation is forced to travel from apex to base by delivery of a stimulus to the apex, the primary wave of excitation, QS in Fig. 15, will be downward. Note that in both instances the wave of excitation (R′ and QS) is longer in duration than the normally propagated waves

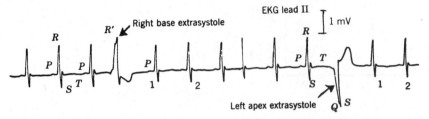

Figure 15 Normal canine ECG, showing induced ventricular basal (R') and apical (QS) systoles.

of excitation because the evoked extrasystoles traveled in myocardium, which has a slower propagation rate than the specialized conduction system of the heart (bundle of His and Purkinje fibers).

The situation of hastened recovery of the tissue under the electrode last to be excited can also be demonstrated experimentally. Figure 16 shows the ECG of a dog recorded with one electrode on the right forelimb and the other applied directly to the apex of the left ventricle. The ventricular electrode (thermode) was a hollow metallic chamber through which cold or warm water could be circulated.

When warm water was circulated through the thermode (Fig. 16, left), local metabolism was increased and recovery was hastened. Under this condition the T wave became large and upright. By circulating cold water through the electrode, recovery was prolonged; hence the T wave became inverted. This sequence of events appears on the right in Fig. 16. In the center of the record it can be seen that at an intermediate temperature the T wave disappeared, indicating that the recovery occurred simultaneously in the regions of the ventricles seen by both electrodes.

Thus it is apparent that the waveform of a bioelectric event is dependent on the time course of depolarization, reverse polarization, and repolarization; the speed with which the depolarization travels in the tissue; the amount of tissue occupied by the wave of excitation; and the orientation of the electrodes with respect to the direction of propagation of the waves of excitation and recovery.

Dipole Theory

Since active tissue is electronegative with respect to an inactive or recovered area, a boundary exists that is characterized by an array of positive and negative charges (see Fig. 17a). The boundary between active and inactive tissue can be represented by a dipole, and because environmental tissues and fluids can conduct current, potential fields will be established, as in Fig. 17b.

The potential field surrounding a current dipole in an infinite volume conductor is represented in Fig. 18. If the dipole moves along its axis, its field will accompany it, and the potential (V_p) at a nearby point (with respect to an indifferent electrode located in a region of zero potential) will start to rise, then fall to zero (when the dipole center is nearest the point), increase in the negative direction, and then

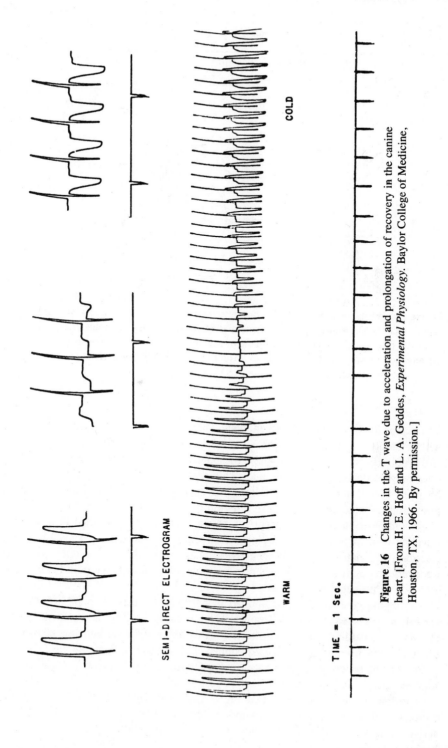

SEMI-DIRECT ELECTROGRAM

COLD

WARM

TIME = 1 SEC.

Figure 16 Changes in the T wave due to acceleration and prolongation of recovery in the canine heart. [From H. E. Hoff and L. A. Geddes, *Experimental Physiology*. Baylor College of Medicine, Houston, TX, 1966. By permission.]

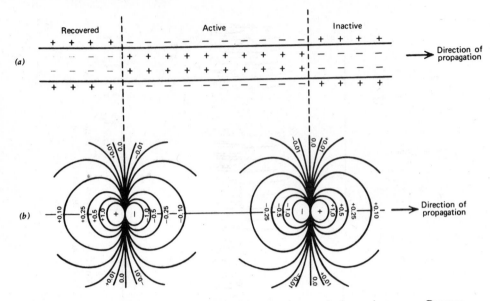

Figure 17   Application of the dipole concept to represent excitation and recovery. Because active tissue is electronegative to inactive and recovered tissue, the boundaries of active tissue can be equated to dipoles. The dipole of excitation travels with its positive pole facing the direction of propagation of excitation. The dipole of recovery travels with its negative pole facing the direction of propagation of recovery.

decrease as the dipole moves farther away. Thus a positive–negative diphasic wave will be described as in Fig. 18b ($d = 1$) as the dipole passes the measuring point. If the point is more distant ($d = 2$), the potential excursion will be in the same direction but decreased in amplitude. This sequence of events describes what is obtained with "monopolar" recording; that is, when one electrode is near active tissue and the other at a distance in a region of no potential change.

According to the dipole concept, propagated excitation is equated to a dipole traveling with its positive pole facing the direction of propagation. Thus a nearby electrode will detect a positive–negative biphasic potential as excitation passes. Recovery (repolarization) is equated to a dipole with its negative pole facing the direction of propagation.

The dipole concept was first applied to nerve by Bernstein's pupil, Hermann (1879); it was later applied by Craib (1927), Wilson et al. (1934), and Macleod (1938a, b) to cardiac muscle. Verification of its applicability to human electrocardiography has been presented by Woodbury et al. (1950). Lorente de Nó (1947), in an elegant series of experiments, mapped out the dipole potential fields surrounding active and recovered regions in frog sciatic nerve.

It is important to recognize that the physiological application of the dipole concept carries some limitations. Although the boundary between active and inactive tissue is sharp enough to allow reasonable use of the dipole concept, the boundary between active and recovering tissue is much more diffuse and irregular;

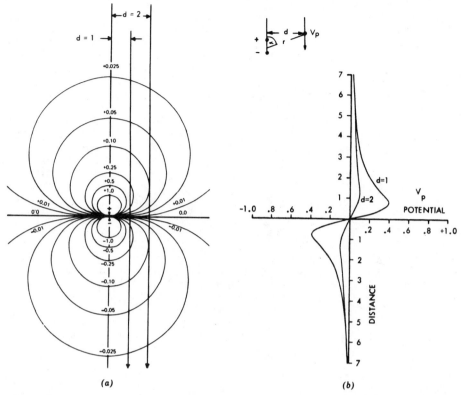

Figure 18   The dipole and its field of potential: (*a*) potential distribution; (*b*) potential encountered by exploring electrode moving along lines (*d* = 1, *d* = 2) parallel to the dipole axis.

hence the dipoles of excitation and recovery do not have the same strength or spatial distribution. Moreover, the dipoles of excitation and recovery increase and decrease in strength temporally, and the amount of tissue occupied by excitation is a property of the type of tissue; hence, the ''separation'' along with the speed of propagation of recovery and excitation. When applying the dipole concept to explain the genesis of a waveform, it is wise to remember these important physiological factors.

POTENTIAL DISTRIBUTION AROUND BIOELECTRIC GENERATORS

After measuring the potential differences between leads placed on various points on the surface of the body, Waller (1889) postulated that the potential distribution at the peak of the R wave due to ventricular activity could be attributed to an equivalent dipole, as in Fig. 19. Since Waller's time, many investigators have plotted the isopotential lines at various instants in the cycle of activity of bioelectric generators. Electrocardiographic isopotential lines appearing on the thorax at dif-

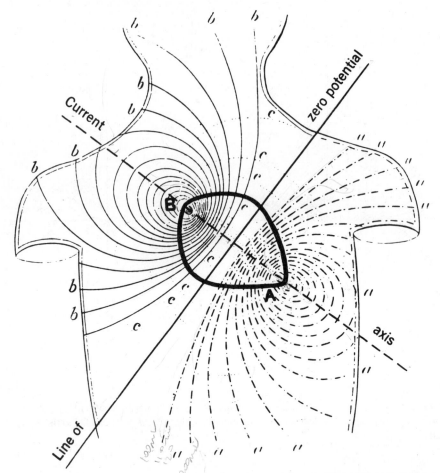

Figure 19   Waller's concept of the distribution of potential on the human thorax resulting from ventricular activity. [From A. D. Waller, *Philos. Trans. R. Soc. London, Ser. B* **180:**169–194 (1889). By permission of the Royal Society.]

ferent instants during atrial and ventricular excitation and recovery were mapped in human subjects by Nahum et al. (1951, 1952–1953), Mauro et al. (1952), Simonson (1952), Frank (1955, 1956–1957), Nelson (1956), Tasaki (1959), Flaherty et al. (1967), Spach et al. (1966); in the dog by Maruo et al. (1952), Taccardi (1962, 1963), Horan et al. (1963), Nelson et al. (1965); and in the monkey and lamb by Nelson et al. (1965).

Such isopotential maps represent the potential distribution during one instant in the cardiac cycle. A complete display of the electrical activity for the whole cardiac cycle would require the plotting of instantaneous potential distributions at each instant in atrial and ventricular activity and recovery, that is, during the P, Tp, QRS, and T waves. Thus, it is apparent that the isopotential lines vary over time. Figure 20 illustrates the time variance of the surface potential distribution during the ventricular depolarization process as described by the QRS wave of the ECG.

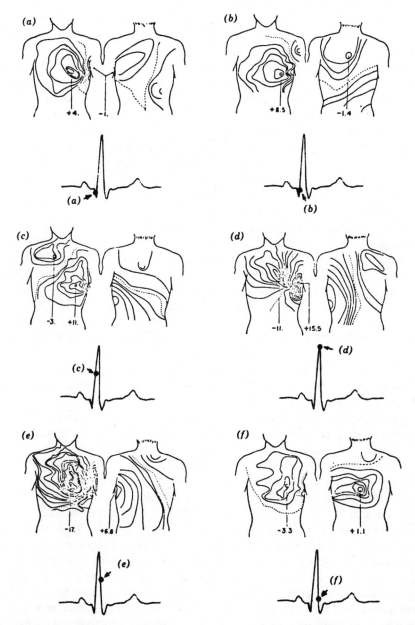

Figure 20 Thoracic potential distribution at various instants in the ventricular depolarization process. Lead I is shown for identification purposes. [From L. H. Nahum, in *Textbook of Physiology*, 17th ed. J. Fulton (Ed.), Saunders, Philadelphia, PA, 1955. By permission of the author and publisher.]

It should be obvious that a temporal series of isopotential maps derived for excitation and recovery of any bioelectric source can be used to identify the source of potential and allow derivation of the voltage–time curve obtained with electrodes located anywhere in the mapped potential field.

Electroencephalographic isopotential lines have been plotted for various cerebral states. Two of the earliest to investigate this method of localizing active regions of the brain were Adrian and Matthews (1934). The study was continued by Brazier (1949), who presented a series of diagrams constructed from the EEG records of normal and abnormal subjects. Two of her diagrams from normal subjects appear in Fig. 21. Figure 21*a* shows the scalp potential distribution during an instant in the development of the alpha rhythm, the normal background activity that characterizes the awake, relaxed subject. Clearly evident is the focal location of this rhythm in the occipital region. Figure 21*b* shows the location of the origin of a low-frequency source in the sleeping subject.

Many penetrating theoretical studies have been carried out on the surface distributions of potentials for dipoles in irregularly shaped volume conductors. Those interested in this aspect of this field should consult the papers by Wilson and Bayley (1950), Frank (1953a), Okada (1956, 1957), Geselowitz (1960), Brody et al. (1961), Hlavin and Plonsey (1963), and Plonsey (1963a, b, c).

THE TRANSMEMBRANE AND EXTRACELLULAR ACTION POTENTIALS

When a strip of irritable tissue in a living organism becomes active, this region is electronegative with respect to the tissue that is inactive (or has recovered). Therefore, current will flow in the anisotropic environmental volume conductor constituted by tissues and fluids, each of which has its own conductance. Consequently, the spatial distribution of current will not resemble that surrounding a dipole in a volume conductor. Nonetheless, a potential field will be established by the current flow, and a voltage can be measured between an exploring (active) electrode placed in the field and another (reference) electrode in a region of zero potential. However, the waveform of the voltage detected by the extracellular active electrode is quite different from the form of the excursion in transmembrane potential when the tissue becomes active and recovers. It would be convenient if there were a simple method to relate the extracellular action potential to the excursion in transmembrane potential. Unfortunately, this relationship can be established only for very simple cases in which the geometry of the active tissue and the environment are simple and the environmental volume conductor is isotropic. Nonetheless, the first steps have been taken to determine the nature of this relationship. In his book on bioelectric phenomena, Plonsey (1969) discusses the difficulties in using the core-conductor (cable) model and in applying field theory to the solution of biological problems based on this model. Excellent papers on the cable analog, which is best applied to a long strip of irritable tissue, were presented by Huxley and Stampfli (1944), Tasaki (1959), Clark and Plonsey (1966), and Geselowitz (1966). The applications of field theory were presented by Lorente de Nó (1947), Clark and Plonsey (1968), and Plonsey (1969). In the application of

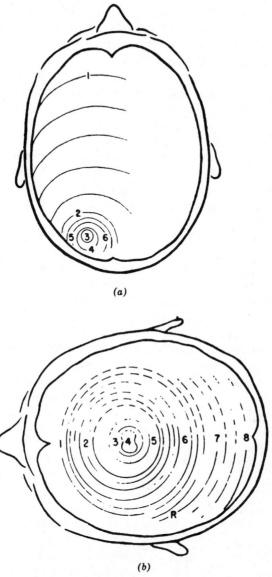

(a)

(b)

Figure 21 Potential distribution on the head due to electrical activity of the brain. (a) Surface potential distribution of an alpha rhythm; (b) surface potential distribution at one instant during sleep. [From M. A. B. Brazier, *EEG Clin. Neurophysiol.* **2**(Suppl.):38–52 (1949). By permission of Masson & Cie, Publisher.]

field theory to determine the extracellular potential distribution, it is necessary to solve the Laplace equation, and the main difficulty centers around specification of the boundary conditions.

Although the solutions of the equations based on the cable analog and those applying field theory are different, both contain a term that is the second derivative of the transmembrane potential. If a simple monophasic waveform for the excursion in transmembrane potential $V(t)$ is chosen, as in Fig. 22, it is possible to differentiate it twice to obtain a waveform that will demonstrate the principal differences between the transmembrane and extracellular potential, recorded with a monopolar electrode. Note that the second derivative is a triphasic wave having an upward wave much shorter in duration than that of the excursion in transmembrane potential.

There is considerable debate regarding the exact relationship between the transmembrane potential and the form of the extracellular action potential, but the work thus far tends to confirm that the form resembles that of a second derivative of the transmembrane potential. Figure 23 presents a compilation of transmembrane potential recordings and extracellular action potentials. The extracellular action potentials have the general appearance of the second derivative of the excursion in transmembrane potential.

While the action potential detected by a local monopolar electrode resembles the second derivative of the excursion in transmembrane potential, the amplitude is small and depends on the distance from the excitable tissue. To illustrate this point, a specimen (2×1 mm) of dog Purkinje fiber was placed in a 3-mL beaker of oxygenated Krebs–Ringer solution and connected to a tiny bipolar stimulating electrode that was connected to a stimulator having an isolated output circuit. A silver–silver chloride reference electrode was placed in the solution about 15 mm distant, and the potential developed in the solution when the specimen was stimulated was measured with a 1-μm micropipet filled with 3 M potassium chloride. Single stimuli were delivered as the tip of the micropipet was brought toward the

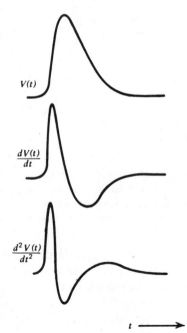

Figure 22 Idealized transmembrane potential excursion $V(t)$, its first derivative $dV(t)/dt$, and its second derivative $d^2V(t)/dt^2$.

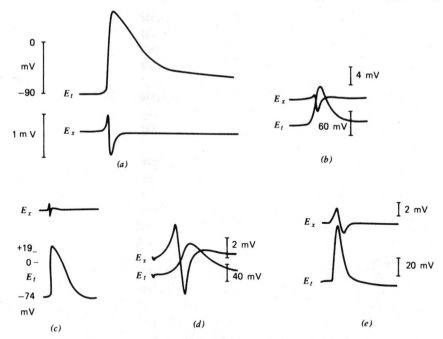

Figure 23 Transmembrane (E_t) and extracellular action potentials (E_x) obtained from different irritable tissues. (*a*) Frog semitendinous muscle. [Redrawn from C. H. Hakansson, *Acta Physiol. Scand.* **39**:291–312 (1957).] (*b*) Toad sartorius muscle. [Redrawn from M. Murakami et al., *Jpn. J. Physiol.* **11**:80–88 (1961).] (*c*) Rabbit atrium. [Redrawn from G. M. V. Williams, *Nature* **183**:1341–1342 (1959).] (*d*) Squid giant axon. [Redrawn from I. Tasaki, *Handbook of Physiology and Neurophysiology*, Vol. I, J. Field, H. W. Magoun, and V. E. Hall, Eds., American Physiological Society, Washington, D.C., 1959.] (*e*) Single spinal motoneurone. [Redrawn from W. H. Freygang and K. Frank, *J. Gen. Physiol.* **42**:749–759 (1959).]

specimen from a distance of about 3 mm (A in Fig. 24) and continuing until the tip of the micropipet penetrated the membrane of a Purkinje fiber (F). An orderly sequence of increase in amplitude was obtained with almost no change in the waveform (A–E) until a cell membrane was penetrated, whereupon the transmembrane potential excursion was recorded (F), revealing a quite different waveform with a much larger excursion in potential. The similarity of the second derivative of the transmembrane potential (G in Fig. 24) to the extracellularly recorded action potentials A–E is striking.

RECORDING BIOELECTRIC EVENTS

Virtually all of the bioelectric events now recorded clinically were well known before the dawn of the twentieth century. However, it was the introduction of the differential amplifier by Matthews (1934) that paved the way for ease in recording

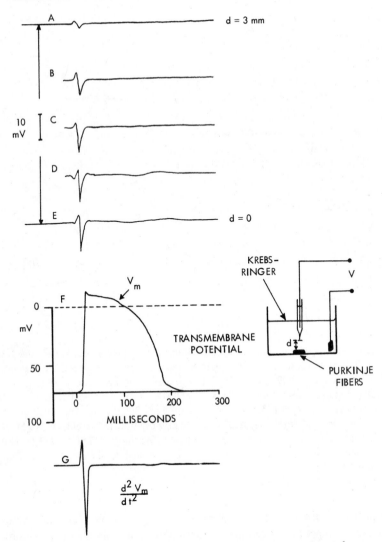

Figure 24 The relation between extracellular potentials (A–E), transmembrane potential (F) and the second derivative of the transmembrane potential G. (Data courtesy of Drs. D. Riopel and R. Vick, 1970.)

without the use of a shielded enclosure for the subject and amplifier. The first differential amplifiers were known as push–pull amplifiers and used triode vacuum tubes. Almost immediately others described their own versions of the differential amplifier; among these were Garceau and Forbes (1934), Adrian and Yamagiwa (1935), and Walter (1936), all of whom were concerned with recording the electrical activity of the nervous system. These amplifiers were symmetrical up to the display device (graphic recorder, oscillograph, or cathode ray tube). The differential-input, single-sided-output amplifier was described by Schmitt (1937) and Toennies (1938). By this time, it was recognized that the most important stage was the input and that a high degree of symmetry between the two halves of the differential amplifier was very important. Toennies showed that a very high degree of symmetry could be obtained by using a high value of resistance in the common cathode circuit. A high effective dynamic resistance was obtained by Goldberg (1944) and Johnston (1947), who used the plate circuit of a pentode as the common-cathode resistor in the input stage. When transistors became available, the collector of the transistor was connected to the common cathode of the input stage. The current–voltage characteristic of the transistor is very similar to that of the pentode. Thus, the early, highly symmetrical (balanced) differential amplifiers employed both vacuum tubes and transistors.

To illustrate the need for the differential amplifier, it is useful to recognize the major source of interference, mainly ground-referred sources such as the 60-Hz, 115-V (rms) power line. It is conventional that one side of the domestic power line is grounded, as shown in Fig. 25. The standard wall outlet has openings for a two-blade-and-rod plug. One of the blades is connected to the cold (ground) side, and the other is connected to the "hot" 115-V supply to deliver current to the device connected to the plug. The rod connects to a separate ground wire that carries no current and is designed to provide a ground for the exposed metal parts of the device connected to the power line. Obviously, a subject touching only the hot side of the power line will receive a shock if he has an adequate conductive and/or capacitive path to ground, as shown in Fig. 25b. Note that although the line voltage is 115 V (rms), the peak-to-peak voltage is $115 \times 2\sqrt{2} = 324$ V.

Now consider the situation of recording a bioelectric event with a single-sided amplifier, that is, one that has one of its input terminals referenced to ground; Fig. 26a illustrates this situation. The 60-Hz power line (E_p) is coupled to the subject

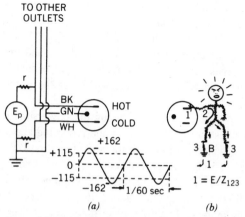

$$Z_{123} = \text{CONTACT RES. (1) + SUBJ. RES. (2) + RES. TO GROUND (3)}$$

Figure 25   Conventional wiring of the two-blade-and-rod power-line (E_p) outlet.

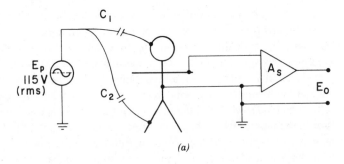

(a)

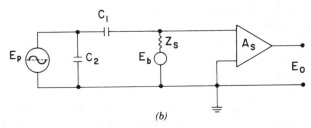

(b)

Figure 26 (a) Recording a bioelectric event (E_b) with a single-sided amplifier (A_S) in the presence of 60-Hz power-line voltage (E_p). (b) The equivalent circuit; Z_S is the electrode–subject impedance.

via two stray capacitances C_1 and C_2; however, it is only C_1 that is important, because no capacitive current through C_2 enters the amplifier input. Figure 26b illustrates the equivalent circuit and shows that the 60-Hz interfering signal is in parallel with the bioelectric event connected to the input of the amplifier (A_s). The electrode–subject impedance is Z_s and a low value of Z_s will decrease the amplitude of the 60-Hz interference because Z_s and C_1 form a voltage divider. The amplitude of the bioelectric signal (E_b) entering the amplifier would not be affected by reducing Z_s. Note that the bioelectric signal may be a millivolt and the 60-Hz interfering signal is 324,000 times as large; therefore, even with a small value for C_1, both the bioelectric signal and the interference will enter the amplifier and will appear on the display.

In addition to reducing Z_s, a method of reducing the power-line interference is to reduce C_1, which involves moving the subject and recording apparatus from the vicinity of the power line, which is difficult if the amplifier is power-line-operated.

Although cumbersome, another method of reducing power-line interference involves placing the subject and recording apparatus in a grounded shielded enclosure and operating the amplifier from batteries within the enclosure. This technique (Fig. 27) was used widely in the early days of electrophysiology, when the shielded room was a standard item in all electrophysiology laboratories.

The differential amplifier made it possible to record bioelectric events in the

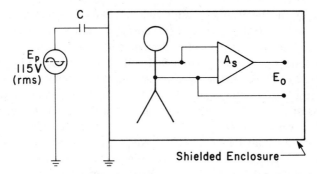

Figure 27 The use of a grounded shielded enclosure to record a bioelectric event with a single-sided amplifier (A_S).

presence of 60-Hz power lines, while at the same time using a ground-referred recording system operated from the power line. Figure 28A illustrates a differential amplifier (A_d) connected to a subject for recording a bioelectric event, for example, the ECG. As before, C_1 and C_2 are the stray capacitances to the power line (E_p). Figure 28B illustrates the equivalent circuit, showing that the 60-Hz interference is coupled to both input terminals (+ and −) by C_1 and C_2. It is important to recognize that the 60-Hz interference appearing on both input terminals is in phase with respect to the ground-reference terminal (R) of the differential amplifier (A_d).

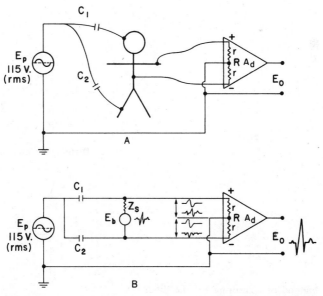

Figure 28 Recording a bioelectric event (E_b) with a differential amplifier (A_d) in the presence of power-line voltage E_p. (A) The connections for recording the ECG (E_b); (B) The equivalent circuit.

However, the bioelectric event (E_b) appearing between the + and R terminals will be out of phase with that appearing between the − and R terminals. Since the differential amplifier can amplify only the difference in the signals between the inputs (+/−) and the reference terminal (R), the ground-referred in-phase interference will not be amplified and will not appear at the output (E_o). The out-of-phase bioelectric signal will be amplified and appear at the output ($A_d E_b = E_o$).

The figure of merit of a differential amplifier is the common-mode rejection ratio (CMRR), which is a measure of the symmetry or equality of the gain of the two sides of the differential amplifier. The CMRR is defined as the differential gain G_d divided by the common-mode gain G_c. Figure 29*A* illustrates the method of measuring the differential gain, and Fig. 29*B* illustrates the technique for determining the common-mode gain. Obviously, a signal generator with an isolated output (i.e., not ground referred) is needed to measure the differential gain using the method shown in Fig. 29*A*. Care must be taken when measuring the common-mode gain to avoid blocking the amplifier by using too large an input signal.

The differential gain can be measured with an unisolated (ground referred) signal generator by connecting one side of the differential amplifier to the common reference terminal, which is also connected to the grounded side of the signal generator. The other side of the differential amplifier is connected to the other terminal of the signal generator. The output of the amplifier divided by the input voltage provided by the signal generator is the differential gain. The common-mode gain is measured as shown in Fig. 29*B*.

Typical differential amplifiers for bioelectric events have a CMRR on the order

A.

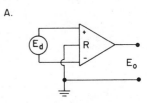

Differential gain $G_d = E_o / E_d$

B.

Common mode gain $G_c = E_o / E_c$
Common-mode rejection ratio
$CMRR = G_d / G_c$

Figure 29   Method of measuring (*A*) the differential gain G_d and (*B*) the common-mode gain G_c and calculating the common-mode rejection ratio CMRR.

of 5000. With care and the use of circuit strategies, it is not too difficult to achieve a CMRR of 50,000 or more.

The use of a differential amplifier does not guarantee immunity from ground-referred (mainly 60Hz) interference. Recall that for no interference to appear at the output, the common-mode rejection ratio must be high and the ground-referred interference must be nearly equal on the two input terminals of the differential amplifier. In Fig. 28A, if C_1 is not equal to C_2, there will be a differential signal that will be amplified. The key to reducing 60-Hz interference is to guarantee that it is symmetrically applied to the input terminals of the differential amplifier. An extremely high common-mode signal may drive the input stage into its nonlinear range and the interference will appear on the output. Another cause for interference to appear in the output is the use of a high and low resistance electrode on the subject.

Magnetically induced interference is not rejected by the differential amplifier. The wires leading from the plus and minus terminals to the subject constitute a single-turn pickup coil. Any nearby changing magnetic field will induce a voltage in this single-turn coil. The method of minimizing this type of interference employs twisted wires to connect the subject to the amplifier. The use of twisted wire cable in a shield to connect the subject to the amplifier offers the best opportunity of minimizing the risk of encountering interference from stray capacitance and magnetic fields produced by nearby power lines.

PRACTICAL DIFFERENTIAL AMPLIFIER

Figure 30 illustrates an easily constructed general-purpose differential amplifier consisting of two high input impedance operational amplifiers (TL062) directly coupled to another operational amplifier (TL061), which provides a single-sided output. The low-frequency response is determined by RC, the product of the input capacitance C and the resistance R, which is the time constant. The sinusoidal low frequency for 70% amplitude is $f_L = 1/2\pi RC$. For recording bioelectric events,

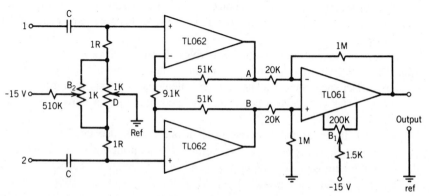

Figure 30 Circuit diagram for a simple differential amplifier. (Courtesy of J. D. Bourland.)

the resistance R is about 2 MΩ, providing an input resistance of $2R$ for the amplifier; C is then selected to obtain the desired low-frequency response.

Certain practical details must be attended to for optimum operation of the differential amplifier shown in Fig. 30A. The first pertains to compensation for the offset present in all operational amplifiers. The offset in the output stage (TL061) is adjusted with potentiometer B_1. With a jumper placed between points A and B, potentiometer B_1 is adjusted so that there is no (dc) voltage at the output. Next, the offset in the input stage is compensated for by first removing the connection between A and B and adjusting the offset potentiometer B_2 until there is no (dc) output voltage. Of course, these settings are made with no signal applied to the input terminals (1, 2).

The common-mode rejection ratio is now adjusted by connecting the two input terminals (1, 2) together and applying a signal generator (e.g., 1 K Hz) between these two terminals and the input reference (Ref). While the amplifier output is measured on an oscilloscope, the input signal is increased to about 1 mV, and the oscilloscope sensitivity is adjusted so that an output can be seen. Then the differential balance potentiometer (D) is adjusted for the minimum amplitude on the oscilloscope. A finer balance can be achieved by increasing the common-mode input signal and repeating the procedure. Care must be exercised to avoid using an input that is too high, otherwise distortion will be encountered. When the best balance has been achieved, the overall common-mode gain is very much less than unity. Then the signal generator is connected between the reference (Ref) and one side of the input (the other amplifier input terminal being connected to the reference). Using a small input to avoid distortion, the differential gain is measured. The common-mode rejection ratio is the differential gain divided by the common-mode gain. Values in excess of 10,000 are typical.

ISOLATED DIFFERENTIAL AMPLIFIER

In many circumstances of bioelectric recording, it is desirable to provide no conducting path and as small a capacitance as possible to ground. In other words, application of the electrodes to the subject and their connection to the amplifying equipment do not provide a path to ground. To achieve this goal, an isolated input stage is employed.

One type of isolated-input amplifier derives its isolation by modulation of a carrier (Fig. 31). After passing through a transformer (T_1) with a low primary-to-secondary capacitance, the modulated carrier is demodulated and the original signal is recovered. The voltage to operate the isolated amplifier is derived from an isolated power supply.

Figure 31a illustrates the principle used in one type of isolated amplifier (A) used as an input stage for bioelectric recording. The amplified bioelectric signal is fed into a modulator (M), the output of which is a high-frequency carrier on which the bioelectric signal rides as shown. This amplitude-modulated carrier is applied to a transformer (T_1) having a low primary-to-secondary capacitance. To the sec-

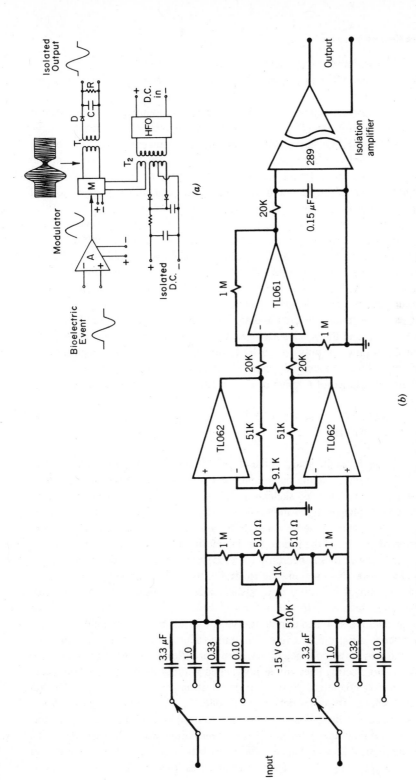

Figure 31 (*a*) Principle employed in one type of isolated-input amplifier, employing amplitude modulation. (*b*) Circuit diagram of a practical isolated differential amplifier based on Analog Devices model 289 isolated amplifier. (Courtesy of J. D. Bourland.)

685

ondary of this transformer is connected a demodulator consisting of a diode (D), integrating capacitor (C), and resistor (R), across which the bioelectric signal appears.

Energy to operate the isolated amplifier (A) and the modulator (M) are derived from a second transformer (T_2), to the primary of which is connected a high-frequency oscillator (HFO), driven by any unisolated dc power supply. The isolated carrier, which is fed directly to the modulator (M), appears across one of the windings of T_2. The high-frequency voltage, which is derived from the other winding on T_2, after rectification and filtering, provides the direct current required to operate the isolated amplifier (A) and modulator (M).

There are many commercially available isolated amplifiers. Typical isolation values are about 20–50 pF capacitance and hundreds of megohms (with respect to the output circuit or dc power supply). Voltage breakdown ratings of 2–5 kV are available. The overall amplification is typically 1:100, with a common-mode rejection ratio (at 60 Hz) of about 1 million (120 dB). The frequency response extends from 0 Hz to typically 5 or 20 kHz.

Figure 31*b* illustrates the circuit diagram of a practical isolated differential amplifier, built around the Analog Devices Model 289 amplifier. This device provides an isolated power supply ($\pm$ 15 V) to operate the differential amplifier consisting of three TL062 operational amplifiers. At the input is shown a selector switch to provide choice of a range of time constant from 3.3 to 0.1 sec.

ELECTROMYOGRAPHY

Electromyography is the study of the electrical activity of muscle; clinical electromyography (or EMG) is the name applied to the investigation of the electrical activity of normal and diseased skeletal muscle with extracellular electrodes. Clinical electromyography provides important information on the physiological status of skeletal muscle and its nerve supply. In cases of muscle paralysis, it allows identification of the site of the lesion, that is, within the brain (upper motor neuron) or spinal cord (lower motor neuron), its axon, the end plate, and muscle fiber. Upper motor neuron dysfunction, due to stroke, hysteria, malingering, trauma, or other causes, although resulting in paralysis, does not produce the same electromyographic signs seen with disease of the spinal motor nerve cell and its associated axon and muscle fibers. When a motor nerve cell or its axon degenerates, or when the nerve fiber to a muscle is severed, the previously innervated muscle fibers are paralyzed and cannot be contracted voluntarily or reflexly. A normally innervated muscle shows no electrical activity at rest; when voluntarily or reflexly contracted it produces action potentials. Following denervation, a muscle is paralyzed; but after a time, which is species-dependent (Table 2), the individual muscle fibers start to contract and relax independently (i.e., to fibrillate), producing a characteristic type of rhythmic action potential called fibrillation waves, which signal that the nerve supply has been interrupted. These random and asynchronous contractions produce no net muscle tension, and they continue as long as there is muscle tissue

TABLE 2   Appearance Time for Fibrillation
Potentials in Denervated Skeletal Muscle

Species	Muscle	Appearance Time (days)
Mouse	Peroneal	3.5
Rat	—	4
Rabbit	—	6
Monkey	Brachioradialis	8
Human	Brachioradialis	18

Source: From G. Weddell et al., *Lancet* **1:**236–239 (1943).

present and denervation persists. If reinnervation does not occur, the muscle fibers atrophy and the fibrillation potentials disappear. If reinnervation occurs, the muscle fibers cease to atrophy, and the fibrillation potentials gradually disappear, being replaced slowly by normal muscle action potentials, which appear when a voluntary effort is made or when the muscle is contracted reflexly. It is important to realize that during reinnervation a characteristic polyphasic (nascent) action potential can be detected with voluntary contraction effort, long before there are visible signs of muscular contraction. Figure 32*a* illustrates a typical normal muscle action potential; Figs. 32*b* and 32*c* show, respectively, fibrillation potentials and a typical electromyographic picture during reinnervation when primitive muscle action and fibrillation potentials are present.

The type of equipment used to record clinical electromyograms merits special consideration because of the small area of the active electrodes and the short duration and rapid rise of the electromyographic signals. Direct graphic recording instruments cannot be employed to obtain recordings of diagnostic significance; instead, a cathode ray oscilloscope is used with an amplifier having a high input impedance (several megohms) and an adequate bandwidth (~2–5000 Hz). The repetition rate of the sweep of the oscilloscope is usually fixed at about 7 sweeps/sec, and the sweep speed is controllable from 20 to 2 msec/cm.

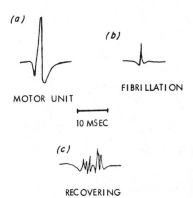

Figure 32   (*a*) Normal motor unit potential and (*b*) normal fibrillation waves; the latter are characteristically present in denervated muscle. (*c*) During early reinnervation, recovering, low-amplitude, short-duration polyphasic action potentials appear during a voluntary contraction effort; at this time muscle contraction is seldom visible.

It is convenient to use a loudspeaker to provide aural monitoring since the diagnostic information is contained in waveform and repetition rate. With very little experience, the ear can be trained to detect normal motor unit action potentials, which produce a thumping sound; fibrillation potentials give a characteristic ticking, clicking, or crackling sound. Although it is easy to recognize these and other characteristic waveforms, considerable skill and experience are needed to assess their significance in terms of the presence of neuromuscular disease or dysfunction.

In general, the clinical electromyographer applies the reference and ground electrodes to the subject, as shown in Fig. 33. Then while the investigator watches the oscilloscope and listens to the loudspeaker, the needle electrode is quickly advanced into the muscle to be examined. Insertion of the needle usually causes mechanical stimulation of subjacent muscle (or nerve) fibers, and a short burst of action potentials will be heard and also seen on the oscilloscope. The character of these insertion potentials depends on the status of the muscle. If normally innervated, the action potentials will resemble normal motor units, which will disappear within a few seconds if the muscle is at rest. Prolonged or absent insertion potentials is a sign of muscle abnormality. When the needle electrode is positioned close to contracting motor units, the action potentials obtained are 1–10 msec in duration and 50–3000 μV in amplitude.

Proper location of the electrode tip is greatly facilitated by the sound in the loudspeaker. As active fibers are approached, the sound becomes characteristically sharper and much more distinct. If the muscle is denervated and enough time has passed (Table 2) for fibrillation potentials to develop, the insertion potentials are a train of short-duration fibrillation waves, which continue at a much slower rate (1–10 per second), thereby providing the diagnostic sign of denervation. Subse-

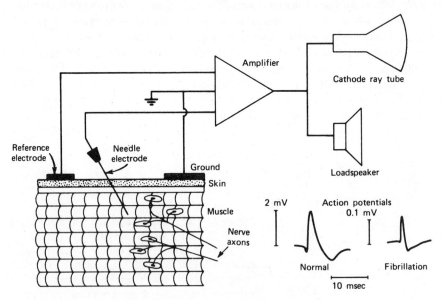

Figure 33   Electromyographic technique.

quent mechanical movement of the needle often sets off a train of positive-wave potentials when the needle electrode is in injured muscle.

To comprehend the various waveforms obtained in electromyographic studies, it is necessary to have an understanding of neuromuscular physiology, which is concerned with the manner in which muscular contraction occurs. The following abbreviated account provides the essential details.

The contractile unit of skeletal muscle is the muscle fiber, which is a single multinucleated cylindrical cell about 50 μm in diameter; when stimulated, the fiber is capable of shortening (contracting) and developing force. A whole muscle consists of parallel bundles (fascicles) of muscle fibers. Each muscle fiber is in turn composed of fibrils, which are bundles of filaments of contractile protein; the filaments are about 150 Å in diameter. The structural arrangement of the contractile filaments causes skeletal muscle to exhibit cross striations visible with a low-power microscope. For this reason it is often called striated muscle.

Activation of each skeletal muscle fiber occurs in response to an action potential traveling along a motor nerve fiber (axon) that innervates the muscle fiber. Depending on the location and function of the muscle, each axon may innervate one muscle fiber (as in the extraocular muscles) or as many as 600–1200 muscle fibers (as in the case of the postural muscles); Fig. 33 illustrates an innervation ratio of 3:1. The combination of the motor nerve cell in the spinal cord, its axon, and the muscle fibers it innervates is the basic functional unit of the muscular system and is called the motor unit. When the nerve action potential reaches the specialized tissue junction between the nerve and muscle (the myoneural junction or motor end plate), a quantum of chemical transmitter (acetylcholine) is released. This transmitter causes a local depolarization of the subjacent polarized membrane of the muscle fiber and initiates an action potential that is propagated over the entire muscle fiber; a single contraction (twitch) follows within about 1 msec. The transmitter is quickly neutralized by acetylcholinesterase, and the end plate is ready to receive another quantum of transmitter. Meanwhile, during the contraction, the membrane of the muscle fiber starts to recover, and recovery is complete even before the full force of contraction is reached. Figure 34 illustrates the temporal relationship between the twitch and the excursion in transmembrane potential. Since recovery is so rapid in skeletal muscle, many closely spaced stimuli can be delivered, and the contractions will fuse into a sustained or tetanic contraction, as in Fig. 34.

The force developed by a muscle is graded in two ways. It is apparent that a single action potential in an axon of the motor nerve will produce a twitch in all the muscle fibers that it innervates. If more axons are activated at the same time, more muscle fibers will be stimulated, and the twitch will develop more force. On the other hand, if a single axon is stimulated more frequently, the twitches will fuse into a tetanic contraction, which develops several times more force than the twitch. Therefore, the force of muscular contraction is graded by controlling the number of axons that are stimulated and the frequency of stimulation in each axon.

In clinical electromyography, muscle action potentials are recorded with a small-area (active) electrode located near a contracting muscle fiber and the reference

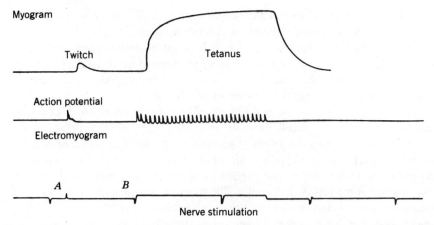

Figure 34   The discontinuous nature of muscle contractions exhibited by a myogram (upper) and an electromyogram (lower) obtained from a frog gastrocnemius muscle by delivering single and repetitive stimuli to the sciatic nerve. A single stimulus (A) provides a single action potential and a twitch; (B) repetitive stimulation at 20 per second evoked an action potential for each stimulus and a sustained (tetanic) contraction. (Time marks, 1 sec.)

electrode located at a distance. Therefore, the waveform obtained with such an extracellular recording method will not resemble the excursion in transmembrane potential because the active electrode measures the potential change caused by extracellular current flow within the muscle, which acts as an inhomogeneous volume conductor. Depending on the medium surrounding the active tissue, the waveform detected approximates the second time derivative of the transmembrane potential. Katz and Miledi (1965) presented an interesting record (Fig. 35) that illustrates this point. Microelectrodes were inserted into frog sartorius muscle immersed in saline at 20°C; one microelectrode was used for stimulation, and the other recorded the transmembrane potential with respect to a reference electrode in the saline. The extracellular recording electrode was about 6 mm from the tendon. The excursion in transmembrane potential is a typical monophasic action potential rising quickly from the resting membrane potential, overshooting (reversing polarization), and slowly returning to the resting membrane potential. The extracellular action potential is triphasic and resembles the second derivative of the transmembrane potential.

The electrical activity of skeletal muscle can be recorded by placing two disk electrodes on the surface of the skin along the axis of a contracting skeletal muscle. The voltage appearing between the electrodes is the algebraic sum of all the action potentials of the contracting and recovering muscle fibers between the electrodes. The frequency and the peak voltage exhibit a nonlinear relationship with the force developed by the muscle. The frequency of the action potentials ranges from zero at rest to several hundred per second during a maximal contraction. Although this noninvasive technique is of value in kinesiology studies, it is too imprecise for the

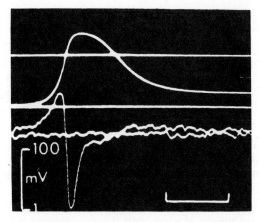

Figure 35   Simultaneous transmembrane potential (upper) and extracellular action potential (lower) recorded from a monopolar electrode near a frog gastrocnemius muscle. The length of the vertical calibration bar represents 100 mV for the transmembrane recording and 1 mV for the extracellular recording. The muscle was stimulated by an intracellular electrode. [From B. Katz and R. Miledi, *Proc. R. Soc. London, Ser. B* **161**:453–482 (1964–1965). By permission.]

diagnosis of neuromuscular diseases that require a needle electrode paired with a surface (reference) electrode (Fig. 33) or a monopolar or bipolar coaxial hypodermic electrode. Using these electrodes, a muscle can be examined for the presence of normal motor units or fibrillation potentials. It is important to understand that the amplitude and duration of the action potentials are dependent on the type of electrode employed and the muscle under investigation.

At the beginning of this section, it was stated that clinical electromyography (in which a needle electrode and a skin-surface electrode are used) provides useful information on the innervation status of skeletal muscle. A few examples are now presented to illustrate how diagnostic information is provided by the EMG. For example, in myasthenia gravis—a condition in which the muscle fibers are normally innervated but transmission of impulses across the myoneural junction is impaired—muscular contraction can be sustained only for short periods. In severe cases there is widespread paralysis involving the respiratory muscles. With this disease, because the muscle fibers are normally innervated, there are no fibrillation potentials at rest. Insertion of the needle electrode produces a train of insertion potentials as in the case of a normal muscle. With voluntary contraction, normal potentials arise but do not persist because of impaired transmission at the myoneural junction. If the disease is severe, the frequency and voltage of the normal motor units are reduced. The diagnosis of myasthenia gravis is confirmed by the administration of a short-acting acetylcholinesterase inhibitor, which temporarily enhances myoneural transmission and provides an essentially normal EMG on voluntary contraction.

Muscular dystrophy is a degenerative disease of muscle in which there is atrophy of some fibers, swelling of others, an increase in sarcolemmal nuclei, and connective tissue separations, with the deposition of fat between other fibers that become hypertrophied. On insertion of the needle electrode, there is a vigorous discharge of low-amplitude, short-duration, high-frequency (dystrophic) potentials. At rest, there are no fibrillation waves because there is usually no nerve damage (see below). With voluntary contraction, the action potentials are low in amplitude, short in duration (1–2 msec), and high in frequency (up to 40/sec); they produce a high-pitched whirring sound in the loudspeaker. As a result of the loss of contractile elements in the motor units, more motor units are brought into action to provide the necessary force; hence, the increased frequency of discharge with voluntary effort is not surprising. On relaxation there is electrical silence. With sustained contraction, the electrical activity alternately increases and decreases as the muscle begins to fatigue, at which time there is a marked reduction in electrical activity. Depending on the severity of the disease, normal motor unit potentials may also be recorded. Fibrillation potentials are rarely seen; if present, they result from nerve interruption due to fibrotic muscle encroaching on nerve fibers within the muscle.

Myotonia is a degenerative disease of muscle in which the individual muscle fibers are hyperexcitable and the whole muscle does not relax readily. Insertion of the needle electrode evokes an intense discharge of regular, high-frequency action potentials that may persist for a few seconds or as long as ~1 min. This pattern of electrical discharge produces a characteristic initial thunderstorm-like sound in the loudspeaker. Similar discharges can be evoked by tapping the muscle or the needle electrode. When relaxation does occur, there is electrical silence and no fibrillation potentials are recorded. During voluntary contraction, normal motor unit activity is recorded along with short-duration discharges from the diseased muscle fibers.

From this brief introductory description of the type of electrical activity recorded in normal skeletal muscles and in several common neuromuscular diseases, it should be evident that if a muscle is denervated, either by disease or by trauma affecting the spinal motor neuron or its axon, paralysis, atrophy of the muscle fibers previously innervated, and fibrillation potentials will occur. In humans, such potentials appear about 2 weeks following denervation; they persist as long as muscle fibers are present. The fibrillation potentials slowly disappear as reinnervation occurs or when the muscle fibers disappear. On the other hand, with diseases that affect muscle fibers (myopathies), fibrillation potentials are absent, and the electrical activity recorded depends on the type of muscle disease.

Readers interested in pursuing the study of electromyography in depth should consult the following original papers: Weddell et al. (1944), Kügelberg (1947), Jasper and Ballem (1949), Denny-Brown (1949), Petersen and Kügelberg (1949), Landau (1951), Lundervold and Li (1953), Buchtal et al. (1954), and Liberson (1962). Among the useful clinical textbooks on electromyography are those by Pearson (1961), Licht (1961), Norris (1963), and Marinacci (1965) and the review of electromyography by Simpson (1973).

ELECTROCARDIOGRAPHY

Regardless of how it is recorded, the electrocardiogram (ECG) merely reflects the propagation of electrical depolarization and repolarization over the various contractile chambers of the heart. Propagation of excitation (depolarization) is the trigger for releasing the stored contractile energy in cardiac muscle. Situations are commonly encountered in which there is an uncoupling of the excitation–contraction mechanism, and excitation can occur without contraction. In addition, a premature ventricular electrical excitation may not be followed by a mechanical contraction strong enough to open the aortic or pulmonic valves. In this circumstance, the number of R waves of the ECG is greater than the number of arterial pulses.

The term electrocardiogram is specifically reserved for a record of the electrical activity of the heart obtained with body-surface electrodes. Cardiac electrogram is the term employed when electrodes are placed directly on or in the heart to detect its electrical activity. A semidirect cardiac electrogram describes a record of the electrical activity of the heart obtained with one direct-heart electrode and one body-surface electrode. These terms are not always used properly, but the correct definitions should be noted. Finally, the English-language abbreviation is ECG, rather than EKG (which derives from the German Elektrokardiogramm). To avoid confusion, electroencephalographers now use ECoG (rather than ECG) to designate the electrocorticogram, which is a recording of the electrical activity of the exposed outer surface (cortex) of the brain.

All hearts consist of a series of contractile chambers suitably equipped with valves that allow blood to be propelled in one direction. Each contractile chamber produces electrical action and recovery potentials associated with mechanical contraction and relaxation (recovery). The general rule is that the bioelectric event precedes the mechanical event. Each contractile chamber, or a region within it, exhibits spontaneous rhythmicity. That special region of the heart with the highest degree of rhythmicity is the pacemaker that normally sets the cardiac frequency; in the mammalian heart this is a region of modified muscle tissue called the sinoatrial (SA) node. The pacemaker rate is affected by temperature and the net neural bias. With these generalizations, it is possible to understand the ECG in many circumstances.

Neither the interference nor the dipole theories explain all the waveforms encountered in clinical electrocardiography. The simplest hypothesis equates the propagation of excitation as the advance of an array of positive charges (dipoles) with negativity trailing. The conventions employed to record this electrical event are given in Figs. 36 and 37; for the polarities indicated, an upward deflection signals the advance of excitation toward the positive electrode. Recovery is indicated by the approach of an array of negative charges (dipoles). If recovery progresses in the same direction as excitation, a downward deflection is obtained in leads shown in Figs. 36 and 37.

A convenient method of studying the cardiac cycle employs the electrocardiogram as a timing reference. This technique will be applied to the cardiac cycle of the mammalian heart, which contains two distinct atria (which contract together)

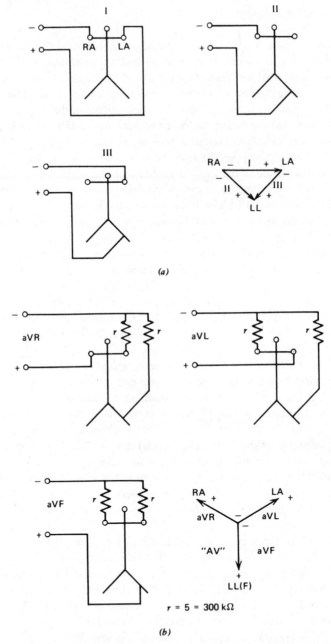

Figure 36 ECG frontal plane leads: (a) limb leads, (b) augmented limb leads.

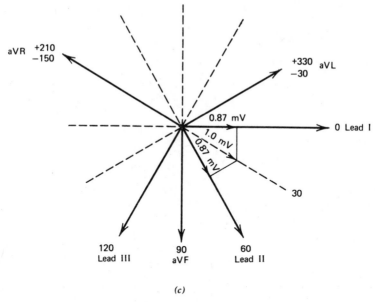

Figure 36 (*Continued*)   (*c*) Frontal plane vectors.

and two separate ventricles, which also contract together shortly after atrial contraction.

Excitation from the atria is propagated to the ventricles by way of a tissue bridge called the atrioventricular (A-V) node, which has a low propagation velocity and therefore delays the spread of excitation to the ventricles. Excitation of the ventricular musculature occurs by way of the A-V node, bundle of His, and Purkinje fibers. It is largely the spread of electrical activity over the surface of the heart that constitutes the electrocardiogram.

The mammalian ECG can be dissected into two major components, one associated with the propagation of excitation and recovery over the atria; the other, with events occurring in the ventricles, the main pumping chambers of the heart. Excitation of the atria gives rise to the P wave, after which atrial contraction propels blood from the atria into the ventricles; this event is sometimes accompanied by the fourth heart sound. An atrial recovery wave exists but is rarely seen because it is obscured by ventricular excitation, which is signaled by the QRS wave. During the latter part of the QRS wave, ventricular contraction commences, which closes the A-V valves (giving rise to the first heart sound). Slightly thereafter, blood is pumped into the lungs by the right ventricle and into the aorta by the left ventricle. Recovery of the ventricles is preceded by the T wave. When ventricular pressure falls below the outflow pressure, the outflow valves (pulmonic and aortic) close suddenly, giving rise to the second heart sound. When ventricular pressure falls below atrial pressure, ventricular filling occurs, which often gives rise to the third heart sound. The evolution of the ECG during movement of the atria and ventricles

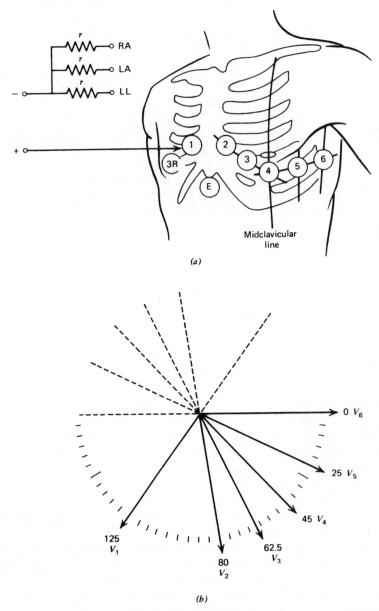

(a)

(b)

Figure 37   The precordial leads. (a) r = 5–300 kΩ. (b) Horizontal plane vectors.

is depicted in Fig. 38; the relationship between the ECG and the events of the cardiac cycle just described appear in Fig. 39. Thus, examination of the various components of the ECG identifies the sequence of excitation and recovery of the heart. The configuration of the ECG and the durations of the various waves carry important physiologic and diagnostic information. The ECG should therefore be viewed as the timing signal for the events of the cardiac cycle.

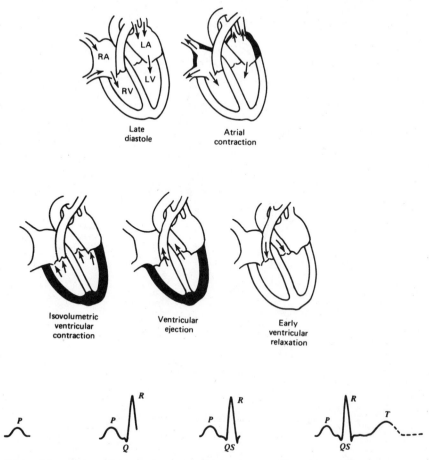

Figure 38   Evaluation of the electrocardiogram during mechanical activity of the heart.

Although Einthoven originally employed the familiar letters P, QRS, and T to designate the waves of the electrocardiogram, considerable confusion soon arose regarding their use in a variety of leads. Pardee (1940) proposed the system that has been adopted universally to describe the intervals and durations of the various waves.

To localize the direction (vectors) of excitation and recovery of the atria and ventricles, and to estimate the extent of injury (such as might result from insufficient coronary circulation), a variety of electrode arrays are employed. The electrode placements are based on easily located anatomical "landmarks"; the most popular of these arrays are illustrated in Figs. 36 and 37. The standard (I, II, III), augmented (aVR, aVL, aVF), and precordial (V) leads are routinely recorded by electrocardiographers. By visual inspection of the recordings and knowledge of the direction represented by each lead, it is possible to locate the mean vectors of excitation and recovery to within 15 degrees. The rule is that the isoelectric lead (or equal positive and negative deflection) is at right angles to the direction of the event (excitation

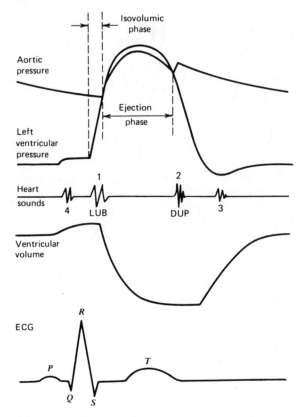

Figure 39   Some events of the cardiac cycle.

or recovery). To identify the direction in which the cardiac vector points, it is merely necessary to look at the polarity in a lead that is orthogonal to the lead with zero net amplitude. If there is no lead array in which the net amplitude is zero, interpolation must be employed by inspection of the leads with the minimum net amplitude.

The concept that underlies the vector representation was proposed by Einthoven et al. (1913), who imagined the heart to be at the center of an equilateral triangle with the apices at the right and left shoulders and the pubis. The leads to these points were placed on the right and left arms and both feet; later only the left foot was used. With this electrode array, it is possible to represent excitation or recovery (of the atria and ventricles) as a vector whose components are amplitudes projected on lead I (RA-LA), lead II (RA-LL), and lead III (LA-LL), as in Fig. 40. Thus if the amplitudes in two of the three leads are known, the magnitude and direction of the cardiac vector is known (see Fig. 40). From this concept of a 120-degree triaxial reference system came Einthoven's law, which states that the amplitude in lead II equals the algebraic sum of the amplitudes in leads I and III. This statement is true only for this triaxial system (Valentinuzzi et al., 1970).

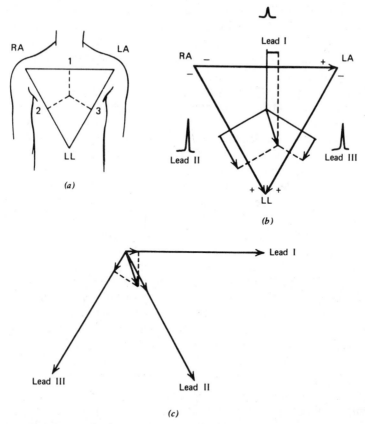

Figure 40 (*a*) Einthoven's triangular representation of the three limb leads, (*b*) their use to locate a cardiac vector, and (*c*) the simplified method of representing the lead axes.

The technique for locating cardiac vectors can be illustrated by referring to Fig. 36*c*, which shows a cardiac vector (which could represent excitation or recovery in either the atria or ventricles) with a magnitude of 1.0 mV and a direction of 30 degrees. Dropping perpendiculars from the tip of the vector to any of the other lead directions will give the amplitude in that lead. Since the vector direction is 30 degrees, its amplitude in lead III is zero, indicating that it is orthogonal to this lead. The amplitude is 0.87 mV in leads I and II, as in Fig. 36. Note that deflections are upward when the perpendicular from the tip of the cardiac vector intersects the solid lines, and downward when the intersection falls on the dashed lines.

This discussion has centered on mean cardiac vectors. However, the maximum and minimum amplitudes do not occur simultaneously in all leads, as was correctly pointed out by Einthoven et al. (1913). Therefore, the technique of obtaining mean amplitudes for the vector components by simple subtraction is merely a practical convenience to allow easy estimation of a mean vector. In reality, at each instant in the cardiac cycle, vector components can be obtained and the instantaneous vectors can be determined. A line joining the extremities of the instantaneous vectors will describe a loop whose major vector usually approximates the mean cardiac vector obtained as described previously. A continuous record of the instantaneous vectors constitutes the study of vector cardiography, which is described in the next section.

In electrocardiographic monitoring, a variety of standard and nonstandard leads (Fig. 41) are used to obtain a large-amplitude QRS wave free from muscle or body-movement artifacts. Thus electrodes are frequently placed on the chest or back. One lead that enjoys considerable popularity is the MX (manubrium–xiphoid) array (Lian and Golblin, 1936; Geddes et al., 1960b) in which the electrodes are located at the ends of the sternum. With this lead, there are no contracting skeletal muscles between the electrodes; in addition, the electrodes are close to the heart, which provides a large-amplitude ECG. Although the MX lead is very convenient for estimating heart rate by counting QRS waves, it is not the best lead for identification of metabolic changes in the ventricles, as revealed by the T wave.

When monitoring bedridden patients, it is not customary to place electrodes on the extremities. Usually self-adhering electrodes are placed on the chest at the left and right shoulders just below the clavicles and on the lower left chest. The ground is sometimes placed on the lower right chest or over the xiphoid process.

Another ECG lead that enjoys some popularity employs one electrode on the thorax just below the right axilla; the other electrode is on the left side of the chest on the midaxillary line and at the level of the fifth or sixth rib. With this transthoracic (TT) array, which approximates lead II (Fig. 41), a large-amplitude ECG can be obtained and the same electrodes can be used for recording respiration by the impedance method (Geddes et al., 1962).

With a single-channel ECG recording, which shows clear P, R, and T waves, it is possible to obtain a considerable amount of valuable information regarding cardiac activity. For example, the presence of an orderly sequence of P, R, and T waves with a normal range of intervals and durations denotes normal cardiac excitation and recovery. The ECG during sudden cardiac slowing in an impaired heart is presented in Fig. 42 along with femoral artery blood pressure. Note that the ECG complex marked X is essentially normal in configuration, yet the force of ventricular contraction was insufficient to open the aortic valve and eject blood. Intermittent interruption of the propagation of excitation between the atria and ventricles is shown in Fig. 43 along with carotid artery blood pressure. At A there is 2:1 atrioventricular block (two P waves for each normal QRS-T complex). Immediately thereafter, total A-V block occurred, as evidenced by the P waves continuing without causing ventricular excitation; however, the ventricles produced two extrasystoles (X_1, X_2) initiating from a focus in the apical region, illustrated by the downward QRS waves, which have no fixed relationship with the P waves. At B, 2:1 A-V block was reestablished. Note that only a minor disturbance in pulse rate and blood pressure accompanied these events. Total A-V block with apical ventricular pacemaker is represented in Fig. 44, which was derived from the same animal. Note that the QRS waves are all inverted and there is no fixed relationship between the atrial P and the ventricular RS waves.

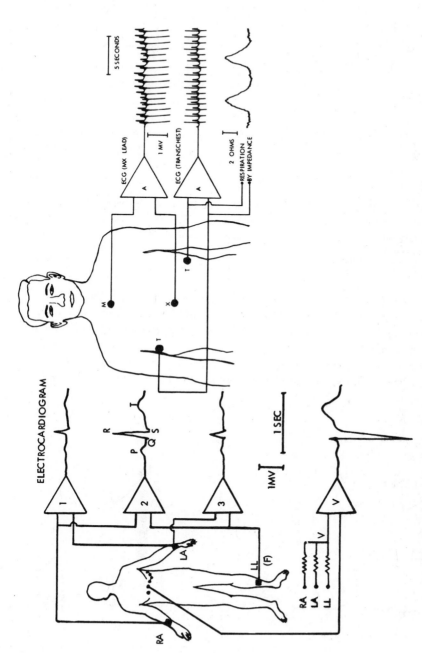

Figure 41 Commonly used ECG lead configurations: left, the standard limb and precordial (V) leads along with typical waveforms; above, two lead systems (MX or manubrium–xiphoid and TT or transthoracic). The MX lead is readily applicable to exercising subjects. With the transthoracic lead, the ECG and respiration can be recorded from the same pair of electrodes. [Redrawn from L. A. Geddes, *IEEE Spectrum* **9:**41–48 (1972).]

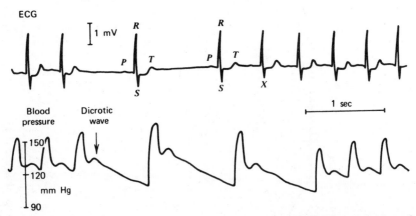

Figure 42 Lead II ECG and femoral artery pressure during sudden vagal slowing of a hypoxic canine heart. Note that during slowing the ECG for beat X exhibited a normal configuration, but the force of ventricular contraction was insufficient to open the aortic valve and eject blood.

Ventricular extrasystoles occurring at the apex and base (just below the atria) are identified in Fig. 45, which displays lead II ECG and femoral artery blood pressure. Note that both the left apical and right basal extrasystole failed to develop enough contractile force to open the aortic valve and produce a blood pressure pulse, as evidenced by the pulse deficit. Also, there is a period of alternating strong and weak beats (pulsus alternans) with a normal ECG following the right basal extrasystole.

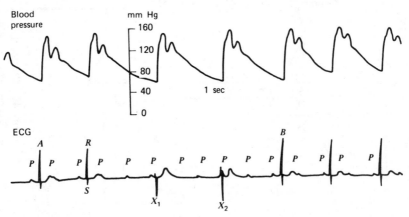

Figure 43 Lead II ECG and carotid artery blood pressure in an anesthetized dog. At A, 2:1 A-V block is present, followed by total A-V block, during which two apical extrasystoles (X_1, X_2) occurred. At B, 2:1 block was reestablished; during this sequence there was minimal change in the blood pressure record.

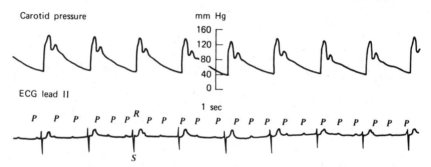

Figure 44   Lead II ECG and carotid artery blood pressure in an anesthetized dog illustrating that total A-V block is present, as shown by absence of fixed relationship between the P and QRS waves. Note that an apical ventricular pacemaker had developed, as evidenced by the downward QRS waves in the ECG. The blood pressure record, of course, gives no clue regarding this disturbed cardiac rhythm in which pacemaker activity is normal, as indicated by the regularly occurring P waves.

As demonstrated earlier, the ventricles have the capability of originating beats with an appreciable degree of automaticity. Figure 46 illustrates one interesting type of arrythmia known as bigeminus rhythm. Note that a ventricular extrasystole (R-S-T) regularly follows each normal beat. The blood pressure shows that the ventricular extrasystoles did not result in ejection of blood, as shown by the carotid artery pressure recording. Thus the ECG shows twice the number of ventricular excitations as blood pressure pulses.

Fibrillation is that condition in a cardiac chamber in which all fibers contract and relax randomly; consequently, there is no pumping action associated with a fibrillating chamber. Since atrial contraction contributes only a small amount to ventricular filling, loss of this component by atrial fibrillation is relatively unimportant in the nonexercising subject. However, the fibrillating atria bombard the

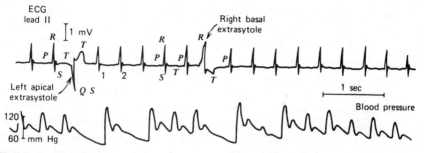

Figure 45   Lead II ECG and femoral artery blood pressure in an anesthetized dog. The induced left apical and right basal extrasystoles failed to result in a ventricular contraction forceful enough to open the aortic valve, as evidenced by the pulse deficits in the blood pressure record. Note the period of pulsus alternans with a normal ECG following the right basal extrasystole and the absence of a pulse following normal beat 2.

ECG lead II

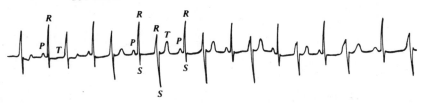

1 sec

Blood pressure

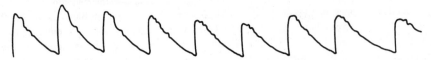

Figure 46   Lead II ECG and carotid artery blood pressure in an anesthetized dog that is exhibiting bigeminus rhythm. Following every normal P, QRS-T complex is a ventricular extrasystole. Since there are twice as many ventricular excitations as blood pressure pulses, it is clear that the extrasystole did not result in an ejection of blood from the left ventricle. In addition, the focus of the extrasystole varied throughout the period of recording.

A-V node with propagated excitations, resulting in a rapid and irregular ventricular rate. In fact, the rate is so high that filling is compromised and cardiac output is reduced because many ventricular contractions do not eject blood, as evidenced by a pulse deficit.

The ECG permits easy identification of the presence of atrial fibrillation. The atrial P waves are absent, being replaced by fibrillation (f) waves. Figure 47 is a record of atrial fibrillation that ceased spontaneously in a dog. The top channel displays a direct atrial electrogram, the second is lead II ECG, and the third is femoral artery blood pressure. While the atria are fibrillating, there are no P waves, and only very small amplitude f waves are visible in lead II. It is quite apparent that there are more ventricular excitations (R waves) than blood pressure pulses during atrial fibrillation. When atrial fibrillation ceased and sinus rhythm was re-tored, the P waves reappeared, as is shown clearly in lead II, and the tachycardia and pulse deficit both disappeared.

Ventricular fibrillation results in the loss of cardiac output and hence in a loss of blood pressure. Asystole of the ventricles exhibits the same condition; however, the ECG allows instant differentiation, for in asystole there are no QRS-T waves, whereas with ventricular fibrillation, the QRS-T waves are replaced by random irregular electrical activity. Figure 48 illustrates the ECG and blood pressure prior to and during the precipitation of ventricular fibrillation.

Ventricular fibrillation is incompatible with life, and if it is not reversed within a few minutes, irreversible damage occurs in the central nervous system. While preparations are made for defibrillation, cardiac compression (open- or closed-

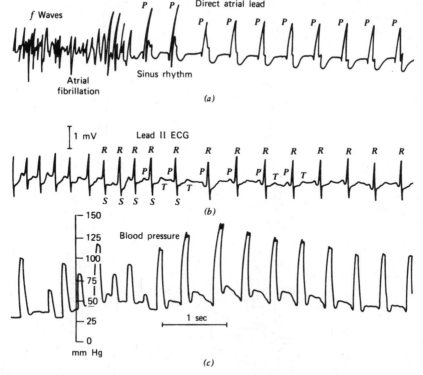

Figure 47 (*a*) Atrial electrogram, (*b*) lead II ECG, and (*c*) femoral artery blood pressure in the dog during atrial fibrillation (left) and normal sinus rhythm (right). Note that during atrial fibrillation there are no P waves in lead II, and there is a tachycardia and pulse deficit. When sinus rhythm returned, the P waves appeared in lead II, and the tachycardia and pulse deficit both disappeared.

chest) and artificial respiration must be applied. Defibrillation is achieved by the passage of a single pulse of current through the ventricles (by transchest or directly applied electrodes) to depolarize the cardiac tissue totally and allow the pacemaker (normally the SA node) to resume pacing.

The ECG shows striking changes when the heart muscle is deprived of an adequate supply of blood, as may occur from narrowing or occlusion of a branch of the coronary arteries. The cells in an area deprived of circulation cannot sustain their metabolic activities, and membrane integrity is lost; this results in the presence of a depolarized area that is electrically negative with respect to healthy tissue. The injured area, which manifests itself as an injury potential in the ECG, is inexcitable and develops no contractile force. With the passage of time the injured area is converted to scar tissue and the injury potential disappears from the ECG.

The type of waveform exhibited by the ECG when myocardial injury is present is often explained by the interference theory, which holds that the voltage appearing between the terminals of the ECG electrodes is due to the summation of the mon-

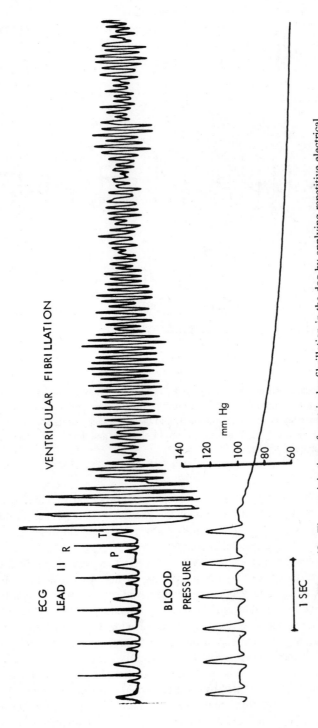

Figure 48 The precipitation of ventricular fibrillation in the dog by applying repetitive electrical stimuli to the right ventricle. Note the replacement of the QRS-T complex by fibrillation waves and the sudden fall in blood pressure.

ophasic myocardial action potentials seen by each electrode, as idealized in Fig. 14. Injury eliminates some of the monophasic action potentials and produces a persistent diastolic depolarization; consequently, the region between the R and T waves is no longer isoelectric, being above or below the baseline, depending on the location of the injury and the polarity for the particular lead.

A typical example of alteration in the ECG due to coronary artery occlusion appears in Fig. 49. On the left is the control electrocardiogram of a dog; one electrode was placed on the left forelimb and the other was on the chest over the apical region. Negativity of the left forelimb electrode is displayed as an upward deflection in the recording. Note that the segment between the end of the R wave (i.e., the S wave) and the beginning of the T wave is isoelectric. A myocardial infarction was created by ligating the left interventricular coronary artery, which resulted in considerable injury (hence persistent depolarization) to the apex of the left ventricle. The absence of excitation in this area reveals itself by an upward displacement in the S-T segment on the right of Fig. 49. This is the classical electrographic sign of early myocardial infarction. However, the upward displacement of the S-T segment is in reality a persistent (diastolic) depression of the baseline due to depolarization of the injured area.

Parenthetically, it is interesting to note that the first evidence of an electrocardiac signal was demonstrated by Koelliker and Mueller in 1856 using the rheoscopic frog; it was first recorded in 1876 by Marey and Lippmann using the capillary electrometer. Human electrocardiograms were recorded by Waller in 1887, also using the capillary electrometer. Dissatisfaction with the capillary electrometer led Einthoven to develop his string galvanometer in 1903. During this time, when cardiology was being born, cardiac action was recorded using pneumatic pulse pickups and the smoked-drum kymograph. Although useful diagnostic information was obtained in this manner, the ability of the electrocardiogram recorded with the

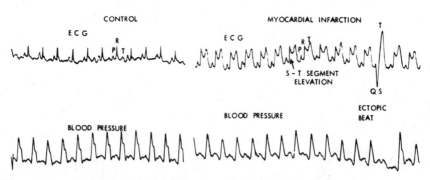

Figure 49 Electrocardiogram obtained from a dog with one electrode (−) on the left forelimb and the other (+) on the left chest wall in the region of the apex beat. On the left is the control record in which the segment between the end of the R wave (i.e., S wave) and the beginning of the T wave is isoelectric. On the right is the ECG after ligation of the left interventricular coronary artery. Presence of apical injury is indicated by the elevation in the S-T segment, which is the classical sign of myocardial infarction.

string galvanometer to demonstrate the sequence of excitation and recovery was soon recognized and pulse recording was abandoned. By the 1920s, string electrocardiographs were in use clinically. Direct-writing recorders started to supplant string galvanometers in the early 1940s. Although the ECG proved very useful in the diagnosis of arrythmias, its greater value in identifying the presence of injury (myocardial infarction) was not established until the late 1930s.

HIS-BUNDLE ELECTROGRAM

With the body-surface ECG, it is only possible to obtain information on the time taken for excitation to travel from the atria to the ventricles, the P-R interval. With His-bundle recording, this time can be divided into three components, P-A, A-H, and H-V, where A refers to atrial, H to His bundle, and V to ventricular excitation. The onset of the A wave occurs slightly after the onset of the P wave; therefore, the P-A interval represents conduction through the atria. The A-H interval represents the time taken for excitation to travel across the atrioventricular (A-V) node. The H-V interval identifies the time taken for excitation to travel from the His bundle to the ventricles, the V wave being the analog of the QRS wave in the ECG. Figure 50 illustrates a typical His-bundle electrogram (HBE) made by passing a catheter electrode through the venous system into the right heart; the ECG is shown for comparison and indicates that the His-bundle (H) wave occurs between the P and QRS waves.

There are normal values for the components of the HBE. Roberts (1975) provided the data for normal subjects.

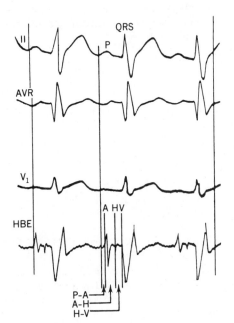

Figure 50 The His-bundle electrogram in relation to body surface electrocardiograms. (Redrawn from Roberts, 1975.)

The autonomic nervous system, pharmacologic agents, congenital abnormalities, and diseases alter the propagation of excitation over the conducting systems of the heart, changing the P-A, A-H, and H-V intervals. Activation of the parasympathetic division of the autonomic nervous system prolongs the A-H interval, while activation of the sympathetic division decreases the A-H and H-V intervals. There are numerous drugs that either prolong or shorten the propagation of excitation across the A-V node. Disease can depress or block conduction in the A-V node and His bundle, and this effect is not only clearly revealed but can also be localized by the HBE.

Sometimes atrial pacing is used to aid in interpreting the HBE. However, when compared to the normal, the A-H interval is increased. The administration of atropine restores the A-H interval to normal. Presumably with atrial pacing, some vagal fibers innervating the A-V node are stimulated.

There are many techniques for recording the HBE; with all a catheter electrode is advanced into the right heart via the venous system. Monopolar, bipolar, and multipolar catheters have been used. However, it is possible to obtain excellent HBEs with the monopolar catheter electrode connected to one terminal of the ECG, with the V terminal constituting the other lead. To obtain a clear HBE, careful adjustment of the catheter electrode is necessary while viewing the recording. Fluoroscopic examination is generally used, and the catheter tip is advanced into the right atrium and across the tricuspid valve into the right ventricle. The catheter is slowly withdrawn across the tricuspid valve until the tip of the electrode is just on the atrial side of the tricuspid valve. At this point the catheter position is adjusted by further withdrawal or advancement or rotation until a satisfactory HBE is obtained. Although the waveform will vary in contour during this procedure, the intervals will vary little. It is important, however, to note that displacement of the catheter electrode by about 1 mm will dramatically reduce the amplitude of the H wave.

VECTORCARDIOGRAPHY

The idea of locating the electrical axis of the ventricles by measuring potential differences appearing between limb electrodes was clearly demonstrated by Waller (1887). Almost a quarter-century later, Einthoven (1913) postulated that in the human thorax the heart was almost in the center of an equilateral triangle in which the apices were the right and left arms (shoulders) and both feet (pubic area). He soon found that only the left foot was necessary and abandoned use of the right foot.

Einthoven knew very well that he was recording only a component of ventricular depolarization in a (frontal) plane parallel to the anterior surface of the body. In addition, on the triangle he plotted only a single line to represent the ventricular (manifest) vector of excitation, reflecting the R wave, although he knew that the R wave reached its peak at different times in the different leads. The notion that a series of instantaneous vectors could be drawn to describe the ventricular depolarization process was due to Williams (1914), who used the Einthoven triangle to plot the synchronous values of the amplitudes during the QRS wave derived from the limb leads.

It remained for Mann (1920) to introduce the concept of the vector loop by plotting the locus of the tips of the instantaneous values of the QRS and T vectors, as recorded by the three limb leads, to obtain loops that he called monocardiograms. Figure 51a illustrates the loop formed by joining the tips of the instantaneous vectors obtained for every 10-msec interval during the QRS wave. Figure 51b gives the derivation of the mean cardiac R wave vector using the net amplitudes for leads I and III. In 1938 Mann built an instrument to record monocardiograms directly. Probably because cathode ray tubes were not readily available, Mann constructed his ingenious galvanometer consisting of a single mirror, which was deflected by three coils mounted with their axes 60 degrees apart, each axis corresponding to one of the leads as represented by the Einthoven triangle. A photographic record of the deflection of a light beam reflected from the mirror produced these early vectorcardiograms, although this name was not to be used until later.

The Braun cathode ray tube was introduced to vectorcardiography by Schellong et al. (1937a, b, c), who used a two-axis tube to obtain vector loops (vector diagrams) in the frontal, horizontal, and sagittal planes. Hollmann and Hollmann (1938) employed a cathode ray tube with three pairs of deflection plates with 60-degree orientation and called the records that they obtained triograms. Sulzer and Duchosal (1938, 1945) used the Braun tube to display what they called planograms derived from electrodes placed to record frontal, sagittal, and horizontal components of the ECG. Studies were carried out by Arrighi (1939) to identify the best electrode placement for the sagittal projection lead. At the same time, Wilson and Johnston (1938) employed a cathode ray tube with their "central terminal" (Fig. 52) to make the Einthoven triangle method practical for clinical vectorcardiography. In this paper Wilson initiated the use of the word vectorcardiogram.

Because the electrocardiograph was in fairly widespread use and provided extremely valuable information on the condition of the heart, the vectorcardiograph was expected to provide more and different data about the functioning of the myocardium. With the availability of the cathode ray tube and high-fidelity voltage amplifiers after 1945, there arose a new interest in multiplane (spatial) vectorcardiography. To record such VCGs, many patterns of electrode location were proposed, most of which could be traced back to the reasoning behind the Einthoven triangle. However, before long it was realized that the basic assumptions in Einthoven's simple equilateral triangle were not entirely valid; for example, the heart is not at the center of an equilateral triangle with apices where the limbs join the trunk, nor is the resistivity of the tissues and fluids surrounding the heart uniform in all directions. Among the first to question the validity of Einthoven's concept were Berger (1929, 1967), Burger and van Milaan (1946, 1947), and Frank (1953b), who constructed a torso model, filled it with copper sulfate, and implanted a dipole generator in it in the position occupied by the heart as determined by X-ray studies on human subjects. Even in this homogeneously conducting model, the potentials of the three limb leads were not those predicted on the basis of Einthoven's triangle.

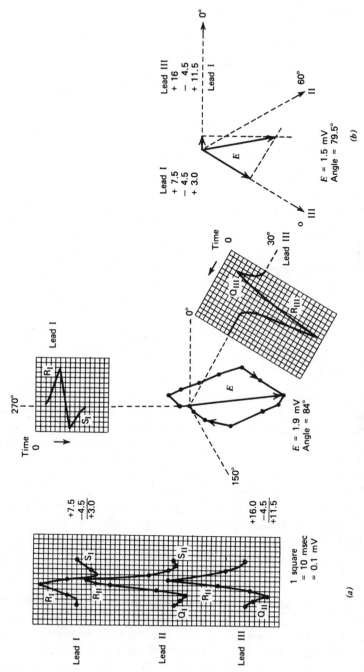

Figure 51 (a) The vector loop for the R wave of the ECG obtained by joining the tips of the instantaneous vectors obtained each 10 msec throughout the QRS wave. (b) The mean QRS vector obtained by using the net amplitude in leads I and III. (Redrawn from L. A. Geddes, *Electrodes and the Measurement of Bioelectric Events*, Wiley, New York, 1972.)

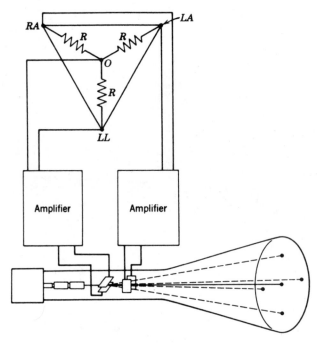

Figure 52   The vectorcardiogram derived from Wilson's central terminal. [From F. N. Wilson and F. D. Johnston, *Am. Heart J.* **16:**14 (1938). By permission.]

These investigators then altered their model by inserting masses of material to simulate the lungs (a bag of moist sand) and spinal column (cork), and showed that the potentials recorded by the limb leads were those represented by a scalene triangle having angles of 96 degrees at the right arm, 56 degrees at the left arm, and 28 degrees at the left leg.

Despite knowledge that the torso is irregular in shape and anisotropic, many body-surface electrode arrangements were developed to obtain voltages from which the ventricular vector loop could be located spatially. The electrode locations were usually chosen on the basis of equal distance from the "center" of the ventricles. The lines joining the electrodes formed the boundaries of a solid figure, which was often used to identify the electrode array. Controversy over the ability of a particular electrode reference frame to locate the "cardiac vectors" has continued to the present time.

Wilson et al. (1947), after studying the potential distribution of an electrically driven dipole placed in a cadaver heart, introduced the equilateral tetrahedral reference frame (Fig. 53). With this system, limb electrodes and the central terminal were used to obtain the frontal plane projection. From a back electrode and the central terminal, the sagittal projection was derived. The relative voltages appearing between the various electrode pairs were in nearly all instances those predicted from the geometry of the torso. With such evidence the tetrahedral system gained considerable support.

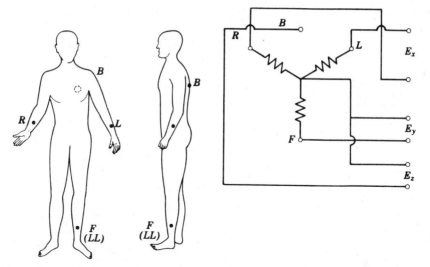

Figure 53   Wilson's tetrahedral reference frame. (Redrawn from G. Burch et al., *Spatial Vectorcardiography*, Lea & Febiger, Philadelphia, PA, 1953.)

Grishman et al. (1951) and Grishman (1952), after obtaining clinical records with the Wilson tetrahedral, the Arrighi (1939) triangle, and the Duchosal (1949, 1952) reference frames, were led to develop a cubic electrode arrangement (Duchosal and Grosgurin, 1952; Duchosal and Sulzer, 1949). With this arrangement the authors claimed that the heart was as equidistant from the electrodes as the thorax allowed and that the electrodes were easily located anatomically.

Although all reference frames provided reasonable VCGs, the QRS and T loops derived from normal subjects exhibited a remarkably wide range of magnitudes and orientations, even when the same vectorcardiographic reference frame was used. In addition, the data obtained with different reference frames were not easily compared. It is not difficult to find possible reasons for this situation. At least two concerted attempts have been made to identify the variables by means of investigations in which electrically driven dipoles were implanted into electrolyte-filled human torso models and the resulting body-surface potential distributions were studied. The investigations by Schmitt and Simonson (1955) and Frank (1956) are fine examples of this technique. From their studies both investigators developed orthogonal lead systems for spatial vectorcardiography. Schmitt's SVEC III system and Frank's VCG lead system are presented in Figs. 54 and 55, respectively. Both systems are used clinically.

In Schmitt's system, 14 active electrodes are employed. The voltage that represents the X component of the cardiac vector is derived from the right- and left-arm electrodes, along with components derived from chest and back electrodes placed at the level of the fifth intercostal space. The Y component is obtained from the head and left-leg electrodes, and the Z component from eight electrodes located on the chest and back at the third and sixth interspace.

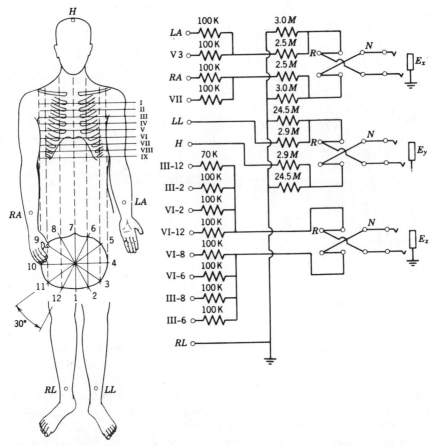

Figure 54   Schmitt's SVEC III orthogonal lead system. [Redrawn from O. H. Schmitt and E. Simonson, *Arch. Intern. Med.* **96**:574–590 (1955), and as reported by H. V. Pipberger and C. R. Wood, *Circ. Res.* **6**:239–224 (1958). The resistor values shown are for an input impedance of 10 MΩ to ground. (By permission of the American Heart Association, Inc.)]

Seven active electrodes are used with Frank's system (Fig. 55). The X component is derived from an array of electrodes that surround the heart approximately at the level of the fifth interspace. The Y component is obtained from the neck and left-leg electrodes, and the Z component from the voltage appearing between an array of three electrodes on the anterior of the chest and one electrode in the back and one on the midaxillary line. To provide more accurate location of the level for the chest and back electrodes, Frank developed a three-electrode exploring tool and presented instructions for its use.

Several comparisons have been made of the data obtained with the various vectorcardiographic reference frames. Frank (1954) presented one of the earliest studies, which examined the validity of the assumptions underlying the Duchosal double cube, the Wilson tetrahedron, and the Grishman cube arrays. Using human

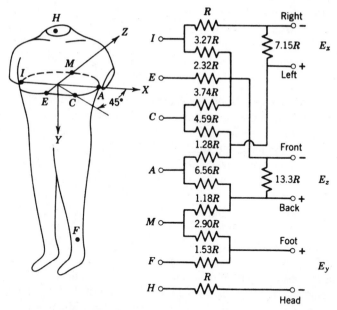

Figure 55 Frank's vectorcardiographic lead system. [From E. Frank, *Circulation* **13:**737–749 (1956). By permission of the American Heart Association.]

torso models filled with an electrolyte and containing a fixed dipole, he measured the potentials at 200 electrode positions and calculated the voltages presented to electrodes placed in the locations specified by the three reference frames. He found that "the scalar lead shapes of the Wilson tetrahedron deviate, on the average, by approximately 15% from the torso dipole variations, but the scalar lead shapes of the systems of Duchosal and Grishman show significantly larger discrepancies." He also found that the standardization factors employed in the Wilson system were too large, particularly with respect to the head-to-foot dipole component (by a factor of 2.3), and added,

"Certain fortuitous features of the Wilson system enable a modification of the standardization factors which leads to results that are fairly satisfactory for a dipole located in the center of the heart. This system which possesses certain other advantages would appear to deserve further study."

The practical value of Wilson's system was also investigated by Abildskov and Pence (1956), who compared data obtained by means of Wilson's tetrahedron with those obtained with the corrected tetrahedron as advocated by McFee and Johnston (1954). In 75 subjects they found that although the data were similar with both methods, the scatter was less with the corrected tetrahedron. Brody (1957) carried out another study on a series of human subjects using the scalene tetrahedron and Wilson's equilateral tetrahedron, discovering that although the scalene tetrahedron was based on sound experimentally determined data, "the mean spatial QRS- and T-vector loci exhibited slightly less scatter and better coefficients of correlation within the uncorrected frame of reference. . . . [The] corrected frame of reference does not appear to possess sufficient merit to warrant its routine application to the analysis of mean QRS- and T-vector orientation."

In another investigation of Wilson's tetrahedral system, Burger et al. (1956) applied their scalene triangle correction and compared data collected on a series of 96 patients with their own reference frame. They found good agreement between the two methods, using the electrode locations advocated by Wilson only when their correction was applied. It is probably because of such studies in which deviations from the "ideal" value turn out to be clinically unimportant that the Wilson method still enjoys support.

The Schmitt, Frank, Helm, and McFee (corrected Einthoven triangle) systems have also been exposed to close scrutiny by Langner et al. (1958). The importance of the differences depends on how critical the reader may be. Langner found that for the Z lead the systems were interchangeable in more than 90% of the cases for the QRS and T loops in regard to shape and orientation. For the X lead, the systems were interchangeable in all cases for the QRS loop and in 90% for the T loop. In another study involving 4 normal and 182 elderly subjects, Simonson et al. (1959) compared the QRS and T loops obtained with eight popular orthogonal-lead systems to find large differences among them. However, they stated, "most types of pathology can be recognized in any of the lead systems." Although their extensive study was carefully executed, they were reluctant to advocate the superiority of one system over another.

Nonogawa (1966) called attention to the important fact that many of the popular electrode reference frames were derived from torso models of Caucasian adults. He wondered whether these frames were applicable to the Oriental torso. Therefore, he constructed Caucasian and Oriental torso models into which he placed electrically excited dipoles and obtained VCG data with the Frank, Schmitt SVEC III, McFee, Polygraph III, and Grishman lead systems. He concluded that in each of the X, Y, and Z axis leads the Schmitt and Frank systems were similar. The other lead systems showed larger differences. However, he also concluded that "these VCG systems, in their original networks, can be applied to the Japanese without appreciable error."

With such variety of reference frames and the lack of clear-cut clinical evidence to indicate the superiority of one reference system over another to identify specific myocardial diseases, it is difficult to set forth criteria that would lead to the adoption of a single method. Information on this interesting field can be found in the monographs by Grant and Estes (1951), Grishman (1952), Goldberger (1953), Burch et al. (1953), Grant (1957), Kowarzykowic and Kowarzykowic (1961), Pozzi (1961), Uhley (1962), Guntheroth (1965), and Lamb (1965). Pozzi's (1961) monograph contains an excellent bibliography of the original papers, which describe the various vectorcardiographic lead systems and potential distributions around the heart of the human subject and in models of the human torso. The bibliography also lists studies in which field mapping was carried out with various dipole models.

The preceding lengthy discussion appears to indicate that the VCG has limited clinical value and will not replace the ECG in routine electrocardiography, particularly since mean cardiac axes can be visually estimated using the six limb and six precordial leads as described in the preceding section. As a teaching device the VCG has much to offer. Its ability to display the rate of depolarization and repolarization is far superior to that of the ECG. Especially well displayed by the VCG are the small, beat-by-beat changes in these quantities. Expanded clinical use of the VCG will depend on the clinical value of the information it produces. So many reference frames are employed, however, that the time when the full usefulness of the VCG is established will probably be delayed.

ELECTROENCEPHALOGRAPHY

The electrical activity of the brain is recorded with three types of electrodes—scalp, cortical, and depth. With scalp electrodes the recording is called an electroencephalogram (EEG). When electrodes are placed on the exposed surface (cortex) of the brain, the recording is called an electrocorticogram (ECoG). Electrodes also may be advanced into the brain, in which case the term depth recording designates the technique. It is interesting that there is surprisingly little damage to the brain with depth recording. Whether obtained from the scalp, cortex, or depths of the brain, the potentials recorded represent the activity of numerous neurons in which fluctuating membrane and action potentials are occurring. These three different techniques are therefore examples of extracellular recording.

The fact that the brain exhibits spontaneous electrical activity was reported by Caton (1875, 1887), who used Thomson's reflecting galvanometer connected to electrodes applied to a variety of animals. His choice of this instrument was fortunate since it had a frequency response (to about 5 Hz) that was adequate for the reproduction of the dominant rhythm of the animals he studied (Geddes, 1987). Caton was not able to make graphic recordings from the animals, although he did provide convincing verbal descriptions of the electrical activity displayed as variations in the position of a luminous spot on a screen. It was about a half-century later when the electrical activity of the human brain was recorded by Berger (1929), who employed a string galvanometer connected to scalp electrodes. Berger's first and succeeding papers were largely unnoticed until Adrian and Matthews (1934) in Great Britain and Jasper and Carmichael (1935) in the United States reviewed them and confirmed Berger's findings, thereby introducing electroencephalography to the English-speaking world. In both investigations, full credit was given to Berger for the discovery. A complete account of the development of electroencephalography was reported under the editorship of Rémond (1971), and an excellent account of Berger's work, including a translation of his papers, was presented by Gloor (1967, 1969).

Electrode Locations

Scalp electrodes are employed in conjunction with both "monopolar" and bipolar recording techniques. Figure 56 illustrates both techniques for connecting a four-channel EEG to a subject. With "monopolar" recording, one side of each

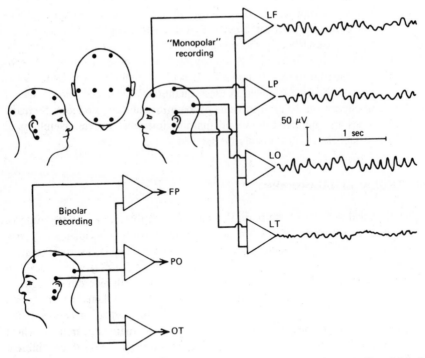

Figure 56 Method of connecting the recording channels for "monopolar" and bipolar recording. With "monopolar" recording, the reference electrode is on the earlobe, chin, or neck.

amplifier is connected to a reference electrode, often located on the earlobe. With bipolar recording, the amplifiers are connected between pairs of scalp electrodes in a regular order. With both types of recording, one-half the number of channels is connected to electrodes on one side of the head; the remaining channels are connected to electrodes on the opposite side of the head. In this way, the electrical activity from homologous areas of the brain can be compared at a glance.

In clinical electroencephalography, 21 electrodes are applied to the head in what is known as the 10-20 system, illustrated in Fig. 57. This array was described by Jasper (1958), who chaired the meeting of the International Federation of EEG Societies, which developed this standard placement.

The 10-20 system employs skull landmarks as reference points to locate the electrodes. In all, 19 scalp and 2 earlobe (auricular, A) electrodes are used to examine the electrical activity of the surface of the brain. To locate the electrodes, the distance from the nasion to inion is first measured along the midline, and five points are marked along this line, as in Fig. 57. The first point locates the frontal pole (F_p), which is 10% of the nasion–inion distance and just above the nasion. No electrode is applied over this reference point, which is used for subsequent measurements. The frontal (F_z), central (C_z), parietal (P_z), and occipital (O_z) mid-

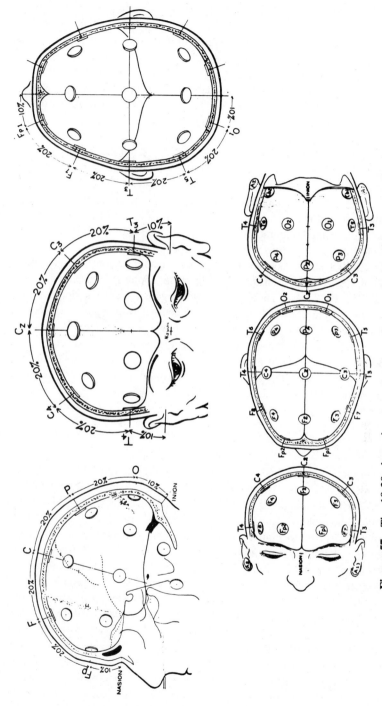

Figure 57 The 10-20 electrode system recommended by the International Federation of EEG Societies. [From H. H. Jasper, *EEG Clin. Neurophysiol.* **10**:371–375 (1958). By permission.]

line electrode points are spaced by 20% of the nasion–inion distance measuring from the frontal pole (F_p), as in Fig. 57. With this technique, the central electrode (C_z) is midway between nasion and inion. A similar method of measurement is used to place two rows of electrodes on the right and left sides of the head. The coronal points are then marked by measuring the distance (through the central point C_z) between the depression just in front of each ear. The depression is easily located anterior to the tragus and is at the root of the zygoma, and 10% of this distance measured up from the depression locates the temporal (T_4, T_3) electrodes on each side of the head. The central electrode positions (C_4, C_3) are marked at 20% of the distance above the temporal points, as in Fig. 57. Then the lowest (temporal) horizontal row of electrode positions is determined by measuring from the frontal pole (F_p) to the inion (see Fig. 57); this procedure locates F_{p2}, F_8, T_4, T_6, and O_2 on the right and F_{p1}, F_7, T_3, and O_1 on the left. The remaining electrodes (F_4, C_4, and P_4 on the right and F_3, C_3, and P_3 on the left) are placed along lines equidistant between the midline and temporal lines and along frontal and parietal coronal lines, respectively, as in Fig. 57. Auricular (A) electrodes are placed on the earlobes.

With the 10-20 system, the even-numbered electrodes are on the right and the odd-numbered electrodes are on the left. Electrodes along the midline are designated by a Z (i.e., F_z, C_z, P_z). There are intentional gaps in the subscript numbering system to allow for the use of other electrode locations, which can be added with the same reference system.

Graphic recording pens are used to display the electrical activity detected by the scalp electrodes. A chart speed of 3 cm/sec and a recording sensitivity of about 7 μV/mm are employed. Step-gain controls and filters are also used; details on the bandwidth for faithful reproduction of the human EEG are presented elsewhere in this chapter.

The Normal EEG

With scalp electrodes applied to the normal relaxed adult human subject, there can be recorded a constantly fluctuating electrical activity having a dominant frequency of about 10 Hz and an amplitude in the range of 20–200 μV. This activity, which is called the alpha rhythm, ranges in frequency from about 8 to 13 Hz and is most prominent in the occipital and parietal areas; it may occupy as much as half the record. The alpha rhythm increases in frequency with age from birth and attains its adult form by about 15–20 years of age. The alpha rhythm is most prominent when the eyes are closed and in the absence of concentration. The frequency of the alpha rhythm is also species-dependent; Fig. 58 illustrates typical alpha rhythm patterns of guinea pig, cat, monkey, and human. Opening the eyes, engaging in patterned vision, or performing such cerebral activity as mental arithmetic diminishes or abolishes the alpha rhythm. Figure 59 presents an outstanding example of this phenomenon in the cat and human.

Although the alpha rhythm is the most prominent electrical activity, other frequencies are present in the normal human subject. For example, there is a considerable amount of low-voltage, higher-frequency (beta) activity present ranging in

GUINEA PIG:

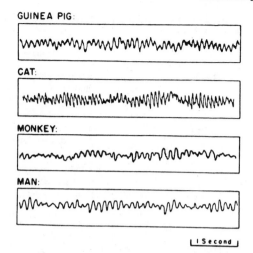

CAT:

MONKEY:

MAN:

|_| Second_|

Figure 58 Typical alpha rhythm patterns of different subjects. (From M. A. B. Brazier, *Electrical Activity of the Nervous System.* Pitman, London, 1951. By permission.)

frequency from 18 to 30 Hz. It is most frequently found in the frontal part of the brain. However, the normal electroencephalogram contains waves of various frequencies (in the range of 1–60 Hz) and amplitudes, depending on the cerebral state. To improve communication between electroencephalographers, a terminology has been developed to describe waveforms and their frequencies; Table 3 presents a glossary of these terms.

The cerebral state profoundly affects the electroencephalogram in the normal subject. Figure 60 illustrates the typical changes that occur with sleep, which is perhaps the best example. As the subject goes to sleep, the higher-frequency activity that is associated with alertness or excitement, and the alpha rhythm that dominates the waking record in the relaxed state, are replaced by a characteristic cyclic sequence of changes that constitute the focus of a new specialty devoted to sleep physiology, in which the EEG is used to identify different stages of sleep.

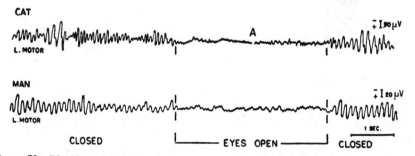

CAT

L. MOTOR

A

$\div I$ 90 μV

MAN

L. MOTOR

$\div I$ 20 μV

1 SEC.

CLOSED |_____ EYES OPEN _____| CLOSED

Figure 59 Blocking of the alpha rhythm in the cat and human by opening the eyes. (From M. A. B. Brazier, *Electrical Activity of the Nervous System.* Pitman, London, 1951. By permission.)

TABLE 3   EEG Waveform Terminology

Waveform	Frequency (Hz)	Remarks
Alpha rhythm	8–13	Parietal-occipital; associated with the awake and relaxed subject; prominent with eyes closed
Beta rhythm	18–30	More evident in frontal-parietal leads; seen best when alpha is blocked
Delta	1–3.5	Associated with normal sleep and present in children less than 1 year old; also seen in organic brain disease
Theta	4–7	Parietal-temporal; prominent in children 2–5 years old
Sleep spindle (sigma)	12–14	Waxing and waning of a sinusoidal wave having the envelope that resembles a spindle; seen during sleep
Lambda	Transient	Visually evoked, low-amplitude, occipital wave, resulting from recognition of a new retinal image
Spike and wave	~3	Sharp wave (spike) followed by rounded wave associated with petit mal epilepsy
V or vertex wave	Transient	Spike about 150–250 msec in duration recorded over the vertex
K-complex	Transient	Vertex wave sometimes followed by a spindle; often seen in sleep and in response to auditory stimulus
Mu (arcade)	8–12	Central dominant, resembling a half-sinusoid (i.e., an arch with the apex downward when recorded with scalp to reference electrode)

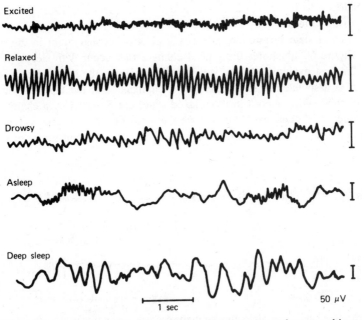

Excited

Relaxed

Drowsy

Asleep

Deep sleep

1 sec

50 μV

Figure 60   The electroencephalographic changes that occur as a human subject goes to sleep. The calibration marks on the right represent 50 μV. [From H. H. Jasper, in *Epilepsy and Cerebral Localization*. W. G. Penfield and T. C. Erickson (eds.). Thomas, Springfield, IL, 1941. By permission.]

An interesting spectrum of cyclic physiological changes occurs during a prolonged period of sleep. In fact, deviation from these normal changes often indicates the presence of brain pathology. There are sleep laboratories where the EEG and several other physiological events are recorded continuously throughout the sleep period. Excellent accounts of the physiological changes that accompany sleep and the criteria for identifying the depth of sleep have been presented by Rechtschaffen and Kales (1968) and Williams et al. (1974).

Sleep Depth

The physiological variables recorded to describe the depth of sleep are the EEG, eye movements (EOG), ECG, and the EMG; respiration is sometimes recorded also. Three monopolar channels of EEG contribute important information regarding the cerebral state. Electrodes are connected to O_2-A_1 to monitor the alpha activity, C_4 (or P_4)-A_1 to detect sleep spindles, V waves, and K complexes; F_4-A_1 is used to monitor slow-wave activity. Note that the three scalp electrodes (even-numbered subscripts) on the right-hand side of the head are paired with one on the contralateral earlobe (A_1). During light sleep, there are slow, disconjugate eye movements; to obtain these, the electrooculogram (EOG) is recorded using two monopolar channels connected to a reference electrode on an earlobe or mastoid process. One of the active electrodes is located 1 cm above and medial to the outer canthus of one eye; the second is 1 cm below and medial to the outer canthus of the other eye. Eye movements that are conjugate appear out of phase; therefore, use of this technique permits easy identification of artifacts in the recording. Other electrode arrays are used in sleep EEG studies, and complete standardization has not been achieved.

The assessment of the degree of muscle relaxation is determined by recording the electrical activity (EMG) of neck muscles. Electrodes are applied to each side of the neck just below the chin. This type of graphic recording, of course, does not faithfully reproduce muscle action potentials. However, the only information desired is assessment of the degree of muscular relaxation.

The electrocardiogram (ECG) is used to determine heart rate by counting the R waves. The electrodes that are applied to the arms serve to detect the ECG and EMG if the arm muscles contract, thereby providing another indicator of muscle activity.

Respiration is sometimes recorded with a thoracic strain gauge or with transthoracic electrodes and an impedance pneumograph. If the latter apparatus is used, the ECG can be obtained from the same pair of transthoracic electrodes (Geddes et al., 1962).

Several scoring systems are applied to the sleep recordings to identify the depth of sleep. Rechtschaffen and Kales (1968) and Williams et al. (1974) have presented detailed accounts of them. The method described by Williams et al. is as follows.

Stage 0. The awake (W) state before the onset of sleep. At least 30 sec of 8–12 Hz occipital activity with a minimum amplitude of 40 μV peak to peak.

Stage 1. Less than 30 sec of 8–12 Hz, 40-μV peak-to-peak occipital activity, and no more than one well-defined spindle or K complex; if an individual does not display clear 8–12 Hz activity, muscle-artifact and eye movement tracings are used.

Stage 2. At least two well-defined spindles, or at least two K complexes, or one of each; no more than 12 sec of 1–3 Hz, 40-μV peak-to-peak, or greater, slow waves.

Stage 3. At least 13 sec of 1–3 Hz, 40-μV peak-to-peak activity, but less than 30 sec of this activity.

Stage 4. At least 30 dominant sec of 1–3 Hz, 40-μV peak-to-peak activity.

As the subject goes from the wakeful (stage 0 or W) relaxed state, in which alpha rhythm dominates the EEG recording, gradual changes occur. With drowsiness (stage 1), alpha activity diminishes and theta (4–8 Hz) activity appears, along with some faster activity. Usually slow eye movements can be recorded. With light sleep (stage 2), the theta activity increases and sleep spindles, V waves, and K complexes appear. Sleep spindles are bursts of waxing and waning 12–14 Hz activity; the V (or vertex) wave is an electronegative sharp wave occurring generally at the vertex and lasting about 150 msec; the K complex is a vertex wave, sometimes followed by a spindle in response to an auditory stimulus. In moderately deep sleep (stage 3), V waves and delta waves (less than 4 Hz) dominate the record. In deep sleep (stage 4) the record is dominated by low-frequency delta waves with a frequency of less than 4 Hz. Throughout the night, periods of rapid-eye-movement (REM) sleep occur, accompanied by body movements. Dreaming has been shown to be associated with REM sleep.

Based on the scoring method just described, the depth of sleep for typical normal adults has been plotted throughout the night. Figure 61 presents an example of how the depth of sleep varies cyclically during a night's sleep. Note that the time spent in deep sleep diminishes after about 2.5 hr, and just before awakening there are many oscillations in the depth of sleep.

Hyperventilation

Rapid, deep breathing, at a rate of about 30/min for about 3 min (hyperventilation), dramatically alters the EEG in normal subjects (Fig. 62). This act reduces

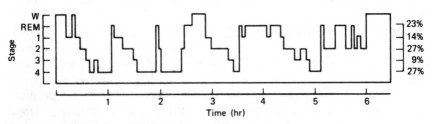

Figure 61 Depth of sleep, expressed in stages, versus duration of sleep, expressed in hours. Depth of sleep varies cyclically throughout the night, becoming very light (REM, or rapid-eye-movement stage) at times. Note that the time spent in the deepest stage of sleep (4) decreases after the first few hours. (Redrawn from L. G. Kiloh et al., *Clinical Electroencephalography*, 3rd ed. Butterworth, London, 1972. By permission.)

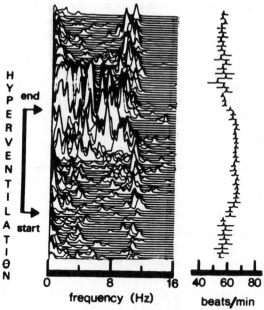

H
Y
P
E
R
V
E
N
T
I
L
A
T
I
Θ
N

end

start

0   8   16   40 60 80
frequency (Hz)   beats/min

Figure 62 Combined compressed spectral array (CSA) of the electroencephalogram and the heart rate (ECG rate) of a subject hyperventilating for 173 sec. The horizontal bars on the ECG rate record indicate the highest and lowest rates during the 4-sec periods of analysis. The heart rate increased just after hyperventilation, and the EEG spectrum did not alter until halfway through the period of hyperventilation. Note that the interbeat variation in heart rate is reduced during the accelerated EEG phase and is markedly increased after the period of hyperventilation. (Record kindly provided by Dr. R. G. Bickford, University of California, San Diego, 1974.)

the venous plasma carbon dioxide (Morrice, 1956). The EEGs of children are especially responsive to hyperventilation. A typical response consists of large-amplitude, bilaterally synchronous, frontally prominent, slow theta activity; the frequency usually decreases with increasing hyperventilation. The lack of bilateral symmetry is an indication of abnormality. Controlled hyperventilation is used as a diagnostic technique to activate irritable and destructive foci, as well as generalized convulsive disorders, including petit mal epilepsy.

Anesthesia

Anesthesia profoundly alters the electroencephalogram in a manner that is dependent on the type and amount of anesthetic employed and the species. The characteristic responses to a variety of anesthetic agents have been reported by Faulconer and Bickford (1960), Brechner et al. (1962), and Sadove et al. (1967). However, despite the differences among the various anesthetic agents, some important similarities accompany anesthesia. The first change that occurs is replacement of the alpha rhythm with low-voltage, high-frequency activity, which accompanies the analgesia and delirium stages. Thus the EEG resembles that of an alert or excited subject, although the subject is not appropriately responsive to stimuli; usually the responsiveness is excessive and/or inappropriate. From this point on, the type of EEG obtained with deepening anesthesia depends on the type of anesthetic and the species. However, when a deeper level of anesthesia is reached, the EEG waveform becomes less dependent on the species and the type of anesthetic. Large-amplitude slow waves begin to dominate the record, and with deepening anesthesia their frequency is reduced and they begin to occur intermittently. With very (dangerously) deep anesthesia, the record is flat (i.e., isoelectric). Complicating interpretation of the EEG in anesthesia are the effects of hypoxia, hypercapnia, and hypoglycemia, all of which mimic deep anesthesia.

Even though in the surgical stages of anesthesia the EEG spectrum is closely dependent on the type of anesthetic and species, it is relatively easy to learn to use the EEG as an approximate indicator of depth of anesthesia by correlating the waveforms with the clinical signs that indicate depth. As an example of the correlation of EEG pattern with anesthesia depth, Bickford (1950) described a servosystem in which the EEG controlled the depth of anesthesia. The technique employed an integrator that summated the EEG activity from one channel; when a critical level of volt-seconds was reached, a thyratron fired, discharging the integrating capacitor and injecting an incremental dose of anesthesia into the vein of an animal that had been anesthetized previously.

The Compressed Spectral Array

Since the physiological state of a subject is reflected in the EEG, attempts have been made to provide bandpass filters and frequency analyzers to display those frequencies in the EEG that correlate best with the status of the subject. A useful display method was described by Bickford et al. (1972), who developed an on-line method of performing an analysis of the EEG frequency components in the 1–16-Hz band. One complete analysis was performed every 4 sec. A small digital computer was used to process the data and generate the display, which is called a "compressed spectral array" (CSA).

The CSA display technique employs an X-Y plotter whose X axis represents the frequency range; the Y axis, for one spectral analysis, represents energy. Immediately after the first 4-sec analysis period, the second begins and the X-Y plotter is advanced by about 1 mm along the Y axis; then it writes out the second 4-sec scan. The process is repeated as long as it is desired to analyze an EEG channel. Thus the X axis of a compressed spectral array represents the frequency range extending from 1 to 16 Hz, and the Y axis indicates the energy of the various components present during one 4-sec scan. Each scan line on the Y axis also represents data analyzed 4 sec later. Hidden-line suppression is used to provide more clarity in the display. A typical compressed spectral array of a subject being monitored during hyperventilation appears in Fig. 62.

Clinical Value of the EEG

The electroencephalogram sees its most valuable service in clinical medicine as a screening test for intracranial pathology. Parenthetically, the clinical correlation of EEG waveforms is much ahead of the rigorous physiological explanation of these phenomena. Thus the utility of electroencephalography rests principally on recognition of patterns of frequency, voltage, and waveform (Gibbs and Gibbs, 1950, 1964; Cohn, 1949; Hill and Parr, 1950, 1963; Hughes, 1961; Kiegler, 1964; Kiloh et al., 1972; Stewart, 1961; Straus, 1952).

The EEG has its greatest value as an aid in the diagnosis and differentiation of the many types of epilepsy, a condition in which groups of neurons in the brain become hyperirritable and, depending on their location, produce sensory, motor, and/or autonomic manifestations. The epilepsies associated with cortical lesions are often detected by the scalp EEG. The EEG in epileptics is usually abnormal between and during attacks. The EEG often provides information on the localization of the area (or areas) of abnormal neuronal activity. In epilepsy the characteristic finding is of spikes (i.e., short-duration waves), alone or in association with other waves. For example, in petit mal epilepsy, in which there is a transient alteration of consciousness (often not easily detected), the EEG shows a characteristic 3-per-second spike-and-wave activity.

Space-occupying lesions, such as tumors, subdural hematomas, and abscesses, give evidence of their presence by slow (delta) waves and depression of normal rhythms in the EEG, which allows localization and an estimate of the extent of the lesion. Such lesions are ideally localized with the bipolar recording technique. If one of the electrodes common to two channels is over the slow-wave focus, there is a phase reversal in the recordings of these two channels.

Injury to the brain accompanies the application of high accelerative and decelerative forces; loss of consciousness and amnesia usually result. The type of posttrauma EEG relates to the extent of neuronal and/or vascular damage. In general, however, a depression in cortical activity and low-frequency activity accompanies such injury. Serial EEGs, taken over a prolonged period, provide useful prognostic information.

It is not the purpose of this section to discuss all the physiologic, pharmacologic, and clinical aspects of electroencephalography. Rather, an attempt has been made to show how recordings of the electrical activity of the brain obtained from scalp electrodes can provide useful clinical information. It is important to be aware that results of the EEG examination are always considered in the context of other clinical findings.

Electroencephalography enjoys a small, but secure, place in clinical medicine, and the interpretation of the EEG for its content of diagnostic information is the province of the well-trained and experienced electroencephalographer, who is aware that an abnormal EEG can be obtained from a normal subject; therefore, he exercises careful clinical judgment when interpreting the EEG.

Sensory Evoked Potentials

An effective stimulus delivered to a sense organ will result in a response detectable on the brain cortex. Although all peripheral sense organs send their information to the cortex, it is easiest to detect the response to auditory, somatosensory, and visual stimuli by locating the electrodes over the appropriate cortical areas; Figs. 63a and b illustrate the areas for the somatosensory system. In reality, the

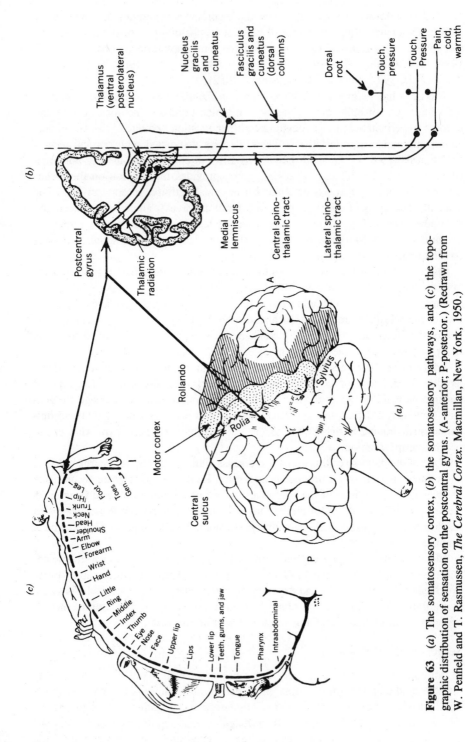

Figure 63 (a) The somatosensory cortex, (b) the somatosensory pathways, and (c) the topographic distribution of sensation on the postcentral gyrus. (A-anterior; P-posterior.) (Redrawn from W. Penfield and T. Rasmussen, *The Cerebral Cortex.* Macmillan, New York, 1950.)

sensory evoked potential reports on the integrity of the sense organ and its neural pathway to the cerebral cortex (Fig. 63c). It should be obvious that the separate parts of the pathway can be studied by applying electrical stimuli to the peripheral nerves and spinal cord.

Figure 63a is a lateral view of the brain showing the two most prominent fissures, the Rollandic and the Sylvian. Anterior to the fissure of Rollando (central sulcus), is the precentral gyrus (bulge), which contains the primary motor areas; behind it is the postcentral gyrus, which is the primary somatosensory area. Sensation from the entire body surface is arrayed along this sensory strip in an interesting manner. Penfield and Rasmussen (1950) determined the topographic distribution of sensation along the postcentral gyrus in humans and represented it as an homunculus (little man). Figure 63c illustrates this representation of sensation (in cross section) along the Rollandic fissure. The body parts of the homunculus are drawn to represent the size of the corresponding cortical sensory areas.

Optimum detection of somatosensory evoked responses requires that electrodes be placed over the appropriate contralateral cortical area. For example, the evoked potential due to stimulation of the right leg is detected with electrodes over the left vertex. Likewise, those from right facial stimulation appear on the left lateral surface of the brain toward the temporal lobe. The response to visual stimuli appears on the posterior (occipital pole) of the cortex. Auditory evoked responses are detected over the superior temporal lobe. Much sensation is bilaterally represented.

Detection of Evoked Cortical Potentials. Recording from electrodes on the cortex over the appropriate area does not provide a clear evoked cortical response because of the background EEG. When the electrodes are placed on the scalp, it is even more difficult to identify the evoked response. For this reason, a special technique called signal averaging is used that assumes that the evoked response is time locked to the stimulus and that the background EEG is a random signal.

Dawson (1951, 1954) introduced signal averaging to reveal evoked cortical responses. In his first study the averaging was performed manually; in the second, an automatic electromechanical averager was used. Dawson recorded the EEG continuously from the scalp while 20 shocks were delivered, 1 sec apart, to the ulnar nerve in the left arm. Figure 64a illustrates the recordings. The records were aligned one below the other, using the stimulus marker (dot). At each 3 msec, the amplitudes were added algebraically (using an arbitrary zero baseline). The summed amplitudes were plotted and are shown in Fig. 64b. Note that because the ongoing EEG approximated random noise, the evoked potential emerged clearly. Note that in the individual records of Fig. 64a the evoked potential can be identified, but its waveform is inconstant due to the superimposed background EEG.

With the easy access to analog-to-digital (A-D) converters and digital computers, signal averaging is now easily performed. The first step in the procedure involves bandpass filtering the EEG so that only the necessary frequency range is sampled. Typically, the bandpass chosen is 0.25–25 Hz. Then the filtered EEG signal is converted to digital form. The sampling rate is dictated by the bandpass selected. Typically, a sampling rate in excess of 100/sec is used. The amplitude resolution

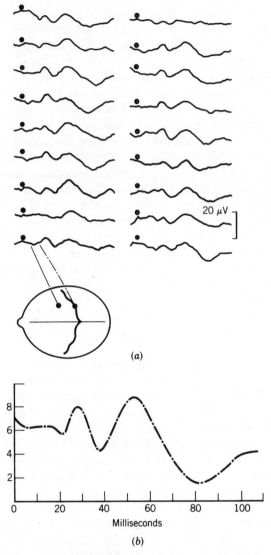

(a)

(b)

Figure 64   (a) Twenty records of EEG showing the stimulus (dot) and the evoked response in the background. (b) The evoked response after signal averaging. [Redrawn from G. D. Dawson, *EEG Clin. Neurophysiol.* **6:**65–84 (1954).]

depends on the number of bits selected. An 8-bit conversion provides an amplitude resolution of $2^8 - 1$, 1 part in 255, or 0.39%.

The averaged evoked potential is processed by aligning the time samples after the stimulus and summing the amplitudes algebraically. The evoked potential emerges from the background in proportion to the number of stimulus-response recordings analyzed. It can be shown that if the evoked response is the signal (S) and the ongoing EEG is the noise (N), then the signal-to-noise (S/N) ratio becomes $\sqrt{n}$ (S/N), where n is the number of stimulus–response sequences analyzed. Typically $n = 100$ or more.

Auditory Evoked Potentials. The response to an auditory stimulus can be recorded from a variety of scalp sites. The acoustic stimulus entering the ear is carried to the brain via the auditory division of the eighth cranial nerve, which enters the spinal cord and synapses in the cochlear nuclei. From here, some fibers ascend uncrossed; others cross and ascend to the quadrigeminal body and medial geniculate in the midbrain. From the medial geniculate, fibers ascend to the auditory cortex, which is located on the superior temporal lobe. Figure 65 illustrates the pathways that participate in carrying the acoustic information to the cortex.

The auditory evoked response to a click is often recorded with one electrode on the vertex and the other over the mastoid process. The response is polyphasic, and a standard nomenclature has been adopted. Figure 66 illustrates typical averaged evoked responses at various times after the stimulus. According to Picton (1974), positive waves I–VII occur in the first 10 msec after a click (Figure 66). The first

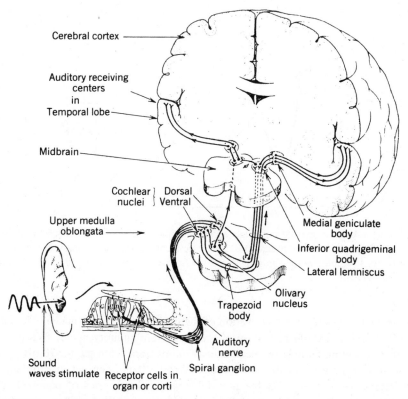

Figure 65 Neural pathway from the inner ear (where the auditory receptors are located) to the auditory cortex (superior temporal lobe).

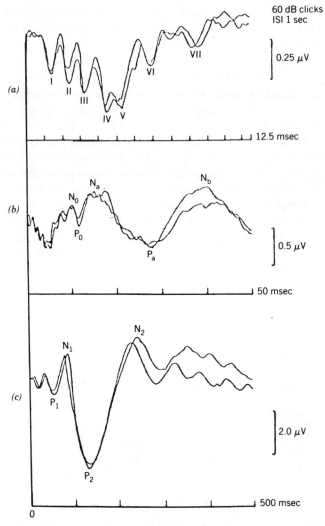

Figure 66 Auditory evoked potentials at various times after the stimulus (60-dB clicks);
(a) 0–12.5 msec, (b) 0–50 msec; (c) 0–500 msec recorded from C_z to mastoid process. A
total of 1024 samples were averaged. [Redrawn from T. W. Picton, *Am. J. EEG Technol.*
14:9–44 (1974).]

and second waves represent activation of the cochlear nerve and nuclei. The later
waves probably identify activation of the brain-stem auditory nuclei. Wave V is
the most easily discernible; its peak latency varies from 5.5 msec for 70-dB clicks
to about 9 msec for near-threshold clicks. Wave VII is often not discernible. In
the interval between 10 and 50 msec after the click, a series of potentials are
recordable over widespread areas of the scalp; these potentials are very difficult to
distinguish from simultaneously occurring reflex scalp muscle potentials. They may
represent thalamic and early cortical potentials. The larger, longer-lasting potentials

(Fig. 66c) elicited by the auditory stimulus are the P1 (50 msec), N1 (100 msec), P2 (170 msec), and N2 (250 msec) components of the vertex potential. This vertex potential is widely distributed over the fronto-central scalp regions and is usually maximally recorded at C_z or F_z (Fig. 67). This vertex potential is altered somewhat by attention to the stimulus, which increases the N1-P2 components, and by sleep, which markedly increases the N2 component. This large N2 component of sleep is homologous to the vertex sharp wave seen during normal sleep electroencephalography.

It was stated earlier that many sensory systems are bilaterally represented. Therefore, it is not surprising that auditory evoked potentials can be recorded from a variety of sites using scalp electrodes. Figure 67 illustrates the widespread distribution of auditory evoked potentials.

Somatosensory Evoked Potentials. Cortical responses can be recorded with scalp electrodes in response to stimuli presented to the surface of the body. Often

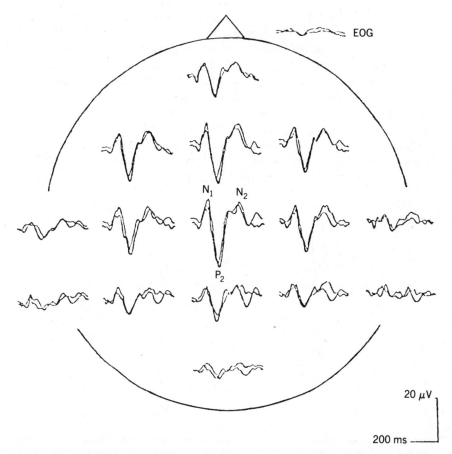

Figure 67 Distribution of auditory evoked response resulting from a 70-dB, 1-kHz tone. Recordings made with monopolar electrodes; 60 samples averaged. [Redrawn from T. W. Picton, *Am. J. EEG Technol.* **14**:9–44 (1974).]

a tactile stimulator is used to deform the skin suddenly; however, it is often more convenient to stimulate sensory nerve trunks electrically with skin-surface electrodes. Figure 68 illustrates the locations for electrodes used to stimulate the median and popliteal nerves. It is important to use a stimulator with an isolated output circuit and to place the subject ground toward the central nervous system and beyond the stimulating electrodes. A constant-current stimulator is preferred.

Figures 68 and 69 illustrate the neural pathway from skin receptors (touch and pressure) to the cortex. The nerve fibers from these receptors enter the dorsal (posterior) spinal cord, cross, and ascend to the thalamus. Some fibers ascend and synapse in the cuneate and gracile nuclei, and then cross and ascend to the thalamus. From the thalamus, fibers ascend to the somatosensory cortex in the postcentral gyrus, the sensory strip (Fig. 63c). Other fibers synapse at the segmental level, cross, and ascend to the thalamus, where they synapse with neurons that send their axons to the sensory cortex (postcentral gyrus).

An easily detected averaged evoked cortical potential can be recorded from scalp electrodes when stimuli are delivered to electrodes on the wrist over the median nerve; Fig. 70 is a typical example. According to Picton (1974), component 0 is an early positive wave peaking at about 15 msec that is widely recorded and probably represents some deep subcortical structure such as the ventrobasal thalamus. Components 1 and 2 at 19 and 26 msec are maximally recorded near the primary somatosensory area and are of opposite polarity on either side of the central sulcus. If the peroneal nerve is stimulated, a similar series of waves are seen; however, they are later and more medially located (over the primary somatosensory cortex for the leg); P1 is at 34 msec, N1 is at 44 msec, and P2 is at 56 msec (Fig. 70). Components 4, 5, and 6 of the median nerve response are of unknown origin; activation of secondary somatosensory areas may generate such potentials. Components 7 and 8 are similar in morphology and distribution to the N1 and P2

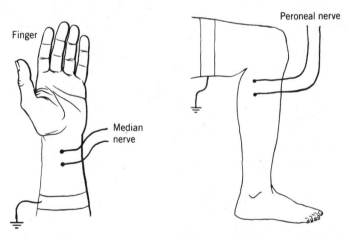

Figure 68 Typical electrode locations for stimulating sensory nerves. An isolated stimulus should be used, and the subject ground should be between the electrode site and the central nervous system. [Redrawn from T. W. Picton, *Am. J. EEG Technol.* **14:**9–44 (1974).]

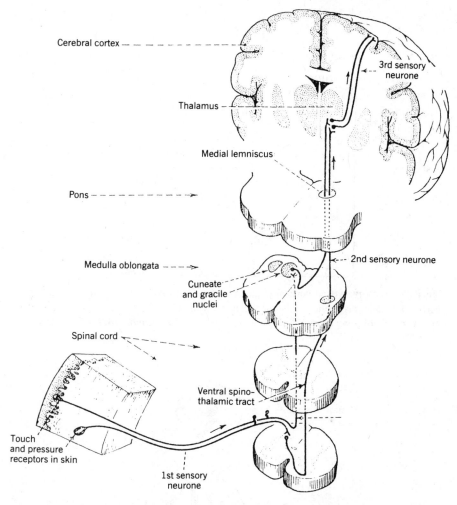

Figure 69   Neural pathways to the cortex for skin (touch and pressure) receptors.

components of the auditory vertex response. Records taken over the spine and lower cranium reveal definite early somatosensory responses; these potentials are probably generated in the posterior columns of the spinal cord and in the medullary relay nuclei, although it is difficult to rule out simultaneous muscle reflex action potentials.

Visual Evoked Potentials. The response to a flash of light or a patterned image can be detected with scalp electrodes placed on the occiput. Visual evoked responses can be recorded from other scalp regions; however, the waveforms differ.

The neural pathway from the retina to the visual cortex is shown in Fig. 71. The retinal receptors send information via the optic nerves, which converge at the

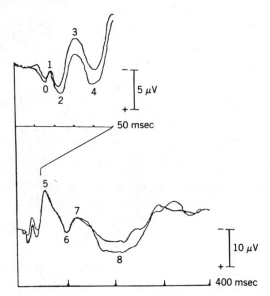

Figure 70 Sensory evoked cortical potentials from C3 to A12, at different times after an electrical stimulus was applied to the median nerve with skin-surface electrodes; 250 samples were averaged. [Redrawn from T. W. Picton, *Am. J. EEG Technol.* **14**:9–44 (1974).]

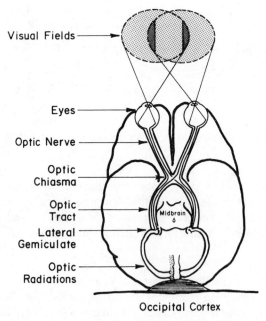

Figure 71 Neural pathway from the retina to the visual (occipital) cortex.

chiasma at the base of the brain. The nerve fibers from the nasal portions of the retinas cross at the chiasma; those from the temporal sides of the retina do not cross. Beyond the chiasma, the fibers become the optic tract, synapse at the geniculate body, and travel to the occipital (calcarine) cortex. On the calcarine cortex is a topographic representation of the retina. Fibers that enter the midbrain synapse and send fibers to other regions of the brain. Therefore, visual evoked responses can be recorded from areas other than the occipital cortex.

Figure 72 is an averaged visual evoked response from the occipital cortex. Designation of the components of the different waveforms is in good agreement. According to Picton (1974), the early positivity (waves I and III) perhaps represents activity in the geniculate or geniculocalcarine tract. The superimposed negative wave II, "the early negative wave," appears to represent early activation of the primary visual cortex. However, there is considerable interindividual variability in the later components of the occipital response, possibly due to individual differences in the structure and orientation of the brain's occipital pole. Components in the latency range of 60–200 msec are quite sensitive to the pattern of visual stimulus. When the evoked response is detected at the vertex (Fig. 73), it resembles the auditory evoked response, so similar nomenclature is used.

Clinical Use of Sensory Evoked Potentials. The ease of acquiring averaged evoked cortical potentials is leading to an increase in clinical applications. Because the evoked potential measures the integrity of the afferent neural circuit, it logically complements the EEG. Perhaps the most popularly used is the evoked auditory response as an aid to evaluating hearing in children too young to be evaluated by conventional hearing tests. The acoustic stimulus consists of tone bursts of different frequencies. By varying the intensity at each frequency, the frequency response of the auditory system can be determined.

Somatosensory evoked potentials are used clinically to evaluate the integrity of

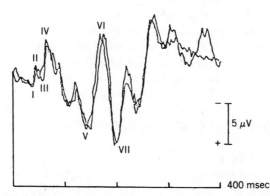

Figure 72   Visual evoked cortical response recorded from O_1 to A_1, using diffuse flashes of light 1–2 sec in duration. Recordings represent 128 responses. [Redrawn from T. W. Picton, *Am. J. EEG Technol.* **14:**9–44 (1974).]

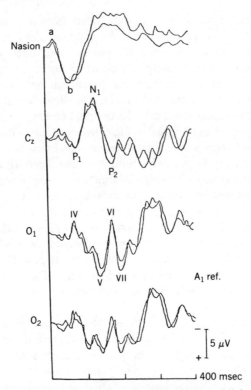

Figure 73   Visual evoked responses due to 128 diffuse flashes of light and recorded from nasion, C_z, O_1, and O_2 sites. [Redrawn from T. W. Picton, *Am. J. EEG Technol.* **14:**9–44 (1974).]

the neural pathway from the periphery to the cortex during spinal surgery. The test is also useful in assessing patients who cannot cooperate and in some neurological diseases, such as multiple sclerosis and peripheral neuropathy.

Visual evoked responses are often recorded in association with electroretinography (ERG), which employs corneal electrodes. The presence of a normal ERG with no vision indicates dysfunction of the visual neural pathway. Each eye and each half of the visual field can be tested separately. The presence of a cortically evoked potential with a very small or undetectable ERG denotes partial retinal damage (e.g., retinitis pigmentosa). The absence of both indicates severe retinal damage.

Visual acuity can be assessed by using a focused and defocused checkerboard stimulus and by using small and large squares on the checkerboard. Such a pattern is usually presented on a television monitor. Various components of the evoked potential are affected by these manipulations. Likewise, glasses can be evaluated using this technique, which is in the early research stage.

Brain maturation can be studied with averaged evoked cortical potentials. As an infant grows, more synaptic connections develop, axons become myelinated, and response times shorten. Studies on the natural history of the evoked cortical potential are ongoing, and this area promises to assume more importance in neonatology.

Evoked cortical potentials are influenced by metabolic status and anesthetic agents. Hypoxia depresses evoked potentials. Sances et al. (1983) showed that some barbiturate anesthetics depress the evoked potential and that halothane abolishes it for some time after it has been withdrawn. It would appear that the study of averaged evoked potentials during anesthesia may lead to another estimator of depth of anesthesia.

In conclusion, the two assumptions underlying the processing of averaged evoked potentials should be recalled: (1) The evoked response is time locked to the stimulus and (2) the background EEG can be equated to a random signal. As would be expected, neither is strictly true, despite the fact that signal averaging raises the response well above the background. The response is not strictly time locked to the stimulus; this time is slightly variable. The background EEG is not always random. Much research is under way to evaluate the limits of the two assumptions.

Motor Evoked Potentials

Whereas the sensory evoked potential (SEP) provides information on the integrity of the neural pathway from the periphery to the cortex, the motor evoked potential (MEP) provides information about the integrity of the neural circuit from the motor cortex to the periphery. These two circuits occupy different places in the spinal cord. Moreover, the blood supply to these two regions is slightly different. The MEP and SEP techniques are beginning to be used clinically during surgical procedures that may apply pressure or strain to the spinal cord or alter its circulation. Figure 74 is a schematic representation of the motor pathways from the cortex to the periphery. The cortical motor area lies in the precentral gyrus of the frontal lobe and has a topographic representation like that of the sensory cortex (see Fig. 63). The representation is contralateral and inverted, with the foot area at the vertex and the face represented on the lower lateral cortex. The large pyramidal motor fibers descend, and about 80% cross (decussate) in the medullary region and descend in the lateral corticospinal tracts and then synapse with an interneuron or a lower motor neuron in the anterior horn of the spinal cord. The remaining fibers descend in the anterior corticospinal tract, crossing and synapsing with an interneuron or a lower motor neuron. It is activation of an anterior horn cell (motor neuron) that causes the innervated muscle to contract.

Adjacent to the motor strip is the suppressor strip (4S); there are other cortical areas (Brodmann's 2, 5, 19, and 24) that, when stimulated, produce inhibition of neurons in the spinal cord. Thus it should be recognized that cortical stimulation can produce both excitation and inhibition.

It has been known since 1870 that electrical stimulation of the motor cortex gives rise to muscle contraction on the opposite side of the body. This great benchmark observation in neurophysiology was made by Fritsch and Hitzig (1870), who stimulated the exposed cortex of the dog. This discovery began the investigation of cortical localization of function.

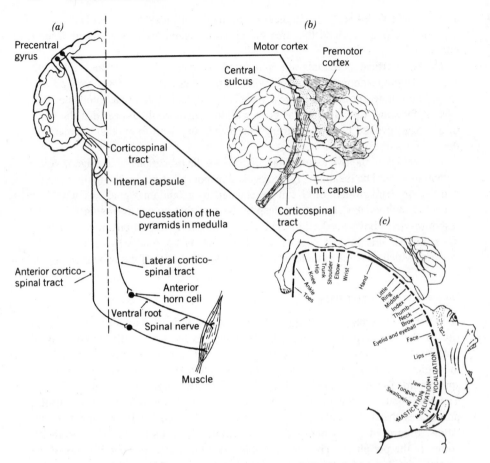

Figure 74   The motor system, showing (*a*) the pathway from the cortex to the periphery, (*b*) its location on the lateral surface of the brain, and (*c*) the topographic distribution on the cortex. (Composed from W. Penfield and T. Rasmussen, *The Cerebral Cortex.* Macmillan, New York, 1950.)

It was shown by Gualtierotti and Paterson (1954) that the motor cortex could be stimulated using scalp electrodes. Employing baboons anesthetized with nitrous oxide and ether, they applied electrodes to the scalp over the motor cortex. With 20–70-mA rectangular or sawtooth stimuli, repeated at rates of 10–150/sec, they obtained contractions in muscles on the opposite side of the body. With frequencies less than 10/sec, the muscle twitches followed the stimuli. However, with continued stimulation, the muscle contractions diminished. After a 2–5-min rest period, the response returned. This study clearly indicated that the technique had potential for human application.

Soon others inquired into the possibility of stimulating the human motor cortex with scalp electrodes Merton and Morton (1980a,b) placed standard EEG electrodes on the scalp over the motor cortex of human subjects. The electrodes were connected across a 100-Ω resistor; a 0.1-μF capacitor, charged to 2 kV, was discharged into the resistor. The stimulus was therefore a 10-μsec capacitor discharge pulse. Twitches in the muscles of the contralateral leg, foot, and toes were obtained for each stimulus. In the same year, Merton and Morton (1980a) discovered that the threshold for stimulation of the motor cortex with scalp electrodes (using the same stimulator) was reduced dramatically if the muscles were contracted slightly by voluntary action. In another paper in the same year, Merton and Morton (1980b) reported phosphenes (light flashes in the visual field) in response to application of the same stimuli to scalp electrodes over the occipital cortex, where vision is represented.

Electrodes were placed on the skin over the spinal column by Merton et al. (1982) to evoke muscle contractions using 10-μsec pulses. Marsden et al. (1983) summarized all of their experiences with scalp electrodes, and to illustrate the method they recorded muscle action potentials in response to the stimuli. Significantly, they reported that their subjects did not complain of pain from the stimulus.

Levy and York (1983) pointed out that the integrity of the efferent spinal cord could be evaluated by placing electrodes over the motor pathways in the lower cord and recording action potentials with headward cord electrodes or with scalp electrodes. In a study using cats, this feat was accomplished with computer-averaged signals; the propagation velocity was 90–110 m/sec in the motor pathways in the spinal cord.

Levy and York (1983) applied the spinal cord stimulation technique to humans. The stimulating electrodes were placed over the lower cord, and the recording electrodes were placed in the cervical region or on the scalp. Computer averaging of 64–256 stimulus–response signals produced very clear recordings in patients undergoing spinal surgery. In the following year, Levy et al. (1984b) applied scalp electrodes over the motor cortex of humans and recorded spinal cord potentials from the motor tracts. With a higher stimulus intensity, potentials could be recorded from peripheral motor nerves.

Figure 75 illustrates a recording of spinal evoked potentials produced with a stimulating electrode (*a*) on the scalp and then (*b*) on the motor cortex. Two successive recordings at each site are shown to illustrate the reproducibility.

A motor cortex evoked cat sciatic nerve action potential is shown in Fig. 76. To make this record, scalp-stimulating electrodes were used, and the averaged sciatic nerve action potential was recorded with a needle electrode. The illustration shows development of the nerve action potential with increasing stimulus intensity. Note that as the intensity is increased, the evoked potential arises slightly earlier.

When a stimulating electrode is placed directly on the motor cortex and a recording electrode is placed over the spinal cord, it is easy to record an averaged motor evoked potential. If a recording electrode is placed on the peripheral nerve that corresponds to the cortical area being stimulated, an averaged action potential is obtained. However, when a scalp-stimulating electrode is used for the same purpose, a larger region of the cortex is stimulated. In this situation it is often more difficult to record an averaged action potential from the peripheral nerve. With

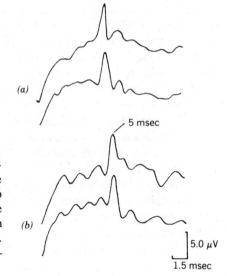

Figure 75 Evoked potential (averaged) detected from the human spinal cord in response to stimulation of the motor cortex using a scalp electrode paired with an indifferent electrode on the hard palate. Two recordings taken from each site are shown to indicate reproducibility. [Redrawn from W. J. Levy et al., *Neurosurgery* **15**:287–302 (1984).]

scalp-stimulating electrodes, it is important to recognize that the current may spread to inhibitory cortical areas, which can result in inhibiting the transmission of impulses across cord synapses preventing the appearance of the expected action potentials from a peripheral nerve even though cord signals are present.

Motor evoked potentials, particularly those from peripheral nerves, are sensitive to both the type and depth of anesthesia as well as metabolic factors. Hypoxia

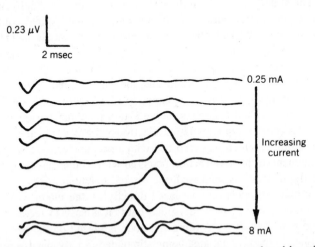

Figure 76 Averaged action potential of the cat sciatic nerve produced by stimulating the motor cortex with a scalp electrode. The different recordings were taken with increasing stimulus intensities, ranging from 0.5 to 8 mA. [Redrawn from M. McCaffrey et al., *J. Neurosurg.* (1986) **19**(2):163–176.]

depresses MEPs, which are best seen with narcotics rather than hypnotic agents. They can be recorded from unanesthetized subjects, but there may be an unpleasant sensation at the site of the scalp electrode.

When recording averaged evoked responses with skin-surface electrodes placed over a peripheral nerve, it is often difficult to identify the nerve signal because it is contaminated by the evoked muscle action potential. In experimental studies it is possible to demonstrate the evoked nerve response by using a myoneural blocking agent.

It is too soon to identify the clinical value of MEPs. The fact that they are present in the spinal cord and peripheral nerves affords a means of testing the continuity of the efferent neural circuit.

ELECTRODERMAL PHENOMENA

Introduction

Skin containing sweat glands (Fig. 77) exhibits two phenomena that arise in response to an attention-getting or alerting stimulus. The two phenomena (Fig. 78) are a decrease in resistance and a change in potential; the accurate measurement of each requires special attention to the type and location of the electrodes, the electrolytes used with them, and the characteristics of the measuring instrument. The change in resistance is referred to as the exosomatic response, and the change in potential is designated the endosomatic response. It is distressing that many different names and symbols are used to describe these two phenomena. Standard-

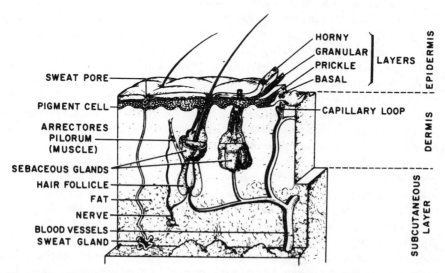

Figure 77   Cross section of facial skin. (From G. L. Sauer, Thomas, Springfield, IL, 1965. By permission.)

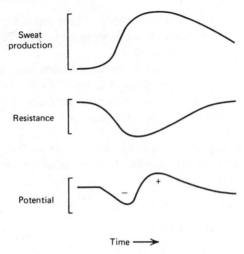

Sweat
production

Resistance

Potential

Time ⟶

Figure 78 Relationship between simultaneously recorded sweat production, skin resistance, and skin potential in response to a strong emotion-provoking stimulus. [Redrawn from C. W. Darrow, *Psychophysiology* **1**:31–38 (1964).]

ization of symbols and terminology is still a subject of considerable debate, even though the phenomena have been investigated for almost a century.

The resistance change (or its reciprocal, conductance), or exosomatic response, was discovered by Féré (1888), who reported a transient decrease in resistance between electrodes applied to the anterior surface of an arm and leg of a hysterical subject who was given a variety of visual and acoustic stimuli. Féré suggested that the phenomenon could be of value in psychophysiological studies. Since Féré's time, the skin has been mapped to identify those regions that provide the maximum change in resistance in response to an alerting stimulus. Table 4 summarizes the data obtained by Edelberg (1967).

The potential change, or endosomatic response, was described by Tarchanoff (1890). This bioelectric event is almost universally called the skin-potential response. Significantly, its measurement requires placement of one electrode over an area supplied with sweat glands (active site) and the other over an area devoid of them (or one that is rendered inactive by skin penetration or abrasion to obtain a reference site). If both electrodes are placed on sites that are equally active (i.e., they produce the same potential change), the potential difference between the electrode terminals will be zero. The relative activity of various body sites has been mapped out by Edelberg (1967), whose data are presented in Table 5. Note that the inner aspect of the earlobe appears to be the least active intact site. Abrasion of the skin, as by a cut, use of a needle electrode, or the application of Shackel's (1959) skin-drilling technique, provides a relatively inactive site. To render a skin site inactive, it is only necessary to penetrate the epidermis down to the stratum malpighi, which is the germinal layer consisting of the basal and prickle cells. No

TABLE 4   Relative Skin Conductance Level and Relative Skin Resistance Response (SRR) for Electrodes Placed at Various Sites on the Body[a]

Site	Number of Subjects	Relative Skin Conductance	Number of Subjects	Relative SRR
Finger				
Palmar	All	1.00	All	1.00
Dorsal	14	0.64	20	0.90
Hand				
Palmar (thenar, hypothenar, and center)	12	1.21	6	1.38
Dorsal	5	0.32		
Wrist				
Volar	11	0.38	5	0.13
Dorsal	5	0.36		
Foot				
Dorsal	14	0.53	9	0.20
Medial, over abductor hallucis muscle	8	1.26	15	1.70
Lateral			5	0.68
Plantar				
Heel	8	1.32	14	0.88
Arch	9	0.91	10	0.60
Ball	8	0.89	14	0.61
Toe	8	1.27	3	0.38

[a]Values expressed with respect to palmar surface of the finger.

Source: R. Edelberg, *Methods of Psychophysiology.* C. Brown (ed.). Williams & Wilkins, Baltimore, MD, 1967. (By permission.)

blood is drawn with Shackel's skin-drilling technique. When so drilled, the site appears shiny at first and soon becomes wetted with tissue fluid.

As stated previously, the electrodermal phenomena have been studied for about a century, yet there is no standardization for the terms used to describe the conductive and voltaic properties of the skin. Terms employing "reflex" and "response" such as galvanic skin reflex or response (GSR), psychogalvanic reflex or response (PGR), skin potential reflex or response (SPR), skin resistance (SR), skin resistance level (SRL), skin resistance response (SRR), skin conductance (SC), skin conductance level (SCL), skin conductance response (SCR), and many others are used, often imprecisely. However, attempts are now being made to encourage psychophysiologists and others to adopt a consistent terminology. Venables and Martin (1967) and Edelberg (1972) (who reported on the terminology recommended by a committee of the Society for Psychophysiological Research) have presented terms that are very reasonable and descriptive. Geddes and Baker have added to this list two terms permitting description of the alternating current properties of the skin; Table 6 presents this terminology. Wang (1957) suggested that "response" be used rather than "reflex," which has a special meaning physiologically. To be consistent with engineering practice, the symbol Z should be used for impedance and Y for its reciprocal, admittance.

TABLE 5   Skin Potential and Relative Skin Potential Response for Electrodes Applied to Various Areas of the Body[a]

Site	Number of Subjects	Skin Potential	Number of Subjects	Relative Skin Potential Response
Finger				
Palmar	25	−39.0	00	1.00
Dorsal	13	−24.8	12	0.57
Forearm				
Over ulner bone, 2 in. from elbow	13	−15.2	12	0.07
Ear				
Inner aspect of earlobe	25	−14.1	24	0.05
Leg				
Over tibial bone, 2 in. above junction with foot	13	−9.2	39	0.18
Foot				
Dorsal			7	0.23
Lateral, near sole			6	1.52
Medial, over abductor hallucis muscle	13	−36.2	12	1.94
Plantar				
Heel			12	3.87
Ball			12	1.89

[a]The "indifferent" or "inactive" electrode was located over a skin-drilled site.

Source: R. Edelberg, in *Methods in Psychophysiology.* C. Brown (ed.). Williams & Wilkins, Baltimore, MD, 1967. (By permission.)

Skin Resistance Response

The transient reduction in skin resistance (or increase in conductance) that accompanies an alerting stimulus can be recorded with one or both electrodes on active sites. Whether linear resistance or conductance changes are recorded depends on the type of circuit employed. Skin resistance level (SRL) and the changes it undergoes (skin resistance response, SRR) are measured with the constant-current circuit. The constant-voltage circuit measures skin conductance level (SCL) and its changes (SCR). Each type of circuit has properties that make it suitable for a

TABLE 6   Terminology for Electrodermal Phenomena

Basal or "Tonic" Level	Abbreviation	Dynamic or "Phasic" Response	Abbreviation	Unit
Skin potential (level)	SP or SPL	Skin potential response	SPR	mV
Skin resistance (level)	SR or SRL	Skin resistance response	SRR	Ω
Skin conductance (level)	SC or SCL	Skin conductance response	SCR	mho
Skin impedance (level)	SZ or SZL	Skin impedance response	SZR	Ω
Skin admittance (level)	SY or SYL	Skin admittance response	SYR	mho

particular application. The advantages and disadvantages of each are discussed subsequently.

Before describing the two types of circuit, it is necessary to recognize the importance of the type of electrode metal and electrolyte employed; as Edelberg et al. (1960; Edelberg and Burch, 1962) have pointed out, both can alter the magnitude of the change in skin resistance. Although lead and zinc, and even aluminum, electrodes have been used in the past with various electrolytes, their suitability is seriously questioned. Edelberg et al. (1960; Edelberg and Burch, 1962) have shown conclusively that calcium chloride, ammonium chloride, potassium sulfate, aluminum chloride, and zinc chloride enhanced the resistance change produced by alerting stimuli. The magnitude of the enhancement at a site was influenced by the direction of the current. Very dilute detergents, acetic acid, and alkali decreased the skin resistance response. In addition, Edelberg (1967) pointed out that standard electrode preparations used for other purposes (e.g., ECG, EEG) are not suitable for recording skin resistance responses. Likewise, attention must be given to the choice of metal, since it can react with the electrolyte to produce a salt that could enhance or depress the resistance response. At present, bare or chlorided silver appears to be the electrode surface preferred by many psychophysiologists. The electrolyte of choice is a weak sodium chloride solution that approximates perspiration (0.1–0.3% NaCl). With this solution, current direction is unimportant. Edelberg (1967) advocated the use of 0.3% NaCl (i.e., 0.05 M) in a starch paste to which was added a preservative. Complete details for preparing two such pastes are presented in his report. For short-term recording, a dilute NaCl solution is satisfactory.

Although mentioned infrequently, the magnitude of the skin resistance response is greatly affected by temperature. Maulsby and Edelberg (1960) and Edelberg (1972) reported that the resistance change decreased by about 5% per degree Celsius reduction in temperature. These authors found considerable individual differences in response; nonetheless, this fact emphasizes the need for controlling or reporting the environmental temperature.

Current Density

In addition to the types of electrode and electrolyte and the temperature of the site, current density is important in determining the magnitude of the skin resistance response. If there were no physiological considerations, increasing the current would produce a larger recordable signal for the same percentage change in resistance or conductance; however, a limit is imposed by important physiological considerations. Edelberg et al. (1960) conducted a series of studies in which a test site was compared with a control site. They found that the skin resistance response increased linearly up to a current density of about 11 $\mu A/cm^2$, but with a current density of 100 $\mu A/cm^2$ the skin resistance response was reduced by about one-quarter. Therefore, as a design figure, a current density of about 10 $\mu A/cm^2$ represents an optimum value.

With a very low current density, the voltage change that represents the endosomatic signal (skin potential response) may be recorded along with that due to the resistance change, if one electrode is on an active site and the other on an inactive site. This point is elaborated in the section dealing with the endosomatic response. Before approaching this subject, it is important to be aware that the current used to obtain the skin resistance response flows through one electrode–subject interface in one direction and through the other in the opposite direction. Therefore, depending on the direction of the current, the potential recorded as the skin potential response could include either series-aiding or series-opposing voltages produced by the potential rise or drop associated with the current flow used to measure the resistance.

Because current flows through the two electrode–electrolyte junctions in opposite directions, two different electrolytic processes may take place if the current density is high enough. In the case of silver–silver chloride electrodes, this situation admits the possibility of adding chloride to the anode and removing it from the cathode. With other metals, consideration should be given to the type of electrolytic products that may be formed, since potentiation or depression of the skin resistance response may occur at either electrode, depending on current direction and the activity of the site over which each electrode is placed. Studies such as those described by Edelberg et al. (1960) and Edelberg and Burch (1962) using control and test sites with forward and reverse current and with one electrode on an active and the other on an inactive site will provide decisive information in a particular recording situation.

Equivalent Circuit

Before the operation of the constant-current and constant-voltage circuits can be discussed, explanations are required regarding the circuit appearing between the terminals of a pair of electrodes used to measure the exosomatic or endosomatic response. Although the equivalent circuit is complex, it consists of three portions, which represent (1) the electrode–electrolyte interface, (2) the skin, and (3) the body tissues and fluids. Figure 79 presents an oversimplified model of these three equivalent circuits as they appear between the terminals (1, 2) of a pair of electrodes placed on the skin.

The electrode–electrolyte interface contains resistive ($R_w R_f$) and capacitive (C_w) components and a half-cell potential ($E_{1/2}$). The magnitude of the resistive component R_w decreases with increasing area and current density; it also decreases as the frequency of the measuring current is increased. The capacitive component (C_w) increases with area, and hence its reactance decreases with area; the reactance of C_w also decreases with decreases in current density and with an increase in the frequency used to measure it. The resistance R_f depends inversely on area; it is usually high, it represents the direct-current resistance of the electrode–electrolyte interface, and it accounts for the electrolytic process. The half-cell potential ($E_{1/2}$) depends on the species of metal, the type and concentration of the electrolyte, and the temperature. A discussion of these factors is presented in Chapter 9.

The equivalent circuit for the skin has been simplified to show a resistance R_{sc}

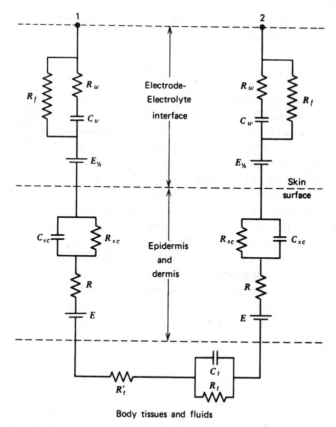

Figure 79 Approximate equivalent circuit for electrodes placed on the skin to record the electrodermal phenomena.

(for the stratum corneum, or dry, horny layer) and a capacitor C_{sc} in which the stratum corneum and subjacent membranes represent the leaky dielectric and the two "plates" are the electrode above and the conducting body tissues and fluids below. The magnitude of R_{sc} is, of course, dependent on the type of electrolyte used and the secretion of sweat. The resistance R represents the resistance of membranes that change their permeability, thus contributing to the skin resistance response. A potential E has been included to represent the voltage that changes to produce the skin potential response. Similar models consisting of variable voltages and variable resistances were proposed by Edelberg (1967) and Lykken et al. (1968). In the case of the skin resistance response, both R and R_{sc} decrease in response to an alerting stimulus; the change in R_{sc} is probably brought about by the secretion of sweat.

Subcutaneous body tissues and fluids can be represented by resistive and capacitive components; the latter is due to cell membranes, and the former is due to intra- and extracellular electrolytes. The origin of this circuit (R'_t-R_t-C_t) was discussed extensively by Cole (1933), and it is attractive because it exhibits an impedance–frequency characteristic quite similar to that of a specimen of living tissue.

Constant-Current Circuit for Resistance Measurement

With the constant-current circuit (Fig. 80a), the voltage e appearing between the electrode terminals (1, 2) is linearly proportional to the skin resistance level R_0 and the skin resistance response ΔR. The essential requirement is that the resistor R_i in series with the voltage source E be much higher (e.g., 100–1000 times) than the equivalent resistive component R_0 of the total impedance Z_{12} appearing between electrode terminals (1 and 2); thus, the magnitude of current that flows will be determined by R_i rather than R_0, even though R_0 may vary among subjects. Figure 80a shows a passive constant-current source obtained by placing a high value of resistance R_i in series with a constant-voltage supply E. Although this technique is convenient and inexpensive, the voltage required to obtain the desired current through the subject is often quite high. There are, however, active constant-current circuits available in which much less supply voltage is needed. For example, the collector circuit of a transistor or the appropriate configuration of an operational

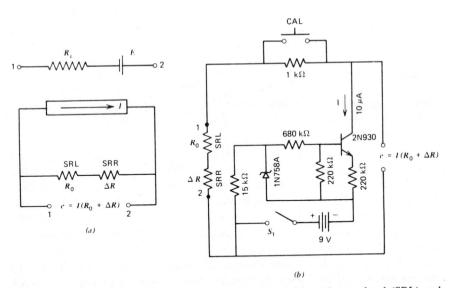

Figure 80 Constant-current circuits for measurement of skin resistance level (SRL) and skin resistance response (SRR). (a) Simple constant-current generator created by using a voltage source E with a resistance R_i, that is high with respect to the skin resistance level R_0, and the changes it exhibits (ΔR), which constitute the skin resistance response (SRR). (b) Constant-current circuit created by placing the subject ($R_0 + \Delta R$) in series with the collector of a transistor (2N930). The current I flowing through the subject is 10 μA and is controlled by the base bias on the transistor derived from the 680- and 220-kΩ resistors arranged in series.

amplifier constitutes excellent constant-current circuits. Figure 80*b* illustrates a simple, low-cost, constant-current circuit used by Geddes et al. (1974). The equivalent impedance of this circuit is 500 MΩ, and it maintains a constant current for a resistance range extending from 0 to 1.5 MΩ. The current value is set by adjusting the resistors that apply bias to the base of the transistor.

With the constant-current circuit, the desired signal is obtained directly from electrode terminals 1, 2 using a recording instrument with an input impedance that is high with respect to R_0. The voltage e across the electrode terminals is given by

$$e = I(R_0 + \Delta R),$$

but

$$I = \frac{E}{R_i} \quad \text{when} \quad R_i \gg R_0 \quad \text{and} \quad \Delta R \ll R$$

$$e = \frac{E}{R_i} R_0 + \frac{E}{R_i} \Delta R.$$

With the constant-current circuit, the voltage across the electrode terminals (1, 2) consists of a large constant voltage ER_0/R_i representing the basal skin resistance, and a smaller one, $E \Delta R/R_i$ that represents the skin resistance response ΔR due to the altering stimulus. If both electrodes are over active sites, ΔR is doubled. As long as R_i is much greater than the total resistance R_0 between the electrode terminals, the change in voltage, which reflects the skin resistance response, is independent of the skin resistance level.

In a typical application, the skin resistance response amounts to from 100 to perhaps 5000 Ω and stands on a constant resistance baseline of 10–50 kΩ. Figures 78, and 83 illustrate typical skin resistance responses. Note that the resistance change is monophasic, consisting of a rapid decrease and a slower increase to the original baseline. A decrease in skin resistance is very frequently displayed as an upward deflection on the record.

Constant-Voltage Circuit for Conductance Measurement

With the constant-voltage circuit (Fig. 81), a low-impedance voltage source E is used. The current I that flows is linearly proportional to the applied voltage and the conductance G_0, which is the basal skin conductance level in the absence of a skin conductance response (SCR). The skin conductance G_0 is the reciprocal of the direct-current resistance component R_0 of the impedance appearing between electrode terminals 1 and 2. Thus $I = EG_0$.

An alerting stimulus will cause a small increase in conductance (ΔG); therefore, the general expression for the current is

$$I = E(G_0 + \Delta G).$$

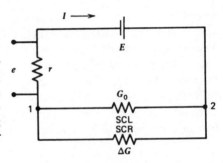

Figure 81 Constant-voltage circuit used for skin conductance measurement. The current due to the skin conductance level (G_0) and its changes (ΔG), which constitute the skin conductance response, are measured by recording the voltage e that appears across the resistor r, which is many times smaller than I/G_0.

Measurement of current is usually accomplished with a current amplifier or by recording the voltage e appearing across a resistance r, which is added to the circuit and is very much smaller than $1/G_0$; in practice, the resistance r is in the range of 10–100 Ω. The voltage across r is therefore

$$e = Ir = rE(G_0 + \Delta G)$$

$$= rEG_0 + rE\,\Delta G.$$

The small conductance-change signal ($rE\,\Delta G$), which is the skin conductance response, stands on a larger skin conductance level signal that amounts to rEG_0. In a practical situation, the actual current that flows through the subject is dependent on G_0, which depends on electrode area and the subject's resistance level; hence, care must be exercised in the choice of a voltage E that will not send excessive current through low-resistance subjects.

In practice, a basal skin conductance of 0.1×10^{-3} mho/cm^2 represents the low resistance range for typical subjects (Edelberg, 1967), with perhaps a value of 0.01–0.002×10^{-3} mho/cm^2 being representative for high-resistance skin. A survey of the published literature on skin conductance was presented by Pfeiffer (1968). For a 1-cm^2 electrode, the voltages that will provide 10 μA of current are 1.0 and 5 V, respectively. Therefore, careful consideration must be given to the choice of voltage with respect to the area of the electrodes if it is desired to maintain the current density at 10 μA/cm^2, the value recommended by Edelberg et al. (1960).

Amplifier Input Impedance

The input impedance of the amplifier connected to record skin resistance or conductance merits special consideration because the requirements are quite different for the two phenomena. In the case of measurement of skin resistance (see Fig. 80a), the amplifier used to record the resistance-dependent voltage e must have an input impedance that is high with respect to the skin resistance level R_0. Note that the output impedance R_i of the constant-current generator is high with respect to R_0. When measuring skin conductance, as in Fig. 81, the conductance-dependent signal e that appears across r must be measured with an amplifier whose input impedance is high with respect to r, which is in turn much smaller than the basal resistance R_0 of the subject, which is $1/G_0$. If a high-sensitivity current-measuring device with a resistive input resistance equal to or less than r is available, it can be substituted for r.

With both the constant-current (resistance measurement) and constant-voltage (conductance-measurement) circuits, the signal due to a resistance or conductance change is very small in comparison with the standing signal representing the basal skin resistance or conductance level. In practice, the standing signal is smaller with the constant-voltage method. With each circuit, the standing signal must be canceled at some point in the system, permitting the much smaller signal produced by the physiological event to be amplified and suitably recorded. Since the insertion of a series-opposing voltage sometimes presents practical problems, the use of an adequately large coupling capacitor is common. The price paid in using a capacitor is the loss of dc or "baseline" information, providing only changes in resistance (SRR) or conductance (SCR). A practical circuit for eliminating the large standing potential at its source is the Wheatstone bridge (Fig. 82). One side of the bridge is constituted by the subject and the series resistance R_i or r, the magnitude of which depends on whether resistance or conductance is to be measured. The other side of the bridge consists of a potentiometer (P); its value is usually chosen so that approximately the same current flows through it as through the subject and the series resistor (R_i or r). When the bridge is balanced for basal values of R_0 or G_0, the voltage $E_{13} = 0$. Changes in E_{13} from the zero value are produced by an appropriate physiological stimulus. This output signal (E_{13}) is connected directly to a differential amplifier, which in turn drives a display device. Adjustment of the potentiometer rotor (3) allows presentation of zero voltage to the amplifier for any resistance or conductance level. The potentiometer is therefore the balance control for the Wheatstone bridge. Whether the bridge circuit provides a signal that represents resistance or conductance depends on the magnitude of the resistance (R_i or r) in series with the subject. With respect to the subject resistance R_0 a high

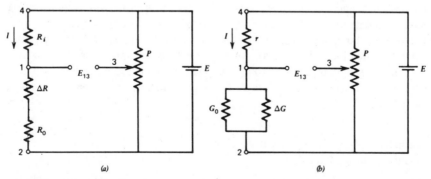

(a)   (b)

Figure 82   Wheatstone bridge circuits arranged for linear indication of skin resistance. (a) Constant-current skin resistance ($R_i \gg R_0 + \Delta R$); (b) constant-voltage skin conductance ($r \ll 1/(G_0 + \Delta G)$).

value of series resistance R_i provides linear resistance recording (Fig. 80); a low value for r provides linear conductance recording (Fig. 81). This important component must be chosen properly. Sufficient attention has not always been given to this point, and in reading some reports it is not possible to tell whether the recordings represent linear resistance or conductance changes.

When using the Wheatstone bridge and a differential amplifier to record skin resistance or conductance, consideration should be given to the need to use an isolated source (E) to supply current to the subject and to the ability of the differential amplifier to tolerate an appreciable common-mode (offset) signal. It is highly desirable to employ a separate source to apply current to the subject and to energize the differential amplifier, to avoid the risk of providing multiple current paths through the subject and input circuit of the amplifier. For example, referring to Fig. 82, the input of the amplifier is connected to points 1 and 3, and in a practical situation it is often necessary to ground point 2 or 4 to reject common-mode signals, such as 60-Hz interference. When this is done, even with the bridge balanced (i.e., $E_{13} = 0$), there is an appreciable standing potential (E_{12} or E_{14}, depending on whether point 2 or 4 is grounded). In operation, the differential amplifier must be able to tolerate this common-mode offset voltage if its common terminal is connected to either 1 or 4.

Bandwidth Requirements

If basal skin resistance or conductance levels are to be recorded, direct-coupled systems are required (i.e., the sinusoidal frequency response must extend to 0 Hz); however, if only changes in skin resistance or conductances are of interest, capacitive coupling with a time constant of 5 sec or longer, as advocated by Edelberg (1967), provides adequate fidelity. This value for the time constant corresponds to a lower sinusoidal frequency limit (for 70% amplitude) of 0.03 Hz.

The high-frequency response required for faithful reproduction of the electrodermal phenomena has not been investigated extensively, possibly because there are so many graphic recording systems that obviously respond much faster than skin resistance and conductance changes. Measurement of the most rapidly changing components of skin resistance and conductance recordings reveals that a rise time (10–90%) of about 0.1 sec is typical. The equivalent sinusoidal high-frequency response is therefore 5 Hz. Thus a bandwidth extending from 0 to above 5 Hz will allow faithful reproduction of skin resistance or conductance levels and their changes. If only changes are of interest, a bandwidth extending from 0.03 to 5 Hz is satisfactory.

Characteristics of Constant-Current and Constant-Voltage Circuits

The type of circuit selected by an investigator depends primarily on the projected use for the data, the size of signal desired, and the electrophysiological model chosen. Extensive discussions on the characteristics and advantages of one method over the other have been presented by Darrow (1964), Wilcott and Hammond (1965, 1966), Edelberg (1967), and Lykken and Venables (1971); selection of the best is by no means a settled issue. If indication of the presence or absence of a response is sufficient, both the constant-current (resistance) and constant-voltage (conductance) circuits are suitable, with the practical exception that the former provides a signal about tenfold larger than the latter. When skin resistance or conductance levels are to be recorded, the size of the bucking voltage required is higher with the skin resistance method. With the constant-current (resistance) circuit, the input impedance of the amplifier must be on the order of many megohms in order to be much higher than the skin resistance level. The input impedance of the amplifier used with the constant-voltage (conductance) system need only be high with respect to the low value of resistance in series with the subject (r in Fig. 81). Alternatively, a current amplifier can be used.

If it is assumed that the secretion of sweat is the major contributor to the decrease in resistance and that the sweat glands are arranged in parallel under the active electrode, the conductance method is the one of choice because the increase in conductance is linearly related to the number of actively secreting sweat glands (Darrow, 1934; Thomas and Korr, 1957). Thus with an increase in number of active sweat glands, current flow through an active site is not changed by other sites becoming active. According to Lykken and Venables (1971), the conductance change is relatively independent of the basal or tonic skin conductance level. With the constant-current circuit, Darrow (1964) has shown that the change in resistance decreases with decreasing skin resistance level. This situation follows from peripheral considerations; however, since a decreased skin resistance is associated with an increase in central response to the stimulus, this effect counteracts the peripheral manifestation.

With the constant-voltage (conductance) method, current is limited only by the skin resistance level of the subject and the internal resistance of the current source, and precautions must be taken to avoid using excessively high current densities ($> 10 \, \mu A/cm^2$) when low skin resistance levels are encountered. With the constant-current (resistance) method, the current is always the same, regardless of the skin resistance level of the subject. However, with a very high skin resistance, the constant-current system may generate a high voltage drop across the skin, which will cause the resistance to fall (Wilcott and Hammond, 1965, 1966).

In some instances it is desirable to use the skin resistance electrodes to detect a bioelectric event, such as the ECG. Use of the conductance method places a short circuit across the electrodes, rendering the pair useless for any other purpose. However, the impedance of a constant-current source is high; therefore, one or both electrodes can be used to record a bioelectric event, providing its amplitude and/or frequency spectrum will allow separation of the skin resistance signal. Use of the same fingertip "dry" silver electrodes for the simultaneous measurement of changes in skin resistance and the ECG was described by Geddes et al. (1974); Fig. 83 presents a typical recording made using this technique in which the subject was asked to take deep breaths to produce large-amplitude skin resistance responses. Figure 84 is a typical recording of skin resistance responses and instan-

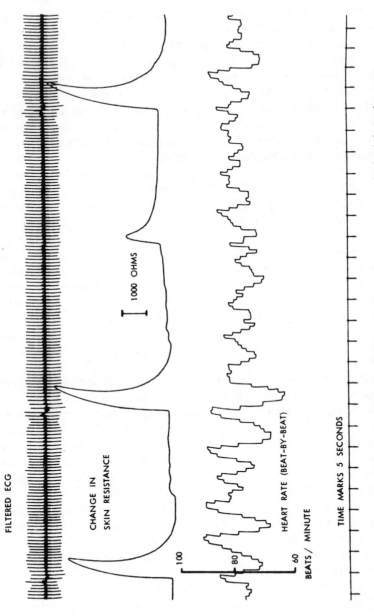

FILTERED ECG

CHANGE IN
SKIN RESISTANCE

1000 OHMS

HEART RATE (BEAT-BY-BEAT)

100

80

60

BEATS / MINUTE

TIME MARKS 5 SECONDS

Figure 83 The electrocardiogram (ECG) and skin resistance response obtained from the same pair of dry silver electrodes applied to the volar surfaces of the tips of the second fingers. The instantaneous heart rate was derived from the ECG. [From L. A. Geddes et al., *Med. Biol. Eng.* **13**:89–96 (1975). By permission.]

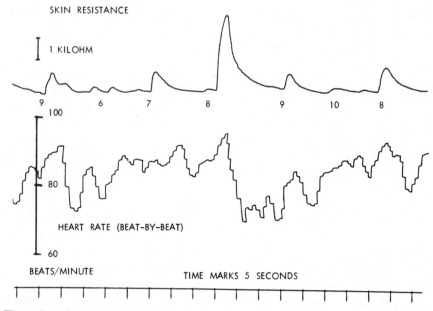

Figure 84 Typical record of changes in skin resistance and beat-by-beat heart rate during a simple lying test in which the subject was asked to concentrate on any number between 6 and 10 and say "no" to each number guessed by the interrogator. Note that the amplitude of the skin resistance change was greatest for number 8. Note also the considerable reduction in heart rate following the first response to number 8.

taneous heart rate, obtained in the same way during a simple lying test. Here the subject was asked to think of a number between 6 and 10 and say "no" to every interrogation. The subject lied about number 8, which was the number he had selected.

Although the skin resistance response is usually recorded using direct current, sinusoidal alternating current has also been employed. Such applications are described in Chapter 11. The studies carried out thus far make it clear that the magnitude of the resistance change decreases with increasing frequency. However, insufficient data exist to indicate the optimum frequency range. There is evidence that use of a frequency of 100 Hz provides a reasonably good skin resistance response and eliminates bothersome galvanic electrode potentials (Edelberg, 1974).

Skin Potential Response

As stated previously, with the endosomatic method one electrode is placed on an active site, the other on an inactive site. The active sites most frequently employed are the sole of the foot, palm of the hand, and the volar surface of a fingertip (often the second finger is employed). Data on the relative activities of the various body sites are presented in Table 5. Chlorided silver electrodes, with a weak electrolyte of known composition approximating that of sweat (~0.3% NaCl), are frequently employed. With one electrode over an area rich in sweat glands (active site) and one on an inactive site, the potential of the active site is negative by an amount that varies from a few to 50 or 60 mV; the actual magnitude depends on many factors. An alerting stimulus produces an initial increase in negativity followed by a decrease (positive wave) and sometimes by a second negative wave (Fig. 78). The first negative and the positive waves were designated the *a* and *b* waves by Forbes (1936); however, this terminology is not widely used.

The skin potential level drifts slowly for about 15 min following application of the electrodes, and the change is believed to be due to hydration of the tissues by the electrolytic preparation. This phenomenon is under active investigation (Edelberg, 1968; Fowles and Venables, 1970) and becomes important when the skin potential level is to be used as a measure of the level of alertness.

Edelberg (1972) pointed out that the several phases of the skin potential response are affected differently by various electrolytes. However, at this time there are insufficient data to permit making strong recommendations. Persumably, weak electrolytes such as those used for skin resistance responses (i.e., 0.3% NaCl) do not enhance or depress the skin potential response.

The temperature of the active site affects the skin potential response; a reduction in temperature decreases the amplitude and affects the negative and positive phases differently. Yokota et al. (1959) showed that the positive phase was absent (with electrodes placed on the palm and dorsum of the hand) when the temperature was decreased to 20°C and reappeared at 30°C. At 40°C the amplitude was increased. The negative phase was most prominent at 20°C (Yokota et al., 1959). These facts suggest that attention should be given to maintaining and reporting the temperature of the site or the environment.

With one electrode on an active site and the other over an inactive site, there are at least two electrode–electrolyte potentials, the skin potential and perhaps an injury potential. If the inactive site has been created by marked abrasion of the skin, the algebraic sum of these voltages appears between the electrode terminals and is presented to the input of the recording apparatus. If it is desired to record this skin potential level (SPL) and the changes it experiences in response to an alerting stimulus (SPR), it is necessary to employ a bucking or canceling voltage in the input circuit of the recording apparatus because the typical change in skin potential is quite small (on the order of millivolts) and the skin potential level (plus electrode and injury potential) may be many tens of millivolts and may therefore block the amplifier. If only changes in skin potential (SPR) are desired, capacitive coupling with an adequately long time constant (~ 5 sec) eliminates the need for using a bucking voltage. In both cases the amplifying apparatus must have an adequately high input impedance for the size of the electrodes employed. In a typical situation, an input impedance greater than 2 MΩ can be used with electrodes having an area of about 1 cm^2.

A typical skin potential response is shown in Fig. 78 along with the change in resistance and secretion of sweat. Note that the waveform of the response is biphasic, the active area becoming initially more negative with respect to the inactive site. The type of waveform is not always symmetrical or biphasic; polyphasic patterns have been reported (Edelberg, 1972).

At this point, a few remarks are in order regarding the endosomatic method. Of paramount importance is the need to locate one electrode on an active site and the other on an inactive site. Since voltage is measured, the technique is easily standardized, calibration being achieved by the application of a step function of voltage on the order of 1 mV. Apart from specifying the electrode type, size, and site, there are no other important variables (presuming that the amplifying system has an adequately high input impedance and adequate bandwidth). If these criteria are met, precise control of electrode area is relatively unimportant unless it becomes so small that R_0 begins to approach the input resistance of the amplifier. If the calibrating signal is maintained for about 20 sec, the time constant of the recording apparatus will be recorded if capacitive coupling is used. Of course, if direct coupling is used, the recorder will remain deflected as long as the calibrating signal is present. If direct coupling is used to obtain the skin potential level, very stable electrodes are required along with provision for an adjustable canceling or bucking voltage. Depending on the electrode locations and suitable separation of component frequencies with appropriate circuitry, one or both of the electrodes can be used to detect another bioelectric event.

Origin of the Electrodermal Phenomena

Although the skin resistance and skin potential responses (SRR and SPR) have been investigated for almost a century, there are insufficient data to formulate an acceptable explanation for them. The many theories and models advanced thus far have been described very fairly by Edelberg (1972), whose review is recommended reading for those wishing to delve further into this subject. Although no single explanation is tenable, certain facts are well accepted. For example, the SRR and SPR both require the presence of active sweat glands (Richter, 1927), which in humans are brought into action by the sympathetic nervous system via the neural transmitter acetylcholine. Thus the sweat glands are sympathetic cholinergic, and their activity is blocked by atropine, which raises the skin resistance level and abolishes both the SRR and SPR. Likewise, interruption of the sympathetic nerve supply to the sweat glands abolishes the SRR and SPR. From this point on, it becomes increasingly difficult to make definite statements. For example, there is no doubt that these two responses reside in the superficial layers of the skin, but the precise level has not been established. Abrasion of the skin down to the granular layer abolishes both responses. Although it is obvious that sweat secretion will lower skin resistance, visible (surface) sweating is not necessary for the production of a skin resistance response. One group of investigators believes that sweat rises in the ducts and spreads laterally, hydrating the stratum corneum and reducing its resistance. However, there appears to be evidence that epidermal membranes become permeable in response to neural stimuli, resulting in a decrease in resistance and a change in membrane potential, and both contribute to the skin resistance and skin potential response. In addition, some investigators believe that there are a presecretory and a secretory potential associated with the activity of a sweat gland and its duct, which, along with sweat expulsion, enhance the detection of a skin potential (and resistance) response. Which of these phenomena dominates or is subordinate in the genesis of the electrodermal phenomena awaits further investigation. However, it is not necessary to have the results of such studies to use the electrodermal phenomena as indicators of activity of the sympathetic nervous system.

ELECTROOCULOGRAPHY

Electrooculography (EOG) is the name given to the technique of recording changes in eye position using circumorbital electrodes. It is well known that placing two orthogonal pairs of electrodes around an eye will permit measurement of potentials that can be used to identify the direction of gaze with respect to the head. The bioelectric event underlying these signals is a standing potential, measurable between the cornea and the posterior pole (fundus) of the eyeball. Thus the eyeball resembles a dipole that can move in an inhomogeneous volume conductor (the head), as illustrated in Fig. 85. The polarity of the potential depends on the type of eye, and the magnitude of the potential increases above a basal value with increasing illumination; this increase forms the basis for electroretinography, which is described in the next section of this chapter.

Apparently the first to report an electrical potential associated with the eye was du Bois-Reymond, who in 1849 made measurements on the tench, a European freshwater fish of the carp family. Marg's (1951) translation of the report is as follows: "With the eye on its side, the cornea and optic nerve could be brought into contact with the electrodes. From this it was shown that an arbitrary point in the surface of the eyeball was positive with respect to the cross-section of the nerve." From this description it is not possible to discover how much the optic nerve injury potential contributed to what is now known to be the standing potential between the cornea and the back of the eyeball. Du Bois-Reymond's experiment was repeated by Dewar and M'Kendrick (1876) and Dewar (1877), using rabbit, cat, dog, pigeon, owl, goldfish, rock fish, stickleback, frog, toad, snake, crab, and lobster eyes connected via du Bois-Reymond's nonpolarizable electrodes to a Thomson reflecting galvanometer. In addition, they observed a change in the standing potential with illumination of the retina. In a postscript to their paper they reported having located Holmgren's (1865–1866, 1870–1871) reports (in Swedish) describing similar studies. These early investigators reported galvanometer deflections rather than voltages, probably because the volt had not been universally adopted as the unit for potential.

Most of the early investigators who had used galvanometers and "nonpolarizable" electrodes to measure the response of the eye to light noted the presence of a steady potential when the retina was not illuminated; this potential was measurable between an electrode on the cornea and one behind the eye, or at an indifferent site on the body. Evidence of the corneoretinal potential in the human

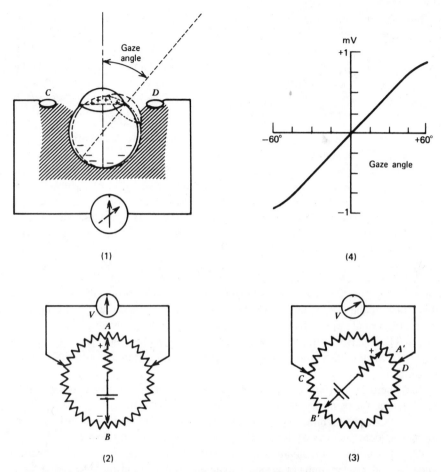

Figure 85 The corneoretinal potential (1) and its representation as an equivalent circuit (2, 3) for forward and right gaze; (4) represents a typical relationship of voltage versus gaze angle. (Redrawn from M. Sosonow and E. Ross, *Electrodes for Recording Primary Bioelectric Signals*, ASD Tech. Rept. 61-437. USAF Wright-Patterson AFB, OH.)

subject came from studies reported by Dewar and M'Kendrick, who were interested in the response of the eye to light. Yet they demonstrated that eye movements could be recorded and stated:

"Having succeeded in detecting the action of light on the retina of the living warm-blooded animal without any operative procedures, it appeared possible to apply a similar method to the eye of man. For this purpose, a small trough of clay or paraffin was constructed round the margin of the orbit, so as to contain a quantity of dilute salt solution when the body was placed horizontally and the head properly secured. Into this solution the terminal of a non-polarisable electrode was introduced, and in order to complete the circuit the other electrode was connected with a large gutta-percha trough containing salt solution, into which one of the hands was inserted. By a laborious process of education it is possible to diminish largely the electrical variation due to the involuntary movements of the eyeball, and by fixing the eye on one point with concentrated attention, another observer, watching the galvanometer, and altering the intensity of the light, can detect an electrical variation similar to what is seen in other animals. This method, however, is too exhausting and uncertain to permit of quantitative observations being made."

Notwithstanding, Dewar and M'Kendrick were the first to demonstrate an eye-position-dependent signal.

Actual measurement of the standing corneofundal potential has been made infrequently. Several authors have reported a magnitude of 6–12 mV, without indicating how the measurement was made. Perhaps the best review of the literature that is concerned with the standing potential was presented by Kohlrausch (1931); a translation and summary of his conclusions were given by Marg (1951), who reported:

"1. In vertebrates the cornea is positive relative to the retina. In invertebrates, however, the anterior of the eye is negative. This corresponds to the difference in orientation of the retinas of subphylum Vertebrata and the retinas of the invertebrates, the visual cells pointing outward in the former and inward in the latter.

"2. The polarity of the standing potential is increased by light (the illumination potential) whether the animal has a positive cornea (vertebrate) or not (invertebrate).

"3. There is a sudden discontinuity in potential at the ora serrata, which is found as one measures the topographic distribution of voltage.

"4. Under certain influences, such as ionic changes or mechanical insults, there are independent changes of the standing and the illumination potential.

"5. One finds a similar alteration in both the standing and the illumination potential under other influences, such as changes in carbon dioxide and oxygen tensions, temperature and electrical stimuli."

Even before the magnitude and true origin of the corneofundal potential were established, it was put to practical use to detect eye position using periorbital electrodes. Schott (1922) and Meyers (1929) appear to have been the first to achieve success using the string galvanometer; Schott employed a wire and a button electrode (both of copper) placed nasally (on the caruncle) and temporally on the conjunctiva in the outer canthus of the cocainized eye. A spectacle frame was used to stabilize the electrodes, and the cocaine diminished electrode irritation. Schott's interest lay in recording nystagmus rather than eye position. Meyers applied a pair of horseshoe-shaped electrodes located bitemporally with the open part facing the eye. He noted that not only were lateral deviations of the eye recorded, but vertical movements could be detected with electrodes above and below one eye. Although he obtained recordings of opposite polarity when the direction of gaze was reversed, he did not study the relationship between recorded amplitude and deviation of the eyes from the central fixation point, probably because his interest was the study of nystagmus. Incidentally, he named the technique "electro-nystagmography" but erroneously attributed the source of the potential to a summation of action potentials of the ocular muscles. Likewise, Jacobson (1930) attributed the electrooculographic signals to the contraction of ocular muscles. Wrong as this was later shown to be, Jacobson appears to have been the first to mention that eye position signals could be obtained with closed eyes.

Up to this time there appear to have been three theories regarding the origin of the signal that reflects eye position. Some thought that contraction of the muscles causing deviation of the eyeball produced action potentials that were summated and detected by the electrodes. Others thought that because string galvanometers were used and there was current flow, a change in interelectrode resistance caused the galvanometer to be deflected as the eyes were deviated. Another group thought that a standing potential existed between the cornea and back of the eyeball and that movement of the eye varied the voltage presented to periorbital electrodes. It was not long before these three theories were subjected to experimental test. In a single paper, Mowrer et al. (1935–1936) clearly showed that the source of the electrooculographic signal was the standing potential that exists between the cornea and fundus of an eye with a functioning retina. The manner by which they dispelled all doubts is interesting for the clear logic of the presentation. For example, the investigators reasoned that if resistance change produced the signal, transtemporal electrodes should detect the same resistance change for deviation of the eyes to the right and left and therefore, the galvanometer should be deviated in the same direction for right and left deviations. Experiment showed that the galvanometer was deflected in opposite directions with left and right deviations of the eyes. To add further proof to the fallacy of resistance change being an important contributor, they recorded the electrooculogram with a high input impedance amplifier connected ahead of a string galvanometer; with this arrangement, virtually no current was drawn from the subject, and left and right gaze produced oppositely directed deflections on the recording.

To prove that summated muscle action potentials were not the basis of the electrooculographic signal, Mowrer et al. (1935–1936) pointed out that contracting muscle is electronegative to resting tissue, and with transtemporal electrodes a gaze to the right produced a positive polarity at the right temporal electrode; if the signal were due to summated muscle action potentials, the polarity should be negative. In addition, summation of action potentials would produce a jagged deflection in the recording; this was never seen. To add even more proof, they placed transtemporal electrodes on a deeply anesthetized cat and deviated the eyes passively by attaching a probe to the anesthetized cornea. The galvanometer showed deflections related to the direction of deviation of the eyeball; under this condition, deviation was produced without muscular contraction. To prove that the electrooculogram so produced was not due to reflex contraction of the ocular muscles, they showed that destruction of the retina, by intraocular injection of a 5% solution of chromic acid, completely abolished the voltage produced by passive movement of the eyes. Finally, they showed that the electrooculogram was produced by a standing potential measurable between the cornea and fundus of the eye by removing the eye and measuring a potential between electrodes in these locations; the cornea was found to be positive with respect to the back of the eyeball; however, they did not report the magnitude of the potential differences.

Now that the existence of a corneofundal potential has been established, it is of value to examine the appropriateness of the model in Fig. 85. If the corneofundal potential is equated to a dipole in a volume conductor, the potential detected by a pair of electrodes placed on the skin, above and below or lateral to an eye, ought to be zero with the gaze directed forward, varying as the sine of the gaze angle measured when the gaze is deflected along the axis of an electrode pair—provided the head does not seriously distort the dipole field. This model can be simplified by considering the electrooculographic generator (the corneofundal potential A–B) to be a battery that moves within a circular resistor. The potential-measuring electrodes are represented by taps (C, D) on the circular resistor (Fig. 85).

Many studies have been carried out to determine the voltage versus gaze angle relationship. In the early days of electrooculography, Fenn and Hursh (1937) reported that the voltage detected by bitemporal electrodes is related to the sine of the angle of deviation from the central fixation point. Since that time, others have sought to confirm or refute this relationship; many have shown that, within limits, the voltage is linearly related to the horizontal angle of gaze. That the electrooculogram did reflect eye position was verified by Hoffman et al. (1939), who used a binocular corneal reflection technique and photographic recording; they concluded that "the electrical method is reliable enough to be used in psychological research." In support of this belief, Halstead (1938) reported being able to detect vertical and horizontal eye movements as small as 1 degree. Even though the potential measured between bitemporal electrodes was found to be related to eye position, Byford (1963) reported that comparisons with an optical eye-tracking device showed that the electrooculographic method was undependable in a few of the subjects being tested.

Among those who have reported a linearity of voltage with angle of gaze are Leksell (1939) for ±40 degrees, Mackensen and Harder (1954) for ±30 degrees, Kris (1957, 1958) for ±5 to ±60 degrees, and Kris (1960) for ± 30 degrees; Mackensen and Harder's data showed a good correspondence with the sinusoidal relationship up to 40 degrees. Law and Devalois (1958) wrote that a linear relationship existed between 0.5 and 15 degrees, and North (1965) stated that the electrooculographic voltage did not follow a sinusoidal relationship with gaze angle; Leksell (1939) and Shackel (1960, 1967) reported that both linear and sinusoidal relationships are good approximations.

In a study by Geddes et al. (1973), a comparison was made between the linear and sinusoidal relationships for horizontal gaze deflection by measuring the potential appearing between a pair of dry silver electrodes located at the outer canthus of each eye. Precise control of gaze direction was obtained by using a semicircular frame (perimeter) equipped with 13 miniature neon lamps, located at every 10 degrees of gaze direction and placed in front of the subject's head (see Fig. 86). The head position was stabilized by a chin support. The subject first directed his gaze at the illuminated neon lamp at the central fixation point (CFP) directly in

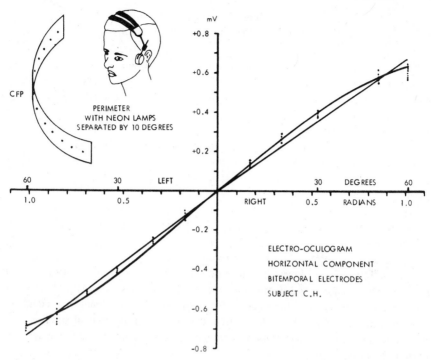

Figure 86 Voltage versus horizontal gaze direction in humans, using bitemporal electrodes. [From L. A. Geddes et al., *Med. Biol. Eng.* **11:**73–77 (1973). By permission.]

front of him. Then the operator extinguished the CFP lamp and illuminated any other lamp; the subject directed his gaze to the newly lit lamp, and afterward the CFP lamp was illuminated. The test was repeated five times for each gaze angle to the left and right from 0 to 60 degrees. The voltage (e) readings obtained for each gaze angle (θ) were plotted versus gaze angle and, for each subject, least-squares fits were obtained for linear ($e = E\theta$) and for sinusoidal ($e = E_m \sin \theta$) representation. A set of data for a typical subject appears in Fig. 86 along with the linear and sinusoidal representations. The data for 22 subjects were analyzed and are summarized in Table 7. This study revealed that for gaze angles up to ± 60 degrees, the sinusoidal representation was superior to the linear representation; the former exhibited a standard error of estimate (SEE) of 0.029, and the latter a value of 0.037. However, for a gaze angle of ± 45 degrees, the linear representation is sufficiently accurate for practical purposes.

Although the dipole concept is very useful for modeling the standing corneofundal potential, it should be mentioned that Kris (1960) showed that whereas electrodes placed lateral to the canthus of the eyes detect only the horizontal component of lateral gaze, an electrode pair placed on the supraorbital margin and the infraorbital ridge do not detect a purely vertical component of gaze direction. In other words, two electrode pairs placed orthogonally around an eye do not detect

TABLE 7 Linear and Sinusoidal Representations for Horizontal Component of the EOG of Each Eye

	Linear Representation[a] $e = E\theta$	Sinusoidal Representation[a] $e = E_m \sin \theta$
Average value	$e = 0.600\theta$	$e = 0.684 \sin \theta$
Maximum value	$e = 1.05\theta$	$e = 1.21 \sin \theta$
Minimum value	$e = 0.364\theta$	$e = 0.413 \sin \theta$

[a]The values of E and E_m are in millivolts; the angle θ is measured in radians (1 radian = 57.3 degrees).

Source: L. A. Geddes et al., *Med. Biol. Eng.* **11**:73–77 (1973).

purely orthogonal eye position signals. Of the two pairs of electrodes, the horizontal pair gives the purest component signal.

In assessing the relationship between voltage and gaze angle, it is important to note that sin θ measured in radians does not differ by more than 10% from θ until an angle of 0.75 radian (43 degrees) is exceeded. For this reason, if a 10% error is acceptable, the linear representation for voltage versus gaze angle is adequate up to this limit. For gaze angles larger than this figure, for theoretical and practical reasons the sinusoidal representation offers a better correlation between voltage and horizontal eye position.

Despite the considerable use made of the electrooculogram, there is no universally agreed-on terminology to describe location of the electrodes about one or both eyes. Two of the pioneer investigators in this field, Miles and Lindsley, proposed the use of lead systems; however, Miles (1939) applied periorbital nasal and temporal electrodes around each eye to record horizontal movements only. Leads 1 and 2 detected the horizontal component of the EOG for the left and right eye, respectively; lead 3 identified the bitemporal (eyes-in-series) electrode pair, lead 4 was recorded between the two nasal electrodes, and lead 5 designated the connection for both eyes in parallel. Lindsley and Hunter (1939) employed lead 1 to designate nasal and temporal electrodes about the right eye, lead 2 to identify the supra- and infraorbital electrodes of the right eye, lead 3 to specify the bitemporal electrode array, and lead 4 to identify a right eye oblique lead employing supraorbital and nasal electrode sites.

Since electrodes are almost always placed lateral to and above and below the eyes to detect horizontal and vertical displacements, it would seem appropriate to create a simple, easily remembered terminology to simplify communication among investigators in this rapidly expanding field. For example, using V and H to designate vertical and horizontal electrodes (hence, eye-movement direction), and L and R as subscripts referring to left and right eyes, the following simple notation may be of assistance; it can be extended readily to designate other less-used electrode arrangements. For example, H_{R+L} would signify addition of the horizontal components of the EOG for both eyes; likewise, H_{R-L} would indicate subtraction of these two signals. Similarly, H_{RLP} could mean the parallel connection of the horizontal electrodes about each eye. Likewise, V_{R+L}, V_{R-L}, and V_{RLP} are designations for the series-aiding, opposing, and parallel connections of the vertical electrodes about the eyes.

ELECTRORETINOGRAPHY

Electroretinography is the study of the potential of the retina of the eye when illuminated. In the dark a standing measurable potential exists across the various layers of the retina. When the retina is illuminated, cyclic changes occur in this potential, a recording of which constitutes the electroretinogram (ERG). Although the bioelectric generators responsible for the phenomenon lie within the various layers of the retina, the ERG can be recorded by placing one electrode on the cornea and the other at the back (fundus) of the eye or at a distance on the surface of the body. Sometimes the reference (body-surface) electrode is placed over the mastoid process, occasionally on the forehead or cheek. The various types of corneal electrodes were described by Sundmark (1959). Figure 87 shows several types that have been used; one of these, the "contact glass" electrode described by Riggs (1941) and Karpe (1945), saw extensive clinical service. Sundmark (1959) presented quantitative data for the optimum design for such electrodes. At present, a contact lens is used to carry the corneal electrode, which often incorporates a chlorided silver wire, a substance that can exhibit its own photoelectric effect (see Chap. 9). Usually a short-acting anesthetic is applied to the cornea to eliminate irritation in response to application of the electrode.

The ERG of the human and animal eye is by no means a simple bioelectric event. Although it arises in the retina, the eye is a complex structure, consisting of photosensitive receptors (rods and cones), nerve cells, and pigment cells, all of which can exhibit bioelectric phenomena. Each human retina has about 120 million rods, 7 million cones, and four types of nerve cells (bipolar, ganglion, horizontal, and amacrine), along with pigment and glial cells. Animals with excellent night (scotopic) vision have retinas dominated by rods (previously designated E retinas); others that see poorly in the dark but well in daylight (photopic vision) have retinas dominated by cones (previously designated I retinas). Most animals, including humans, have mixed retinas.

The type of ERG recorded with one electrode on the cornea and one on the surface of the body depends on many factors; perhaps the most important relates to the environmental conditions (i.e., whether the eye has been light- or dark-adapted). A typical ERG obtained in response to a 2-sec burst of high-level illumination of the retina with white light is shown in Fig. 88. The letter designations (a, b, c) for three of the four waves were provided by Einthoven and Jolly (1908). In the vertebrate eye, retinal illumination causes the corneofundal potential to first decrease slightly (a wave); then it exhibits a marked increase, which describes the prominent b wave. The combination is often designated the "on effect." With sustained illumination of the retina, the potential falls and then rises slowly to describe the c wave. When the illumination is removed, a d wave or "off effect"

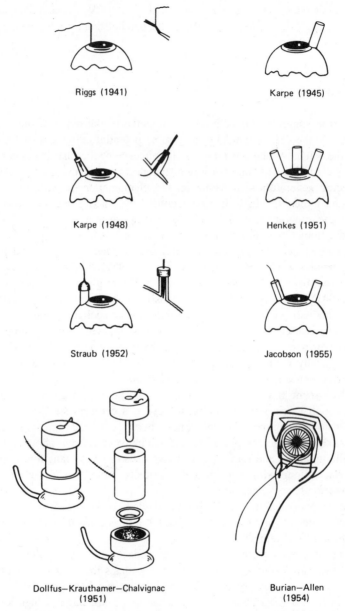

Riggs (1941)

Karpe (1945)

Karpe (1948)

Henkes (1951)

Straub (1952)

Jacobson (1955)

Dollfus–Krauthamer–Chalvignac
(1951)

Burian–Allen
(1954)

Figure 87   Various types of corneal electrodes used to detect the electroretinogram. [From E. Sundmark, *Acta Ophthalmol.* **37**:8–40 (1959). By permission.]

is frequently recorded. The relative magnitudes of these waves depend on the illumination intensity, the degree of light or dark adaptation, and the type of retina. In response to a brief flash (~ 50 msec) of light, only the a and b waves are recordable.

Granit (1962) presented a most comprehensive description of the ERG for dark-

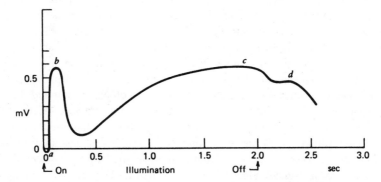

Figure 88   Typical human electroretinogram in response to a long-duration (2-sec) light stimulus of high intensity. (Redrawn from M. Sosonow and E. Ross, *Electrodes for Recording Primary Bioelectric Signals*, ASD Tech. Rept. 61-437 (1961). USAF Wright-Patterson AFB, OH.)

and light-adapted cone- and rod-dominated retinas; Fig. 89 is his illustration. From numerous experimental techniques that used light and dark adaptation, variation of light intensity, color and duration, anesthesia, hypoxia, and drugs, it has been possible to show that the complex cornea–body surface photobioelectric potential is made up of at least three components designated PI, PII, and PIII, which reflect

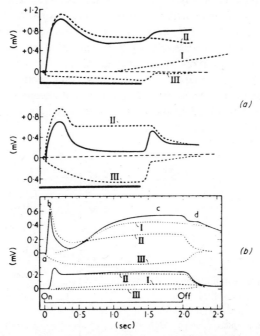

Figure 89   (*a*) The I (cone) electroretinogram of dark-adapted (upper) and light-adapted (lower) eyes. (*b*) The E (rod) electroretinogram in response to two intensities (upper, 14; lower, 0.14 mL). The PI, PII, and III, components appear as dashed curves. [From R. Granit, in *The Eye*. H. Davson (ed.). Academic Press, New York, 1962. By permission.]

different slow and fast retinal processes. Readers interested in pursuing study of the meanings of these components are directed to Granit's review (1962).

As stated earlier, the ERG is often recorded in response to a short-duration (~ 50 msec or less) stimulus, and in this situation only the a and b waves are obtained. It was also stated that most retinas contain two types of photoreceptors, rods and cones; the former are receptors for night (scotopic) vision and the latter for day (photopic) vision. Each type of receptor has a different spectral sensitivity, the rods being primarily blue-green-sensitive and the cones being primarily orange-red-sensitive. Adrian (1945) presented an excellent study demonstrating the separate ERGs of the rods and cones. Using himself as the subject, he recorded the ERG using a corneal–cheek electrode array. Single flashes (25 msec) of light of different colors were used to illuminate the retina, which was first light-adapted and then dark-adapted. Adrian's results (Fig. 90) indicate that in the light-adapted eye, which yields a cone-dominated response, the ERG was maximum for orange-red light and no response was obtained for blue light. In the dark-adapted eye, which yields a rod-dominated response, the ERG was maximum for blue-green light, and the smallest amplitude was obtained for deep red light. Note that the amplitudes and time courses of the ERGs for light- and dark-adapted eyes are different.

The degree of contribution of each of the retinal cell types in the genesis of the ERG is by no means settled. There is agreement that the photoreceptors (rods and cones) and the bipolar cells play important roles. It is therefore apparent that since the presence of an ERG is indicative of a functioning retina, the ERG ought to be of value as a diagnostic tool. However, before discussing this topic, a few comments are in order regarding the manner in which visual information reaches the cortex where light and form are discriminated.

As stated previously, the retina of a human eye contains about 120 million rods and 7 million cones; thus there are 127 million photoreceptors. These receptors are complexly interconnected in the retina and synapse, first with bipolar cells,

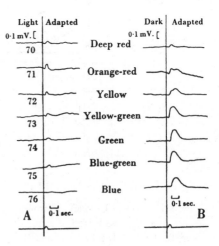

Figure 90 The electroretinograms of humans in response to single flashes of light of various colors presented to the (A) light-adapted and (B) dark-adapted eye. Bottom tracings show the duration of the flash of light. [From E. D. Adrian, *J. Physiol.* **104**:84–104 (1945). By permission.]

then ganglion cells. Axons of the ganglion cells exit the globe and constitute the optic nerve, which contains only about a million fibers. Most of the fibers of the optic nerve synapse again with neurons in the geniculate nucleus of the thalamus. Fibers arising from this structure project to the visual (occipital) cortex, the primary processing area for visual information. How, in the presence of more receptors than centrally communicating pathways, visual acuity is so good, remains a mystery.

Despite the close linkage of the ERG with the visual process and despite the ease of recording the ERG in the human, clinical use of the ERG for diagnosis is slow to emerge, and several studies have been carried out to demonstrate its clinical usefulness. For example, Sachs (1929) found that the ERG amplitude was smaller in response to red-light stimulation in subjects who are color-blind to red light (protanopes). Karpe (1945) conducted a carefully controlled study of the ERG in patients with known visual defects. The technique employed a bright flash of light, about 40 msec in duration, and recorded the ERGs from dark-adapted eyes using a saline-filled cup (contact glass) electrode paired with one on the forehead. With this technique he found a reduced ERG amplitude in subjects with diseases that affected the rods. He also reported that a difference in ERG amplitude greater than 25% between the eyes is indicative of retinal pathology; a difference of 10% is within normal limits. According to Ito (1973), the ERG amplitude is remarkably decreased in subjects with retinal pigment degeneration and with retinal detachment. He stated that the ERG is often recorded before and after the surgical removal of congenital cataracts to confirm retinal function.

Perhaps the clinical use of the ERG is limited because applying the technique to the human subject is time-consuming and not without some risk to the subject since it is necessary to desensitize the cornea by the topical application of an anesthetic and the protective reflex is temporarily depressed. Because the retina can be examined visually with an ophthalmoscope, the changes produced by disease are often quite obvious to the trained observer. Moreover, the subject can be interrogated, and the history often provides the necessary diagnostic information.

MAGNETOGRAPHY

Magnetography is the term used to describe a recording of the magnetic field that accompanies a bioelectric event. The movement of electric charge gives rise to a magnetic field. During excitation (depolarization) and recovery (repolarization) in excitable tissue there is a translocation of ions across cell membranes. This charge movement gives rise to a magnetic field that can be detected with suitable equipment. Because electrograms, i.e., recordings of bioelectric events, and magnetograms have a common origin, they reflect the same event. However, each provides a different type of information. Because magnetic fields pass freely through living tissue, there is little attenuation of the magnetic field produced by active and recovering tissue. With skin-surface electrodes, the voltage detected is a highly attenuated (and modified) version of the bioelectric event. Importantly, the location of an active bioelectric source can be specified because the magnetic field is directional. There is no need for contact with the body to record magnetograms; therefore, the method can be called electrodeless recording. However, the magnetic fields produced by excitable tissues are very small; Fig. 91 presents a summary of intensity versus frequency spectrum of a variety of biomagnetic signals. Because of the low intensity, it is often necessary to use magnetic shielding and/or signal averaging to obtain an adequate signal-to-noise ratio. Prior to the early 1970s the magnetic fields produced by active and recovering tissues were measured by the voltage induced in a search coil of very many turns. With such a detector, the magnetogram resembles the first derivative of the bioelectric event. In the early 1970s, the superconducting quantum interference device (SQUID), which has the ability to detect very feeble magnetic fields, became available (see review by Doyle, 1971). This device, which soon was produced commercially, became the standard tool for investigating biomagnetic fields. Use of the SQUID and signal averaging to enhance the signal-to-noise ratio makes it possible to display very clean magnetograms.

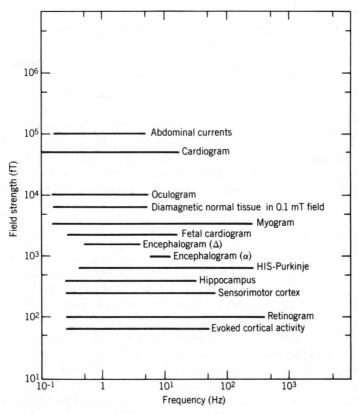

Figure 91   Field strength versus frequency spectrum of biomagnetic events. [Redrawn from G. R. Romani et al. *Rev. Sci. Instrum.* **53**(12):1815–1845 (1982).]

Magnetograms from isolated frog nerve were recorded by Seipel and Morrow (1950), who used a 3000-turn coil of fine wire; the coil measured 2 mm × 3 mm × 6 mm. With the coil placed alongside a stimulated, isolated sciatic nerve, the magnetic field of the action potential was recorded. Stratbucker et al. (1963) measured the changing magnetic field associated with the beating of an isolated guinea pig heart by recording the voltage induced in a coil of 17,640 turns wrapped on a toroid that was concentric with the heart located in a volume conductor. The voltage induced in the coil resembled the first time derivative of the ECG, which was detected by apex–base electrodes in the volume conductor. The human mangeto-cardiogram was recorded by Baule (1965) and Baule and McFee (1963, 1970), who introduced the parallel-coil technique (Fig. 92a) that was employed by many later workers. The coils used by Baule were 30 cm long and 9 cm in diameter and were placed normal to the thorax. Each coil contained 1 million turns wound on a ferrite core. The coils were connected in series and provided a peak voltage (~ 30 μV) proportional to the rate of change of the magnetic field (Fig. 92b). Safonov et al. (1967) employed a similar technique, except that they placed the detector and subject in a magnetically shielded iron enclosure with walls 1.5 in. thick. Cohen (1967a, b) described an improved magnetically shielded enclosure for magnetography that employed Molypermalloy. A layer of aluminum 0.19 in. thick was applied to the inner shell. The cubical housing measured 86 in. × 88 in. × 88 in. Subjects from whom magnetograms were to be recorded were placed in this enclosure. The magnetic detector comprised several coils (each 200,000 turns, 5 cm long and 8 cm in diameter) placed on a ferrite core and covered with a brass cylinder to provide electrostatic shielding. The detector was mounted securely in front of the thorax of the subject. With an overall bandwidth extending to 30 Hz, quite acceptable magnetocardiograms were recorded.

SQUID. In 1962, Brian Josephson, then a graduate student at Cambridge University, predicted that if two superconductors were weakly coupled, current would flow between them without any external potential being applied. He also stated that if a bias were applied to the junction, an alternating current would be developed having a frequency proportional to the bias level. Within a year his prediction was verified, and the device is now called the Josephson junction. When used to detect a magnetic field it is called a SQUID (superconducting quantum interference device).

The simplest configuration of the SQUID consists of a ring of superconducting material (e.g., niobium) in which there is a weak link that constitutes the junction (typically an oxide layer). The superconducting property is achieved by operation at very low temperature (e.g., 4 K). Figure 93 illustrates the voltage–current (V–I) curve of a typical junction. The voltage for the current transitions depends on Planck's constant and the charge on an electron. The no-voltage current I_c depends on the strength of the magnetic field (ϕ) presented to the device.

There are many methods for using the Josephson junction to detect a feeble magnetic field; however, the two illustrated in Fig. 94 are typical. In Fig. 94a, two junctions are biased with direct current; Fig. 94b, radiofrequency bias current,

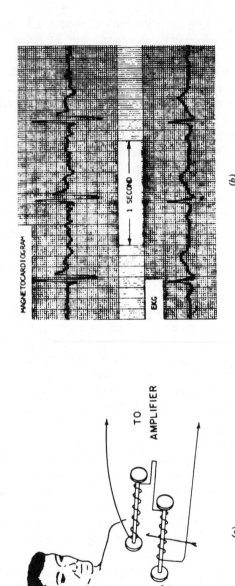

(a)

(b)

Figure 92 (a) Method first employed to detect the magnetic component of the cardiac action potential; (b) magnetocardiogram and electrocardiogram. Each of the two pickup coils consisted of 2 million turns of wire wound on a dumbbell-shaped ferrite core about 1 ft long. [From G. Baule and R. McFee, *Am. Heart J.* **66**:95–96 (1963). By permission.]

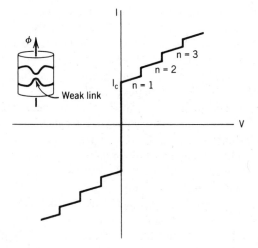

Figure 93   The Josephson junction, represented as a ring with a weak link and the current–voltage (I–V) characteristic. ϕ is the magnetic field. [Redrawn from O. Doyle, *Electronics* **49**(5):33–42 (1971).]

typically 20 MHz, is used. These bias currents are applied by appropriately designed feedback circuits that use the unprocessed SQUID output as inputs. The signal proportional to magnetic field strength is derived from the voltage across a resistor in the feedback circuit.

In a practical embodiment, the coil that senses the magnetic field is coupled to

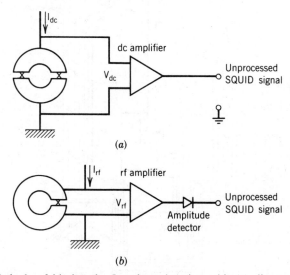

Figure 94   Methods of biasing the Josephson junction with (*a*) direct current and (*b*) radiofrequency current.

the SQUID, and the whole assembly is submerged in liquid helium contained in a Dewar flask that is magnetically, electrically, and thermally shielded. Figure 95 is a cutaway view of one model. A variety of detecting coils are available for special purposes. The detecting coil and the coupling transformer are made of superconducting materials. It is the lower part of the assembly containing the detecting coil that is placed over the biomagnetic source.

Cohen was one of the first to use the SQUID for magnetography (Cohen et al., 1971; Cohen, 1972). Using it with a subject in a magnetically shielded room, he first recorded the magnetoencephalogram of humans (Fig. 96). He then used the same equipment to obtain magnetocardiograms of dogs during experimental myocardial infarction created by inflating a cuff around a coronary artery branch. With an effective bandwidth of 0–40 Hz, control and infarction MCGs were obtained. Figure 97 is a typical example of the canine MCG before and after producing the infarct by occlusion of the left anterior descending coronary artery. Note the change that resembles the S-T segment shift characteristically seen in the electrocardiogram with myocardial infarction.

Saarinen et al. (1978) recorded the MCG of normal human subjects and provided

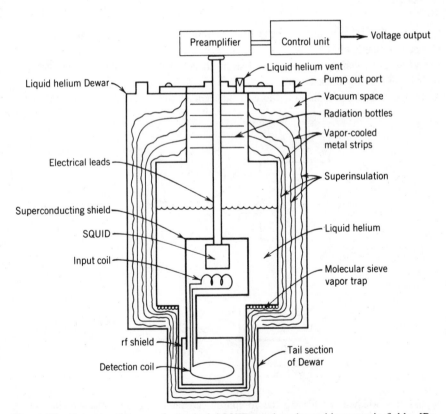

Figure 95 Cutaway diagram of a typical SQUID used to detect biomagnetic fields. [Redrawn from G. R. Romani et al., *Rev. Sci. Instrum.* **53**(12):1815–1845 (1982).]

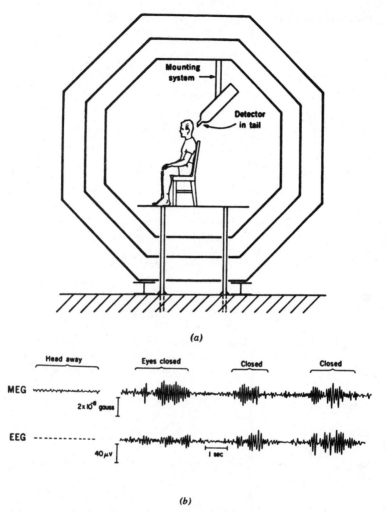

Figure 96 (*a*) Method of obtaining magnetoencephalograms by enclosing a subject in a triply shielded enclosure and using a superconducting magnetometer as a detector. (*b*) Typical magnetoencephalogram (MEG) and electroencephalogram (EEG) from a human subject. [From D. Cohen, *Science* **175**:664–665 (1972). By permission.]

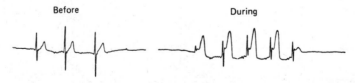

Figure 97 Magnetocardiograms obtained from the dog by use of a superconducting magnetometer placed in front of the chest. The control (before) and during occlusion of the left anterior descending coronary artery are shown. Note that injury is indicated by the equivalent of an S-T segment elevation. This illustration can be compared with the ECG in myocardial infarction shown in Fig. 49. (Courtesy of D. Cohen, Frances Bitter National Magnet Laboratory, Massachusetts Institute of Technology.)

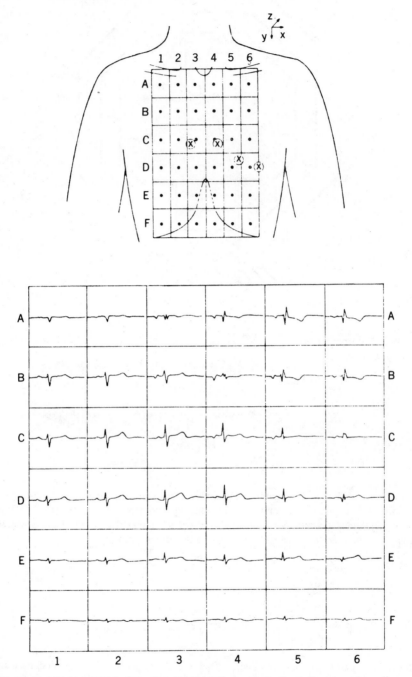

Figure 98 (Top) Frontal-plane sites for recording and (bottom) the magnetocardiograms obtained from these sites. [Redrawn from M. Saarinen et al., *Ann. Clin. Res.* **10:**1–22 (1978).]

a frontal plane map of the amplitudes accorded with the SQUID placed over the thorax; Fig. 98 is a reproduction of their results, showing that the maximum QRS amplitude occurs over the apex-beat area. Typically the MCG field strength is on the order of 50 picotesla (pT).

The first fetal MCG was recorded by Kariniemi et al. (1974); Fig. 99 presents one of their recordings, which also shows the maternal ECG. To make this record, the patient was taken to a nearby cottage where the magnetic interference was less than in the hospital. Especially noticeable in Fig. 99 is that the maternal (M) and fetal (F) MCGs are oppositely directed. The author reported that it was often possible to obtain the fetal MCG without the maternal MCG. If this turns out to be a frequent occurrence, then the fetal MCG could be of considerable value in monitoring heart rate during labor.

Averaged sensory evoked fields (SEFs) over the left hemisphere due to contra-lateral median nerve stimulation using 1-msec pulses at a rate of 1.9/sec were recorded by Okada et al. (1981). Figure 100 illustrates the responses at different sites over the scalp along and slightly posterior to the Rollandic fissure. The records were made starting at the vertex and moving 1 cm downward. Cortical localization exhibited by the SEF is similar to that for the somatosensory evoked potential.

Averaged auditory evoked magnetograms from humans were reported by Hari et al. (1980), along with the auditory evoked potential. Figure 101a illustrates the auditory evoked potential (AEP) recorded from an electrode at P_z. The auditory evoked field (AEF) was measured at two sites, P_3 and F_7, on the left side of the head. The stimulus consisted of a 1000-Hz tone burst lasting 800 msec presented to both ears. The time between bursts was 4 sec. The magnetograms show three components at 100 and 180 msec and the steady-field (SF) component. The polar-ities for these components were studied at various sites over the right hemisphere; Fig. 101b shows polarities for the three components with a phase reversal along

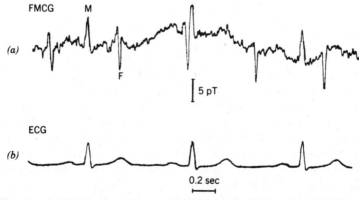

Figure 99   (a) Fetal magnetocardiogram and (b) maternal electrocardiogram. Note that in the fetal MCG, the maternal (M) and fetal (F) ventricular waves are inverted. [Redrawn from V. Kariniemi et al., *Perinat. Med.* **2**:214–216 (1974).]

Contralateral magnetic field

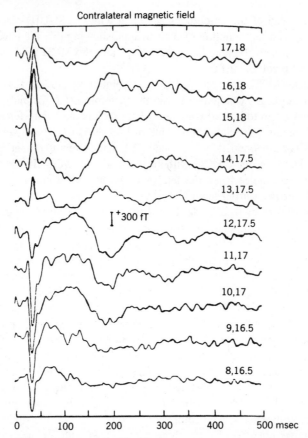

Figure 100   Somatosensory evoked fields (SEFs) from the right hemisphere in response to contralateral median nerve stimulation. The tracings were made along and posterior to the Rollandic fissure at 1-cm increments starting at the vertex. [Redrawn from Y. C. Okada et al., in *Biomagnetism.* S. N. Erne et al. (eds.). de Gruyter, Berlin, 1981.]

the Sylvian fissure; the open circles represent inward fields, and the closed circles represent outward fields. It is clear that although the auditory area lies along the temporal lobe, there are widespread cortical responses as in the case for the auditory evoked potential described earlier in this chapter.

Despite the fact that magnetography has been practical for only about a decade, there is a considerable literature on the subject. Much of this information was presented at a meeting sponsored by NATO and includes basic and applied topics ranging from physiology to technical instrumentation. The proceedings were published in a volume edited by Williamson et al. (1983).

The future of magnetography cannot be predicted at this time. As a research tool, it is extremely useful for its ability to locate active and recovering bioelectric sources, but it is far too soon to predict its value in clinical medicine.

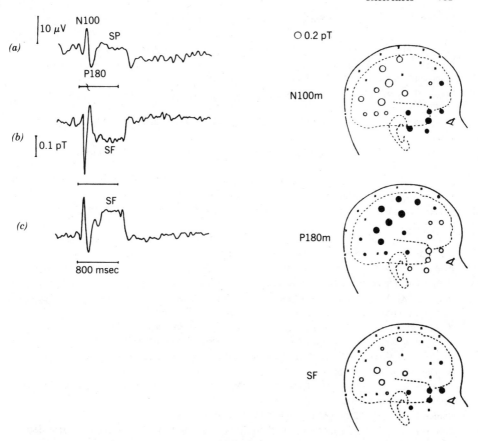

Figure 101 (*a*) Auditory evoked potential (AEP) from F_2; auditory evoked fields (AEFs) from (*b*) P_3 and (*c*) F_7 in response to an 800-msec tone burst of 1 kHz. Diagrams at right show distribution of AEFs over the right hemisphere; the open circles indicate an inward field. [Redrawn from R. Hari et al., *Exp. Brain Res.* **40**:237–240 (1980).]

REFERENCES

Abildskov, J. A., and E. D. Pence. 1956. Comparative study of spatial vectorcardiograms with the equilateral tetrahedron and a corrected system of electrode placement. *Circulation* **13**:263–269.

Adrian, E. D. 1945. The electric response of the human eye. *J. Physiol.* **104**:84–104.

Adrian, R. H. 1956. The effect of external and internal potassium concentration on the membrane potential of frog muscle. *J. Physiol.* **133**:631–658.

Adrian, E. D., and B. H. C. Matthews. 1934. The Berger rhythm: Potential changes from the occipital lobes in man. *Brain* **57**:355–385.

Adrian, E. D., and K. Yamagiwa. 1935. The origin of the Berger rhythm. *Brain* **55**:323–351.

Arrighi, F. P. 1939. El eje electrico del corazon en el espacio. *Prensa Med. Argent.* **26**:253–283.

Baule, G. M. 1965. Instrumentation for measuring the heart's magnetic field. *Trans. N. Y. Acad. Sci.* **27**:689–700.

Baule, G. M., and R. McFee. 1963. Detection of the magnetic field of the heart. *Am. Heart J.* **66**:95–96.

Baule, G. M., and R. McFee. 1970. The magnetic heart vector. *Am. Heart J.* **79**:223–236.

Bennett, A. L., F. Ware, A. L. Dunn, and A. R. McIntyre. 1953. The normal membrane resting potential of mammalian skeletal muscle measured *in vivo*. *J. Cell. Comp. Physiol.* **42**:343–357.

Berger, H. 1929. Über das Elektronkephalogramn des Menschen. *Arch. Psychiatr. Nervenkr.* **87**:527–570.

Berger, H. 1967. On the electroencephalogram of man. (trans. by P. Gloor). *EEG Clin. Neurophysiol.*, *Suppl.* **28**:1–350.

Bickford, R. G. 1950. Automatic electroencephalographic control of general anesthesia. *EEG Clin. Neurophysiol.* **2**:93–96.

Bickford, R. G., T. W., Billinger, N. I. Fleming, and L. Stewart. 1972. The compressed spectral array (CSA)—A pictorial EEG. *Proc. San Diego Biomed. Symp.*

Brazier, M. A. B. 1949. A study of the electric fields at the surface of the head. *EEG Clin. Neurophysiol.* **2** (Suppl.):38–52.

Brechner, V. L., R. D. Walter, and J. B. Dillon. 1962. *Practical Electroencephalography for the Anesthesiologist*. Thomas, Springfield, IL, 107 pp.

Brody, D. A. 1957. An analysis of the plane and spatial electrocardiographic indices of normal subjects as referred to an orthogonalized lead system. *Am. Heart J.* **53**:125–131.

Brody, D. A., J. C. Bradshaw, and J. W. Evans. 1961. A basis for determining heart lead relations of the equivalent cardiac multipole. *IRE Trans. Bio-Med. Electron.* **BME-8**:139–143.

Buchtal, F., C. Guld, and P. Rosenflack. 1954. Action potential parameters in normal human muscle and their dependence on physical variables. *Acta Physiol. Scand.* **32**:200–229.

Burch, G., J. A. Abildskov, and J. A. Cronvitch. 1953. *Spatial Vectorcardiography*. Lea & Febiger, Philadelphia, PA, 173 pp.

Burdon-Sanderson, J., and F. J. M. Page, 1879. On the time relations of the excitatory process in the ventricle of the heart of the frog. *J. Physiol.* **2**:384–435.

Burger, H. C., and J. B. van Milaan. 1946. Heart vector and leads. *Br. Heart J.* **8**:157–161.

Burger, H. C., and J. B. van Milaan. 1947. Heart vector and leads. Part II. *Br. Heart J.* **9**:154–160.

Burger, H. C., J. B. van Milaan, and W. Klip. 1956. Comparison of two systems of vectorcardiography with an electrode to the frontal and dorsal sides of the trunk respectively. *Am. Heart J.* **51**:26–33.

Byford, G. H. 1963. Non-linear relations between the corneo-retinal potential and horizontal eye movements. *J. Physiol.* **168**:14P–15P.

Caton, R. 1875. The electric currents of the brain. *Br. Med. J.* **2**:278.

Caton, R. 1887. Researches on the electrical phenomena of cerebral gray matter. *Trans. 9th Int Med. Congr.* **3**:247–249.

Clark, J., and R. Plonsey. 1966. A mathematical evaluation of the core conductor model. *Biophys. J.* **6**:95–112.

Clark, J., and R. Plonsey. 1968. The extracellular potential field of the single active nerve fiber in a volume conductor. *Biophys. J.* **8**:842–864.

Cohen, D. 1967a. A shielded facility for low-level magnetic measurements. *J. Appl. Phys.* **38**:1295–1296.

Cohen, D. 1967b. Magnetic fields around the torso: Production by electrical activity of the human heart. *Science* **156**:652–654.

Cohen, D. 1968. Magnetoencephalography: Evidence of magnetic fields produced by alpha-rhythm currents. *Science* **161**:764–786.

Cohen, D. 1972. Magnetoencephalography. *Science* **175**:664–666.

Cohen, D., and L. Chandler. 1969. Measurements and a simplified interpretation of magnetocardiograms from humans. *Circulation* **39**:395–402.

Cohen, D., and D. McCaughan. 1972. Magnetocardiograms and their variation over the chest in normal subjects. *Am. J. Cardiol.* **29:**678-685.

Cohen, D., J. C. Normann, F. Molokhia, and W. Hood. 1971. Magnetocardiography of direct currents: S-T segment and baseline shifts during experimental myocardial infarction. *Science* **172:**1329-1332.

Cohn, R. 1949. *Clinical Electroencephalography.* McGraw-Hill, New York, 639 pp.

Cole, K. S. 1933. Electrical conductance of biological systems. *Cold Spring Harbor Symp. Quant. Biol.* **1:**107-116.

Coombs, J. S., J. C. Eccles, and P. Fatt. 1955. The electrical properties of the motoneurone membrane. *J. Physiol.* **130:**291-325.

Craib, W. H. 1927. A study of the electrical field surrounding active heart muscle. *Heart* **14:**71-109.

Darrow, C. W. 1934. Quantitative records of cutaneous secretory reactions. The significance of skin resistances in the light of its relation to the amount of perspiration. *J. Gen. Psychol.* **11:**435.

Darrow, C. W. 1964. The rationale for treating the change in galvanic skin resistance response as a change in conductance. *Psychophysiology.* **1:**31-38.

Dawson, G. D. 1951. A summation technique for detecting small signals in a large irregular background. *J. Physiol.* **115:**2P-3P.

Dawson, G. D. 1954. A summation technique for the detections of small evoked potentials. *EEG Clin. Neurophysiol.* **6:**65-84.

Denny-Brown, D. 1949. Interpretation of the electromyogram. *Arch. Neurol. Psychiatry* **61:**99-128.

Dewar, J. 1877. The physiological action of light. *Nature* **15:**433-435.

Dewar, J., and J. G. M'Kendrick. 1876. On the physiological action of light. *Trans. R. Soc. Edinburgh* **27:**141-166.

Donders, F. C. 1872. De secondaire contracties onder den involed der systolen van het hart, met en zonder vagus-prikkfung. *Utrecht Rijksuniv. Phys. Lab. Onder Zoekinjen* **1** (Suppl. 3):246-255.

Doyle, O. 1971. Josephson junctions leave the lab—But only a few at a time. *Electronics* **44:**38-45.

Draper, M. H., and S. Weidmann. 1951. Cardiac resting and action potentials recorded with an intracellular electrode. *J. Physiol.* **115:**74-94.

du Bois-Reymond, E. R. 1849. Utersuchungen über Thierische Electrizität. G. Reimer, Berlin.

Duchosal, P., and J. R. Grosgurin. 1952. The spatial vectorcardiogram obtained by use of a trihedron and its scalar comparisons. *Circulation* **5:**237-248.

Duchosal, P. W., and R. Sulzer. 1949. *La Vectorcardiographie.* Karger, Basle, Switzerland and New York, 172 pp.

Durnstock, G., M. E. Holman, and C. L. Prosser. 1963. Electrophysiology of smooth muscle. *Physiol. Rev.* **43:**482-528.

Eccles, R. M. 1955. Intracellular potentials recorded from a mammalian sympathetic ganglion. *J. Physiol.* **130:**572-584.

Edelberg, R. 1967. Electrical Properties of the Skin. In *Methods in Psychophysiology.* C. Brown (ed.). Williams & Wilkins, Baltimore, MD.

Edelberg, R. 1968. Biopotentials from the skin surface: The hydration effect. *Ann. N. Y. Acad. Sci.* **148:**252-262.

Edelberg, R. 1972. Electrical activity of the skin. In *Handbook of Psychophysiology.* N. S. Greenfield and R. D. Sternback (eds.). Holt, Rinehart & Winston, New York.

Edelberg, R. 1974. Personal communication.

Edelberg, R., and N. R. Burch. 1962. Skin resistance and galvanic skin response. *Arch. Gen. Psychiatry* **7:**163-169.

Edelberg, R., T. Greiner, and N. R. Burch. 1960. Some membrane properties of the effector in the galvanic skin response. *J. Appl. Physiol.* **15:**691-696.

Einthoven, W. 1903. Ein neues Galvanometer. *Ann. Phys.* **4** (Suppl.):1059-1071.

784 The Bioelectric Events

Einthoven, W., and W. A. Jolly. 1908. The form and magnitude of the electrical response of the eye to stimulation by light at various intensities. *Q. J. Exp. Physiol.* **1**:373–416.

Einthoven, W., G. Fahr, and A. de Waart. 1913. Über die Richtung und die manifeste Grosse der Potentialschwankungen in menschlichen Herzen und über den Einfluss der Herzlage auf die Form des Elektrokardiogramms. *Arch. Gesamte Physiol.* **150**:275–315.

Einthoven, W., G. Fahr, and A. de Waart. 1950. On the direction and manifest size of the variations of potential in the human heart and on the influence of the position of the heart on the form of the electrocardiogram. Translated by H. E. Hoff and P. Sekeli. *Am. Heart J.* **40**:163–211.

Faulconer, A., and R. G. Bickford. 1960. *Electroencephalography in Anesthesiology.* Thomas, Springfield, IL, 90 pp.

Fenn, W. O., and J. B. Hursh. 1937. Movements of the eyes when the lids are closed. *Am. J. Physiol.* **118**:8–14.

Féré, C. 1888. Note sur des modifications de la résistance électrique sous l'influence des excitations sensorielles et des émotions. *C. R. Soc. Biol.* **40**:217–218.

Flaherty, J. T., M. S. Spach, J. P. Bonneau, R. V. Canent, R. C. Barr, and D. C. Sabiston. 1967. Cardiac potentials on body surface of infants with anomalous left coronary artery (myocardial infarction). *Circulation* **36**:345–358.

Forbes, T. W. 1936. Skin potential and impedance responses with recurring shock stimulation. *Am. J. Physiol.* **117**:189–199.

Fowles, D. C., and P. H. Venables. 1970. The reduction of palmar skin potential by epidermal hydration. *Psychophysiology* **7**:254–261.

Frank, E. 1953a. Theoretical analysis of the influence of heart dipole eccentricity on limb leads, Wilson central-terminal voltage and the frontal plane vectorcardiogram. *Circ. Res.* **1**:380–388.

Frank, E. 1953b. A comparative analysis of the eccentric double-layer presentation of the human heart. *Am. Heart J.* **46**:364–378.

Frank, E. 1954. A direct experimental study of three systems of spatial vectorcardiography *Circulation* **10**:101–113.

Frank, E. 1955. Absolute quantitative comparison of instantaneous QRS equipotentials on a normal subject with dipole potentials on a homogeneous torso model. *Circ. Res.* **3**:243–251.

Frank, E. 1956. An accurate, clinically practical system for spatial vectorcardiography. *Circulation* **13**:737–749.

Frank, E. 1956–1957. Spread of current in volume conductors of finite extent. *Ann. N.Y. Acad. Sci.* **65**:980–1002.

Freygang, W. H., and K. Frank. 1959. Extracellular potentials from single spinal motoneurones. *J. Gen. Physiol.* **42**:749–759.

Fritsch, G., and E. Hitzig. 1870. Ueber die elektrische Erregbarkheit des Grosshirns. *Arch. Anat., Physiol. Wiss. Med.* **37**:300.

Garceau, E. L., and T. W. Forbes. 1934. A direct coupled amplifier for action currents. *Rev. Sci. Instrum.* **5**:10–13.

Geddes, L. A. 1987. What did Caton see? *EEG Clin. Neurophysiol.* (in press).

Geddes, L. A., H. E. Hoff, D. M. Hickman, and A. G. Moore. 1960a. Exercising subjects. *J. Appl. Physiol.* **15**(2):311–312.

Geddes, L. A., M. Partridge, and H. E. Hoff. 1960b. An EKG lead for exercising subjects. *J. Appl. Physiol.* **15**:311–312.

Geddes, L. A., H. E. Hoff, D. M. Hickman, M. Hinds, and L. Baker. 1962. Recording respiration and the electrocardiogram with common electrodes. *Aerosp. Med.* **33**:791–793.

Geddes, L. A., J. D. Bourland, G. Wise, and R. Steinberg. 1973. Linearity of the horizontal component of the electro-oculogram. *Med. Biol. Eng.* **11**(1):73–77.

Geddes, L. A., J. D. Bourland, R. W. Smalling, and R. B. Steinberg. 1974. Recording skin resistance and beat-by-beat heart rate from the same pair of dry electrodes. *Psychophysiology* **11**:394–397.

Geselowitz, D. B. 1960. Multipole representation for an equivalent cardiac generator. *Proc. IRE* **48**:75–79.

Geselowitz, D. B. 1966. Comment on the core conductor model. *Biophys. J.* **6**:691–692.

Gibbs, F. A., and E. L. Gibbs. 1950. *Atlas of Electroencephalography*, Vols. 1 and 2. Wesley Press, Cambridge, MA.

Gibbs, F. A., and E. L. Gibbs. 1964. *Atlas of Electroencephalography*, Vol. 3. Wesley Press, Cambridge, MA.

Gloor, P. 1967. Trans. of Berger's papers. *EEG. Clin. Neurophysiol., Suppl.* **28**:1–350.

Gloor, P. 1969. Hans Berger; on the electroencephalogram of man. *EEG Clin. Neurophysiol., Suppl.* **28**.

Goldberg, H. 1944. Bioelectric-research apparatus. *Proc. IRE* **32**:330–336.

Goldberger, E. 1953. *Unipolar Lead Electrocardiography and Vectorcardiography*. Lea & Febiger, Philadelphia, PA, 601 pp.

Granit, R. 1962. Neurophysiology of the retina. In *The Eye*, Vol. 2. H. Davson (ed.). Academic Press, New York.

Grant, R. P. 1957. *Clinical Electrocardiography—The Spatial Vector Approach*. McGraw-Hill, New York, 225 pp.

Grant, R. P., and E. H. Estes. 1951. *Spatial Vector Electrocardiography*. Blakiston Co., Philadelphia, PA, 145 pp.

Grishman, A. 1952. *Spatial Vectorcardiography*. Saunders, Philadelphia, PA, 217 pp.

Grishman, A., E. R. Borun, and H. L. Jaffe. 1951. Spatial vectorcardiography. *Am. Heart J.* **41**:483–493.

Grundfest, H. 1947. Bioelectric potentials in the nervous system and in muscle. *Annu. Rev. Physiol.* **9**:477–506.

Grundfest, H. 1966a. Comparative electrobiology of excitable membranes. *Adv. Comp. Physiol. Biochem.* **2**:1–116.

Grundfest, H. 1966b. Heterogeneity of excitable membranes: electrophysiological and pharmacological evidence and some consequences. *Ann. N. Y. Acad. Sci.* **137**:901–949.

Gualtierotti, T., and A. S. Paterson. 1954. Electrical stimulation of the unexposed cerebral cortex. *J. Physiol.* **125**:278–291.

Guntheroth, W. G. 1965. *Pediatric Electrocardiography*. Saunders, Philadelphia, PA, 150 pp.

Hakansson, C. H. 1957. Action potentials recorded intra and extracellularly from the isolated frog muscle fiber in Ringer's solution and in air. *Acta Physiol. Scand.* **39**:291–312.

Halstead, W. C. 1938. A method for the quantitative recording of eye movements. *J. Psychol.* **6**:177–180.

Hari, R., K. Aittoniemi, M. I. Jarvinen, T. Katila, and T. Varpula. 1980. Auditory evoked transient and sustained magnetic fields of the human brain. *Exp. Brain Res.* **40**:237–240.

Hecht, H. H. 1956–1957. Normal and abnormal transmembrane potentials of the spontaneously beating heart. *Ann. N.Y. Acad. Sci.* **65**:700–740.

Helm, R. A. 1957. An accurate lead system for spatial vectorcardiography. *Am. Heart J.* **53**:415–424.

Hermann, L. 1879. Allgemeine Muskelphysik. *Handb. Physiol. Bewegunsapparate* **1**:1–260.

Hill, D., and G. Parr. 1950. *Electroencephalography: A Symposium on Its Various Aspects*. Macdonald & Co., London, 438 pp.

Hill, D., and G. Parr, 1963. *Electroencephalography: A Symposium on Its Various Aspects*. Macmillan, New York, 509 pp.

Hlavin, J. M., and R. Plonsey. 1963. An experimental determination of a multipole representation of a turtle heart. *IEEE Trans. Bio-Med. Electron.* **BME-10**:98–105.

Hodgkin, A. L. 1951. The ionic basis of electrical activity in nerve and muscle. *Biol. Rev. Cambridge Philos. Soc.* **26**:339–409.

Hodgkin, A. L., and P. Horowicz. 1957. The differential action of hypertonic solutions on the twitch and action potential of a muscle fiber. *J. Physiol.* **136:**17P-18P.

Hodgkin, A. L., and A. F. Huxley. 1939. Action potentials recorded from inside a nerve fiber. *Nature* **144:**710-711.

Hoff, H. E., and L. A. Geddes, 1962. *Experimental Physiology,* 2nd ed. Baylor College of Medicine, Houston, TX.

Hoffman, A. C., B. Wellman, and L. Carmichael. 1939. A quantitative comparison of the electrical and photographic techniques of eye-movement recording. *J. Exp. Psychol.* **24:**40-53.

Hoffmann, B. F., and E. E. Suckling. 1953. Cardiac cellular potentials: Effect of vagal stimulation and acetylcholine. *Am. J. Physiol.* **173:**312-320.

Hollmann, H. E., and W. Hollmann. 1938. Das Einthovensche Druckschema als Grudlage neuer elektrokardiograpischen Registriermethoden. *Z. Klin. Med.* **134:**732-753.

Holman, M. E. 1958. Membrane potentials recorded with high resistance micro-electrodes. *J. Physiol.* **141:**464-488.

Holmgren, F. 1865-1866. Method at objektivera effekten of liusintryck po retina. Upsala Lakareforenings Forhanklingar, 1865-1866. *Acta Soc. Med. Ups.* **1:**177-184 (in Swedish).

Holmgren, F. 1870-1871. On the retinal current *Acta Soc. Med. Ups.* **6:**419 (in Swedish).

Horan, L. G., N. C. Flowers, and D. A. Brody. 1963. Body surface potential distribution. *Circ. Res.* **13:**373-387.

Hughes, R. R. 1961. *An Introduction to Electroencephalography.* J. Wright, Bristol, 118 pp.

Huxley, A. F., and R. Stampfli. 1944. Evidence for saltatory conduction in peripheral myelinated nerve fibers. *J. Physiol.* **108:**315-339.

Huxley, A. F., and R. Stampfli. 1951. Direct determination of membrane resting potential and action potential in single myelinated nerve fibers. *J. Physiol.* **112:**476-495.

Ishitoya, J. T. Sakurai, I. Aita, and K. Sasaki. 1965. A new type of spatial vectorcardiograph *Tohoku J. Exp. Med.* **85:**1-8.

Ito, H. 1973. Personal communication.

Jacobson, E. 1930. Electrical measurement of neuromuscular states during mental activity. *Am. J. Physiol.* **95:**694-702.

Jasper, H. H. 1958. International Federation of Societies for Electroencephalography and Clinical Neurophysiology. Appendix IX. The ten-twenty electrode system of the International Federation. *EEG Clin. Neurophysiol.* **10:**371-375.

Jasper, H. H., and G. Ballem. 1949. Unipolar electromyograms of normal and denervated human muscle. *J. Neurophysiol.* **12:**231-244.

Jasper, H. H. and L. Carmichael. 1935. Electric potentials from the intact human brain.

Johnston, D. L. 1947. Electro-encephalograph amplifier. *Wireless Eng.* **24:**237-242.

Kariniemi, V., J. Ahopelto, P. J. Karp, and T. E. Katila. 1974. The fetal magnetocardiogram. *J. Perinat. Med.* **2:**214-216.

Karpe, G. 1945. The basis of clinical electroretinography. *Acta Ophthalmol.* **23**(Suppl. 23-24):1-116.

Katz, B., and R. Miledi. 1965. Propagation of electric activity in motor nerve terminals. *Proc. R. Soc. London, Ser. B* **161:**453-482.

Kerwin, A. J. 1953. The effect of frequency response of electrocardiographs on the form of electrocardiograms and vectorcardiograms. *Circulation* **8:**98-110.

Kiegler, J. 1964. *Electroencephalography in Hospital and General Consulting Practice.* Elsevier, Amsterdam, 180 pp.

Kiloh, L. G., A. J. McComas, and J. W. Osselton. 1972. *Clinical Electroencephalography,* 3rd ed. Butterworth, London, 239 pp.

Koelliker, R. A., and J. Mueller. 1856. Nachweis der negativen Schwankung des Muskelstroms am natürlich sich contrahirenden Muskel. *Verh. Phys.-Med. Ges. Wurzburg* **6:**528-533.

Kohlrausch, A. 1931. Elektrische Erscheinungen am Auge. *Handb. Norm. Pathol. Physiol.* **12**(2):1394–1496.

Kowarzykowic, H., and Z. Kowarzykowic. 1961. *Spatial Vectorcardiography.* Pergamon; Oxford, 254 pp.

Kris, C. 1957. Electrical measurement of eye movement during perception. *Proc. Int. Congr. Psychol., Amsterdam, 1957* pp. 247–249.

Kris, C. 1958. A technique for electrically recording eye position. WADC Tech. Rep. 58–60 (ASTIA Doc. AD 209385). USAF Wright-Patterson AFB, OH, 33 pp.

Kris, C. 1960. Vision: Electro-oculography. In *Medical Physics.* Vol. 3. O. Glasser (ed.). Year Book Publishers, Chicago, IL pp. 692–700.

Kügelberg, E. 1947. Electromyograms in muscular disorders. *J. Neurol., Neurosurg. Psychiatry* **10**:122–136.

Lamb, L. E. 1965. *Electrocardiography and Vectorcardiography.* Saunders, Philadelphia, PA, 1954. 609 pp.

Lambert, E. H. Committee on Instrumentation and Technique of the American Association for Electromyography and Electrodiagnosis. 1954, 11 pp. (Personal communication.)

Landau, W. M. 1951. Comparison of different needle leads in EMG recording from a single site. *EEG Clin. Neurophysiol.* **3**:163–168.

Langner, P. H. 1952. The value of high fidelity electrocardiography using the cathode ray oscillograph and an expanded time scale. *Circulation* **5**:249–256.

Langner, P. H., R. Okada, S. R. Moore, and H. C. Fies. 1958. Comparison of four orthogonal systems of vectorcardiography. *Circulation* **17**:46–54.

Law, T., and R. L. Devalois. 1958. Periorbital potentials recorded during small eye movements. *Pap. Mich. Acad. Sci., Arts Lett.* **43**:171–180.

Leksell, L. 1939. Clinical recording of eye movements. *Acta Chir. Scand.* **82**:262–270.

Levy, W. J., Jr. 1983. Spinal evoked potentials from the motor tracts. *J. Neurosurg.* **58**:38–44.

Levy, W. J., Jr., and D. H. York. 1983. Evoked potentials from the motor tracts in humans. *Neurosurgery* **12**(4):422–429.

Levy, W. J., Jr., M. McCaffrey, D. H. York, and F. Tanzer. 1984a Motor evoked potentials from transcranial stimulation of the motor cortex in cats. *Neurosurgery* **15**(2):214–227.

Levy, W. J., D. H. York, M. McCaffrey, and F. Tanzer. 1984b. Motor evoked potentials from transcranial stimulations of the motor cortex in humans. *Neurosurgery* **15**:287–302.

Lian, C., and V. Golblin. 1936. Intérêt nosographique et pratique de la derivation precordiale auriculaire s 5. *Arch. Mal. Coeur Vaiss.* **29**:721–734.

Liberson, W. T. 1962. Report on the standardization of reporting and terminology in electromyography. *EEG Clin. Neurophysiol.* **22**:107–172.

Licht, S. H. 1961. *Electrodiagnosis and Electromyography.* E. Licht, New Haven, CN, 470 pp.

Lindsley, D. B., and W. S. Hunter. 1939. A note on polarity potentials from the human eye. *Proc. Natl. Acad. Sci. U.S.A.* **25**:180–183.

Lorente de Nó, R. 1947. *A Study of Nerve Physiology* Part 2. Rockefeller Institute, New York, Chap. 16.

Lundervold, A., and C.-L. Li. 1953. Motor units and fibrillation potentials as recorded with different kinds of needle electrodes. *Acta Psychiatr. Neurol. Scand.* **28**:201–212.

Lykken, D. T., and P. H. Venables. 1971. Direct measurement of skin conductance: A proposal for standardizations. *Psychophysiology* **8**:656–672.

Lykken, D. T., R. D. Miller, and R. F. Strahan. 1968. Some properties of skin conductance and potential. *Psychophysiology* **8**:253–268.

Mackensen, C., and S. Harder. 1954. Untersuchunger zur elektrischen Aufzeichnung von Augenbeiwegungen. *Albrecht von Graefes Arch. Ophthalmol.* **155**:397–412.

Macleod, A. G. 1938a. The electrogram of cardiac muscle: An analysis which explains the regression or T deflection. *Am. Heart J.* **15:**165-186.

Macleod, A. G. 1938b. The electrocardiogram of cardiac muscle. *Am. Heart J.* **15:**402-413.

Mann, H. 1920. A method of analyzing the electrocardiogram. *Arch. Intern. Med.* **25:**283-294.

Mann, H. 1938. The monocardiograph. *Am. Heart J.* **15:**681-689.

Marey, E. J. 1876. Des variations electriques des muscles du coeur en particulier étudiées au moyen de l'électromètre de M. Lippmann. *C. R. Hebd. Seances Acad. Sci.* **82:**975-977.

Marg, E. 1951. Development of electro-oculography. *Arch. Ophthalmol.* **45:**169-185.

Marg, E., and G. G. Heath. 1955. Localized electroretinograms from isolated poikilothermic retinas. *Science* **122:**1234-1235.

Marinacci, A. A. 1965. *Clinical Electromyography.* San Lucas Press, Los Angeles, CA, 199 pp.

Marsden, C. D., P. A. Merton, and H. B. Morton. 1980. Maximal twitches from stimulation of the motor cortex in man. *J. Physiol.* **312:**5P.

Marsden, C. D., P. A. Merton, and H. B. Morton. 1982. Percutaneous stimulation of spinal cord and brain. *J. Physiol.* **328:**6P.

Marsden, C. D., P. A. Merton, and H. B. Morton. 1983. Direct electrical stimulation of corticospinal pathways through the intact scalp in human subjects. In *Control Mechanisms in Health and Disease.* J. E. Desmedt (ed.), Raven Press, New York.

Matthews, B. H. C. 1934. A special purpose amplifier. *J. Physiol.* **81:**28-29.

Maulsby, R., and R. Edelberg. 1960. The interrelationship between the galvanic skin response, basal resistance and temperature. *J. Comp. Physiol. Psychol.* **53:**475-479.

Mauro, A., L. H. Nahum, R. S. Sikand, and H. Chernoff. 1952. Equipotential distribution for the various instants of the cardiac cycle of the body surface of the dog. *Am. J. Physiol.* **168:**584-591.

Mauro, A., L. H. Nahum, and R. Sikand. 1952-1953. Instantaneous equipotential distribution on the thoracic surface of human subjects with cardiac pathology. *J. Appl. Physiol.* **5:**698-704.

McCaffrey, M., W. J. Levy, and D. York. 1986. The motor evoked potential in acute spinal cord surgery in the cat. *J. Neurosurg.* **19**(2):163-178.

McFee, R., and F. D. Johnston. 1954. Electrocardiographic leads. III. Synthesis. *Circulation* **9:**868-880.

Merton, P. A., and H. B. Morton. 1980a. Electrical stimulation of human motor and visual cortex through the scalp. *J. Physiol.* **305:**9-10P.

Merton, P. A., and H. B. Morton. 1980b. Stimulation of the cerebral cortex in the intact human subject. *Nature* **285:**227.

Merton, P. A., H. B. Morton, D. K. Hill, and C. D. Marsden. 1982. Scope of a technique for electrical stimulation of human brain, spinal cord and muscle. *Lancet* **2:**597-600.

Meyers, I. L. 1929. Electronystagmography. *Arch. Neurol. Psychiatry* **21:**900-918.

Miles, W. R. 1939. The steady polarity potential of the human eye. *Proc. Natl. Acad. Sci. U.S.A.* **25:**25-36.

Morrice, J. K. W. 1956. Slow wave production in the EEG with reference to hyperpnoea, carbon dioxide and autonomic balance. *EEG Clin. Neurophysiol.* **8:**49-72.

Mowrer, G. H., T. C. Ruch, and N. E. Miller. 1935-1936. Corneo-retinal potential differences as basis of galvanometer method of recording eye movements. *Am. J. Physiol.* **114:**423-428.

Murakami, M., K. Watanabe, and T. Tomita. 1961. Effect of impalement with a micropipette *Jpn. J. Physiol.* **11:**80-88.

Nahum, L. H., A. Mauro, H. M. Chernoff, and R. J. Sikand. 1951. Instantaneous equipotential distribution on surface of the human body for various instants in the cardiac cycle. *J. Appl. Physiol.* **3:**454-464.

Nahum, L. H., A. Mauro, H. Levine, and D. G. Abrahams. 1952-1953. Potential field during the S T segment. *J. Appl. Physiol.* **5:**693-697.

Nastuk, W. 1953. The electrical activity of the muscle cell at the myoneural junction. *J. Cell. Comp. Physiol.* **42**:249–272.

Nelson, C. V. 1956. Human thorax potentials. *Ann. N.Y. Acad. Sci.* **65**:1014–1050.

Nelson, C. V., E. T. Angelakos, and P. R. Gastonguay. 1965. Dipole moments of dog, monkey and lamb hearts. *Circ. Res.* **17**:168–177.

Nonogawa, A. 1966. Comparison of five different vectorcardiographic systems. *Jpn. Circ. J.* **30**:1009–1016.

Norris, F. H. 1963. *The EMG.* Grune & Stratton, New York, 134 pp.

North, A. W. 1965. Accuracy and precision of electro-oculographic recording. *Invest. Ophthalmol.* **4**:343–348.

Okada, R. H. 1956. Potentials produced by an eccentric current dipole in a finite-length circular conducting cylinder. *IRE Trans. Bio-Med. Electron.* **BME-7**:14–19.

Okada, R. H. 1957. An experimental study of multiple dipole potentials and the effects of inhomogeneities in volume conductors. *Am. Heart J.* **54**:567–571.

Okada, Y. C., L. Kaufman, D. Brenner, and E. J. Williamsson. 1981. Application of a SQUID to measurements of somatically evoked fields. In S. N. Erne, H. D. Hahlborn, and H. Lubbig (eds.). *Biomagnetism.* de Gruyter, Berlin.

Pardee, H. E. B. 1940. Nomenclature and description of the electrocardiogram. *Am. Heart J.* **29**:1–12.

Pearson, R. B. 1961. *Handbook of Clinical Electromyography.* Meditron Co., El Monte, CA, 72 pp.

Penfield, W., and T. Rasmussen. 1950. *The Cerebral Cortex.* Macmillan, New York. 1950

Petersen, I., and E. Kügelberg. 1949. Duration and form of action potential in the normal human muscle. *J. Neurol., Neurosurg. Psychiatry.* **12**:124–128.

Pfeiffer, E. A. 1968. Electrical stimulation of sensory nerves with skin electrodes for research, diagnosis, communication and behavioral conditioning. A survey. *Med. Biol. Eng. Comput.* **6**:637–651.

Phillips, C. G. 1955. The dimensions of a cortical motor point. *J. Physiol.* **129**:20P–21P.

Picton, T. W. 1974. Evoked cortical potentials, how? what? and why? *Am. J. EEG Technol.* **14**(4):9–44.

Plonsey, R. 1963a. Current dipole images and reference potentials. *IEEE Trans. Bio-Med. Electron.* **BME-10**:1–8.

Plonsey, R. 1963b. Reciprocity applied to volume conductors and the ECG. *IEEE Trans. Bio-Med. Electron.* **BME-10**:9–12.

Plonsey, R. 1969. *Bioelectric Phenomena.* McGraw-Hill, New York.

Pozzi, L. 1961. *Basic Principles in Vector Electrocardiography.* Thomas, Springfield, IL, 292 pp.

Rechtschaffen, A., and A. Kales (eds.). 1968. *A Manual of Standardized Terminology, Techniques and Scoring System for Sleep Stages of Human Subjects,* Nat. Inst. Health Publ. No. 204. U.S. Govt. Printing Office, Washington, D.C.

Remond, A. (ed.). 1971, *Handbook of Electroencephalography and Clinical Neurophysiology,* Vol. 1. Elsevier, Amsterdam.

Richter, C. P. 1927. A study of the electrical skin resistance and the psychogalvanic reflex in a case of unilateral sweating. *Brain* **50**:216–235.

Riggs, L. A. 1941. Continuous and reproducible records of the electrical activity of the human retina. *Proc. Soc. Exp. Biol. Med.* **48**:204–207.

Roberts, N. K. 1975. *The Cardiac Conductive System and His-Bundle Electrogram.* Appleton-Century-Crofts, New York.

Saarinen, M., P. Siltanen, P. J. Karp, and T. F. Katila. 1978. The normal magnetocardiogram I. Morphology. *Ann. Clin. Res.* **10**(Suppl. 21):1–22.

Sachs, E. 1929. Die Aktionsstrome des menschlichen Auges, ihre Beziehung zu Reiz und Empfundung. *Klin. Wochenschr.* **8**:136–137.

Sadove, M. S., D. Becka, and F. A. Gibbs. 1967. *Electroencephalography for Anesthesiologists and Surgeons.* Lippincott, Philadelphia, PA, 95 pp.

Safonov, V. M., V. M. Provotorov, V. M. Lube, and L. I. Yakimenkov. 1967. Method of recording the magnetic field of the heart (magnetocardiography). *Bull. Exp. Biol. Med.* **64:**1022–1024.

Sances, A. D., J. B. Myklebust, S. J. Larson, J. F. Cusick, and R. C. Weber. 1983. The evoked potential. In *Impact Injury of the Head and Spine.* S. J. Larson (ed.). Thomas, Springfield, IL, Chap. 7.

Schellong, F., and E. Schwingel. 1937. Das Vektordiagramm. II. *Z. Kreislaufforsch.* **29:**596–607.

Schellong, F., S. Heller, and E. Schwingel. 1937a. Das Vektordiagramm. 1. *Z. Kreislaufforsch.* **29:**497–509.

Schellong, F. E. Schwingel, and C. Hermann. 1937b. Die praktisch-klinische Methode der Vektordiagraphie und des normale Vektordiagramm. *Arch. Kreislaufforsch.* **1:**1.

Schmitt, O. H. 1937. A simple differential amplifier. *Rev. Sci. Instrum.* **8:**126–127.

Schmitt, O. H., and E. Simonson. 1955. The present status of vectorcardiography. *AMA Arch. Intern. Med.* **96:**574–590.

Schott, E. 1922. Über die Registrierung des Nystagmus und anderer Augenbewegungen vermittels des Saitengalvanometers. *Dtsch. Arch. Klin. Med.* **140:**79–90.

Seipel, J. H., and R. D. Morrow. 1950. The magnetic field accompanying neuronal activity. *J. Wash. Acad. Sci.* **50:**1–4.

Seipel, J. H., and R. D. Morrow. 1960. The magnetic field accompanying neuronal activity. *J. Wash. Acad. Sci.* **50:**1–4.

Shackel, B. 1959. Skin-drilling: A method of diminishing galvanic skin potentials. *Am. J. Psychol.* **72:**114–121.

Shackel, B. 1960. Pilot study in electro-oculography. *Br. J. Ophthalmol.* **44:**89–113.

Shackel, B. 1967. In *A Manual of Psychophysiological Methods.* P. H. Venables and I. Martin (eds.). North-Holland Publ., Amsterdam, pp. 300–334.

Simonson, E. 1952. The distribution of cardiac potentials around the chest in one hundred and three normal men. *Circulation* **6:**201–211.

Simonson, E., O. Schmitt, and H. Nakagawa. 1959. Quantitative comparison of eight vectorcardiographic lead systems. *Circ. Res.* **7:**296–302.

Simpson, J. A. 1973. Electromyography: Neuromuscular diseases. *Handb. EEG Clin. Neurophysiol.* **16B:**5–162.

Spach, M., W. P. Silberg, J. P. Borneau, R. C. Barr, E. C. Long, T. M. Gallie, J. B. Gabor, and A. G. Wallace. 1966. Body surface isopotential maps in normal children. *Am. Heart J.* **72:**640–652.

Stewart, L. 1961. *Introduction to the Principles of Electroencephalography.* Thomas, Springfield, IL, 55 pp.

Stratbucker, R. A., C. M. Hyde, and S. E. Wixson. 1963. The magnetocardiogram—A new approach to the fields surrounding the heart. *IEEE Trans. Bio-Med. Electron.* **BME-10:**145–149.

Straus, H. 1952. *Diagnostic Electroencephalography.* Grune & Stratton. New York, 282 pp.

Sulzer, R., and P. W. Duchosal. 1938. Applications de la planographie. *Arch. Mal. Coeur Vaiss.* **31:**682–685, 686–696.

Sulzer, R., and P. W. Duchosal. 1945. Principes de cardiovectorgraphie. *Cardiologia* **9:**106–120.

Sundmark, E. 1959. The contact glass in human electroretinography. *Acta Ophthalmol.* **37** (Suppl. 52–58):8–40.

Taccardi, B. 1962. Distribution of heart potentials on dog's thoracic surface. *Circ. Res.* **11:**862–869.

Taccardi, B. 1963. Distribution of heart potentials on the thoracic surface of normal human subjects. *Circ. Res.* **12:**341–352.

Tarchanoff, J. 1890. Über die galvanischen Erscheinungen in der Haut der Menschen bei Reizungen der Sinnesorgan und bei verschiedenen Formen der psychischen Thatigkeit. *Arch. Dtsch. Ges. Physiol.* **46:**46–55.

Tasaki, I. 1959. Conduction of the nerve impulse. In *Handbook of Neurophysiology*, Vol. 1. J. Field, H. W. Magvien, and V. E. Hill (eds.). American Physiological Society, Washington, DC, pp. 75–121.

Thomas, P. E., and I. M. Korr. 1957. Relationship between sweat gland activity and electrical resistance of the skin. *J. Appl. Physiol.* **10:**505–510.

Toennies, J. F. 1938. Differential amplifier. *Rev. Sci. Instrum.* **9:**95–97.

Uhley, H. N. 1962. *Vector Electrocardiography.* Lippincott, Philadelphia, PA, 339 pp.

Valentinuzzi, M. E., L. A. Geddes, H. E. Hoff, and J. Bourland. 1970. Properties of the 30° hexaxial (Einthoven-Goldberger) system of vectocardiography. *Cardiovasc. Res. Cent.Bull.* **9:**64–72.

Venables, P. H., and I. Martin. 1967. Skin resistance and skin potential. In *A Manual of Psychophysiological Methods.* P. H. Venables and I. Martin (eds.). North-Holland Publ., Amsterdam.

Waller, A. D. 1887. A demonstration on man of electromotive changes accompanying the heart's beat. *J. Physiol.* **8:**229–234.

Waller, A. D. 1889. On the electromotive changes connected with the beat of the mammalian heart and of the human heart in particular. *Philos. Trans. R. Soc. London, Ser. B.* **180:**169–194.

Walter, W. G. 1936. The location of cerebral tumors by electroencephalography. *Lancet* **2:**305–308.

Wang, G. H. 1957. The galvanic skin reflex: A review of old and recent works from a physiologic point of view. *Am. J. Phys. Med.* **36:**295–320.

Weddell, G., B. Feinstein, and R. E. Prattle. 1943. The clinical application of electromyography. *Lancet* **1:**236–239.

Weddell, G., B. Feinstein, and R. E. Prattle. 1944. The electrical activity of voluntary muscle in man under normal and pathological conditions. *Brain* **67:**178–257.

Wilcott, R. C., and L. J. Hammond. 1965–1966. On the constant-current error in skin resistance measurement. *Psychophysiology* **2:**39–41.

Williams, E. M. V. 1959. Relation of extracellular to intracellular potential records from single cardiac muscle fibers. *Nature* **183:**1341–1342.

Williams, H. B. 1914. On the cause of the phase difference frequently observed between homonymous peaks of the electrocardiogram. *Am. J. Physiol.* **35:**292–300.

Williams, R. L., I. Karacan, and C. J. Hursh. 1974. *The EEG of Human Sleep.* Wiley, New York, 169 pp.

Williamson, S. J., G. L. Romani, L. Kaufman, and I. Modena (eds.). 1983. *Biomagnetism.* Plenum, New York, 706 pp.

Wilson, F. N., and R. H. Bayley. 1950. The electric field of an eccentric dipole in a homogeneous spherical conducting medium. *Circulation* **1:**84–92.

Wilson, F. N., and F. D. Johnston. 1938. The vectorcardiogram. *Am. Heart J.* **16:**14–28.

Wilson, F. N., F. D. Johnston, A. G. Macleod, and P. S. Barker. 1934. Electrocardiograms that represent the potential variations of a single electrode. *Am. Heart J.* **9:**447–458.

Wilson, F. N., F. D. Johnston, and C. E. Kossman. 1947. The substitution of a tetrahedron for the Einthoven triangle. *Am. Heart J.* **33:**594–603.

Woodbury, L. A., J. W. Woodbury, and H. H. Hecht. 1950. Membrane resting and action potentials of single cardiac muscle fibers. *Circulation* **1:**264–266.

Yokota, T., T. Takahashi, M. Kondo, and B. Fujimori. 1959. Studies in the diphasic waveform of the galvanic skin reflex. *EEG Clin. Neurophysiol.* **11:**687–696.

13

Radiant Energy Devices

INTRODUCTION

Many different instruments that produce one or another form of energy are used for measurement, diagnosis, and therapy. Some are optical, producing visible, infrared, or ultraviolet radiation. Still others employ radiofrequency current. Perhaps the first energy-producing device was the X-ray machine. In this chapter the types of generators of energy and selected biomedical applications of them will be described.

LIGHT-EMITTING DIODES

It is frequently necessary to have a light source with a specified spectral output and a long life. In many physiological applications the color of the light is important, and filtering the output of an incandescent lamp to obtain the desired color reduces the light output for a given power input to the light source. The light-emitting diode (LED) is an ideal candidate for such applications and is being used increasingly in a large number of colorimetric and noncolorimetric transduction applications.

Certain semiconductor diodes emit light when they are forward biased because the electrons in the material are raised to the conduction energy level and then fall back to recombine with holes. When the electrons fall back, energy is released as radiation. The color (wavelength) of the radiation is a property of the material. In the design of LEDs, the materials are carefully chosen to obtain the desired radiation. Light-emitting diodes are available that emit infrared, red, orange, yellow, green, and blue light; a large number emit infrared radiation. The current–voltage characteristic for several LEDs and their radiation spectra, along with the spectral sensitivity of the average human eye, are illustrated in Fig. 1.

Table 1 summarizes the wavelengths produced by the various semiconductor emitters. Some manufacturers employ wave-changing techniques to obtain a color other than that emitted by the semiconductor material. With this technique, the emitted radiation is used to excite a phosphor that produces light of the desired color; this technique is employed in conventional fluorescent lighting.

Light-emitting diodes are available in a variety of configurations and are best

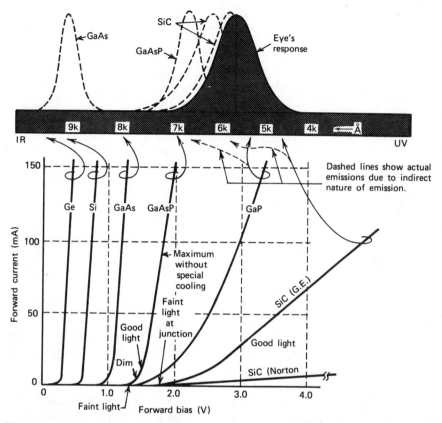

Figure 1   Current–voltage characteristics of various light-emitting diodes and their spectral emission characteristics. Such devices are commercially available from Monsanto, Electronic Special Products, 800 N. Lindberg Blvd., St. Louis, MO 63166; Hewlett-Packard, 620 Page Mill Rd., Palo Alto, CA 94304; General Electric, Miniature Lamp Dept., Nela Park, Cleveland, OH 44112; Norton Research Corp., 70 Memorial Dr., Cambridge, MA 02142; RCA Electronic Components, Harrison, NJ 07029; and Texas Instruments Incorporated, Semiconductor Components Div., Box 5012, Dallas, TX [From *Electronic Design News* October:54 (1968).

seen head-on. In some models a hemispherical lens is applied to focus the beam; in others the light is emitted from a bright, pointlike source. Some LEDs emit light in the form of a bright bar. LEDs must be classed as low-power devices (typically 100 mW); higher power units are available, but a heat sink is usually required for cooling. Over a limited range, the light output varies linearly with current.

The current–voltage curve of a typical LED reveals that it is a low-impedance device (Fig. 2). In addition, the range of voltage over which the device can be operated safely is quite narrow. Figure 2*b* indicates the range over which light output is linear with current, and Fig. 2*c* shows the light output (ϕ) (relative to

TABLE 1   Solid-State Emitters

Material	Wavelength (nm)
GaAs	900
Si–GaAs	940
GaP–Zn,O	698
GaP–N	565
GaP–Zn	553
$GaAs_{1-x}P_x$	670
	660
	610
	500
$Ga_{1-x}Al_xAs$	688
SiC	590
SiC	450
GaP	560
$Ga_xAs_{1-x}P$	650–700
$In_xGa_{1-x}As$	850–3150
InAs	3150
$Pb_xSn_{1-x}Te$	6100

the output at 20 mA) with increasing current. Because the typical LED has a steep current–voltage curve, it must be driven by a current source so that the correct operating point can be maintained easily.

The LED is a rapidly responding (microseconds to nanoseconds) light emitter in which the light output is linear with applied current over a limited range. Therefore, precautions must be taken when using it as an analog device; it sees its best service in digital circuits (i.e., when the information is carried by an off-on sequence of light flashes).

The relationship between the spectral output of light-emitting diodes to that produced by other light sources is plotted in Fig. 3. Also shown are the transmission characteristics of a variety of materials through which radiant energy must often pass. In viewing this chart, it should be recalled that the visible spectrum ranges

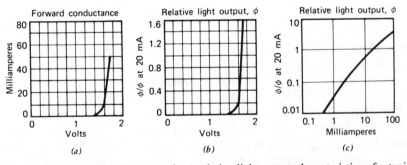

Figure 2   (*a*) Forward conductance; (*b, c*) relative light output characteristics of a typical gallium arsenide phosphide light-emitting diode (LED).

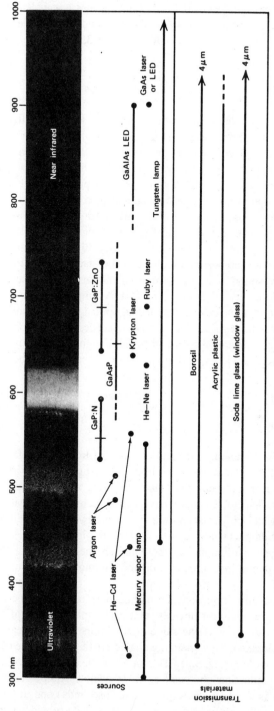

Figure 3 Spectral emission characteristics of light emitters and absorption characteristics of various materials. The visible spectrum extends from 350 to 700 nm. [Redrawn from H. E. Hardeman, *Electronics* **46**:109–114 (1973).]

from 350 to 700 nm (mμ) or 3500–7000 Å. Red light has a wavelength of about 600 nm, the infrared spectrum is beyond 700 nm, and the wavelength of the ultraviolet spectrum is shorter than blue light, or about 350 nm.

OPTOELECTRONICS

Many circuit design problems are readily solved by the use of light-emitting devices and light sensors, and a specialty has developed that is concerned with the use of light detectors and electrically driven emitters of electromagnetic radiation. The term optoelectronics designates the activities in this field. The combination of a light source and miniature photodetectors for reading punched cards and tape is a familiar example of optoelectronics. More sophisticated is the use of laser beams for fiberoptic communication, distance measurement, surgery, and the production of holographic images. In fact, the whole field of television and motion pictures might well become a part of this new area of specialization. Another area in optoelectronics deals with the design and use of solid-state letter and number displays. The numerical displays in most electronic calculators are constituted by light-emitting diodes and liquid crystal displays (LCDs). A simple optoelectronic device consisting of a light emitter and detector, called an optical isolator, allows coupling information from one circuit to another without electrical connection, the information being carried by a beam of visible or invisible light. There is no doubt that the field of optoelectronics will expand, and from it we can expect the creation of many new devices.

OPTICAL ISOLATORS

The combination of a photodetector and a source of light constitutes an optical isolator; sometimes it is called a photon coupler. At first glance it might seem that an excessively inefficient route has been taken by using a signal to produce light and then using a photodetector to detect the light and recover the signal. However, this technique provides electrical isolation between the two circuits, allowing both to be at quite large differences in potential. In fact, the insulation in some optical isolators will withstand a difference in potential in the kilovolt range. Optical isolation is also used to eliminate ground-loop and common-mode signals that arise in many circuits.

Desirable as the benefits from optical isolation may be, it must be recognized that optical couplers are nonlinear devices; that is, the presentation of a signal to the light emitter will not provide the same signal from the photodetector unless special precautions are taken. This operating characteristic is due to the components of most optical isolators—namely, an LED to produce the photons (electromagnetic radiation) and a photojunction photocell as the detector. Although the response time of both devices is short (microseconds to nanoseconds) and the response of the detector is linear with light intensity, the emitter (LED) provides a linear light output only over a limited range of current applied to it. Thus, optical isolators see their most value in digital circuits (e.g., those in which information is carried by a sequence of on–off pulses). The wavelength of the radiant energy is not an important consideration beyond the need to provide the appropriate detector, and many optical isolators employ infrared radiation as the coupling agent.

Although optical isolators are designed primarily for digital systems, it is possible to use them as analog devices because there is a region in which the output of the light emitter is linear with applied current. Figure 4 illustrates a method that employs two optical isolators (LED1, 2; PJ1, PJ2) to obtain linear operation. The input signal (E_{in}) is amplified by a unity-gain amplifier, which provides a signal for the LED-driving amplifier. The output of amplifier A_1 is fed into a similar amplifier (A_2) connected for unity-gain operation and provides an inverted signal to drive a second LED-driving amplifier. Therefore, the light emitted by one LED increases and that from the other decreases. The operating points of the LEDs are chosen for linear operation (i.e., light output is linear with current). The light output, detected by the junction photocells (PJ1, PJ2), is applied to a differential amplifier (A_3), which enlarges the photon-coupled signal. It should be apparent that the system just described uses the two LEDs in push–pull, class A operation. The system will exhibit a bandwidth extending from zero to a high frequency which need be limited only by the response time of the optical isolator (LED1, 2 and PJ1, 2).

One very practical use for the combination of a light emitter and detector is in resistance–capacity coupled amplifiers with long time constants, as are frequently

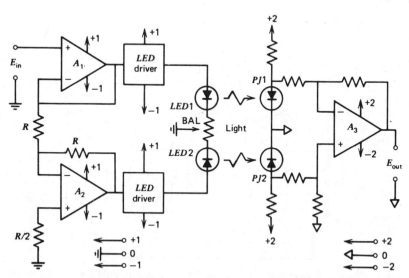

Figure 4 The use of an optical isolator (LED1, LED2, and PJ1, PJ2) to provide coupling without direct electrical connection. The signal is coupled by modulating the light output of the light emitting diodes (LED1, LED2) and detecting the light by two junction photocells (PJ1, PJ2).

used in the life sciences. Large-amplitude signals block such amplifiers, and it is necessary to wait many seconds until the voltages on the coupling capacitors return to their quiescent operating points. Quick return to the operating point can be accomplished by the use of shorting switches to reestablish the voltage levels. Switch contacts bounce, often causing undesired transients. The wiring associated with switches would add considerable capacitance and thereby reduce the high-frequency response of the amplifier. Rapid reestablishment of the operating point can be attained without penalty by using a photoconductive cell mounted in front of a controllable light source.

It will be recalled that the dark resistance of a typical photoconductive cell is extremely high (hundreds of megohms), and when illuminated the resistance drops to a few hundred ohms. Thus, by mounting a photoconductor in front of a small pilot light or LED (and with the whole assembly placed in a lightproof case), a high-quality, remote-controlled switch can be obtained. When the photoconductive cells in several such devices are connected across the input terminals of differential resistance–capacitance coupled amplifiers as in Fig. 5, the voltages on the coupling capacitors can be quickly restored to the operating values by depressing a push-button (TR), which illuminates all the light bulbs (L) in front of the photoconductive cells (PC).

This brief discussion of optoelectronic techniques is designed to make the reader aware of a few methods of solving some unusual problems. The widespread availability of miniature, low-cost photoemitters and photodetectors provides the researcher with an array of components that can be applied to solve a wide variety of problems.

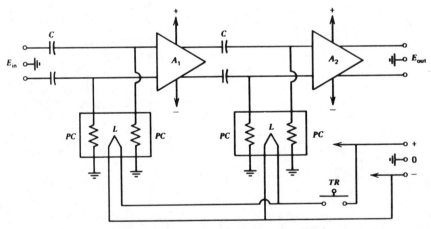

Figure 5   The use of photoconductive cells (PC) adjacent to light sources (L) to provide quick trace restoration (TR) in capacitively (C) coupled amplifiers. Depression of the trace restore switch (TR) illuminates the photoconductors and reduces their resistance to a few hundred ohms, thereby shortening the coupling time constants.

BLACKBODY RADIATION

All objects at a temperature above absolute zero (0 K) emit radiant energy as a consequence of their temperature. By measuring this radiant energy, it is possible to determine the temperature of a heated object. The fundamental physical law that underlies this phenomenon is contained in the Planck equation

$$W_\lambda = \frac{\epsilon C_1}{\lambda^5} \left[e^{C_2/\lambda T} - 1 \right]^{-1} \tag{1}$$

In this expression T is the absolute temperature (kelvin) of the radiating object, and W_λ is the spectral emissive power density at the wavelength λ. The emissivity ϵ is an experimentally determined property of the surface of the radiator at the wavelength λ. A perfect radiator is a standard blackbody, which has an emissivity of 1.0. A perfect reflector has an emissivity of zero. A polished reflecting surface will have an emissivity of 0.01–0.05. C_1 and C_2 are the first and second radiation constants, which have the values

$$C_1 = 2\pi h c^2 = 3.74 \times 10^{-12} \text{ W-cm}^2$$

and

$$C_2 = \frac{hc}{k} = 1.44 \text{ cm-K},$$

where h = Planck's constant,
$\quad c$ = the velocity of light, and
$\quad k$ = Boltzmann's constant.

The spectral emissive power W_λ has a finite value only as it applies to a finite bandwidth $\Delta\lambda$. In calculating and plotting values for W_λ, it is useful to express the result in watts per square centimeter per micrometer bandwidth as shown in Fig. 6.

It is of some interest to observe that the total power radiated by a blackbody for all wavelengths ($\lambda = 0$–∞) can be calculated by integrating the Planck equation from zero to infinity. Performing this operation provides the Stefan–Boltzmann law,

$$W_T = \epsilon \sigma T^4, \tag{2}$$

where W_T is the total radiated power in watts, ϵ is the emissivity of the radiator, σ is the Stefan–Boltzmann constant [5.67×10^{-12} W/(cm^2)(K^4)], and T is the absolute temperature.

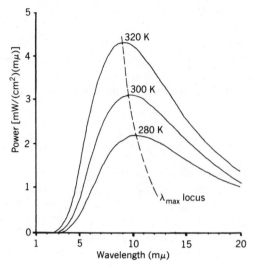

Figure 6   The power radiated at different wavelengths for an ideal blackbody at different temperatures.

As stated by the Planck equation, the power W emitted by an object is a function of the absolute temperature T. Figure 6 illustrates the wavelength distribution of power for an ideal radiator (blackbody) raised to various temperatures. Note that when the temperature is raised, two effects are produced: (1) the radiant power increases and (2) the wavelength for maximum power (λ_{max}) becomes shorter.

The wavelength for the maximum radiated power is described by Wien's displacement law, which was derived by differentiating the Planck equation, equating the result to zero, and solving the resulting equation. The solution identifies the wavelength (λ_{max}) for maximum radiated power:

$$\lambda_{max} = 2898/T. \qquad (3)$$

In this expression λ_{max} is in micrometers, and T is the absolute temperature (K).

At this point it is important to recall that the spectral region for visible light extends from about 350 to 700 nm. Figure 7 illustrates the relative spectral sensitivity of the human eye for day (photopic) and night (scotopic) vision. It is clear that the infrared wavelengths, which are longer than 700 nm, are invisible to the human eye. It is interesting to note that Fig. 6 demonstrates that when a blackbody radiator is raised to higher and higher temperatures, the wavelength for maximum radiated power moves toward the visible spectrum. Heated bodies may emit considerable light in the visible spectrum, although the spectral peak may be in the infrared region; this is particularly true for the incandescent tungsten-filament lamp as shown in Fig. 7.

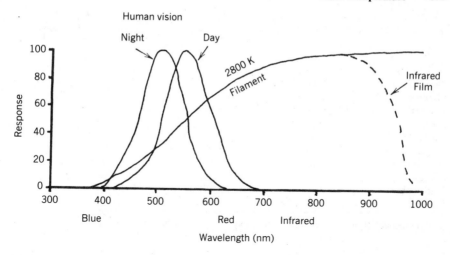

Figure 7   The visible and infrared spectra showing the relative sensitivity of the human eye and the light emitted by a tungsten-filament lamp operating at 2800 K. The eye sensitivity data have been normalized to show equal-amplitude night and day vision spectra. In point of fact, at night much lower light levels can be perceived than in daytime.

COLOR TEMPERATURE

When a blackbody is heated to above 773 K (500°C) it emits appreciable visible light. For this reason it has become customary to specify color in terms of temperature. Color temperature is the temperature at which the light from a blackbody radiator matches the light from the heated radiator.

The term color temperature pertains to visible light and is used frequently in illuminating engineering and photography. When a tungsten filament is heated by the passage of current, a faint red glow appears at about 500°C; at about 850°C it is bright red, and at 1500°C it appears nearly white. It is noteworthy that in the case of an incandescent lamp, which operates with a filament temperature of about 2800 K, although white light is emitted, about 80% of the radiated power is in the infrared region. From Wien's displacement law, λ_{max} for a 2800-K lamp is 1.03 μm, which is well in the infrared spectrum.

Various light sources are described in terms of their color temperatures. The concept is useful in matching illumination to photographic film and to television cameras to obtain the correct color reproduction. Table 2 presents a typical listing of color temperatures, along with the wavelength λ_{max} for maximum energy emitted by a blackbody radiator at that color temperature, as calculated from Wien's displacement law. Note that λ_{max} and the color may not agree because the energy distribution of most heated radiators is broad enough to provide a substantial amount of energy in the visible spectrum.

TABLE 2 Color Temperature for Radiators

Item	Color	°C	K	λ_{max} (nm)
		Temperature		
Blackbody	Dull red	700	973	2,978
Blackbody	Cherry red	900	1,173	2,470
Blackbody	Orange	1,100	1,373	2,110
Blackbody	White	>1,500	1,773	1,634
Candle flame	Yellow	1,700	1,973	1,489
Tungsten lamp	White	2,527	2,800	1,147
Tungsten lamp	Daylight	3,727	4,000	724
Sunlight[a]		4,727	5,000	580
Northern sky	Blue	9,727	10,000	290
Northern sky	Bright blue	25,727	26,000	111

[a]About one-third of the spectral energy emitted by the sun is in the visible spectrum.

UNITS

Figures 1, 3, and 7 illustrate the infrared, visible, and ultraviolet spectra, along with the sensitivity of the human eye for day and night vision. Unfortunately, there are at least four units presently used to describe the wavelength of radiant energy. In the early days the angstrom (Å) was used to describe the visible spectrum, which ranges from 3000 to 7000 Å. (Angstrom was the Swedish professor who first measured the wavelength of visible light.) Later the millimicron ($1 \text{ m}\mu = 10^{-9}$ meter) was used; $10 \text{ Å} = 1 \text{ m}\mu$. With international adoption of SI (Système International) units the term micrometer (μm) has become more widely used than micron for 10^{-6} meter, and nanometer is displacing millimicron. (The prefixes micro and nano denote 10^{-6} and 10^{-9}, respectively.) Thus, visible light extends from about 3500 to 7000 Å or from 300 to 700 nm (or mμ).

RADIATION FROM THE HUMAN BODY

The temperature of the body core is typically 37°C. Thermography measures the temperature of the surface of the skin, which is about 5°C cooler than body temperature. On the Kelvin scale, skin temperature (32°C) is 305 K. From Wien's displacement law, the wavelength λ_{max} for maximum radiation is

$$\lambda_{max} = \frac{2898}{305} = 9.50 \ \mu\text{m} \quad \text{or} \quad 9500 \text{ nm.}$$

Therefore the peak of radiant energy from the human body is in the infrared region. However, in order to use the radiated power as a measure of skin temperature, it is necessary to know the emissivity of skin.

The emissivity of the human skin has been investigated fairly extensively in vivo and in vitro. Hardy was one of the first to provide such data when he reported a value of 0.980 ± 0.01 in the wavelength range extending from 4 to 20 μm (Hardy and Muschenheim, 1934; Hardy, 1939). He also stated that more than 70% of the radiated energy from human skin falls in this region. Mitchell et al. (1967) reported a value within 1% of unity for human skin; they also reviewed the data reported to date. Watmough and Oliver (1968a,b) reported a value within 2% of unity for the 2–5.4-μm region and later a value that increased monotonically from 0.95 at 2–6 μm. From all of these data it can be concluded that the emissivity of human skin (black or white) is very nearly unity in the region around 9.5 μm where the maximum amount of energy is radiated. Lloyd-Williams (1964) stated, "the human skin, whether white or black is, in a thermal sense, an almost perfect blackbody radiator and painting or blackening its surface cannot increase its radiation." Therefore, measurement of the radiant energy from human skin provides an indication of its temperature. Thermography, which deals with thermal mapping of the skin is discussed in Chapter 5.

GAS-DISCHARGE LAMPS

Within the past decade, a remarkable variety of gas-discharge lamps have become available. Although the common denominator in all of these is the passage of current through a plasma (a cloud of ions and electrons), the operating conditions and design are dictated by the type of radiation desired. The ions in the gas are produced by high-velocity electrons that collide with electrons in the atoms of the gas, raising the energy levels. Radiation is emitted when the electrons fall back to their lower energy levels. The high-velocity electrons are produced by an electric field created by application of a potential to two electrodes in the discharge chamber. However, the electric field can be produced without electrodes by placing the discharge tube in a radiofrequency field. Radiation is also produced when high-velocity electrons are slowed by passing through a medium. This process is called Bremsstrahlung (braking radiation); it is one of the mechanisms by which X-rays are produced and is characterized by rather broad-band radiation.

The wavelength of the radiation from a gas-discharge tube depends on the atomic species, the pressure, and the current. Of course, the glowing gas heats the discharge chamber and the electrodes, producing blackbody radiation that underlies the gas-emission spectrum. However, the energy from this source is usually much less than that produced by the gas discharge.

The current through a gas-discharge tube is a nonlinear function of the applied voltage. Starting with a low voltage, the current is low and depends on the voltage applied to the electrodes. This current is due to electron flow to the anode and is called the dark current. In Fig. 8, 0–A illustrates this region in which the equivalent resistance is high. When the voltage is raised further, the electrons are accelerated and collide with gas molecules, producing ions; consequently the current is increased; curve A–B illustrates this condition. With a further increase in voltage, a self-sustaining discharge occurs (at B in Fig. 8) and the voltage drops. The equiv-

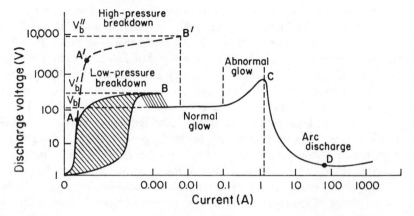

Figure 8 Idealized voltage–current characteristics of a gas-discharge lamp. From 0 to A, electrons are collected and accelerated. The accelerated electrons produce ions by collision with gas molecules. Soon, enough ions are created to cause a breakdown B, resulting in a glow discharge, at which the voltage drops to the glow value (V_b). Over a considerable range of current, the voltage is constant, but it rises as more current is caused to flow in the abnormal glow region. At C an arc discharge occurs; the current increases markedly and the voltage decreases. (Redrawn from J. D. Cobine, *Gaseous Conductors*, Dover, New York, 1958.)

alent resistance decreases, demonstrating the need to use a current source (or ballast) with such devices. As the current is increased further, the voltage across the electrodes is constant over a fairly wide range; this is the normal glow region, which can be used to create a constant-voltage source as was employed in voltage-regulator tubes of the VR series. With increasing current, the voltage starts to rise, identifying the abnormal glow region, which terminates with the arc discharge at C. At this point the voltage decreases considerably. With increasing current, the voltage continues to decrease, soon reaching a minimum, as shown by D in Fig. 8. Note that the region from C to D represents a negative resistance characteristic and for stability a ballast must be used. The sequence of events shown in Fig. 8 is highly idealized and is pressure-dependent.

In addition to the atomic species, the major difference among gas-discharge tubes is the operating pressure. Figure 9 presents a summary of the events for an air discharge (right), and the pressure range for different types of gas-discharge tubes (left). The arc lamps operate at relatively high pressures, and the glow lamps at low pressures. The neon lamp is perhaps the most familiar of the glow lamps; some contain neon, while others contain neon and a small amount of argon. Such devices operate at about 20 mmHg. Yellow-orange light is produced.

The sodium vapor lamp, which is common, is a low-pressure gas-discharge lamp, although there are high-pressure units. The discharge chamber contains sodium vapor and a trace of argon to aid in starting the glow. It is used for highway lighting because of its extremely high efficiency (about 300 lumens per watt) and

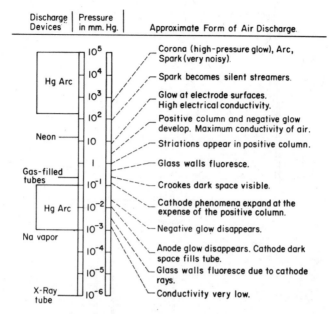

Discharge Devices	Pressure in mm. Hg.	Approximate Form of Air Discharge.
Hg Arc	10^5	Corona (high-pressure glow), Arc, Spark (very noisy).
	10^4	Spark becomes silent streamers.
	10^3	Glow at electrode surfaces. High electrical conductivity.
	10^2	Positive column and negative glow develop. Maximum conductivity of air.
Neon	10	Striations appear in positive column.
	1	Glass walls fluoresce.
Gas-filled tubes	10^{-1}	Crookes dark space visible.
Hg Arc	10^{-2}	Cathode phenomena expand at the expense of the positive column.
	10^{-3}	Negative glow disappears.
Na vapor	10^{-4}	Anode glow disappears. Cathode dark space fills tube.
	10^{-5}	Glass walls fluoresce due to cathode rays.
X-Ray tube	10^{-6}	Conductivity very low.

Figure 9 Pressures used in various gas-discharge tubes (left) and characteristics of an air-filled discharge tube at different pressures. (Redrawn from data in J. D. Cobine, *Gaseous Conductors.* Dover, New York, 1958.)

because of its spectral output (589.0 and 589.6 nm). This bright yellow light has a wavelength that is close to that for the maximum sensitivity of the dark-adapted human eye (520 nm) and light-adapted eye (560 nm).

Probably the most important type of gas-discharge lamp is the mercury vapor unit, which is at the heart of a host of commonly encountered lamps. The discharge can be operated under either high- or low-pressure conditions, depending on the desired result. Perhaps the most important property of the discharge is the considerable amount of ultraviolet radiation produced at 253.7 nm. Figure 10 illustrates the mercury vapor spectrum when the discharge tube is operated at (*a*) low pressure and (*b*) high pressure. Note that with the higher pressure, the energy in the visible region exceeds that in the ultraviolet.

The ultraviolet radiation produced by the low-pressure mercury vapor lamp (operating at a few millimeters of mercury with a little argon to aid starting) is used in all fluorescent lamps. The ultraviolet radiation excites the phosphor coating the inner surface of the tube, which emits the visible light. The color of the light is dictated by the choice of phosphor.

Sometimes ultraviolet radiation is known as black light, the radiation peaking at 365 nm and extending from about 340 to 400 nm (50% points). This type of ultraviolet source consists of a mercury vapor discharge in a tube with an inside coating of cerium-activated calcium phosphate. The ultraviolet excites the calcium

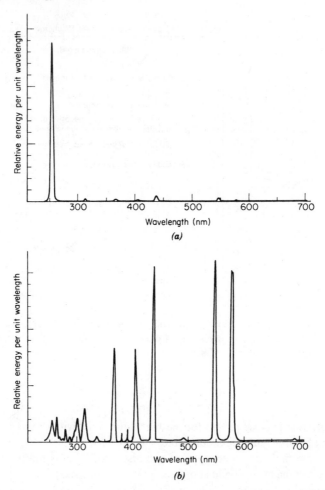

Figure 10   Energy spectrum of mercury vapor discharge at (*a*) low and (*b*) high pressure. (Redrawn from *Electric Discharge Lamps*. J. F. Waymonth, M.I.T. Press, Cambridge, MA, 1971.)

phosphate, which emits the radiation. The envelope is chosen to transmit this radiation but not the 253.7-nm radiation. Such black-light sources are used to excite fluorescent materials.

The mercury arc is the backbone of the newer metal halide (halogen) lamps. In such devices, the mercury and a metal halide (usually an iodide of indium, thallium, sodium, lithium, or thorium) is contained in a quartz discharge tube. The light emitted by halogen lamps is mainly in the visible region, the different metal halides producing stronger radiation at different given wavelengths. For example, the indium lamp emits more blue, the thallium more green, the sodium more yellow, the lithium more red, and the thorium more white light. This technology permits tailoring the light output as desired by choosing the appropriate metal halide.

The strong ultraviolet radiation at 253.7 nm produced by the low-pressure mercury vapor lamp is of considerable importance in biomedical applications. However, to make this radiation available, it is necessary to contain the discharge in a quartz chamber, which is transparent to ultraviolet radiation. Ordinary glass is opaque to such radiation.

In physical therapy, several terms are used to describe the ultraviolet spectrum. The long-wavelength region (340–360 nm) is called ultraviolet A (UVA). The middle range (which includes radiation at 253.7, 280, and 290–320 nm with a peak at 296.7 nm) is called ultraviolet B (UVB). The short-wavelength ultraviolet (90% of the energy at 253.7 nm) is called ultraviolet C (UVC). Two other terms are used to describe the ultraviolet generators: hot quartz (HQ) and cold quartz (CQ). These terms pertain to the operating temperature of the quartz capsule that contains the radiating gas. Cold quartz refers to the mercury vapor lamp that emits about 90% of its radiation at 253.7 nm. Hot quartz refers to radiation ranging from 253.7 to 320 nm, with a peak around 296.7 nm.

Biomedical Applications

Ultraviolet radiation exhibits photochemical properties; it reacts with cells and microorganisms to alter their function. It is therefore not surprising that this type of radiation has bactericidal properties. Ultraviolet radiation is used extensively in dermatology for a variety of purposes.

Germicidal Applications

Hart and Sharp (1947) clearly demonstrated the bactericidal property of ultraviolet radiation (253.7 nm) in studies using intensities of 20,000–60,000 ergs/cm^2. They found a range of susceptibility among commonly encountered bacteria. Koller (1952) subsequently tabulated the energy levels required to kill a large variety of microorganisms; his data appear in Table 3. It is interesting to note that the wavelength for maximum bactericidal effect is 260 nm, very close to that (253.7 nm) produced by the mercury vapor lamp.

Armed with their information, Hart and Sharp studied the number of deaths due to infection in operating rooms for 5 years before the use of ultraviolet to purify the air and for the first 5 years of its use. In the 5-year period before its use, there were 17 deaths due to infection in 14,885 operations. In the 5 years during which ultraviolet was used, there was only one infection-caused death in 37,121 operations.

Pigment Augmentation

Ultraviolet radiation in the sun's rays or from a discharge lamp will cause skin tanning (pigmentation), which is a photochemical response involving the release of the skin pigment melanin. In the basal skin layer are located the melanocytes that contain melanin. On exposure to ultraviolet radiation the melanocytes take up

**TABLE 3   Energy Level at 253 7 nm to Inhibit Colony
Formation in 90% of the Organisms**

Organism	Inhibiting Energy Level (ergs/cm^2) ($\times 10^{-2}$)
Bacillus anthracis	452
B. megatherium sp. (veg.)	113
B. megatherium sp. (spores)	273
B. paratyphosus (avg. of 3 strains)	320
B. subtilis (mixed)	710
	600
B. subtilis (spores)	1200
Corynebacterium diphtheriae	337
Dysentery bacilli (avg. of 5 strains)	220
Eberthella typhosa	214
Escherichia coli	300
Micrococcus candidus	605
M. piltonensis	810
M. sphaeroides	1000
Neisseria catarrhalis	440
Phytomonas tumefaciens	440
Proteus vulgaris	264
Pseudomonas aerugenosa	550
Ps. fluorescens	350
Salmonella enteritidis	400
S. typhimurium (avg. of 3 strains)	800
Sarcina lutea	1970
Serratia marcescens	242
	220
Shigilla paradysenteriae	168
Spirillum rubrum	440
Staphylococcus albus	184
	330
	184
Staph. aureus	218
	260
	495
Streptococcus hemolyticus	216
Strep. lactis	615
Strep. viridans	200

Source: L. F. Koller, *Ultraviolet Radiation*. Wiley, New York, 1952.

tyrosine from the circulation to synthesize melanin. The preexisting melanin in the skin also darkens; both contribute to skin darkening. It should be recognized that skin pigmentation is also affected by hormones. Melanocytes are not uniformly distributed over the skin surface, being about three times as dense on the face as on the thigh. Thus the response to the same amount of ultraviolet radiation will be different on different parts of the body.

Melanin strongly absorbs ultraviolet radiation and provides protection for the deeper skin layers. About 80% of the radiation is absorbed in the first 0.2 mm of the skin, i.e., the epidermis is the major site of absorption. In regions where the skin is thick, such as the palms of the hands and soles of the feet, very little of the radiation reaches the melanocytes. Consequently, these sites pigment very little. It is important to note that pigmentation is a delayed process, requiring about 0.5 day for the pigment to be released from the melanocytes. Suntan protection preparations act as filters that absorb the ultraviolet radiation so that less reaches the melanocytes.

In using ultraviolet radiation to induce pigmentation, it is essential that the eyes be protected. Exposure can cause conjunctivitis and temporary or permanent blindness. Ordinary glass is virtually opaque to ultraviolet radiation, and eyeglasses afford protection. However, they should fit snugly.

Rickets

The photochemical effect of ultraviolet radiation is used in the treatment of rickets, a disease characterized by depressed calcium absorption due to a deficiency of vitamin D. In rickets, there is depressed calcification of the bones and teeth. The bones are swollen at their ends and easily deformed, and the teeth are subject to decay. Diet and the administration of vitamin D often solve the problem. However, in many cases, whole-body ultraviolet radiation is used. The ultraviolet radiation converts provitamin D in the skin to vitamin D.

Dermatology

Dermatologists often use ultraviolet radiation to treat psoriasis and acne. The former is characterized by intense itching of the skin. In its treatment, ultraviolet radiation is often combined with drugs that sensitize the skin to ultraviolet radiation. In acne, there occurs a red swelling around the facial hair shafts associated with infection that responds to ultraviolet radiation. Sometimes ultraviolet radiation is effective in enhancing wound healing; the mechanism is due to the bactericidal effect of ultraviolet radiation.

Jaundice

Blue light (400–500 nm) is used in the treatment of jaundice in neonates and premature infants. Jaundice is a yellow coloration of the skin due to the accumulation of bilirubin, the end product of heme metabolism. Heme, the iron pigment, comes from the breakdown of red blood cells; the liver cleans the circulation of bilirubin. An excess of heme or depressed liver function results in excess bilirubin deposition in the skin. The photochemical effect of blue light (400–500 nm) produces an oxidative reaction on bilirubin, resulting in water-soluble end products that are excreted in the urine and bile, thus clearing the skin of its yellow hue. The treatment involves irradiating the whole body with blue light at 400–500 nm.

OZONE

A by-product of the generation of ultraviolet is the production of ozone (O_3), a very powerful oxidizing agent. The amount produced depends on the intensity of the ultraviolet radiation and increases with decreasing wavelength below 253.7 nm. Because the olfactory receptors are very sensitive to ozone, one can detect a concentration as little as 0.01 part per million (ppm). A concentration of 10 times this amount is irritating to the mucous membranes of the nose and throat. One to ten parts per million produces headache and respiratory distress.

The amount of ozone produced by the typical low-pressure mercury vapor ultraviolet lamp operating at 253.7 nm is small. However, if the envelope of the lamp is transparent to 184.9 nm, the ozone production will be more. According to Koller (1952), with such a lamp in a room with ordinary ventilation, the concentration is unlikely to exceed a few hundredths of a part per million.

An ozone generator can be created by enclosing an ultraviolet-producing mercury vapor lamp (radiating at 184.9 nm) in ordinary glass and passing oxygen through it. Koller (1952) reported that about 10 g of ozone is produced per kilowatt-hour of operation.

LASERS

A laser is a device that produces radiant energy with special properties. The term laser is an acronym for *l*ight *a*mplification by *s*timulated *e*mission of *r*adiation. Laser radiation is monochromatic and coherent, i.e., the waves are all in phase across the beam. Laser radiation can be absorbed, refracted, reflected, polarized, converged, diverged, and split. The monochromatic and coherent character of laser radiation makes it possible to focus the beam very sharply, and hence the energy density can be extremely high. These characteristics make it possible to create many novel devices.

The laser principle was first proposed in a paper by Schawlow and Townes (1958), who suggested the use of a gas of alkali metal excited by strong ultraviolet light. The first working laser was described by Maiman (1960), who used a synthetic ruby (aluminum oxide) containing a small amount of chromium. The ruby rod was excited by a discharge lamp. Since then, numerous other types of lasers have been described. Lasers are widely used in industry; their use in medicine is increasing rapidly. Although the stimulated emission phenomenon can be produced in solids, liquids, and gases, laser efficiency is not as high in liquids.

The laser principle is perhaps best explained using the solid-state ruby laser, which consists of a rod of aluminum oxide containing 0.05% chromium. The ends of the rod are perpendicular to the axis and are highly polished. On each end is a reflecting surface, one being virtually 100% reflecting, the other slightly less so; special coatings are used to achieve this condition. An energy source (pump), such as a high-intensity flash from a mercury vapor discharge lamp, emits radiation into the ruby rod. This radiation displaces electrons from the chromium atoms, which

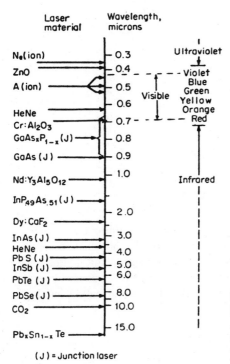

Laser
material

Wavelength,
microns

Ne(ion)   — 0.3   Ultraviolet
ZnO   — 0.4 — — — — Violet
A (ion)   — 0.5   Blue
                              Visible   Green
                           — 0.6   Yellow
HeNe   Orange
Cr:Al2O3   — 0.7 — — — — Red
GaAsxP1−x (J)   — 0.8
GaAs (J)   — 0.9
                           — 1.0
Nd:Y3Al5O12   Infrared
InP.49As.51(J)
                           — 2.0
Dy:CaF2
InAs(J)   — 3.0
HeNe   — 4.0
Pb S (J)   — 5.0
InSb (J)   — 6.0
PbTe (J)
PbSe(J)   — 8.0
CO2   —10.0
                           —15.0
PbxSn1−x Te

(J) = Junction laser

Figure 11 Laser materials and the wave-
lengths that they produce. [Redrawn from
Handbook of Components for Electronics.
C. A. Harper (ed.). McGraw-Hill, New
York, 1977, Chap. 5.]

produces photons of energy when they fall back. The photons release more electrons as they are reflected back and forth within the rod—more electrons, more
photons, and more reflections. The rod behaves as a resonant cavity. Some of the
energy emerges from the partially coated end as the laser beam.

As stated previously, the laser phenomenon can be produced in gases and liquids. In gases, the pumping is achieved by the application of a voltage to electrodes
in the gas. In the case of liquids (dye lasers), the pump is another laser. There are
also PN junction (diode) lasers in which energy pumping is achieved by the passage
of a current through the PN junction.

Figure 11 and Table 4 list many of the popular types of lasers and the wavelength
of the radiation produced. Note that the radiation produced extends from the ultraviolet to the infrared; both continuous-wave and pulsed-energy lasers are available,
the latter permitting fine control of the energy output.

Biomedical Applications

All biomedical applications of laser energy depend on tissue absorption. However, the particular response depends on where the absorptions occurs. Cornelius
(1980) presented an informative chart (Fig. 12) that summarizes the effects of laser
radiation on living tissue. Observe that the three ranges of radiant energy (infrared,
visible, and ultraviolet) produce different tissue responses. Infrared induces molec-

TABLE 4   Characteristics of Lasers

Material	State	Wavelength (nm)
Ruby	Solid	694.3
CO_2	Gas	10,600
NdYAG	Solid	1,060
Ar^+	Gas	514.5
He-Ne	Gas	632.8
GaAs	Solid	840
Xe	Gas	3,507
Kr	Gas	476.1–647
N_2	Gas	337

ular vibration, leading to heat and, if intense enough, to burning and tissue vaporization. Infrared energy, to a lesser degree, can produce photochemical effects and molecular bond dissociation. Visible light produces photochemical effects and, if the energy level is high enough, heat. Ultraviolet radiation can produce molecular bond dissociation, as well as skin burns. Ultraviolet has germicidal effects; high-intensity radiation can vaporize tissue.

Surgery

The intense, small-area beams of the CO_2 (gas) and the NdYAG (solid-state) lasers lend themselves well to the creation of a laser scalpel. The CO_2 laser pro-

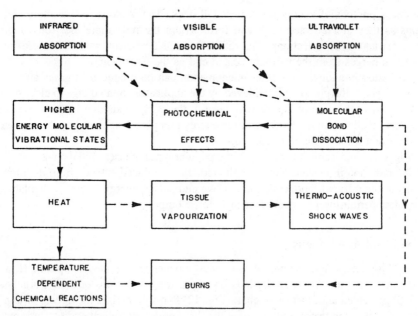

Figure 12 Effects of infrared, visible, and ultraviolet radiation. [Redrawn from W. A. Cornelius, *Australas. Phys. Eng. Sci. Med.* **6**(3):106–114 (1983).]

duces radiation at 10.6 μm in the far infrared. At this wavelength, tissue absorption is high; hence the beam penetrates little and heats superficial tissue. Since the process is thermal, tissue is cut by vaporization; the heating in tissue adjacent to the cut produces coagulation, and small blood vessels are sealed. Although perhaps ideal for surgery, the CO_2 laser beam is difficult to direct to the operative site. Because there are no optical fibers now available that can carry radiation at this wavelength, the energy must be directed by mirrors.

NdYAG laser, which produces infrared energy at 1060 nm, is also used to create a laser scalpel. At this wavelength, the tissues do not absorb as well (compared to 10.6 μm), and the penetration (laterally and in depth) is greater. Thus slightly more tissue destruction and more extensive hemostasis can be achieved. In addition, this radiation is easily directed to the operative site via flexible fiber-optic waveguides.

An NdYAG surgical laser was described by Deutsch et al. (1980). This device consisted of a 100-W laser that delivered its infrared radiation (1060 nm) to a sharpened quartz scalpel blade via a fiber-optic cable. They reported successful cutting and coagulation in animal and human studies but indicated that higher power would be desirable. They also stressed the need to wear protective glasses to prevent retinal damage to the surgical team.

Heimbach et al. (1980) reported preliminary studies with an argon laser coupled to a bundle of glass fibers (3 m long), terminating on a quartz scalpel blade. The visible blue-green radiation (488 and 514 nm) was used to excise burns on pig skin. They reported surgical ease, good hemostasis, and the need for the surgical team to wear protective glasses to prevent retinal damage.

Interestingly, one of the first medical uses for laser energy was in ophthalmology. The excellent coagulation properties of the argon ion laser (500 nm) has been used to spot weld detached retinas and to seal leaking blood vessels in eyes of patients with diabetic retinopathy. The fact that the radiation is visible allows carefully controlled delivery of the laser energy and monitoring of the result.

Dermatology

Laser energy has been used with success to destroy skin blemishes. In this application, the wavelength chosen should be such that high absorption (and little penetration) is achieved. The argon (500 nm) and NdYAG (1060 nm) lasers are frequently used to destory tattoo marks and port wine nevi.

Miscellaneous Uses

Because of its unique properties, laser radiation is used in a variety of ways. For example, violet and ultraviolet radiations have a photochemical effect on cells. The narrow laser beam is used to assist alignment of X-ray therapy machines. Blood flow has been measured with laser-Doppler techniques. Perhaps the most valuable use of the properties of the laser beam is in the creation of holograms, which are three-dimensional images.

X-RAYS

Introduction

X-rays are penetrating, ionizing radiation with wavelengths extending from about 200 to 10 pm (1 pm = 10^{-12} m); thus X radiation lies below the ultraviolet spectrum. X-rays can be absorbed, diffracted, and scattered but are not focused or deflected by an electric or magnetic field. They travel in straight lines from their source, which is usually a metal with a high atomic number (e.g., tungsten) bombarded by high-velocity electrons. X-rays have many uses in diagnosis and therapy; some examples will be presented subsequently.

In the late 1800s many scientists were preoccupied with the passage of current through gases at low pressure. The standard procedure involved the application of a high voltage to electrodes in a glass chamber containing the gas at the desired pressure. Such (Crookes) discharge tubes (Fig. 13), were not sealed; they were connected to a vacuum pump so that the pressure in the tube could be varied. Wilhelm Conrad Roentgen, professor of physics at Wurzburg, was one of those engaged in such research in November 1895. His experiments, which led to the discovery of X-rays, are beautifully recounted by Dibner (1963). [The history of radiology is well documented by Glasser (1933), that of the X-ray tube is covered by Coolidge (1930).]

Roentgen covered a Crookes discharge tube with black cardboard and applied a high voltage to it using a Ruhmkorff coil (which produces a high alternating voltage). In a darkened room he noticed a glow emanating from nearby fluorescent crystals. The crystals were later replaced by a plate of barium platinocyanide. (Such plates were commonly used to display fluorescence produced by cathode rays, i.e., a stream of electrons.) Roentgen immediately realized that he had discovered invisible rays and set about to study their properties. Using the fluorescent screen as the indicator, he found that a book of 1000 pages, blocks of wood, and a sheet of tinfoil had negligible effects on the rays. Sheets of gold, platinum, or lead provided different absorptions. It required a sheet of lead 1.5 mm thick to block the rays, which he called X (for unknown) rays. His epoch-making discoveries included the fact that X-rays affected photographic film in the same way as visible light. Among

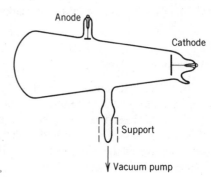

Figure 13 Typical Crookes tube, which contained gas at a low pressure. It was a tube of this type that Roentgen used to discover X-rays.

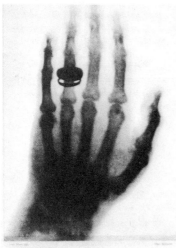

Hand des Anatomen Geheimrath von Kölliker in Würzburg.

Figure 14 X-ray picture of Kolliker's hand taken by Roentgen. (From B. Dibner, *The New Rays of Professor Roentgen.* The Burndy Library, Norwalk, CT, 1963. By permission.)

the absorbers that Roentgen investigated was the human hand, which, when placed on the fluorescent plate, provided an errie shadow of the bones. The first public demonstration of an X-ray picture (later called a roentgengram) is undoubtedly that of the left hand (Fig. 14) of Roentgen's colleague Kolliker, anatomist at the University of Wurzburg. On January 23, 1896, at a demonstration at the university, Kolliker placed his hand on a photographic plate, which when developed revealed the bone structure of his hand and the ring on his third finger. Parenthetically, such pictures soon became numerous and appeared often in the public press.

X-Ray Tubes

The first X-ray tubes were gas-filled diodes (Crookes tubes) in which the gas pressure was critical for the efficient production of X-rays. Because Crookes tubes, induction coils, and electrostatic generators were everywhere, Roentgen's experiments were easily duplicated, and X-rays were put to use almost immediately. However, these gas-filled tubes were fickle and required constant attention to keep them operating. Introduction of the heated-filament, high-vacuum (a few hundredths of a micrometer) tube by Coolidge (1913) made the production and control of X-rays practical. Electrons from the filament are focused and accelerated to the tungsten anode by a high potential. X-rays are produced by two mechanisms: (1) electron dislodgment from the inner shells of the atoms in the target (anode) and (2) slowing down of the electrons by the target (Bremsstrahlung). The X-rays spread radially from their point of origin on the anode, as shown in Fig. 15a. It was soon found that the high-speed electrons from the filament struck the anode with such energy that it melted at the point of impact. To dissipate the heat better, the tungsten anode was mounted on a heavy copper block within the tube. Finally, the rotating anode was proposed by Thompson in 1914 (Coolidge, 1930). Rotation of the anode

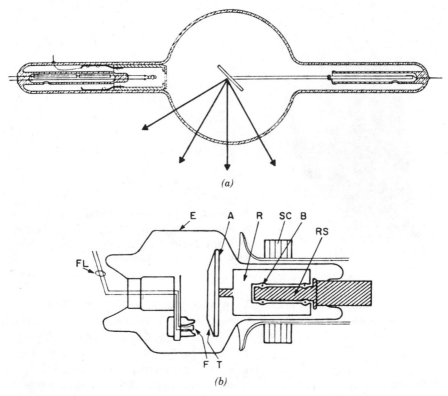

Figure 15 X-ray tubes. (*a*) Hot cathode type, (*b*) rotating anode type (showing hot cathode F, anode T).

(at 3000–3500 rpm) was accomplished by the use of a rotating magnetic field (as used in induction motors) produced by stator windings outside the tube. Thus, when a voltage pulse is applied to the rotating anode, the electron beam is very unlikely to strike the anode at the same spot each time the tube is used to produce X-rays. The whirring sound heard when an X-ray machine is turned on is produced by the rotating anode. Figure 15*b* illustrates the rotating-anode X-ray tube, which also contains a heated cathode to provide the electron beam.

Output of the X-Ray Tube

The output of an X-ray tube is described in terms of the applied voltage (in kilovolts) and the current (in milliamperes) that flows through it. With a direct voltage, X-rays are produced as long as the voltage is applied. Observe in Fig. 16 that above a certain voltage range the current in the X-ray tube is mainly dependent on the filament current. Thus, it is possible, in part, to separately control the current and voltage to obtain the desired result. If an alternating voltage is applied to the anode, X-rays will be produced only when the anode is positive. In this circum-

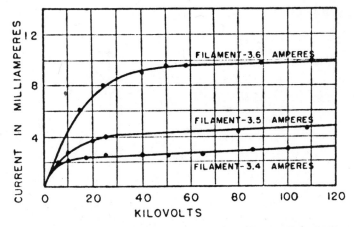

Figure 16   Current–voltage characteristics of an X-ray tube with different filament currents.

stance, it is the peak voltage (kilovolts peak, kVp) that is specified. Typically full-wave rectification is used and the X-ray beam occurs with twice the power-line frequency.

The wavelength and intensity of the X-rays are related to the type of target, the applied voltage, and the anode current. The radiation is broad-band, as shown in Fig. 17 for the same anode current at 50 and 100 kVp. The wavelength for the peak energy shifts toward the shorter wavelengths with increasing applied voltage. The wavelength (in picometers) for maximum energy is equal to 1860/kV. Observe in Fig. 17 that at 50 kV the wavelength for maximum intensity is 37.2 pm; at 100 kV the wavelength is 18.6 pm.

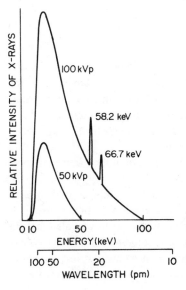

Figure 17   Energy spectra for a tungsten anode for the same anode current and for 50 and 100 kVp. (Redrawn from W. R. Hendee, E. L. Chaney, and R. P. Rossi, *Radiologic Physics.* Year Book Publishers, Chicago, IL, 1977.)

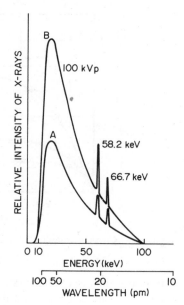

Figure 18   Energy spectra for a tungsten target with 100 KVp and (*A*) low and (*B*) high anode currents. (Redrawn from W. H. Hendee, E. L. Chaney, and R. P. Rossi, *Radiologic Physics*. Year Book Publishers, Chicago, IL, 1977.)

   The intensity of the X-ray beam at a fixed anode voltage depends on the filament current as shown in Fig. 18. Note that because the voltage is fixed at 100 kV, the peak occurs at the same wavelength. Therefore, the intensity of the X-ray beam depends on the applied anode voltage and the filament current. However, the wavelength for peak intensity decreases with increasing anode voltage, as shown in Fig. 17. The X-ray spectrum of diagnostic machines was reported by Epp and Weiss (1966).

Filtering

   Much of the output from an X-ray tube lies in the longer wavelengths and contributes little to diagnostic techniques, and if it were all retained it would unnecessarily increase the exposure to the patient. To avoid this situation, filters are used. Although the glass envelope of the X-ray tube absorbs some of the long-wavelength X-rays, metal filters are used in addition. For diagnostic X-ray purposes (below 120 kV), aluminum is used. With therapeutic techniques [120–1000 kV (1 MV)], copper is used. Above 1 MV, lead is employed. Often the filter consists of one or more metal sheets.

   It should be noted that different tissues have different coefficients of absorption at different wavelengths. Figure 19 presents this information, which is useful in guiding the use of X-rays to visualize the different tissues. It means also that the emergent spectrum is different from the spectrum presented to the tissues. Tissues obey Beer's law of absorption; i.e., the ratio of emergent intensity I_e to the incident intensity I_0 is of the form $I_e/I_0 = e^{-\mu t}$, where μ is the linear attenuation coefficient and t is the tissue thickness.

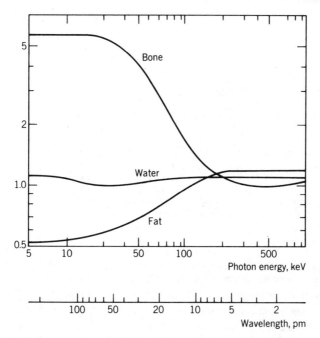

Figure 19   Relative attenuation coefficient of tissues to X-rays referred to air. (From B. Jacobson and J. Webster, *Medicine and Clinical Engineering*. Prentice-Hall, Englewood Cliffs, NJ, 1977.)

Units

Three units are used to describe radiation intensity; the roentgen (R), the rad, and the rem (radiation equivalent man). Table 5 presents a compilation of the definitions of these units.

Diagnostic Techniques

In diagnostic procedures, the anode voltage ranges from 20 to 120 kVp. After passing through the subject, the radiation may be displayed on film, a fluoroscopic

TABLE 5   Definitions of Radiation Units

roentgen (R)	2.58×10^{-4} C per kilogram of air, as measured by a standard ionization chamber, 3R liberates 1.610×10^{12} ion pairs per gram of air; 1 R = 0.869 rad.
rad	Unit of absorbed dose equal to 100 erg per gram of air; rad = 0.869 R. (The unit is not restricted to air and corresponds to an energy absorption of 0.01 J/kg.)
rem	Unit of equivalent dose. The number of rems is equal to the dose in rads multiplied by a quality factor that depends on the nature of the radiation. (The quality factor for X-rays is 1.0.)

Source: Adapted from H. E. Johns and J. R. Cunningham, *The Physics of Radiology*, 3rd ed. Thomas, Springfield, IL, 1969.

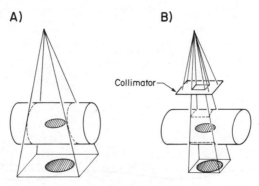

Figure 20   X-ray beam (*A*) without a collimator and (*B*) with a collimator to confine the X-ray beam to include only the desired target.

screen, or an image amplifier, often coupled to a video monitor. Each of these modalities will now be described. However, before discussing them, it is important to recognize that the most important points pertaining to the use of diagnostic (and therapeutic) procedures is to confine the beam so that only the region of interest is illuminated by the X-ray beam. In Fig 20*A* the beam illuminates much more than the region of interest (darkened circle), causing unnecessary irradiation of adjacent tissues. The extent of the beam is reduced by using strips of lead arranged to provide just enough beam width to allow examination of only the area of interest, as shown in Fig. 20*B*. Most X-ray machines provide an optical means to adjust the collimator.

Film

X-ray film is similar to photographic film. The photosensitive emulsion can be composed of fine grains of silver halide, in which case the picture has high resolution but the emulsion is not very sensitive; when a coarse-grained emulsion is used, the resolving power is not as good, but the sensitivity is higher and a shorter exposure time is required. The former type of film is called slow; the latter, fast. The choice is the trade-off that pertains to visual photography. To increase the sensitivity of X-ray film, intensifying screens are used; these are films containing fluorescent salts. A screen is placed on each side of the photographic film in the cassette. The X-ray beam causes the fluorescent material to emit light, which exposes the film.

The response of X-ray film is described by its characteristic curve, which is a plot of optical density (blackness) versus the logarithm of the exposure. The optical density is defined as log (1 /transmission). For example, if 10% of the incident radiation is transmitted, the optical density is 1; if 1% is transmitted, the optical density is 2. Figure 21*a* illustrates a typical optical density versus log exposure curve. The slope of the curve is dependent on the type of film. The rating of the film is its gamma value, being defined as the slope $(D_2 - D_1)/(X_2 - X_1)$ in the

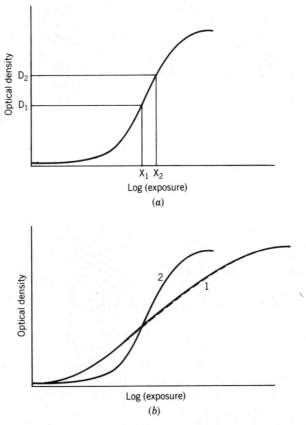

Figure 21 (a) Characteristic curve for X-ray film. Gamma is defined as the slope $(D_2 - D_1)/(x_2 - x_1)$. (b) Typical curve for (1) low- and (2) high-gamma films.

linear region. The gamma value describes the contrast capability; a high-gamma film provides high contrast. However, it should be realized that a high-gamma film has a narrower exposure range, as shown by curve 2 in Fig. 21b.

Grids

Primary radiation passing through a subject produces the desired shadow image on the photographic film. However, some of the radiation is scattered by the subject's tissues and emerges traveling in many different directions, thereby causing a loss of detail in the image. Therefore, it is desirable to block the scattered radiation; this is the function of the grid that is placed over the X-ray film. Bucky (1915) appears to have been the first to describe such a device, which was developed by Potter (1916). Three types of grids are used: parallel (linear), focused, and crossed. In all three, alternate strips of lead are used to block the scattered X-rays. A typical linear grid is shown in Fig. 22a. The lead strips are typically 50

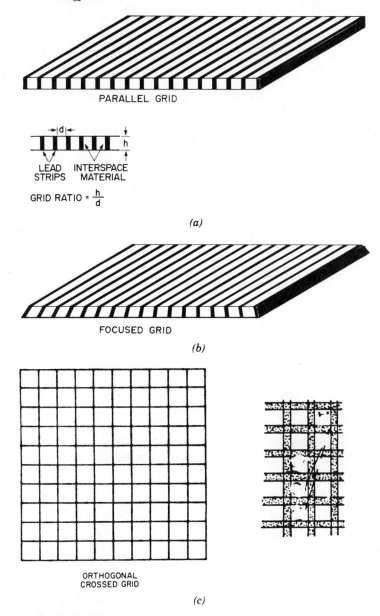

Figure 22   Grids. (*a*) Linear, (*b*) focused, and (*c*) crossed.

μm thick and are spaced by radiotransparent strips 250 μm thick; the strips are about 2.5 mm high. Thus the X-ray image is composed of 83 lines to the inch. In some models, the dimensions are chosen so that there are 100 lead strips to the inch. This line structure is often visible on the X-ray film; however, ingenious techniques have been developed to move the grid during the exposure.

The focused grid, shown in Fig. 22b, is constructed similarly to the linear grid, except that the lead strips are tilted so that they are parallel to the collimated X-ray beam. Obviously, the distance from the X-ray tube must be standardized with the focused grid.

Figure 22c illustrates a typical crossed grid. Essentially this device consists of two linear grids placed orthogonally. The crossed grid eliminates scattered radiation in both directions, thereby improving the resolution of the image.

Although the various types of grids improve image resolution by eliminating scattering, the grid absorbs X-rays. Therefore, the exposure must be increased by a factor of 3–5.

Fluoroscopy

Roentgen was the first to use a fluoroscopic screen and to create a hand-held fluoroscope. These early devices became popular for viewing the hand bones; one is shown in Fig. 23a. They were also widely used to study the motion of internal organs illuminated by X-rays. Fluoroscopic screens, measuring up to 14 in. × 17 in. for placement behind the patient (Fig. 23b) replaced the hand-held screens by the 1930s. The newer screens contained zinc and cadmium sulfides with a trace of silver to increase their sensitivity to X-rays. The fluorescent material was supported by leaded glass, which faced the viewer, affording some protection since the fluorescent coating absorbs only about 7% of the X-rays.

The fluoroscopic image is dim, and the viewer's eyes require time dark adap-

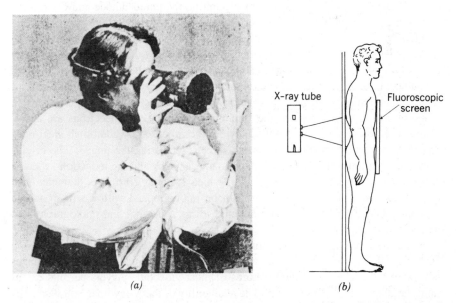

(a)   (b)

Figure 23 (a) Early hand-held fluoroscope, which preceded the larger fixed conventional screen shown in (b).

tation, a procedure that requires about 20 min. In addition, goggles must be worn to protect the eyes and a leaded apron to protect the body. Despite these inconveniences, such fluoroscopic images were valuable for viewing the passage of radio-opaque barium salts through the gastrointestinal tract. Of course, X-ray photographs could be taken at any time.

The early fluoroscopic techniques were by no means safe. Operators often did not take the time to dark adapt the eyes, resulting in the use of higher tube voltages and currents, thereby increasing exposure to the patient and operator. Many operators did not wear protective goggles or an apron, believing they were not needed because the viewing time was short. However, X-ray dosage is cumulative, and X-ray operators soon acquired dangerous doses of radiation.

Fluoroscopy gained considerable public appeal in the 1930s. At that time, many large shoe stores installed fluoroscopes so that the patrons could view the bones in the feet while wearing their new shoes, thereby assuring themselves of a good fit. However, this practice only lasted a few years.

Image Intensifier

The device that made fluoroscopy safe and practical was the image-intensifier tube, sometimes called the image amplifier. The first of such devices was introduced by Coolidge (1939). This device, called an image reproducer, was used with a conventional fluoroscopic screen, the light from which was focused onto a photocathode in a tube. The electron image from the photocathode was accelerated and focused electronically and caused to strike a small fluorescent screen within the tube, thereby producing a small, bright image. Langmuir (1940) eliminated the optical lenses used by Coolidge by incorporating the photocathode and fluorescent screen and enclosing both in the tube, giving birth to the modern image intensifier.

Figure 24a illustrates a cross-sectional view of a typical image-intensifier tube, which is an evacuated chamber containing a large input fluorescent screen at one end and a small fluorescent viewing screen at the other end. X-rays passing through the subject produce a visible image on the input fluorescent screen, which is coated with a photoemissive surface of cesium and antimony that releases electrons in proportion to the brightness of the impinging radiation. The electrons are accelerated by a potential of 25–35 kV. They are then focused by additional electrodes and strike the small viewing fluorescent screen, recreating the image. The brightness amplification results from the electron acceleration and the reduction in image size (about 1/10). The viewing screen, which is about 20 mm in diameter, can be viewed with a lens system, or it can be photographed with a still or movie camera. Alternatively, with a half-silvered mirror, viewing and photography can be accomplished simultaneously.

Since the early 1960s, image-intensifier tubes have been used with television cameras and video monitors as shown in Fig. 24b. Tape recording of such images is now routine. The stop-frame features of most videotape players permits examining serial images 1/30 sec apart. The availability of the X-ray image on videotape permits easy application of computer techniques to enhance the image.

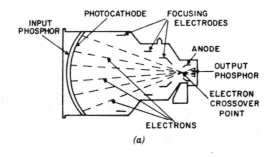

(a)

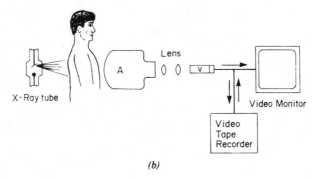

(b)

Figure 24 (a) Image-intensifier tube and (b) its use with a video camera, monitor, and tape recorder.

Computerized Tomography

A computerized tomogram (CT) (also called a computed tomogram) is a two-dimensional, reconstructed display of tissue attenuation to an X-ray beam. There are many different ways of creating such tomograms (tome = slice); the rotary system will be used to explain the principle, which has added a new dimension to X-ray visualization of tissue. Whereas a conventional X-ray image is a shadowgram at right angles to the X-ray beam, a tomogram is an image that describes the attenuation (absorption) along the path of the X-rays.

Hounsfield (1973) described the first practical instrument for making cross-sectional X-ray images. Early efforts along these lines were described by Kak (1979), who also presented the basic theory underlying the various methods of acquiring enough information to reconstruct a tomogram.

The X-ray tube emits a narrow (collimated) beam of X-rays, typically 100 kVp, which travel in a straight line through the subject's tissues (Fig. 25). The emergent attenuated ray is measured by the detector as shown. The output of the detector is inversely proportional to the total attenuation experienced by the beam. The total attenuation is a function of all of the absorbers in the path. If the tissue is homogeneous, the emergent radiation I_e is related to the incident radiation I_0 by Beer's law:

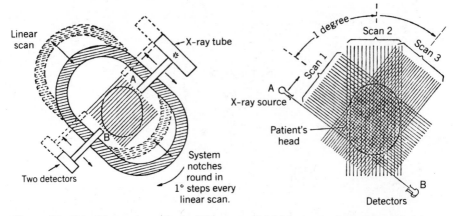

Figure 25 Principle employed in the CT scanner. Multiple scans of the object (circle) are obtained with the X-ray tube: and detector at one angular position. Then other scans are made with the X-ray tube and detector rotated at 1-degree intervals. From the multiple absorption measurements the cross-sectional absorption image (tomogram) is constructed. [Redrawn from G. N. Hounsfield, *Br. J. Radiol.* **41:**1014-1022 (1973).]

$$\frac{I_e}{I_0} = e^{-\mu t},$$

where μ is the absorption coefficient and t is the absorbing path length.

The scanning principle developed by Hounsfield is shown in Fig. 25. With one angular position of the X-ray tube and detector, 160 measurements of attenuation were made by moving the X-ray tube and detector incrementally to scan the subject. The angular position was incremented by 1 degree, and another scan taken, as shown in Fig. 25. Note that as multiple views and scans are taken, a total of 160 × 180 absorption measurements are made. In this way, the object is viewed from different angles, and from the 28,800 measurements of absorption data the cross-sectional attenuation picture is reconstructed.

Living tissue is not homogeneous, and each type has its own attenuation coefficient; moreover, the tissues are spatially distributed. If the spatial distribution is described by x and y coordinates, the attenuation is a function of x and y, and the ratio of the emergent to incident radiation is

$$\frac{I_e}{I_0} = \exp\left(-\int \mu(x, y)\, ds\right),$$

where ds is the differential path length along the ray and the integral is evaluated along the path from the X-ray tube to the detector. Taking the negative natural logarithm,

$$\ln \frac{I_e}{I_0} = \int \mu(x, y) \, ds.$$

This is the fundamental equation of the CT process. By taking multiple scans, $\mu(x, y)$, the spatial distribution of attenuation, can be determined.

In the rotary CT instrument (Fig. 26), multiple views (scans) of the tissues are obtained by indexing the X-ray tube and detector to new positions and making a measurement. The indexing may amount to a few degrees or more. Thus each element of the tissue is viewed from multiple directions. It takes only a few minutes to acquire the data, which are displayed by a video monitor as the tomogram. The computer analysis is usually complete in about 1 min or less. The computed tomogram represents a slice of tissue 5–10 mm thick and is typically composed of 160 $\times$ 320 or 256 $\times$ 256 picture elements, depending on the design of the instrument.

Since the absorption data are in computer storage, many useful techniques can

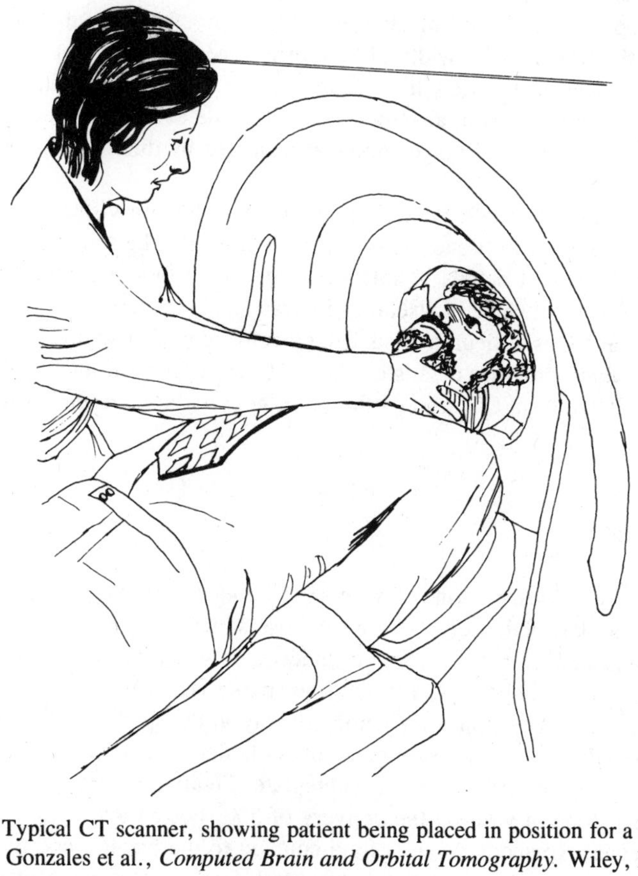

Figure 26 Typical CT scanner, showing patient being placed in position for a brain scan. (From C. F. Gonzales et al., *Computed Brain and Orbital Tomography*. Wiley, New York, 1976.)

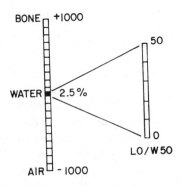

Figure 27   Absorption scale in which air is assigned a value of −1000, water zero, and bone +1000. Within this range it is possible to select a level and range for displaying the tomogram. The example shows choice of level 0 and range (width) 50, designated L0/W50.

be applied to increase the value of the display. For example, a level and range of absorption can be selected to represent the scale from white to black. The scale for attenuation ranges from +1000 to −1000; the value assigned to air is zero. The absorption for water is −1000 and for bone +1000. Within this range, the level L and display width W can be selected for reproduction on the video monitor. In Fig. 27 the level 0 and a width of 50 (corresponding to 2.5% of the range) were selected. The designation for this choice is L0/W50. By using this strategy, extremely small differences in absorption can be made evident. In addition, the various levels in the selected range can be represented by different colors on a video monitor.

Whereas conventional X-ray techniques are excellent for visualizing hard tissues and contrast media, soft tissues do not show up as well. The ability of computerized tomography to reveal details in soft tissue make it a most valuable tool. Perhaps CT has had the most value in visualizing intracranial structures. The brain is housed in dense bone and is difficult to visualize by conventional X-ray; CT has eliminated this problem and provides details on tissue structure hitherto impossible to obtain. Figure 28 illustrates a CT scan of the brain near its base, revealing the skull and soft tissues.

LITHOTRIPSY

Lithotripsy (*lithos* = stone, *tripsis* = grinding or rubbing) is the term used to designate the destruction of stones by the use of an extremely steep pressure gradient. Ultrasound or energy from an underwater spark discharge can provide the required pressure gradient. At present, the spark discharge appears to be the more convenient for kidney stones. When the energy in the spark-gap shock is focused, an extremely high local pressure gradient is obtained. Absorption of the energy in the shock wave causes the stone to disintegrate. Figure 29 illustrates the destruction of a kidney stone in vitro by the delivery of 500 shock waves.

In practice, the shock wave is fluid-coupled to the patient, and the focal point of the energy is the site of the stone. The small fragments of the disintegrated stone pass out in the urine. As yet the technique is not well suited to destroying gallstones, because of their different physical properties.

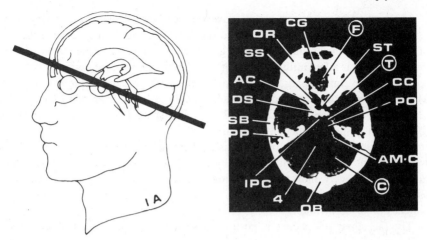

Figure 28   Normal CT scan bone structures of skull base: crista galli (CG), anterior clinoid processes (AC), orbital roof (OR), sphenoid sinus (SS), dorsum sella (DS), sella turcica (ST), petrous pyramids (PP), internal occipital protuberance (OB). Parenchymal structures: gyrus rectus and medial orbital gyrus frontal lobe (F), temporal lobe (T), cerebellar hemisphere (C), pons (PO). CSF-containing structures: fourth ventricle (4) approximately 8 mm in diameter appearing almost square, midline and immediately posterior to the pontomedullary junction. Interpeduncular (IPC), crural (CC), and ambient (AM-C) cisterns. (From C. F. Gonzalez et al., *Computed Brain and Orbital Tomography.* Wiley, New York, 1976. By permission.)

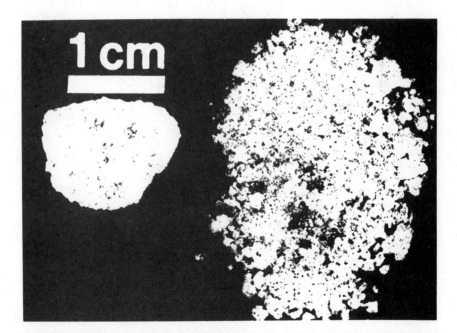

Figure 29   A kidney stone (left) and its destruction in vitro (right) by 500 shock waves. (From C. Chaussey, *Extracorporeal Shock Wave Lithotripsy.* Karger, New York, 1982. By permission.)

The method of generating shock waves and delivering them to a urinary stone is shown schematically in Fig. 30. The shock wave is generated between the tips of two 4-mm-diameter tungsten-tipped electrodes having a 20-degree taper to form the gap, which is a few millimeters long. The longer the gap, the higher the voltage required to develop a spark, and the higher the peak pressure in the shock wave. The spark is generated by discharging a 2-μF (C) capacitor charged to 27 kV (E). The energy per pulse is $0.5CE^2$, or 729 J. The spark is caused to occur at the focus of an elliptical reflector, measuring 6.5 × 11.5 cm for its semiaxis. The stone is caused to be at the other focus of the ellipse. The duration of the shock wave is about 1 μsec, and its peak intensity is about 1.5 kbar. The pressure rises to its peak in a very short time, resulting in an extremely steep pressure gradient. Efficient coupling of the energy in the shock wave is accomplished by having the patient immersed in water.

The (anesthetized) patient is positioned so that the stone is at the other focal

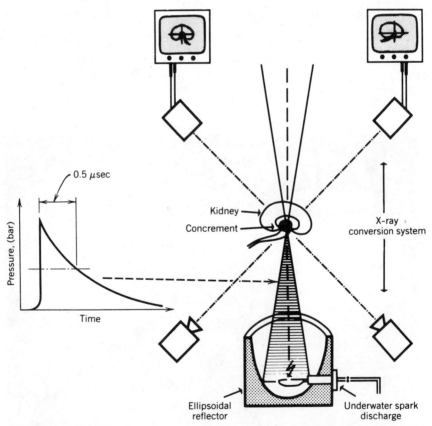

Figure 30   Method of focusing shock waves (from an underwater spark discharge) to reach a kidney stone. (Redrawn from C. Chaussey, *Extracorporeal Shock Wave Lithotripsy.* Karger, New York, 1982.)

point of the ellipse indicated by two crossing X-ray beams. Image intensifiers are used to display the images on video monitors, as shown in Fig. 30. The spark gap in the elliptical reflector is under the subject in the water-filled tank. The apparatus is arranged so that when the focal point coincides with the stone, it is at the center of the cross lines on both video monitors.

A treatment procedure consists of placing the patient in the water tank and inducing anesthesia with a short-acting narcotic. Many pulses of energy, triggered by the R wave of the ECG, are delivered. A loud thump is heard when each shock wave is delivered. Typically, the destruction of a stone requires the delivery of a few to perhaps 2000 pulses. The stone's disintegration can be seen on the video monitor, thereby allowing efficient control of the therapy.

The lithotripter has profoundly altered the way kidney stones are treated. Prior to its use, surgery was the only certain method of removing the larger stones. Chaussey (1982) reviewed 2 years' experience with 206 patients with kidney stones, about one-third of whom had prior surgical treatment. Of the total patient population, following lithotripsy 99% were free from symptoms (intense pain) and of these 10.5% had small residual concretions. The remaining 1% required surgical treatment for stone removal.

DIATHERMY

Introduction

Diathermy embraces the use of radiofrequency (rf) energy to produce heat in living tissue. Table 6 summarizes the frequencies (and wavelengths) used. The targets for the heat are the subcutaneous tissues, mainly muscles and joints. Figure 31 illustrates the overlying tissues, and Table 7 lists the electrical properties of some tissues.

The term diathermy (dia = through; thermy = heat) was introduced by Nagelschmidt (1907) and now refers to the use of three different frequency ranges (and wavelengths): long-wave, short-wave, and microwave. Long-wave (or d'Arsonval) diathermy uses electrodes in ohmic contact with the subject and employs frequencies ranging from 500 kHz to 2 MHz. This mode is little used today. Short-

TABLE 6 Diathermy Characteristics

Modality	Frequency (MHz)	Wavelength	Applicator
Long wave	1[a]	300 m	Electrodes in ohmic contact with the skin
Short wave	13.56	21.1 m	Insulated electrodes and induction coil
	27.12	11.06 m	
Microwave	2450	12.2 cm	Radiator placed above the tissue surface
	900	33.3	

[a]May vary between 0.5 and 2 MHz.

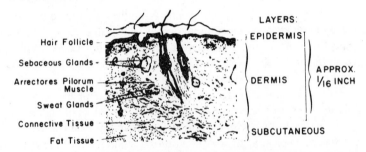

LAYERS:

Hair Follicle -
Sebaceous Glands -
Arrectores Pilorum Muscle -
Sweat Glands -
Connective Tissue -
Fat Tissue -

EPIDERMIS
DERMIS
SUBCUTANEOUS

APPROX.
$1/16$ INCH

Figure 31   Cross section of the skin. Each layer has different electrical and thermal properties. (Redrawn from G. L. Sauer, *Teen Skin*. Thomas, Springfield, IL, 1965. By permission.)

wave diathermy employs frequencies ranging from 10 to 100 MHz (typically 27.12 MHz) and insulated electrodes; i.e., the subject is capacitively coupled to the radiofrequency generator. Occasionally, short-wave currents are induced into living tissue with a coil placed over the skin. Microwave diathermy employs frequencies ranging from 900 to 2450 MHz, with the latter being the most popular in the United States. The radiofrequency energy is coupled into the subject by a radiator or antenna that resembles an optical reflector, being hemispherical or sometimes V-shaped. The radiator is placed several centimeters above the skin.

As stated previously, the major goal is to produce a temperature rise in deep tissues. An elevation in temperature increases metabolic rate and profoundly increases blood flow due to heat-induced vasodilation. The therapeutic benefit derives from these two responses.

Coupling to the Tissues

Two techniques for coupling short-wave radiofrequency current to tissue are shown in Figs. 32 and 33. With the capacitance method (Fig. 32), the tissue to be

TABLE 7   Properties of Tissues

	Electrical	Thermal	
Tissue	Frequency (MHz)	Resistivity (Ω-cm)	Dielectric constant
Skin	0.05	350	—
	25	150	95
	3000	37–50	40–45
Fat	0.05	1200–5000	—
	25	1500–3000	15
	3000	440–900	4–7
Muscle	0.05	400–500	
	25	150	100–115
	3000	43–45	45–48

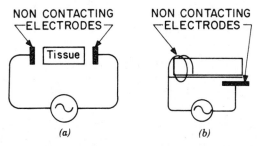

Figure 32   Capacitive coupling of radiofrequency energy to living tissue. Although two insulated plate electrodes (a) are typical, occasionally (b) one electrode is a few turns of heavily insulated flexible wire.

heated forms part of the dielectric between the two insulated electrodes (Fig. 32a). Thus, the insulation, tissue, and air form the dielectric between the two metallic electrodes. Although insulated plate electrodes are typical, occasionally one electrode is constituted by a few turns of heavily insulated wire, as shown in Fig. 32b. This technique is employed to create an insulated electrode that surrounds a member (leg or arm); the other insulated plate electrode is usually placed at the end of the member, e.g., back or buttocks. The energy is capacitively coupled into the tissue. In the rf generator there is a means to bring the circuit to resonance (tuning) at the frequency employed.

Two methods of inductive coupling are shown in Fig. 33. The inductor can be formed by a heavily insulated wire wrapped around the tissue (Fig. 33a), or it can consist of a helix (spiral or pancake coil) as shown in Fig. 33b. Typically, with a 10-cm diameter coil, the tissue is 2 cm from the coil.

The inductive method of heating is produced by eddy currents induced in the tissues, which are reasonably good conductors because of their electrolyte content.

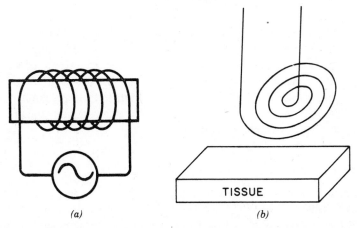

Figure 33   The induction method of coupling radiofrequency energy into living tissue (a) with a solenoid coil and (b) with a helical (pancake) coil.

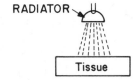

Figure 34   Coupling radiofrequency energy into living tissue with a microwave radiator.

Figure 34 illustrates the method by which microwave (900- and 2450-MHz) energy is coupled into living tissue. Because the wavelength is short (33.3 and 12.2 cm), the dimensions of the radiators are relatively small. The distances from the radiator to the subject are short, typically a few centimeters, and quite important.

It is useful to recognize that the depth of penetration of current and therefore the heating produced by long-wave, short-wave, and microwave diathermy are markedly different. Moreover, the regions of the body to which the radiofrequency energy is coupled vary in their electrical properties. These facts make it difficult to provide simple rules for obtaining uniform heating. This important aspect of diathermy will be discussed after some information is presented on the temperature range for pain and tissue damage.

Thermal Responses of Tissues

When radiofrequency (rf) current is applied to living tissue, there is the chance that the temperature will rise excessively. In a few instances skin burns have been produced in the routine use of diathermy. For a time it was thought that there were beneficial nonthermal effects to rf current. Accordingly, treatments were applied with field strengths that did not produce heating. This technique was soon abandoned, and it is now well established that the beneficial effects of diathermy are due solely to heat. However, it still is argued by some that there are nonthermal effects of microwave energy on cells.

It is important to establish the maximum safe temperature for living tissue and to understand tissue sensitivity to heat. It has been fairly well established that a sustained temperature of 45°C is close to the threshold for denaturation of many proteins, frank tissue damage occurs with a slightly higher temperature (Moritz and Henriques, 1947; see Fig. 59). A thermal stimulus just below 45°C, applied to skin, which is typically at 32°C (89.6°F), is painful. In fact, a controlled thermal stimulus applied to the skin comes close to being a standard pain stimulus, useful for testing the potency of analgesic drugs.

Short-Wave Diathermy

Both capacitive and inductive coupling are used with short-wave diathermy; D'Arsonval (1892, 1893, 1897) introduced both techniques. Because of the availability of power vacuum tubes to generate substantial radiofrequency power, use of the capacitance method became the most popular, being championed by Schereschewsky (1926). A few years later, books on the technique were published by de Cholnoky (1937) and Schliephake (1938). Surprisingly, the techniques of application have changed little since then.

The most frequently used electrodes employed with the capacitive technique are metal disks 10–20 cm in diameter. In some cases the electrodes are completely contained in a glass chamber (shoe), the front surface of which is in contact with the skin. Sometimes electrodes insulated with a rubber or plastic cover are connected to the rf generator by wires with very thick insulation because the voltages used are in the kilovolt range.

The thermal pattern between the electrodes is not uniform and depends on the distance from the tissue, the electrical properties of the tissue, the blood flow in the heated region, and the power output from the generator. The heating pattern is determined by the electric field between the electrodes. Figure 35a illustrates a typical electrostatic field pattern of a capacitor and demonstrates that the field is

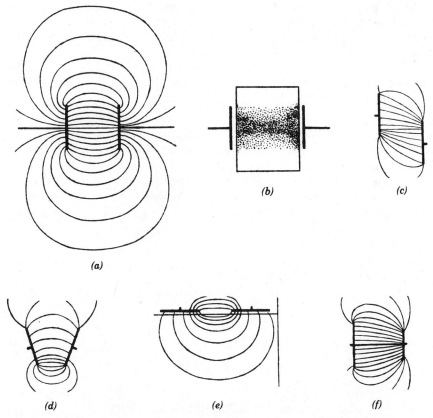

(b)

(c)

(a)

(d)   *(e)*   *(f)*

Figure 35   (a) Capacitive field and (b) heating pattern for parallel-plate electrodes. (c–f) Field patterns for asymmetrically placed capacitive electrodes. (Redrawn from B. O. Scott, *The Principles and Practices of Diathermy.* Thomas, Springfield, IL, 1957.)

most concentrated between the electrodes and decreases markedly beyond their boundaries. When the electrodes are placed to encompass a uniformly conducting medium, such as a tissue phantom, the heating pattern depends on the electrical properties of the phantom, its size, and the distance to the electrodes. With closely placed electrodes, the heating is greatest immediately below the electrodes and decreases toward the center of the phantom (Fig. 35*b*). When the electrodes are not aligned, but still parallel (Fig. 35*c*), there will be more heating under the regions of the electrodes that are closest to each other. If the electrodes are opposite each other, but not parallel (Fig. 35*d*), there will be maximum heating under the regions of the electrodes that are closest to each other. When the electrodes are on the same side of the tissue and closely spaced (Fig. 35*e*), there will be hot regions in the tissue where the electrodes are closest. Finally, if one electrode is smaller than the other, maximum heating will occur under the smaller electrode (Fig. 35*f*).

When the electrodes are placed a short distance from the surface of the phantom, the superficial and deep heating are decreased, but the ratio of surface heating to deep heating is reduced over that with closely spaced electrodes; Fig. 36 makes this point. Because the overall heating is less with widely spaced electrodes, the output of the generator must be increased.

Informative as these simple models are as a guide, in practice the situation is slightly different. Radiofrequency current is applied to a body region that is a stratified conductor, consisting of skin, fat, muscle, and bone, each with different electrical properties (Table 7). Modeling studies have been carried out on the relative heating in the skin, fat, and muscle layers by Scott (1953b), Guy et al. (1974), and Yang and Wang (1979). The data developed in these studies are not in complete accord. Nonetheless there is some agreement that the superficial layers in the models are heated more than the deeper layers. With electrodes on the same side of a member, Guy et al. (1974) pointed out that the current distribution is affected by the distribution of blood vessels, which provide many small, low-resistance pathways through the fat layers. He proved his point by constructing two double-layer phantoms, one with and one without channels to simulate blood vessels. In the phantom without channels, there was virtually no heating in the simulated fat layer.

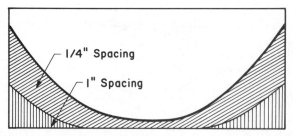

Figure 36   Diagram showing the distribution of power dissipation between two capacitive electrodes with $\frac{1}{4}$-in. and 1-in. spacing. Note that the power dissipation gradient is steeper with the closer spacing. [Redrawn from B. O. Scott, *Proc. R. Soc. Med.* **46**:331-335 (1953).]

The steep thermal gradients predicted by theory appear to be diminished in vivo by the enhanced blood flow that results from the vasodilation induced by the elevated temperature. Despite the controversy over the thermal distribution, it appears that most investigators believe that with capacitively coupled electrodes the superficial tissues become hotter than the deeper tissues.

Perspiration. With the passage of time as the subcutaneous tissues are being warmed, the skin also becomes warm, and perspiration can accumulate and run over the skin surface. Perspiration is a relatively low-resistivity electrolyte that can provide a good shunt path for the rf current around the body segment being warmed. Therefore considerable localized superficial heating can arise if the perspiration is allowed to accumulate. In practice, a thick layer of toweling is often used to absorb the perspiration. However, it should be noted that toweling acts as a good thermal insulator, and careful monitoring of the patient is necessary to avoid overheating.

Metal Implant. The presence of a metal implant is an important consideration with shortwave diathermy. Scott (1957) analyzed this situation and reported several important observations. For example, he showed that if a wire was placed lengthwise between the insulated electrodes and held at the middle, it did not become heated when the field was present. He then constructed a phantom using agar gel to which a double iodide of mercury and silver was added. At room temperature this gel is lemon yellow; at 45°C it is brick red. He then placed a conductor lengthwise in the gel and applied the electrodes and the rf current. The gel turned brick red at both ends of the wire, indicating heating. He pointed out that the wire provided a shunt path that carried considerable current, and the high current densities at the ends of the wire caused the heating.

Figure 37 illustrates the important point regarding the heating of a metallic implant. The amount of heating depends on the degree of current shunting. The three wires (A, B, C) are all in the field, and the heating will be maximum at the ends of the longest wire (A). If it is removed, heating will occur at the ends of B, by an amount that is less than occurred at the ends of A. With only wire C in the field, heating will occur, but it will be less than that at the ends of B; the shorter the piece of wire, the smaller the current flowing through it.

If the metallic implant is covered with an insulator, the current-concentrating effect will be related inversely to the thickness of the insulation and to the length of the implant in the field. An insulating layer on a metallic implant merely adds

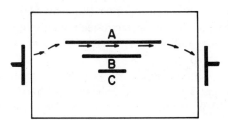

Figure 37 The effect of a metal implant in a volume conductor exposed to short-wave diathermy using capacitive electrodes. The longest metal implant (A) provides a shunt path for the current, and a high current density occurs at its ends. (Redrawn from B. O. Scott, *The Principles and Practice of Diathermy*. Thomas, Springfield, IL, 1957.)

a capacitor in series with the conductor. Because the frequency is high, the reactance of the capacitive covering will be low, especially if the insulation is thin. Therefore, current concentration will still occur with an insulated implant, and some concentrations can be expected at its extremities.

The conclusion to be drawn from the foregoing discussion is that the greater the length of the highly conducting path in the direction of the field, the greater the heating at its ends. To minimize heating in an implant, the field should be oriented at right angles to the long axis of the implant.

Inductothermy. A conductor placed in an alternating magnetic field will have a current induced in it. The intensity of the current depends on the magnetic field strength and its frequency, and inversely on the resistivity of the conductor. Because living tissues are rich in electrolytes, which are reasonably good conductors, tissue heating is easily produced by eddy currents induced by an alternating magnetic field. Moreover, magnetic fields pass through tissues very easily; therefore the distribution of heating is different with inductothermy than with capacitive coupling of rf current with insulated electrodes.

Two types of coils are used with inductothermy; Fig. 33a illustrates the solenoid with which the tissue to be heated is placed inside the coil. The helical (pancake or spiral) coil (Fig. 33b) has been called the monode or drum. When the coil is formed by winding heavily insulated wire around the body segment, thick toweling is first wrapped around the region to absorb perspiration. Toweling is also employed when the helical coil is placed at the specified distance from the skin. In both cases, the geometrical arrangement of the coil with respect to the tissues affects the distribution of induced current and therefore the thermal pattern.

The solenoid form of inductor is infrequently used, probably because of practical difficulties. Scott (1953a,b) presented important recommendations on the proper use of the solenoid form of coil. Figure 38 illustrates correct (B, D) and incorrect (A, C) application of the solenoid to body segments. When two solenoids are used, the turns of the coils must be arranged so that the electromagnetic fields are additive as shown in Figs. 38B and D.

The helical coil is used frequently and offers unique characteristics for depositing heat in muscle. Guy et al. (1974) pointed out that when a helical coil is placed at a specified distance from the skin, a substantial current can be induced in muscle as shown in Fig. 39: Lehmanm et al. (1968, 1969) carried out thermal mapping studies with helical coils on the thighs of pigs and human volunteers. To measure temperature, they used high-resistance insulated microthermistors advanced into small-diameter (0.024 in.) Teflon catheters placed at various depths in the thighs. Each thermistor was connected to a simple radiofrequency filter (for removal of the diathermy current), ahead of its connection to the temperature-recording equipment. Careful tests were made to validate the ability of the microthermal probes to measure temperature in the presence of the rf field.

Spatial temperature mapping was carried out (Guy et al., 1974) along two axes and at different depths in the thighs under the 11.4-cm-diameter helical coil (monode) placed 3 cm above the skin. About 70 W of power was delivered for 5 min

INCORRECT   CORRECT

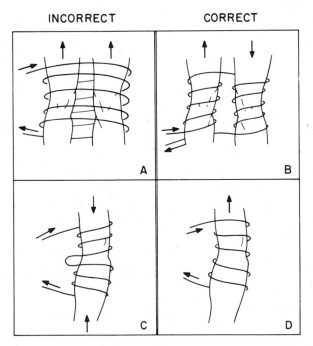

Figure 38 (*A*, *C*) Incorrect and (*B*, *D*) correct methods of using a solenoid to produce tissue heating by inductothermy. [Redrawn from B. O. Scott, *Proc. R. Soc. Med.* **46**:331-335 (1953).]

to the pig tissue. The results, shown in Fig. 40, demonstrate that the heating was maximum under the coil perimeter, and although a substantial temperature rise occurred in the muscle, the maximum temperature rise occurred at the fat–muscle interface.

In the human studies, the same insulated microthermistor probes were inserted to various depths in the thighs for temperature measurement. The surface of the 11.4-cm-diameter monode was placed 2 cm above the skin, and the locations of the temperature probes and the thickness of the fat layer were determined in each subject using radiography. The power used was 200 W applied for about 20 min. During the period of exposure to the energy, a blood pressure cuff was inflated quickly to arrest blood flow for 5 min and then deflated. Figure 41 presents a typical record of temperature and time at the different depths and reveals that the temperature rise was higher in the muscle than in the superficial tissues. The plateau in temperature was attributed to the increased blood flow from vasodilation due to the heating. Arresting blood flow with the blood pressure cuff increased the heating rate; release of the cuff pressure caused rapid cooling.

Lehmann et al. (1969) then measured the temperature rise at various depths in the thighs of the human volunteers without and with toweling wrapped around the thigh. The surface of the monode was placed 2 cm above the thigh. Figure 42

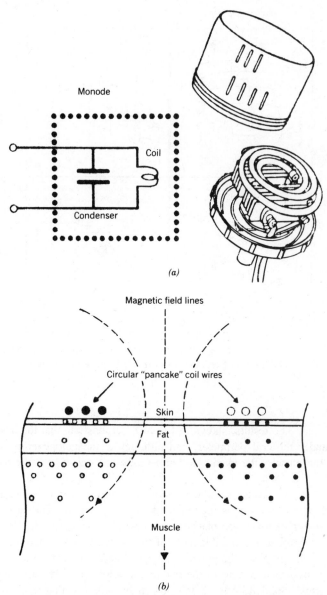

Monode

Coil

Condenser

(a)

Magnetic field lines

Circular "pancake" coil wires

Skin

Fat

Muscle

(b)

Figure 39   (*a*) The induction coil and (*b*) the field it produces in cross section. Dark spots indicate current-density vectors directed into the paper, and open circles indicate vectors out of the paper. [Redrawn from A. W. Guy et al., *Proc. IEEE* **62:**55-75 (1974).]

illustrates the temperature–time data for both experimental situations and reveals that the temperature rose more rapidly and to a slightly higher value when the skin was wrapped with toweling. The characteristic temperature plateau, due to thermally induced vasodilation, was evident in both studies.

In the same human study, Lehmann et al. (1969) measured the temperature in

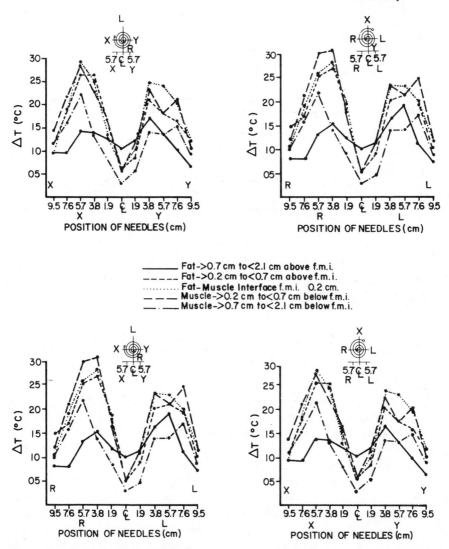

Figure 40 Thermal patterns in pig thigh specimens produced by a helical coil above the skin. [Redrawn from A. W. Guy et al., *Proc. IEEE* **62**:55–75 (1974).

muscle in subjects with 1- and 2-cm thick layers of subcutaneous fat. They found that the higher muscle temperature occurred in subjects with the thinner layer of fat.

These studies by Guy et al. (1974) and Lehmann et al. (1968, 1969) with models, pig specimens, and human volunteers indicate that induction heating with the helical coil provides good heating in the muscle with a broad maximum in the region of the fat–muscle boundary. Finally, muscle heating is less in the presence of a thick layer of overlying fat. It should be noted that the area that was heated was dependent on the area of the helical coil, which has a toroidal field pattern.

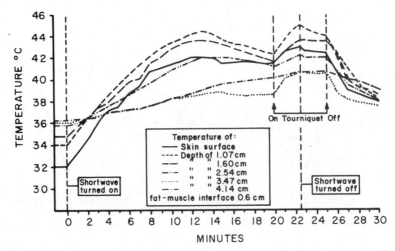

Figure 41 Temperature recorded in human thigh during application of short-wave radio-frequency energy with occlusion of blood flow after 20 min. [Redrawn from J. F. Lehmann et al., *Arch. Phys. Med. Rehabil.* **50:**117–123 (1969).]

Microwave Diathermy. The use of microwaves for tissue heating had to await the availability of microwave generators capable of delivering about 100 W continuously. Krusen et al. (1947) reported on having been interested in microwave heating a decade earlier; however, the necessary technology had not been available at that time. The first tissue microwave heating studies were conducted by Leden working with Krusen. They had obtained a 3000-MHz (10-cm) generator in 1945 and directed its output into dog limbs using a hemispherical radiator, 3.5 in. in diameter, placed 5 cm above the skin. About 65 W was applied for 20 min; this thermal dose produced a temperature rise of 3–5°C.

Microwaves share many of the properties of light: they can be reflected, refracted, diffracted, and absorbed. Coupling of this type of electromagnetic radiation to tissues is accomplished by a radiator (director) that is a type of antenna. Microwave energy is led to the radiator by a coaxial cable or a waveguide that is a metallic tube, usually with a rectangular cross section. The power delivered to the radiator can be varied as desired; usually 400 W is the maximum available.

Radiators used to couple the microwave energy to tissue are hemispherical or corner reflector. Figure 43 illustrates these types. The hemispherical radiators (Fig. 43*A,B*) differ only in their diameters. The corner reflector (*C*) was introduced by Krusen (1951) and was designed to heat large areas. With each, the energy is directed into the tissue with a beam that has essentially the dimensions of the reflector. However, the field intensity across the face of the reflector is not uniform. In the case of the hemispherical radiators, the field intensity at the center is approximately one-half of that near the perimeter. In the case of the corner reflector, the field is slightly oval, with the maximum intensity in the central area. With a homogeneous medium in front of the radiator, the heating is maximum where the

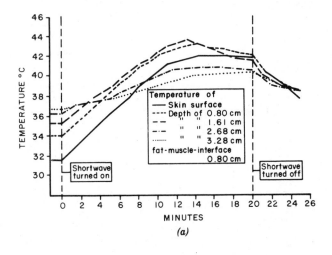

(a)

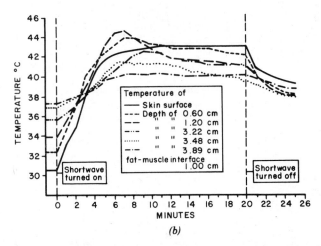

(b)

Figure 42 Temperature in human thigh (*a*) with 2-cm air space and (*b*) with 3 mm of towel between the electrodes and skin. [Redrawn from J. F. Lehmann et al., *Arch. Phys. Med. & Rehabil.* **50**:117–123 (1969).]

field strength is maximum, i.e., at the surface. However, in a multilayered medium with differing electrical and thermal properties, the heating pattern is complex, as will be demonstrated.

Schwan and Piersal (1954) and Schwan (1965) measured the resistive and dielectric properties of a variety of tissues and pointed out that the relative heating depends on the tissue properties, the thickness of the several layers (skin, fat, and muscle), and the frequency used to produce heating (see Table 7).

Johnson and Guy (1972) assembled these facts into two illustrations derived from calculations (Fig. 44) that show the absorbed power in a simulated fat–muscle

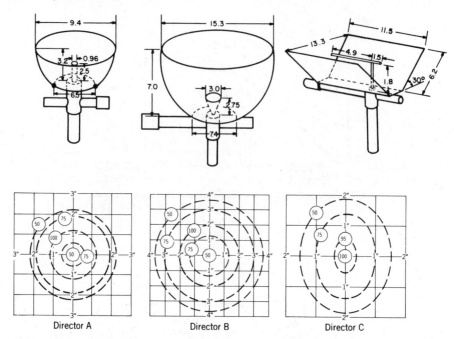

Figure 43   Radiators: (*A*, *B*) small and large hemispherical; (*C*) corner reflector. The temperatures measured on an excised specimen of skin are graphed below them. [Redrawn from J. W. Rae et al., *Arch. Phys. Med. Rehabil.* **30**:119–214 (1949).]

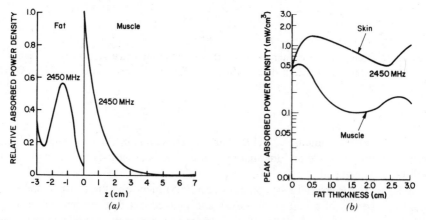

Figure 44   (*a*) Relative absorbed microwave power in simulated fat and muscle and (*b*) peak absorbed power with varying fat thickness. [Redrawn from C. C. Johnson and A. W. Guy, *Proc. IEEE* **60**:692–720 (1972).]

layer (Fig. 44a) and the absorbed power in skin (2 mm) and muscle as the thickness of the fat layer was varied (Fig. 44b). Absorbed power was used to indicate the expected maximum heating, but it must be remembered that tissue thermal properties (and blood flow) play an important role. These model studies predicted that the temperature rise throughout the tissues would be uneven.

The measured temperature rise in human tissue under a corner radiator (Fig. 43C) emitting 2450-MHz energy was measured by Lehmann et al. (1965). The radiator was 2 cm from the skin, and the subcutaneous fat was 8 mm thick. The power used (17 W) corresponded to a power density of 160 mW/cm^2, a value in the discomfort zone. Figure 45 illustrates the temperature rise over a 30-min period and demonstrates the general predictions from the model studies, that the temperature rise is less with increasing tissue depth. Figure 45 also shows that the temperature reaches a maximum first in the superficial tissues and later in the deeper layers. The decrease in temperature is due to the increased blood flow produced by thermally induced vasodilation; the increased blood flow carries away the heat. From the model studies and those carried out in human subjects, it is clear that the temperature rise with 2450-MHz energy is uneven.

To achieve a more even temperature distribution, the use of lower microwave frequencies for diathermy was investigated by Lehmann et al. (1962, 1965), Guy and Lehmann (1966), Johnson and Guy (1972), and Yang and Wang (1979). Lehmann et al. (1962) calculated and measured the temperature rise in excised pig thighs at room temperature and exposed to 900- and 2450-MHz energy, using a

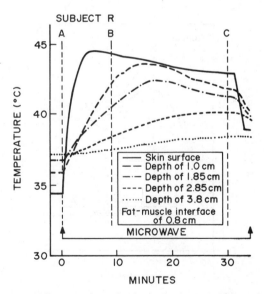

Figure 45 Temperature rise at various depths in the human thigh exposed to 2450-MHz electromagnetic energy using a corner radiator. [Redrawn from J. F. Lehmann et al., *Arch. Phys. Med. Rehabil.* **47**:307–314 (1965).]

waveguide as a radiator. The temperature distribution in skin, fat, and muscle were measured for two thicknesses of fat (2 and 4 cm). The measurements, which supported the predictions, showed that muscle heating was better at 900 MHz when the specimen contained a thin fat layer. With a thick fat layer, relatively high temperatures were encountered with both microwave frequencies.

Lehman et al. (1965) compared the tissue heating with 900- and 2450-MHz energy applied to the lower anterior thighs of human volunteers using a waveguide radiator. A treatment period ranging up to 30 min was used. With both frequencies, the temperature increased and reached a peak in 10–11 min. Thereafter the temperature decreased slightly. Figure 46 illustrates the results, which should be compared with the data in Fig. 45. Note the superiority of earlier deep heating by the 900-MHz energy.

In order to reveal the superiority of 900-MHz energy in producing deeper and more uniform heating, the data were represented in terms of the percentage of skin temperature. Figure 47 illustrates these comparisons made using waveguides to deliver the 2450-MHz (Fig. 47A) and 900-MHz (Fig. 47B) energy. It is clear that a slightly more uniform and deeper temperature distribution was obtained at 900 MHz. Subsequent studies by Guy and Lehmann (1966), Johnson and Guy (1972), and Yang and Wang (1979) all provide the same type of information, namely 900-MHz energy gives slightly more even heating.

Although 900-MHz energy appears to produce slightly more uniform tissue

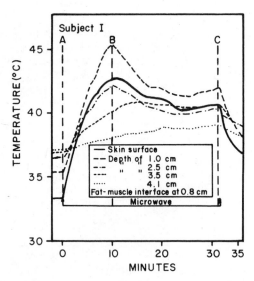

Figure 46 Temperature rise in human thighs exposed to 900-MHz electromagnetic energy delivered by a waveguide. [Redrawn from J. F. Lehmann et al., *Arch. Phys. Med. Rehabil.* **47:**307–314 (1965).]

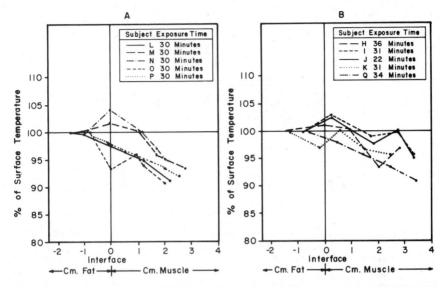

Figure 47 The distribution of temperature in the human subjects exposed to (*A*) 2450 MHz and (*B*) 900 MHz using waveguides as radiators. The temperatures at different times are expressed in terms of the skin temperature. [Redrawn from J. F. Lehmann et al., *Arch. Phys. Med. Rehabil.* **47**:307–314 (1965).]

heating, the radiators for frequencies lower than 2450 MHz are larger, so it becomes difficult to heat small areas of tissue. However, if large areas are the desired targets, or if whole-body heating is desired, the lower frequencies are more desirable. Although some of the lower frequency bands are legally assigned for industrial and medical use outside of the United States, only 2450 MHz has been assigned for such use in the United States.

Conclusion

There is no better way to conclude this discussion than to point out that the ultimate goal of all diathermy techniques is to produce uniform tissue heating. Despite the fact that the deposition of heat is nonuniform, uniformity of tissue heating is increased by the increased blood flow due to the thermally induced vasodilation. An elegant portrayal of the importance of blood flow is shown in Fig. 48, which was presented by Guy and Johnson (1974). It is clear that diathermy is contraindicated in regions where increased blood flow cannot occur. Regarding the studies carried out with physical models that predict steep thermal gradients, this finding is not normally encountered in vivo because the thermally induced vasodilation and consequent increased blood flow dramatically reduce the thermal gradients.

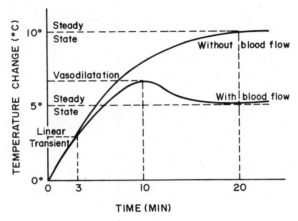

Figure 48   The general nature of tissue heating with diathermy with and without blood flow. [Redrawn from A. W. Guy and C. C. Johnson, *Proc. IEEE*, **62**:55–75 (1974).]

ELECTROSURGERY

Introduction

Electrosurgery employs 0.5–2-MHz (alternating) radiofrequency current applied to a small-area (active) electrode to produce dessication, coagulation, and cutting in living tissue. Although Cushing and Bovie (1928) are usually credited with popularizing electrosurgery, it was in use much earlier. In 1911, Clark, in the United States, developed a spark-gap generator and used its alternating current to remove skin blemishes. However, Doyen (1909), in France, had used a similar unit to excise skin blemishes. By 1930, the advantages of electrosurgical techniques were recognized; among these are the saving of time, assurance of asepsis, absence of bleeding, and elimination of the transfer of infection from diseased to normal tissue that sometimes occurred with a scalpel. Wound healing with electrodissection is almost the same as with scalpel cuts. These features were testified to by a panel of eminent surgeons who were convened on the occasion of the Conference on Electrosurgery at the Clinical Congress of the American College of Surgeons (1931). The enthusiasm in these reports, which cover a wide range of surgical procedures, shows how quickly surgeons embraced the new techniques. At this conference there was only one report on wound healing (Ellis, 1931), in which it was shown that, except for skin incisions, there is little difference between scalpel and electrosurgical cutting methods. Shortly thereafter, the first American textbook on electrosurgery was published by Kelly and Ward (1932); in it there is a good review of the histologic changes in tissue in response to electrosurgical currents. Earlier Doyen (1917) had published his text that outlined his experience with the spark-gap electrosurgical unit.

The electrosurgical instrument is a generator of controlled radiofrequency (rf) current that is applied to an active point, blade, or loop electrode to produce

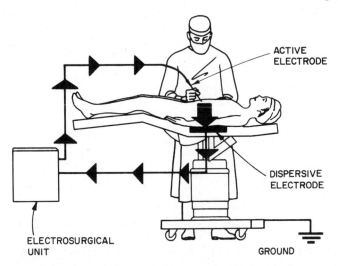

Figure 49 Essential features of electrosurgery. The cutting, coagulation, dessication, or fulguration occurs at the tip of the active electrode held by the surgeon. The return path for the current is provided by the large-area dispersive electrode, which is located at a convenient site on the patient.

dessication, fulguration, coagulation, and cutting. The return path for the current is via a large-area dispersive, reference, indifferent, or ground electrode placed at a convenient location on the subject, as shown in Fig. 49. The tissue responses are produced at the active electrode because of the high current density there. The function of the dispersive electrode is to provide a return path for the current with a negligible rise in skin temperature.

The different tissue responses depend on (1) the method of applying the active electrode and (2) the type of current employed. With some techniques, the active electrode is held above the tissue before the current is applied; with others, it contacts the tissue before current application. Continuous and interrupted currents are employed to achieve the desired tissue response. These factors will be discussed subsequently.

Current Waveforms

Several types of generators are used to provide the rf current used in electrosurgical techniques. The fundamental frequency ranges from 0.5 to 2 MHz. Figure 50 illustrates the spectrum of waveforms used in electrosurgery. The simplest, and the first to be used, was the damped sine wave (Fig. 50A), generated by a spark-gap oscillator. The waveform consists of short bursts of 0.5–1-MHz rf current delivered at a rate of 120/sec when a 60-Hz power line is used to energize the oscillator. Each pulse of current consists of a short train of damped sine waves and lasts a fraction of a millisecond. Such a waveform produces excellent coagulation and fair cutting under the active electrode.

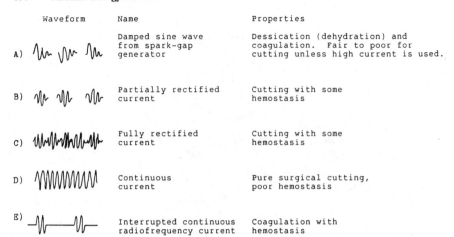

Waveform	Name	Properties
A)	Damped sine wave from spark-gap generator	Dessication (dehydration) and coagulation. Fair to poor for cutting unless high current is used.
B)	Partially rectified current	Cutting with some hemostasis
C)	Fully rectified current	Cutting with some hemostasis
D)	Continuous current	Pure surgical cutting, poor hemostasis
E)	Interrupted continuous radiofrequency current	Coagulation with hemostasis

Figure 50   Current waveforms used in electrosurgical techniques.

When power vacuum tubes became available (in the 1920s), they were used to generate rf current for electrosurgery. The first vacuum tube oscillators produced what became known as partially rectified radiofrequency current. This waveform, which is shown in Fig. 50*B*, consists of bursts of rf current delivered at a rate of 60/sec, with the envelope being a half sinusoid. Such a waveform provided good cutting with fair coagulating characteristics. Soon thereafter, fully rectified rf current as shown in Fig. 50*C* was used. In this case the rf current was delivered at a rate of 120 pulses/sec. Cutting with this type of current was good, but coagulation was only fair.

It was soon found that the use of continuous-wave rf current, as shown Fig. 50*D*, produced a pure cutting effect. With this type of uninterrupted current, the tissues vaporize and part easily in advance of the active electrode. However, the edges of incision bleed freely because the coagulating effect is poor.

Experience has shown that the use of continuous rf current (Fig. 50*D*) provides pure cutting, and the use of short-duration pulses of current (Fig. 50*A*) produces excellent coagulation with poor cutting. Therefore, electrosurgical instruments were constructed in which a spark gap was used to deliver the coagulating (damped sine wave) current and a vacuum tube was used to deliver a more or less constant cutting current. To provide cutting and coagulation at the same time, a technique of controlled mixing (blending) of the two types of currents was developed. Figure 50*E* illustrates short-duration bursts of coagulating current produced by modern solid-state electrosurgical units.

Tissue Responses

The simplest tissue response is dessication or drying (Fig. 51*A*), which is accomplished by placing the active electrode in contact with the tissue and then applying low-intensity rf current. The waveform of the current is relatively un-

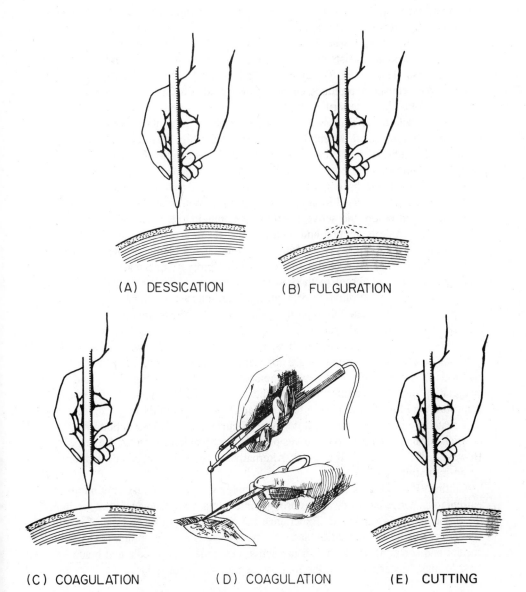

(A) DESSICATION   (B) FULGURATION

(C) COAGULATION   (D) COAGULATION   (E) CUTTING

Figure 51 (*A*) The technique for dessicating (drying) tissue by placing the active electrode in contact with the tissue and applying the radiofrequency current. (*B*) Fulguration (spark-ing), which employs short-duration bursts of rf current applied with the electrode above the tissue to provide superficial (spray) coagulation. (*C*) Coagulation, in which short-duration bursts of rf current are employed. (*D*) Coagulation of a blood vessel. (*E*) Pure cutting by application of continuous (unmodulated) rf current, which vaporizes the tissue as the active electrode is advanced.

important, since the mechanism involves resistive heating. The amount of dessication is related to the electrode area and to the intensity and duration of current application. Superficial tissue destruction can be achieved by fulguration (fulgur = lightning), which consists of drawing sparks from the active electrode held just above the tissue (Fig. 51B). To achieve this effect, interrupted (damped sinusoidal) or interrupted constant-amplitude current is delivered. The sparking or fulguration from the active electrode strikes the tissue at different points each time the pulse of current is delivered. Thus, with the electrode held in one place over the tissue, the area of tissue heated depends on the current intensity and its duration of application. Fulguration is used to destroy superficial skin growths and blemishes. With higher intensity current, coagulation is achieved. When the electrode is held above the tissue, the term spray coagulation is often used to describe the procedure.

Two techniques are used to achieve coagulation. With one, the electrosurgical unit is activated before the active electrode is applied (Fig. 51B); with the other, the active electrode is applied and then the electrosurgical unit is activated (Fig. 51C). In the former case (spray coagulation), there is the likelihood of stimulation of nearby nerves and muscles due to the rectifying property of the arc (see later in this chapter). The preferred method is shown in Fig. 51C. For coagulation, the intensity of current and duration of application are chosen to attain a temperature rise sufficient to coagulate tissue protein (above 45°C). The thermal lesion extends radially from the electrode site.

A blood vessel can be coagulated very easily by grasping it with a forceps or hemostat so that the vessel edges are apposed. Then, before activation, the active electrode is touched to the forceps or hemostat, as shown in Fig. 51D, and the coagulating current is applied for a second or so. On removal of the forceps or hemostat, the blood vessel is seen to be sealed. Bleeding in fairly large vessels can be arrested by this technique, and the type of current used is less important since no arc is formed. The surgeon's gloves provide electrical insulation for the surgeon. However, thick gloves must be used. Alternatively, the hemostat can be supported on an insulating block.

Cutting (Fig. 51E) is accomplished by applying a more or less continuous rf current to an active electrode as it is brought into contact with and advanced through the tissue which is vaporized. Experience has shown that for each type of active electrode, which can be needle, blade, or loop, there is an appropriate intensity of current and speed of movement of the active electrode. The needle and blade are used to make linear incisions; the loop is used to scoop out tissue.

Electrosurgical Current Levels

The intensity of current used for the various techniques varies widely. Table 8 lists typical magnitudes. The lowest intensity of current is used to destroy superficial skin blemishes. The highest currents are used to remove growths within the bladder, which contains urine, the most highly conducting of the body fluids. With the aid of a cystoscope it is possible to view the interior of the bladder while cutting or coagulating current is applied to an electrode on the cystoscope, as shown in Fig. 52.

TABLE 8   Current Levels and Duration of Typical Electrosurgical Procedures

I   Summary of Results of Emergency Care Research Institute Studies

Procedure	Average Voltage (V)	Average Current (mA)	Average Resistance (Ω)	Average Power (W)	Minute Duty Cycle Avg.	Max.
Transurethral resection						
Cut	370	680	540	250	15%	45%
Coag.	290	480	630	140		
Laparascopic tubal ligation						
Cut	230	520	520	110	12%	40%
Coag.	100	370	310	40		
General Surgery						
Cut	260	320	1240	70	1.4%	20%
Coag.	120	240	640	30		

II   Summary of Results of Studies by the NDM Corporation

Procedure	Current[a] (mA) Min.	Max.	Avg.	Duration of Activation[a] (sec) Min.	Max.	Avg.
Transurethral resection						
Cut	239 (162)	407 (297)	297 (200)	1.6 (.68)	3.8 (2.3)	2.1 (.69)
Coag.	179 (78)	419 (400)	256 (88)	1.4 (.5)	5 (7.6)	1.9 (.7)
Laparoscopic tubal ligation						
Cut	126 (120)	430 (290)	239 (135)	1.7 (.58)	5.4 (4.9)	2.6 (3.2)
Coag.	61 (57)	118 (80)	86 (70)	3.2 (.31)	26 (20)	10 (7.4)
General surgery[b]						
Cut	238 (188)	340 (101)	281 (147)	2 (2)	7.6 (11)	2.2 (1.8)
Coag.	146 (94)	267 (157)	198 (114)	4.7 (5.2)	11 (7.8)	6.5 (5.2)

[a]Numbers in parentheses are standard deviations.
[b]General surgical procedures include prostatectomy, laparotomy, thoracotomy, hip pinning, hysterectomy, nephrectomy, and D & C.
Source: Part I Data excerpted form *Health Devices* **2** (8–9) (June–July) (1973).
Source: Part II: J. De Rosa, personal communication, 1986.

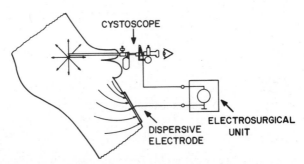

Figure 52   Use of the cystoscope with an electrosurgical instrument. [Redrawn from G. Flachenecker, *J. Urol.* **122:**336–341 (1979).]

Dispersive Electrodes

In the early days of electrosurgery, no dispersive electrode was used; the return path for the electrosurgical current was provided by the distributed capacitance between the subject and ground. This technique worked because one side of the electrosurgical generator was grounded. However, if a small area of the subject came into contact with a grounded object, a high current density occurred at this site and often a severe burn resulted. It was soon recognized that provision of a large-area return path electrode for the current eliminated the risk of burns. Accordingly, several types of dispersive electrodes were developed to be applied to the subject (i.e., on the buttocks, shoulder, etc.) to establish a definite return path for the current. At present there are four types of dispersive electrodes in use. The simplest is a large, dry, metal plate (Fig. 53A). More frequently, an electrolyte-coated metal plate is used (Fig. 53B). Another type consists of an electrolyte-soaked foam pad backed by a metal electrode (Fig. 53C). Recently, conducting adhesives have been used to hold the metal plate to the skin. The capacitive electrode (Fig. 53D) consists of a metal foil that is completely covered with a thin film

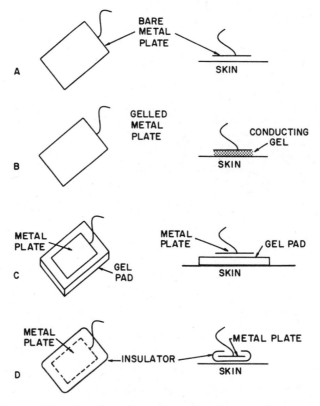

Figure 53 Types of dispersive electrodes (A) Dry metal plate; (B) metal plate coated with a conducting gel; (C) gelled foam pad; and (D) capacitive electrode.

of insulating material, which prevents ohmic contact between the metal electrode and skin.

With the dry electrode (Fig. 53A), it is often difficult to obtain uniform contact with the skin unless the subject lies on the electrode. The use of a conducting electrode paste, gel, or conducting adhesive permits low-resistance uniform contact with the subject. With the capacitive electrode, there is no conducting (ohmic) path with the subject; the current flows through the reactance of the capacitor, which is constituted by the metal electrode, the dielectric, and the conducting fluids under the skin. The dielectric (insulator) in this type of capacitor is the insulating film covering the metal electrode and the dry outer layers of the skin.

There are some subtleties relating to capacitive dispersive electrodes that merit careful consideration. For example, initially the dielectric (insulator) of the capacitive electrode is constituted by the thickness of the insulating film covering the metal electrode plus that of the dry outer layer of the skin (stratum corneum). With the passage of time, the electrode prevents the evaporation of perspiration, and the stratum corneum becomes hydrated. When this occurs, the thickness of the dielectric becomes only that of the insulating material on the metal electrode.

Electrosurgical current I passing through the capacitive electrode results in the development of a voltage across the dielectric. The voltage V across the dielectric is equal to the current multiplied by the reactance X of the capacitive electrode; therefore,

$$V = IX.$$

Now the reactance $X = 1/2\pi fC$, where f is the frequency of the electrosurgical current and C is the capacitance, which can be calculated from the area A of the electrode and the thickness t and dielectric constant k of the insulating material covering the electrode. The expression for the capacitance of a parallel-plate capacitor in picofarads (1 pF $= 10^{-12}$ F) is

$$C = 0.0885kA/t,$$

where A and t are the area and thickness in centimeters and k is the dielectric constant. The expression for capacitance when A and t are in inches is

$$C = 0.2244kA/t.$$

The electrosurgical current I flows through this capacitance and produces a voltage drop V, which is

$$V = IX = \frac{I}{2\pi fC}.$$

At this point it is informative to calculate the capacitance of a typical capacitive dispersive electrode and the voltage across it as it carries electrosurgical current.

Consider an electrode measuring 6 in. × 4 in. with a 5-mil (0.005-in.) thick dielectric of a typical polyester such as polypropylene. At 1 MHz the dielectric constant is 2.55. Therefore the capacitance in picofarads (pF) is

$$C = \frac{0.2244 \times 2.55 \times 24}{0.005} = 2747 \text{ pF}.$$

The reactance X at 1 MHz is

$$X = \frac{1}{2\mu f C} = \frac{1}{6.28 \times 10^6 \times 2747 \times 10^{-12}}$$

$$= 57.97 \ \Omega.$$

The rms voltage drop V across this electrode for a 300-mA cutting current is

$$V = IX = 0.3 \times 57.97 = 17.4 \text{ V}.$$

The dielectric must withstand the peak-to-peak voltage, which is 2.82 times the rms voltage or 49.1 V. A 1-mil thick (0.001 in.) noninsulating film can withstand 650 V; therefore the 5-mil film can withstand 3250 V. Obviously, the film will not break down.

Note that the foregoing calculations were based on the use of 300 mA (rms) of unmodulated sinusoidal (cutting) current. The situation is far different when damped coagulating current is used in which the duty cycle (percent of time of current flow) is very small. Thus the peak-to-peak value will be many, many times the rms value that is indicated by typical (rms) radiofrequency ammeters. Thus the dielectric film must be designed to withstand the high peak-to-peak voltages produced by coagulating current.

Skin-Temperature Rise. Skin-temperature rise studies have been carried out on most types of dispersive electrodes (i.e., dry metal foil, electrolyte-coated metal foil, electrolyte-soaked foam pad, and capacitive electrode). Geddes et al. (1980) conducted skin-temperature rise studies on human subjects to whom dry aluminum and copper foil electrodes were applied. Calibrated thermography was used to measure the skin temperature before applying the electrodes and at the instant of their removal when the flow of electrosurgical current was arrested. Figure 54a illustrates the result and indicates that the temperature rise is by no means uniform under a dry electrode. Geddes et al. also reported that dry metal-foil electrodes were found to be variable and unpredictable in their performance. Some who use large-area dry metal electrodes cannot confirm these observations. However, in these cases, the patient is lying on the large metal-plate electrode, which ensures good contact.

The skin-temperature rise under electrolyte-coated metal-foil electrodes applied to human subjects was reported by Silva et al. (1977), Aubry-Frize et al. (1978),

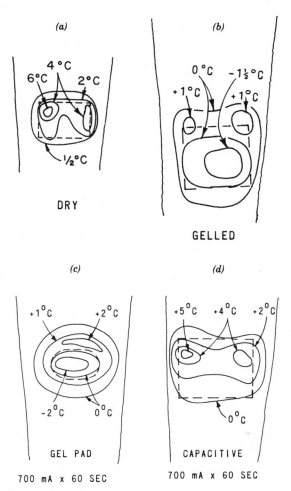

(a)

DRY

(b)

GELLED

(c)

GEL PAD

700 mA x 60 SEC

(d)

CAPACITIVE

700 mA x 60 SEC

Figure 54 Temperature-rise isotherms for (*a*) dry, (*b*) gelled metal-foil, (*c*) gelled foam pad, and (*d*) capacitive electrodes applied to human subjects (700 mA of cutting current flowed for 60 sec).

and Pearce et al. (1979). Figure 54*b* illustrates Pearce's typical temperature-rise map. It is interesting to note that the temperature rise is less than that found with dry electrodes. In both studies the same current–time program was used (700 mA for 1 min). Observe the perimeter heating with the electrolyte-coated metal-foil electrode. The decrease in skin temperature is due to evaporative cooling by the electrolytic paste.

The thermal performance of the thick electrolyte-soaked gelled foam-pad electrode was reported by Allen et al. (1982). Figure 54*c* illustrates a typical skin-temperature rise map obtained on human subjects. Interestingly enough, although this foam-pad electrode has only about one-fourth the area of conventional metal-plate electrodes, the temperature rise is similar for the same current–time program. Perimeter heating is also evident.

Pearce and Geddes (1980) reported preliminary skin-temperature rise data under capacitive electrodes. These studies on human subjects, using 700 mA for 60 sec, have shown (Fig. 54d) that capacitive electrodes produce a much more uniform but slightly higher skin-temperature rise than electrolyte-coated metal-foil electrodes. In addition, the impedance is slightly higher than that encountered with standard electrolyte-coated electrodes. The most striking difference, however, is the relative absence of a hot perimeter.

Current-Density Distribution. The lack of temperature uniformity on the skin under conductive dispersive electrodes merits comment. It indicates that the current-density distribution is nonuniform. An ingenious method measuring current-density distribution was reported by Nelson et al. (1975), who used a multi-element electrode and measured the current in each element. They found that the current density varied about threefold over the surface of the electrode. In computer-based modeling studies, Overmeyer et al. (1979), Caruso et al. (1979) and Wiley and Webster (1982) calculated the current-density distribution under a metal electrode placed on a uniform conducting medium that simulated the skin. They found that the current density at the electrode perimeter is about three times that existing under the center of the electrode (Fig. 55). Since heating depends on the square of the current density, it is reasonable to expect perimeter heating with this type of electrode.

Standards for Dispersive Electrodes

Many international standards-promulgating groups are working to develop performance standards for dispersive electrodes. In the early days of electrosurgery it

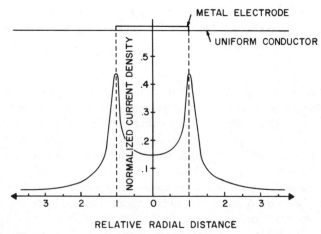

Figure 55 Current-density distribution under a dispersive electrode on a uniformly conducting medium. [Redrawn from Overmeyer et al. (1979) and Caruso et al. (1979).]

was believed that area was the all-important factor in distributing current and thereby controlling the rise in underlying skin temperature. The Association for the Advancement of Medical Instrumentation (AAMI) (1984) is now drafting a performance standard for dispersive electrodes. The 1984 draft (4.2.3.1) reads in part,

"Tests of compliance with the maximum temperature criterion shall be conducted on human volunteers or on a suitably-structured surrogate medium.

"The human subjects pool must consist of at least four males and four females, of which at least two must be identifiable as 'thermally sensitive.' (Thermally sensitive persons are defined as persons having an apparent tissue composite resistivity greater than 1200 ohm-cm at the electrode site when measured at 50 kHz with a 5-cm [outside diameter] annular tetrapolar electrode . . .)

"If surrogate media are used, the tester must demonstrate that the phantom structure is electrically and thermally similar to a 'thermally sensitive' person. Both the long-term and short-term tests must be performed a minimum of four times on each human subject.

"The temperature measurement method used must have an overall accuracy of better than 0.5°C and a spatial resolution of at least 1 sample per square centimeter of the electrode thermal pattern. The measurement apparatus must scan the entire electrode thermal pattern in less than 15 seconds. In both tests, the preapplication electrode temperature must be 23°C ± 1°C.

"1. (1) Short-Term Test. In the short-term test, the electrode under test will carry a minimum current of 700 mA RMS (+10, −0 percent) for 60 seconds. The maximum temperature rise in any of the short-term tests shall not exceed 6°C. The test current of 700 mA shall be attained within 5 seconds of the beginning of the test. In the short-term test, the electrode shall have been resting on the skin for 30 minutes prior to the application of current.

"2. (2) Long-Term Test. The electrode under test will carry a minimum current of 300 mA RMS (+10, −0 percent) at a duty cycle of not less than 33 percent with a minimum of one activation per minute for a total period of 1 hour. The maximum temperature rise in any of the long-term tests shall not exceed 10°C. No more than one long-term test should be conducted on a person in a 4-hour period.

"4.3.2. *Electrode Contact Impedance.* The contact impedance is to be measured by placing the dispersive electrode under test at some convenient site on a human volunteer, in accordance with the manufacturer's instructions. The test shall be conducted at a current of 200 mA RMS and at frequencies of 500 kHz and 2.3 MHz. The RMS potential difference between the electrode cable connection and a reference point located outside of the primary current field is divided by the RMS total electrode current to determine the contact impedance.

NOTE: The reference electrode for the potential measurement must be essentially non-current-carrying (the voltmeter must have an input impedance greater than 2 kohms at the frequency of measurement).

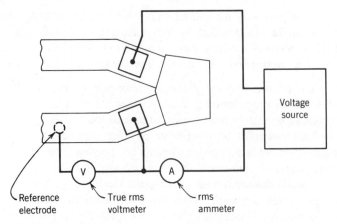

Figure 56 Method for measuring electrode contact impedance. (Redrawn from the Association for the Advancement of Medical Instrumentation (AMMI) *Standard for Electrosurgical Devices*. AAMI, Arlington, VA, 1984. By permission.)

"In the example shown [Fig. 56] the electrode under test was placed on the thigh and the potential reference electrode consisted of an ECG monitoring electrode placed on the calf muscle (out of the primary current field).

"The test must be repeated for at least 10 randomly chosen electrodes applied to at least two 'thermally sensitive' human volunteers."

Burns under Dispersive Electrodes

When carefully applied, virtually all presently used dispersive electrodes provide a low enough power density to prevent burns. However, when an electrode is misapplied or becomes dislodged when a patient is repositioned, the area of contact may be reduced and the stage is set for a burn. Battig (1968) discussed this topic extensively. Moreover, if the wire from the dispersive electrode to the electrosurgical unit is broken or becomes disconnected, the return path for the current will be that for the lowest impedance from the patient's body to ground. The path may include any part of the body adjacent to the metal parts of an operating table or monitoring electrodes for electrocardiography or any other electrodes connected for special purposes. Because the area of contact with the body will be small, high current densities and burns can occur at these sites. Such alternate current pathways constitute the major source of electrosurgical mishaps—and lawsuits. Becker et al. (1973) surveyed the available literature on burns associated with the use of electrosurgical instruments. They found that the burns in nine patients were due to a broken wire to the dispersive electrode, defective ground-sentry circuitry, capacitive coupling between the electrosurgical leads and ECG monitoring leads, and misuse of equipment.

In Becker's paper there are data to indicate the current intensity, duration of flow, and electrode area that will produce skin damage. Table 9 presents a summary of the data that represent current flow through small-area electrodes. Note that the

TABLE 9   Thermal Effects of Radiofrequency Current

Current mA (rms)	Duration (sec)	Electrode Area (cm^2)	Current Density (mA/cm^2)	Power Density[a] [W/(cm^2)/(Ω)]	Energy Density Factor[b] [(mA/cm^2)^2 sec]	Tissue Response
200	30	3.8	52.6	0.011	8.3 × 10^4	Reddening of surrounding tissue
300	20	3.8	78.9	0.024	12.5 × 10^4	Pain and blistering
400	10	3.8	10	0.042	11 × 10^4	Unbearable pain
400	20	1.0	400	0.16	320 × 10^4	Second-degree burn

[a]Power density is expressed on a per-ohm basis due to unknown contact impedance at the dispersive electrode. Note that very low power densities (on a per-ohm basis) show a wide range of physiologic responses. This suggests that the criteria suggested in 76 C-M (see Table 1) have not included enough variables.
[b]The energy-density factor multiplied by resistivity is a measure of the number of calories applied to the tissues under the dispersive electrode. With appropriate scaling and use of the specific heat of the tissues, it is possible to calculate the temperature rise under the dispersive electrode.
Source: C. M. Becker, et al., *Anesthesiology* **38**(2):106–122 (1973).

severity of skin response is related to the power density and to the energy density factor; the latter quantity appears to correlate better with the severity of skin response.

When electrosurgical current returns via typical electrocardiograph electrodes, skin burns can occur. De Rosa and Gadsby (1979) conducted studies to demonstrate this point. Figure 57 illustrates the temperature rise versus duration of current flow for different electrode current densities.

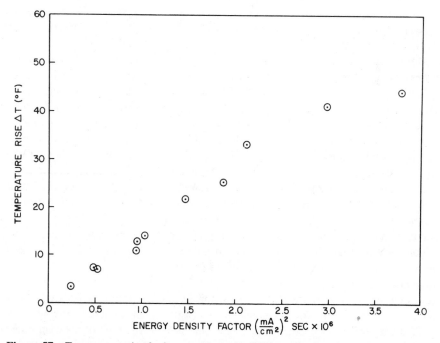

Figure 57   Temperature rise for human skin under ECG-monitoring electrodes for different energy density factors. Calculated from De Rosa and Gadsby (1979).

To provide skin-temperature rise data based on electrosurgical current intensity and time factors, Pearce et al. (1983) conducted studies on pigs. Electrodes were applied to the back with conducting gel. Temperature rise was measured using high-speed calibrated thermography. Figure 58a illustrates the temperature rise versus energy density factor; $[(A/(cm^2)t]$ Fig. 58b illustrates the burns. These data are fairly consistent with those obtained by De Rosa on humans shown in Fig. 57. Table 10 summarizes the data from Pearce's paper. It should be recalled that the current density under an electrode is not uniform and that the tissue response may be dependent on electrode geometry.

Perhaps the most important factor in producing skin burns is contained in the burn strength–duration curve, originally presented by Moritz and Henriques (1947). This study showed that the burn severity was related to temperature and the duration of exposure to that temperature on the skin. Using metal chambers heated by circulating hot water, Moritz and Henriques plotted curves that related temperature to the duration of exposure to that temperature required to produce irreversible epidermal injury and to produce necrosis in porcine skin, which is an excellent analog for human skin; Fig. 59 presents their data. It is clear that a high temperature can be tolerated for a short time. It is also clear that a skin burn will occur at a much lower temperature if that temperature is maintained for a long period. It is generally assumed that a skin temperature of 45°C can cause a burn if it persists.

Output Circuits

In order to understand how electrosurgical burns can occur, it is necessary to recognize that the alternate current pathways depend partly on the type of output circuit in the electrosurgical unit.

An electrosurgical current generator is illustrated in Fig. 49 as a box with two wires connected to the patient. One wire conducts the current to the active electrode, the other provides a return path for the current via the dispersive electrode. However, within the box is one of three types of output circuit. Although the type of output circuit is irrelevant to normal operation of the device with properly connected electrodes, it assumes considerable importance in abnormal circumstances, which, unfortunately, are not rare. The type of output circuit largely determines the current intensity under fault conditions.

The three types of output circuits are illustrated in Fig. 60. An electrosurgical generator is a potent source of high-frequency alternating current in series with an output impedance Z_o, which amounts to a few hundred ohms. Figure 60A illustrates the grounded-output circuit that was used in the earliest electrosurgical generators. Figure 60B illustrates the ground-referred output circuit; the ground reference is provided by a capacitor (C), which has a low reactance for the radiofrequency current and a high reactance for 60-Hz current. Use of this type of circuit minimizes shock hazard from 60-Hz leakage current. Figure 60C illustrates the isolated output circuit, in which neither output conductor has a direct connection to ground. Any ground path for either conductor is dependent on the magnitude of the distributed capacitance (C_d) from each output lead to ground, plus the capacitance of the electrode cables to ground. The isolation is often provided by a transformer.

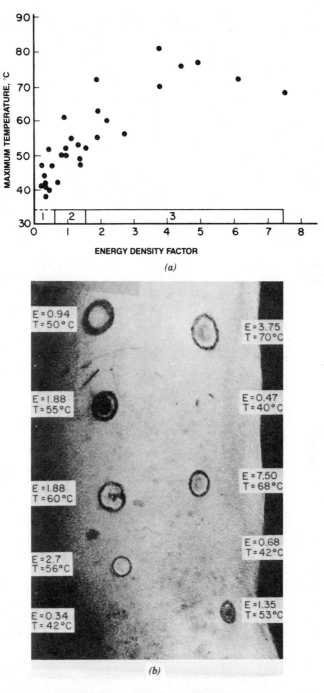

(a)

(b)

Figure 58 (a) Maximum temperature rise versus energy-density factor of circular electrodes on pig skin. The numbers 1, 2, and 3 refer to the burn classification. (b) Burns on pig skin under circular electrodes with different energy-density factors (E). [From J. A. Pearce et al., *Med. Instrum.* **17**:225–231 (1983). By permission.]

TABLE 10   Experimental Conditions and Results

Expt. No.	Current (mA)	Time (sec)	Electrode Size (cm²)		$\bar{J}^2t$ [A²(cm⁴)(sec⁻¹)]		Max. Temp. (°C)		Burn Severity Index	
			L	R	L	R	L	R	L	R
68-A1	500	60	4	2	0.94	3.75	50	70	2.36	7.44
A2	500	30	2	4	1.88	0.47	55	40	4.28	0.1
A3	500	30	2	1	1.88	7.50	63	68	6.32	7.81
A4	300	30	1	2	2.70	0.68	56	42	7.1	0
A5	300	60	4	2	0.34	1.35	42	53	0	1.18
68-B1	500	60	2	4	3.75	0.94	70	49	11.7	2.75
B2	450	30	1	2	6.08	1.52	72	52	7.75	4.27
B3	600	60	4	2	1.35	5.40	—	—	—	12.49
B4	700	40	2	8	4.90	0.31	77	44	6.55	0.01
B5	650	30	8	4	0.20	0.79	41	50	0	0.31
B6	300	60	2	4	1.35	0.34	47	38	0.20	0.01
68-C1	500	60	2	4	3.75	0.94	81	52	14.87	4.32
C2	700	60	8	4	0.46	1.84	52	72	1.84	7.43
C3	700	30	4	8	0.92	0.23	61	47	4.81	0.31
C4	380	60	2	4	2.17	0.54	60	47	4.90	0.20
C5	540	60	2	4	4.37	1.09	76	55	9.99	4.02
C6	300	60	4	2	0.34	1.35	41	49	0	2.36

L = left site; R = right site; $\bar{J}^2t$ = relative energy density factor.
Source: Pearce et al. (1983).

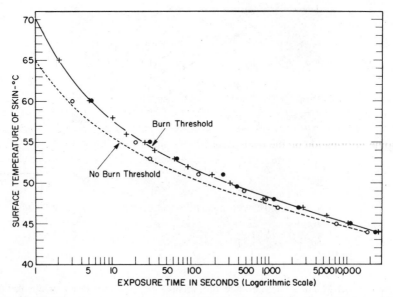

Figure 59 Temperature versus exposure time for burns. [Redrawn from Moritz and Henriques (1947).]

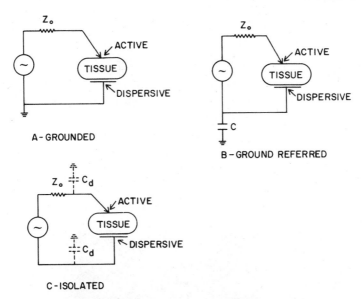

Figure 60 Typical output circuits for electrosurgical generators. (*A*) Grounded output; (*B*) ground-referred; (*C*) isolated output circuit.

Each of the three types of output circuit has its own characteristics under fault conditions, typically breakage of the conductor from the dispersive electrode, failure to apply the dispersive electrode, or accidental operation of the electrosurgical unit with the active electrode short-circuited to ground. These fault situations create a variety of alternate current pathways that can cause severe burns. Only by careful analysis is it possible to identify the cause of a burn in an accident.

Radiofrequency Interference

Because of the transient nature of the current pulses used in electrosurgery, the energy emitted covers a wide frequency band. Patient monitoring and radio reception in the environment are blanked out when an electrosurgical unit is used. There is some information on the energy spectra emitted by electrosurgical units. Dobbie (1969) reported that the frequency spectrum of coagulating current extended beyond 30 MHz. A detailed study of the energy spectra of cutting and coagulating current delivered by solid-state, vacuum tube, and spark-gap electrosurgical units was undertaken by Pearce (1984), who measured the energy spectra for current without an arc and with an arc at the electrode–tissue interface. A summary of these results will now be presented.

Figure 61*a* illustrates the cutting waveform from a solid-state electrosurgical unit with a frequency of 500 kHz. The energy spectrum for 200-mA (rms) current without an arc is shown in Fig. 61*b* and with an arc at the electrode–tissue interface in Fig. 61*c*. It is clear that the presence of the arc greatly augments the higher-frequency components.

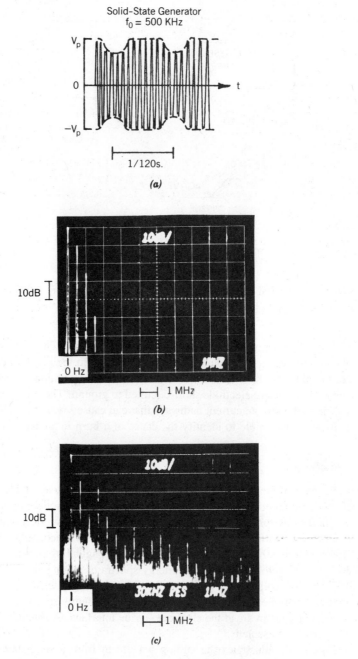

Figure 61 (*a*) Cutting current waveform from a solid-state electrosurgical unit. (*b*, *c*) Current frequency spectra at 200 mA (rms) (*b*) with no arc and (*c*) with an arc at the electrode–tissue interface. [Courtesy of J. A. Pearce (1984).]

Figure 62*a* illustrates the cutting current waveform from a vacuum tube electrosurgical unit operating at 2.5 MHz. The energy spectrum at 200 mA (rms) is shown without an arc (Fig. 62*b*) and with an arc (Fig. 62*c*) at the electrode–tissue interface. Establishment of the arc greatly enhances the high-frequency components.

The waveform for coagulating current from a solid-state electrosurgical unit is shown in Fig. 63*a*. The energy spectrum (at 200 mA rms) is shown without an arc in Fig. 63*b* and with an arc in Fig. 63*c* at the electrode–tissue interface. As with the cutting current, the presence of an arc augments the high-frequency spectrum.

Figure 64*a* illustrates the waveform for coagulation delivered by a spark-gap electrosurgical unit. Figure 64*b* shows the energy spectrum (at 200 mA rms) with no arc at the electrode–tissue interface. The spectrum when an arc is present is shown in Fig. 64*c*.

The foregoing clearly demonstrates that the energy spectrum from an electrosurgical unit is extremely broad. To date, it has not been possible to create filters for the electrosurgical unit or a bioelectric recorder to allow recording during electrosurgery.

It is clear that with both cutting and coagulating current, the frequency spectrum is broadened when an arc is struck at the active electrode. This fact has been confirmed by Tucker et al. (1984), who found that more low-frequency components are produced with coagulating current, as shown by Figs. 63 and 64. The significance of this fact is that coagulating current is more likely to produce tissue stimulation. The mechanism will be described in the following paragraphs.

Tissue Stimulation

It is not uncommon to encounter muscle stimulation in tissue near the active electrosurgical electrode. Such stimulation would not be predicted on the basis of the short period (1/frequency) of one cycle of electrosurgical current. The stimulating capability of electrosurgical current was demonstrated by Hungerbuhler et al. (1974) and Geddes et al. (1975); in both cases, ventricular fibrillation was produced. In Hungerbuhler's report, an intravascular catheter was applied to a human subject. In the study by Geddes et al., a catheter electrode was in a dog heart. Figure 65 illustrates the precipitation of ventricular fibrillation with a catheter electrode in the right ventricle and connected to an electrocardiograph. The return path for the electrosurgical current was interrupted, and the active electrode was applied to the chest. The result was immediate ventricular fibrillation.

The circumstances under which electrosurgical current can stimulate were investigated by Foster and Geddes (1986) in two types of experiments in which the current could be passed through a subject with and without an arc in the circuit. Figure 66 illustrates the arrangement of equipment for the study. The electrosurgical instrument was connected via an ammeter to a dispersive electrode on the dog's back. The sciatic nerve stimulating electrode consisted of a saline-soaked

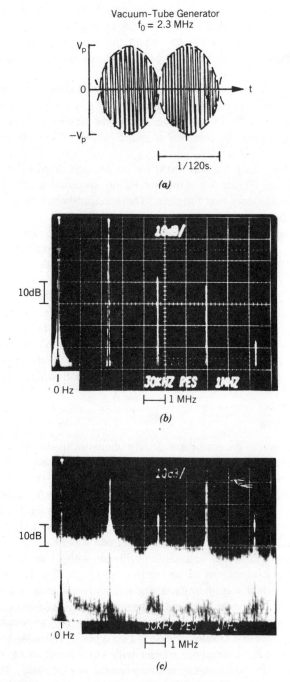

Figure 62   (*a*) Cutting current waveform of a vacuum tube electrosurgical unit. (*b*, *c*) Current frequency spectra at 200 mA (rms) (*b*) with no arc and (*c*) with an arc at the electrode–tissue interface. [Courtesy of J. A. Pearce (1984).]

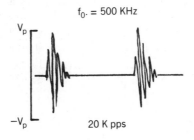

$f_{0.} = 500$ KHz

V_p

$-V_p$

20 K pps

Solid-State Generator

(a)

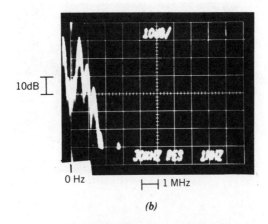

10dB

0 Hz

⊢—⊣ 1 MHz

(b)

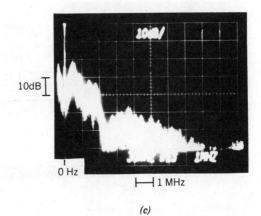

10dB

0 Hz

⊢—⊣ 1 MHz

(c)

Figure 63   *(a)* Coagulating current waveform of a solid-state electrosurgical unit. *(b, c)* Current frequency spectra at 200 mA (rms) *(b)* without and *(c)* with an arc at the electrode-tissue interface. [Courtesy of J. A. Pearce (1984).]

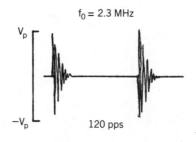

Spark-Gap Generator

(a)

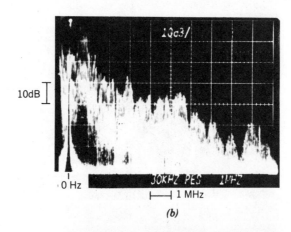

(b)

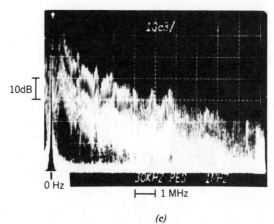

(c)

Figure 64   (*a*) Coagulating current waveform of a spark-gap electrosurgical unit. (*b*, *c*) Current frequency spectrum at 200 mA (rms) (*b*) without and (*c*) with an arc at the electrode-tissue interface. [Courtesy of J. A. Pearce (1984).]

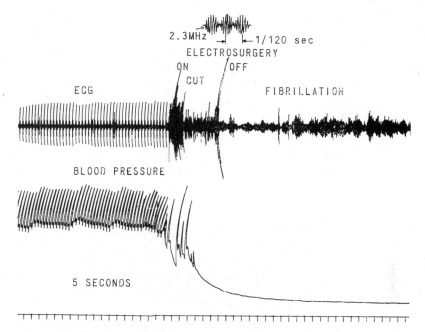

Figure 65   Ventricular fibrillation induced in the dog by electrosurgical current.

gauze pad covering a $\frac{1}{2}$-in. ball electrode, which was in series with a saline-soaked sponge in a metal dish. The active electrosurgical electrode could be plunged into the sponge before current was applied or advanced toward the sponge with the electrosurgical unit activated. In the former case, no arc was formed; in the latter case, an arc was struck. Arc and no-arc studies were performed with two of the most popular electrosurgical instruments. One was a solid-state type; the other contained vacuum tubes and spark gaps. In the former, the cutting current consisted of unmodulated 0.5-MHz current; for coagulation, this current was delivered in

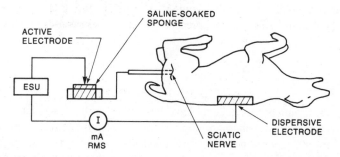

Figure 66   Arrangement of equipment to demonstrate the stimulating capabilities of electrosurgical current with an arc and no arc at the active electrode–sponge interface. [From K. S. Foster and L. A. Geddes, *Med. Instrum.* **20**(6):335–336 (1986). By permission.]

TABLE 11   The Stimulating Capabilities of Cutting and Coagulating Current

Instrument	Mode	Current [mA(rms)]	Contraction Arc	Contraction No Arc
1	Coag.	200	Yes	No
	Cut	500	Yes	No
2	Pure cut	200	Yes	No
	Spark gap coag.	600	—	No
	(moderate hemostasis)	200	Yes	—
	Spark gap coag.	500	—	No
	(marked hemostasis)	• 100	Yes	—
	Spark gap coag.	250	—	Trace
	(max. hemostasis)	< 100	Yes[++]	—

Source: Foster and Geddes, *Med. Instrum.* **20**(b): 335–336(1986).

20-kHz bursts (see Fig. 63). The second instrument produced 2-MHz current modulated at twice the power-line frequency. The coagulating (hemostasis) current was provided by the spark gaps, which delivered short-duration damped sine waves at twice the power-line frequency (see Fig. 64).

Table 11 summarizes the results for the arc and no-arc conditions for both electrosurgical units. Note that in every case when an arc was struck, the sciatic nerve was stimulated and muscle contraction occurred. In only one case when spark-gap current was applied with no arc was a slight muscular contraction produced.

As shown earlier in this chapter and by Pearce (1986), the presence of an arc at the active electrosurgical electrode results in a broadening of the frequency spectrum of the electrosurgical current. Both low- and high-frequency components are produced. It is probably the low-frequency components that provide the stimulus.

The study just described has certain implications. If coagulation (hemostasis) is to be produced without stimulation, good practice would indicate that the active electrode should be applied to the tissue before the electrosurgical unit is activated. If muscular contractions are to be avoided when using cutting current, the active electrode should not be used in the presence of large nerve trunks or plexuses.

Pacemakers

An increasing number of patients have implanted cardiac pacemarkers. These devices are becoming much more sophisticated and programmable by external signals. There are reports indicating that presently available demand pacemakers are inhibited by electrosurgical current. Many revert to a fixed-rate mode of operation. There is the possibility that some of the newer programmable units might be reprogrammed by the rapid intermittent use of electrosurgical current.

REFERENCES

Allen, J., L. A. Geddes, J. A. Pearce, and J. C. Mullikin. 1982. The effect of adipose tissue on the thermal performance of electrosurgical electrodes. *Clin. Eng.* **6**(4):313-318.

Association for the Advancement of Medical Instrumentation (AAMI). 1984. *Standard for Electrosurgical Devices.* AAMI, Arlington, VA.

American College of Surgeons. 1931. Conference on electrosurgery. *Surg. Gynecol. Obstet.* **52**:502-520.

Aubry-Frize M., A. Leduc, R. Marsolais, and R. Carrier. 1978. Assessment of skin temperature elevation due to electrosurgical current. *Proc. 13th Annu. Meet. Assoc. Adv. Med. Instrum., 1978.*

Babbs, C. F., and De Witt, D. P. 1981. Physical principles of local heat therapy for cancer. *Med. Instr.* **15**(6):367-373.

Battig, C. G. 1968. Electrosurgical burns and their prevention. *JAMA* **204**:1025-1029.

Becker, C. M., I. V. Malhotra, and J. Hedley-White. 1973. The distribution of radiofrequency current and burns. *Anesthesiology* **38**(2):106-122.

Bucky, G. 1915. German Patents DRP 284,371, 287,653, and 287,657.

Caruso, P., J. A. Pearce, and D. P. DeWitt. 1979. Temperature and current density distributions at electrosurgical dispersive electrode sites. *Proc. 7th N. Engl. Bioeng. Conf. 1979* pp. 373-374.

Chaussey, C. 1982. *Extracorporeal Shock Wave Lithotripsy.* Karger, New York, 112 pp.

Clark W. L. 1911. Oscillatory dessication in the treatment of accessible growths and minor surgical conditions. *J. Adv. Ther.* **29**:169-183.

Cobine, J. D. 1958. *Gaseous Conductors.* Dover, New York, 606 pp.

Cobine, J. D. 1980. Introduction to vacuum arcs. In *Vacuum Arcs.* J. M. Lafferty (ed.). Wiley, New York, 372 pp.

Coolidge, W. D. 1913. Powerful roentgen ray tube with a pure electron discharge. *Phys. Rev.* **2**:429.

Coolidge, W. D. 1930. The development of modern roentgen-ray generating apparatus. *Am. J. Roentgenol. Radium Ther.* **24**:605-620.

Coolidge, W. D. 1939. Image reproduction. U.S. Patent 2,158,853, May 16.

Cornelius, W. A. 1983. Application of lasers in medicine. *Australas. Phys. Eng. Sci. Med.* **6**:106-114.

Cushing, H., and W. T. Bovie. 1928. Electrosurgery as an aid to the removal of intracranial tumors. *Surg., Gynecol. Obstet.* **47**:751-784.

d'Arsonval, A. 1892. Sur les effets physiologiques de l'état variable et des courants alternatifs. *Bull. Soc. Int. Electr.*

d'Arsonval. A. 1893a. *Arch. Physiol. Norm. Pathol.* **5**:401-408, 789-790.

d'Arsonval, A. 1893b Influences de la fréquencie sur les effets physiologiques des courants alternatifs. *C. R. Hebd. Seances Acad. Sci.* **116**:630-633.

d'Arsonval, A. 1897. Action physiologiques des courants alternatifs à grande fréquence. *Arch. Electr. Med.* **7**:133.

de Cholnoky, T. 1937. *Short Wave Diathermy.* Columbia Univ. Press, New York, 310 pp.

De Rosa, J., and P. D. Gadsby. 1979. Radiofrequency heating under ECG electrodes. *Med. Instrum.* **13**:273-276.

Deutsch, M. B., J. C. Stothert, B. Ashleman et al. 1980. Laser scalpel for solid organ surgery. *Am. J. Surg.* **139**:665-668.

Dibner, B. 1963. *The New Rays of Professor Roentgen.* The Burndy Library, Norwalk, CN, 55 pp.

Dobbie, A. K. 1969. The electrical aspects of surgical diathermy. *Biomed. Eng.* **4**:206-216.

Doyen, E. 1909. Sur la destruction des tumeurs cancéreuses accessibles. *Arch. Elect. Med. Physiol.* **17**:791-795.

Doyen, E. 1917. *Surgical Therapeutics and Operative Techniques.* William Wood & Co., New York 746 pp.

Ellis, J. D. 1931. The rate of healing of electrosurgical wounds. *JAMA* **96**(1):16–18.

Epp, E. R., and H. Weiss. 1966. Experimental study of photon energy spectrum of primary diagnostic x-rays. *Phys. Med. Biol.* **11**:(2):225–238.

Foster, K. S., and L. A. Geddes. 1986. The cause of stimulation with electrosurgical current. *Med. Instrum.* **20**(6):335–336.

Geddes, L. A., W. A. Tacker, and P. Cabler. 1975. A new electrical hazard associated with the electrocautery. *Med. Instrum.* **9**:112–113.

Geddes, L. A., J. A. Pearce, J. D. Bourland, and L. Silva. 1980. Thermal properties of dry metal foil electrodes. *Clin. Eng.* **5**:13–18.

Glasser, O. (ed.). 1933. *The Science of Radiology.* Thomas, Springfield, IL., 450 pp.

Gonzalez, C. F., C. B. Grossman, and E. Palacios. 1976. *Computed Brain and Orbital Tomography.* Wiley, New York, 276 pp.

Guy, A. W., and C. C. Johnson. 1974. *Proc. IEEE* **62**:55–75.

Guy, A. W., and J. F. Lehmann. 1966. On the determination of optimum microwave diathermy frequency for a direct contact applicator. *IEEE Trans. Biomed. Eng.* **BME-13**:76–87.

Guy, A. W., J. R. Lehmann, and J. B. Stonebridge. 1974. Therapeutic applications of electromagnetic power. *Proc. IEEE* **62**:55–75.

Hardy, J. D. 1939. The radiating power of human skin in the infrared. *Am. J. Physiol.* **127**:454–462.

Hardy, J. D., and C. Muschenheim. 1934. The radiation of heat from the human body. IV. *J. Clin. Invest.* **13**:817–831.

Hart, D., and D. G. Sharp. 1947. Surgery: Asepsis. In *Medical Physics,* Vol. 1. O. Glasser (ed.). Year Book Publishers, Chicago, IL.

Heimbach, D. M., D. Neal, J. D. Doty, et al. 1980. The use of the argon laser assisted quartz scalpel in burn wound excision to fascia. *J. Trakima* **20**(2):123–126.

Hounsfield, G. N. 1973. Computerized transverse axial scanning (tomography). *Br. J. Radiol.* **41**:1014–1022.

Hungerbuhler, R. F., J. P. Swope, and J. G. Reeves. 1974. Ventricular fibrillation associated with the use of electrocautery. *JAMA* **230**:430–436.

Johnson, C., and A. W. Guy, 1972. Nonionizing electromagnetic wave effects in biological materials and systems. *Proc. IEEE* **60**:692–720.

Kak, A. 1979. Computerized tomography with x-ray, emission and ultrasound sources. *Proc. IEEE* **67**(9):1245–1272.

Kelly, H. A., and G. E. Ward. 1932. *Electrosurgery.* Saunders, Philadelphia, PA, 305 pp.

Koller, L. R. 1952. *Ultraviolet Radiation.* Wiley, New York, 270 pp.

Krusen, F. H. 1951. New microwave diathermy director for heating large regions of the human body. *Arch. Intern. Med.* **32**:695–698.

Krusen, F. H., J. F. Herrick, U. Leden, and K. G. Wakim. 1947. Microkymatotherapy. *Proc. Staff Meet. Mayo Clin.* **22**:209–224.

Langmuir, I. 1940. Image reproduction. U.S. Patent 2,198,479, April 23.

Lehmann, J. F., A. W. Guy, V. C/ Johnston, G. D. Brunner, and J. W. Bell. 1962. Comparison of relative heating patterns produced in tissues by exposure to microwave energy frequences of 2450 and 900 megacycles. *Arch. Phys. Med. Rehabil.* **43**:69–76.

Lehmann, J. F., V. C. Johnston, J. A. McMillan, D. R. Silverman, G. D. Brunner, and L. A. Rathburn. 1965. Comparison of deep heating by microwaves at frequencies 2456 and 900 megacycles. *Arch. Phys. Med. Rehabil.* **49**:307–314.

Lehmann, J. F., A. W. Guy, B. J. DeLateur, J. B. Stonebridge, and C. G. Warren. 1968. Heating patterns produced by short-wave diathermy using helical induction coil applicators. *Arch. Phys. Med. Rehabil.* **49**:193–198.

Lehmann, J. F., B. J. DeLateur, and J. B. Stonebridge. 1969. Selective muscle heating by shortwave diathermy with a helical coil. *Arch. Phys. Med. Rehabil.* **50:**117–123.

Lloyd-Williams, K. 1964. Pictorial heat scanning. *Phys. Med. Biol.* **9:**433–456.

Maiman, T. H. 1960. Stimulated optical radiation in ruby. *Nature* **187:**493–494.

Mitchell, D., C. H. Wyndham, T. Hodgson, and P. R. N. Nabarro. 1967. Measurement of the total normal emissivity of skin without the need for measuring skin temperature. *Phys. Med. Biol.* **12**(3):359–366.

Moritz, A. R., and F. C. Henriques. 1947. The relative importance of time and surface temperature in the causation of skin burns. *Am. J. Pathol.* **23:**605–720.

Nagelschmidt, F. 1907. *Verh. Ges. Dtsch. Naturforsch. Aerzte* **79:**58.

Nelson, J. A., L. C. Gogliano, and D. D. Clements. 1975. Current distribution at electrosurgical ground sites. *Proc. 28th Annu. Conf. Eng. Med. Biol.* **25:**12.

Overmeyer, K., J. A. Pearce, and D. P. DeWitt. 1979. Measurements of temperature distribution at electrosurgical dispersive electrode sites. *Trans. ASME* **101:**66–72.

Pearce, J. A. 1984. Personal communication, June.

Pearce, J. A. 1986. *Electrosurgery.* Chapman & Hall, London, 270 pp.

Pearce, J. A., and L. A. Geddes. 1980. The characteristics of capacitive dispersive electrodes. *Proc. 5th Annu. Meet. Assoc. Adv. Med. Instrum., 1980* **15:**162.

Pearce, J. A., L. A. Geddes, J. D. Bourland, and L. F. Silva, 1979. The thermal behavior of electrolyte-coated metal-foil dispersive electrodes. *Med. Instrum.* **13:**298–304.

Pearce, J. A., L. A. Geddes, J. VanVleet, K. Foster, and J. Allen. 1983. Skin burns from electrosurgical electrodes. *Med. Instrum.* **17:**225–231.

Potter, H. E. 1916. Diaphragming roentgen rays, studies and experiments. *Am. J. Roentgenol.* **3:**142–145.

Schawlow, A. L., and C. H. Townes. 1958. Infrared and optical masers. *Phys. Rev.* **112:**1940–1949.

Schereschewski, J. W. 1926. Physiological effects of currents of very high frequency. *Public Health Rep.* **41:**1939–1963.

Schliephake, E. 1938. *Les ondes électriques courtes en biologie.* Gauthier-Nidlars, Paris, 96 pp.

Schwan, H. P. 1965. Biophysics of diathermy. In *Therapeutic Heat.* S. Licht, New Haven, CT, 593 pp.

Schwan, H. P., and G. M. Piersal. 1954. The absorption of electromagnetic energy in body tissues. I. *Am. J. Phys. Med.* **33:**371–404.

Scott, B. O. 1953a. The effects of metal on short-wave field distortions. *Ann. Phys. Med.* **1:**238–244.

Scott, B. O. 1953b. Discussion of the present position of short-wave diathermy and ultrasonics. *Proc. Soc. Med.* **46:**331–335.

Scott, B. O. 1957. *The Principles and Practice of Diathermy.* Thomas, Springfield, IL, 103 pp.

Silva, L. F., D. DeWitt, J. A. Pearce, F. J. Bohac, and L. A. Geddes. 1977. Temperature distribution under electrosurgical dispersive electrodes. *Proc. 12th Annu. Meet. Assoc. Adv. Med. Instrum., 1977* **25:**160.

Tucker, R. D., O. H. Schmitt, C. E. Sievert, and S. E. Silvis. 1984. Demodulated low-frequency currents from electrosurgical procedures. *Surg. Gynecol. Obstet.* **159:**39–43.

Watmough, D. J., and R. Oliver. 1968a. Emissivity of human skin in the wavelength between 2μ and 6μ. *Nature* **214:**622–634.

Watmough, D. J., and R. Oliver. 1968b. Emissivity of human skin in vivo between 2.0 μ and 5.4 μ measured at normal incidence. *Nature* **214:**885–886.

Wiley, J. D., and J. G. Webster. 1982. Analysis and control of the current distribution under circular dispersive electrodes. *IEEE Trans. Biomed. Eng.* **BME-29:**381–389.

Yang, W. T., and T. H. Wang. 1979. Shortwave and microwave diathermy for deep tissue heating. *Med. Biol. Eng. Comput.* **17:**518–523.

14

Ventilation and Ventilators

INTRODUCTION

In physiology, the term ventilation refers to the delivery of oxygen to the lungs. When the respiratory system becomes impaired or ceases to function, it is necessary to use an artificial means to move air into and from the lungs. In general, there are three ways to accomplish this goal: (1) the application of intermittent negative pressure to the body (excluding the head) or the application of localized force to the body surface, (2) the application of intermittent positive pressure to the airway, and (3) electrical stimulation of the nerves and muscles that produce inspiration.

BODY RESPIRATORS

Devices that cause air to flow in and out of the trachea by the application of force to the body are often called body respirators. There are at least four different types: the tank or chamber (iron lung), the chest respirator (cuirass), the rocking bed, and the abdominal belt. Each of these devices has a specific use. The first two can provide the total ventilatory needs of a patient; the others are designed to augment the ventilatory capabilities of a patient.

Chamber (Iron Lung) Respirator

Lung ventilation by the intermittent application of negative pressure to the body (excluding the head) was reported by Sauerbruch (1904). Thus was born the principle of the modern iron lung, which solved the pneumothorax problem for surgeons and also eliminated the need for tracheal intubation. Some applications of the principle indicate that the body was in very large chambers with the head in another. Sometimes the subject was entirely in the negative-pressure chamber with a tube leading from the face mask to the outside of the chamber. Fairly widespread use of the modern iron lung occurred in the 1930s. According to Emerson (1979), he had developed and provided for commercial sale an iron lung in which the negative pressure was produced by the to-and-fro motion of a large leather diaphragm at

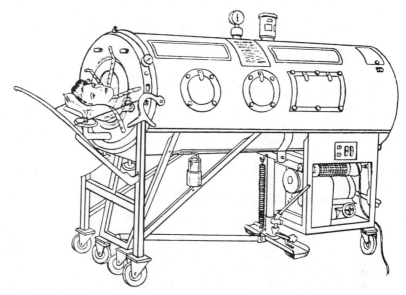

Figure 1   Iron lung for applying intermittent negative pressure to the exterior of the body, excluding the head. (Courtesy of J. H. Emerson Co., Cambridge, MA.)

the end of the chamber. His advertising literature indicates that noisy suction pumps were used prior to that time.

The tank, cabinet, or iron lung respirator (Fig. 1) consists of a chamber in which the subject is placed with the head excluded. Intermittent negative pressure is applied to the chamber, causing the thorax and abdomen to exand. A soft airtight seal surrounds the neck. Air is drawn into the lungs via the nose and mouth, and lung inflation is accomplished. The chamber is then returned to atmospheric pressure (or slightly above); the chest and abdomen recoil, and air passes out of the lungs via the nose and mouth. The negative pressure is created in some models by the movement of a large flexible diaphragm at the end of the chamber. In other models, the negative pressure is created by a valved suction pump (often a vacuum cleaner).

The negative pressure applied to the chamber need not be high to accomplish inspiration. Several tens of centimeters of water are adequate to move a tidal volume. The overall compliance of a typical iron lung with a patient in it is expressed in terms of the number of liters of air moved divided by the peak pressure required to move this volume. In a typical situation, a tidal volume (500 mL) is moved by a negative pressure of about 20–30 cm of water. Sometimes at the end of inspiration, a slight positive pressure is applied to assist expiration.

In the iron lung, the patient is usually supine; however, some models permit posturing the patient in the prone position. In some units provision is made for a 15-degree head-down position to facilitate drainage of the respiratory tree.

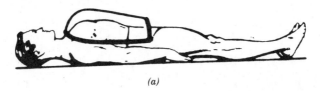

(a)

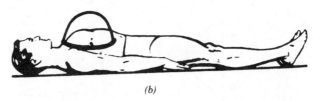

(b)

Figure 2   The chest (cuirass) respirator. (*a*) The chest–abdomen model; (*b*) the chest model. Intermittent negative pressure applied to the cuirass draws the chest into the device, causing inspiration. Expiration occurs when the negative pressure is removed.

Chest (Cuirass) Respirator

The first chest-fitting shells (partial iron lungs) appeared just before the 1920s. Such a device, called a cuirass or chest respirator (Fig. 2), consists of a shell that fits snugly around the anterior chest, usually from the shoulders to the abdomen. A soft gasket (sponge rubber or air bladder) provides an airtight seal with the body. Two straps passing around the back hold the cuirass in place. Intermittent negative pressure is applied to the space between the shell and thorax. The negative pressure causes the chest to expand, and air enters the lungs by way of the nose and mouth. Expiration is brought about when the negative pressure is removed and passive recoil of the thorax occurs. In some instances a slight positive pressure is applied to assist expiration.

The cycling rate of the cuirass can be set to match the patient's spontaneous breathing, if present. The volume of air inspired is related to the peak negative pressure applied to the cuirass. In a typical case, a pressure of about 30 cm H_2O will provide a tidal volume of about 500 mL.

Cuirass respirators were widely used as total or partial respiratory support devices for polio patients. An excellent comparison of their capabilities with those of the iron lung was presented by Collier and Affeldt (1954). Figure 3 illustrates the volume of air moved (expressed as percent of total lung volume) versus negative pressure for the iron lung (tank), chest cuirass, and chest–abdomen cuirass.

Rocking Bed Respirator

If a patient is strapped to a bed that can pivot at its center, as shown in Fig. 4, the weight of the abdominal organs can be used to move the diaphragm. For example, if the bed is rocked through an angle of ±45 degrees from the horizontal,

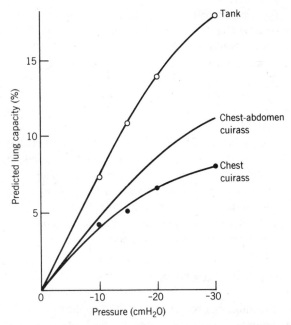

Figure 3   Comparison of the ventilatory efficacy of the iron lung (tank) and chest–abdominal and chest cuirass respirators. The volume of air moved is expressed as percent of total lung capacity. [Redrawn from C. Collier and J. Affeldt, *Appl. Physiol.* **6:**531–538 (1954).]

in the head-down position air will be expelled, and in the head-up position the diaphragm will be pulled down and air will be drawn into the lungs. This motion is sufficient to move an appreciable fraction of the required tidal volume. Usually, the rocking bed is used as a respiratory assist, the rocking frequency being set to match the patient's spontaneous respiratory rate. Synchronization turns out to be remarkably easy.

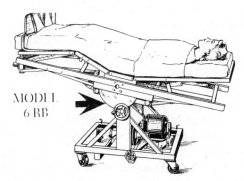

Figure 4   The rocking bed. The patient is secured to the bed, which can be adjusted to move up to ±45 degrees from the horizontal. In the head-down position, the abdominal organs press the diaphragm headward and expel air. In the foot-down position, the abdominal organs draw the diaphragm downward and effect inspiration. (Courtesy J. H. Emerson Co., Cambridge, MA.)

According to Emerson (1979), the idea that a rocking bed could be used as a ventilator was offered by Eve in the United Kingdom. Around 1949, Dr. J. Wright had the McKesson Co. motorize a bed to make it rock. In 1950, the Emerson Co. started to provide rocking beds commercially. The device was used by many polio patients.

Abdominal Belt Respirator

By placing a suitably large inflatable bladder around the abdomen and applying rhythmic pressure to it, the abdominal contents can be pressed against the diaphragm, thereby expelling air from the lungs. When the bladder is deflated, the abdominal contents resume their normal position, and inspiration occurs.

One model of the pneumobelt described by Adamson et al. (1959) consisted of a large flat bladder built into a girdle. The cycling of pressure was synchronized with the patient's breathing to provide respiratory assistance.

POSITIVE-PRESSURE VENTILATORS

Ventilation of the lungs can be achieved by the application of intermittent positive pressure to the trachea via a cuffed endotracheal tube or a snugly fitting face mask. For convenience, devices that ventilate the lungs in this way will be designated airway ventilators.

The idea of applying positive-pressure air to the mouth to ventilate the lungs is by no means new. Fisher (1947) reported that midwives were the first to apply positive pressure to the lungs using the now-familiar mouth-to-mouth technique to start breathing in newborn infants as early as the sixteenth century. Positive pressure has been used to ventilate the lungs of animals since the mid-1660's, but the technique was late in entering clinical medicine, despite the fact that Good's textbook of medicine (1836) offers ample evidence that the value of artificial respiration was well recognized. Good wrote: "The lungs (of a subject) should be inflated with the warm breath of a healthy man, or which is better, oxygen gas."

Apparently the first lung ventilator was the Fell–O'Dwyer instrument introduced about 1898 (Mushin et al., 1969). It consisted of a tracheal tube connected to a T tube, one side of which was connected to a foot-operated bellows. The other side of the T tube was covered by the thumb during lung inflation and then opened to allow deflation of the lungs.

To be effective, mechanical ventilators must have four operating features: (1) a means for inflating the lungs with air (or a mixture of gases), (2) a means of arresting lung inflation, (3) a means of allowing expiration to take place by elastic recoil of the lungs and thorax, and (4) a means for repeating these processes. Many different techniques are used to accomplish these four tasks.

Mechanical and Electrical Analogs of the Airway

To appreciate the demands placed on a ventilator, it is useful to understand the nature of the pneumatic circuit of the airway. In its simplest form, the lung–trachea circuit can be equated to a resistance R and a compliance C. Figure 5A illustrates a simple first-order model for the lumped resistance and compliance that constitute the mechanical components of the respiratory system. The respiratory gas must flow through a resistance to expand the compliant chamber that models the lungs. A typical value for airway resistance is 5–10 cm $H_2O/(L/sec)$. A typical value for compliance is 0.05 L/cm H_2O.

The temporal aspect of lung inflation can best be understood by the application of a constant pressure P to the airway as shown in Fig. 5B. Immediately flow F occurs and the lungs start to expand. The magnitude of the instantaneous flow (Fig. 5C) depends directly on the pressure and inversely on the resistance. The initial flow is therefore 15 cm H_2O divided by the airway resistance, which is approximately 6 cm $H_2O/(L/sec)$. Therefore the initial flow is $15/6 = 2.6$ L/sec. As the lungs expand (Fig. 5D), the flow F diminishes exponentially as shown in (Fig. 5C). If the pressure is maintained constant, the flow will decrease to zero as the lungs become fully inflated (Fig. 5D). If the compliance is 0.05 L/cm H_2O, and a pressure of 15 cm H_2O were applied, the lungs would ultimately inflate to a volume of $0.05 \times 15 = 0.75$ L, and the alveolar pressure would reach 15 cm

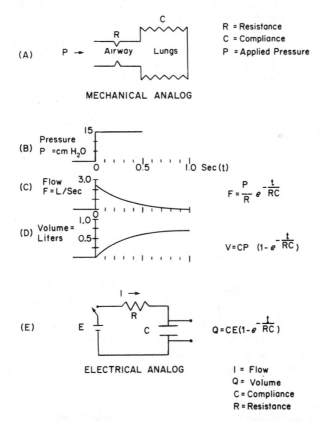

Figure 5 (A) Simple mechanical analog of the airway–lung–thorax. (B) Application of constant pressure P, (C) the flow and (D) volume that result. (E) A simplified electrical analog.

H_2O when the flow has fallen to zero. If the pressure is increased, the initial flow (P/R) will be increased, and the volume of gas entering the lungs will be increased. When the lungs are fully inflated and the flow is zero, the alveolar pressure will be the applied pressure P.

The simple mechanical analog of the lungs has the electrical analog shown in Fig. 5E. The resistance R represents the airway resistance, and the capacitance C represents the compliance of the lungs and thorax. When a constant-pressure ventilator is applied, its pressure is equivalent to the battery voltage E. The analog of airflow F is the current, and the charge Q on the capacitor is the analog of air volume V delivered to the lungs. Since the voltage on the capacitor is proportional to the charge, this voltage is a scaled analog of volume. The ventilator has been equated to a battery that really models a constant-pressure ventilator.

Another option for modeling the ventilator employs a constant-flow generator. In this case, the voltage source is replaced by a constant-current source, which is like a voltage source in series with a very high resistance.

There are six major quantities associated with lung ventilation: (1) minute volume (the volume delivered to the lungs in a minute), (2) tidal volume (the volume delivered to the lungs with each cycle of lung inflation), (3) ventilatory rate (the number of lung inflations per minute), (4) inflation pressure (end-inflation airway pressure), (5) airway compliance (which describes the elastic nature of the lungs and thorax), and (6) airway resistance. These qualities are interrelated by the following equations:

$$\text{Minute volume (L/min)} = \text{ventilation rate (per min)}$$
$$\times \text{tidal volume (L)}$$
$$\text{Tidal volume (L)} = \text{Inflation pressure (cm } H_2O)$$
$$\times \text{compliance (L/cm } H_2O)$$

This product assumes that the lungs inflate to the applied pressure.

$$\text{Initial flow (L/sec)} = \frac{\text{pressure (cm } H_2O)}{\text{resistance } [\text{cm } H_2O/(L/\text{sec})]}$$

In practice, all but two of the six quantities can be controlled by the ventilator setting. The compliance and resistance of the lung and thorax are determined by the subject. Inflation pressure and the duration of inflation, along with resistance and compliance, determine the tidal volume. The minute volume will then depend on the cycling rate of the ventilator. Recall that in a normal resting subject breathing air, the tidal volume is about 0.5 L and the respiratory rate is about 12/min. Therefore the minute volume is about 6 L. From this minute volume, the oxygen uptake is about 250 mL/min.

The linear model just presented for the lung and thoracic system is highly idealized. In point of fact, the volume–pressure characteristic is sigmoidal. More-

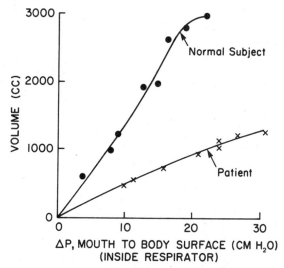

Figure 6 Volume–pressure curves for a normal subject and a poliomyelitis patient, the latter obtained with negative intrathoracic pressure provided by an iron lung.

over, the curve for inspiration is slightly different from the curve for expiration. Thus the complete pressure–volume curve forms a loop, the area of which is the energy lost during the respiratory cycle. However, it is only in research studies that this aspect of respiration is examined.

In the practical domain, volume–pressure curves for normal subjects are good indicators of lung compliance. Figure 6 illustrates a normal static volume–pressure curve and a curve obtained from a poliomyelitis patient with a stiff rib cage, that is, one with a low compliance. The difference is quite striking and points out the difficulty in ventilating subjects with stiff chests.

VENTILATOR OPERATION

Basically, there are four types of ventilators that apply intermittent gas pressure to the airway to inflate the lungs. They are the pressure-cycled, volume-cycled, time-cycled, and flow-cycled. In addition, some ventilators permit patient cycling, i.e., a beginning inspiratory effort triggers the ventilator to apply gas pressure to the trachea.

Pressure-Cycled Ventilator

In the pressure-cycled ventilator (Fig. 7), the airway pressure is sensed at the mouth while a high positive pressure P_v is developed in the ventilator as shown in Fig. 7a(1). As the lungs inflate [Fig. 7a(3)], the sensed pressure at the mouth [Fig. 7a(4)] starts to increase toward the applied pressure P_v, which may amount to 40

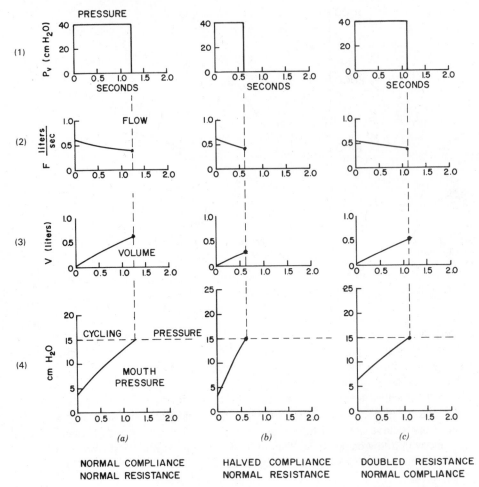

Figure 7 Operating conditions for the pressure-cycled ventilator (*a*) with normal airway compliance and resistance, (*b*) with halved compliance and normal resistance, and (*c*) with doubled resistance and normal compliance. Only the lung-inflation phase is illustrated. P_v is the ventilator pressure.

cm H_2O. Note that P_v is measured in the ventilator and the tubing between the ventilator and subject's airway provides a resistance to flow. With this high pressure P_v applied to the ventilator–subject–airway circuit, the flow of air [Fig. 7*a*(2)] into the lungs is almost constant and the volume delivered rises almost linearly with time [Fig. 7*a*(3)], because the first portion of a rising exponential curve is nearly linear. When the sensed pressure at the mouth reaches the preset cycling pressure (e.g., 15 cm H_2O as shown in Fig. 7*a*(4), lung inflation is arrested and provides an inflation volume of 0.65 L [Fig. 7*a*(3)], after which the expiratory phase begins. The next lung inflation occurs in response to the setting on the ventilatory rate control. Note, however, that lung inflation takes a finite time, as does deflation, and the cycling rate must be chosen adequately low so that expiration can be completed before the next lung inflation is initiated.

Changes in airway compliance and resistance can affect the operation of a pressure-cycled ventilator. Suppose that the compliance decreased by half—i.e., the lung–thorax system becomes stiffer—and this change occurs in the absence of any alteration in airway resistance (Fig. 7b). The initial gas flow would be the same. However, since the mouth pressure for cycling is preset, the decreased compliance results in a dramatic decrease in time to reach the preset pressure. Therefore the inflation (tidal) volume will be considerably less, as shown in Fig. 7b(3).

If a doubling in airway resistance occurs with normal compliance (Fig. 7c) the preset pressure will be reached slightly later, and the tidal volume will be decreased slightly, as shown in Fig. 7c(3).

It can be seen that with the pressure-cycled ventilator a decrease in compliance or an increase in airway resistance decreases the tidal volume. Both situations can occur together, dramatically reducing the tidal volume.

Clearly, if the ventilator pressure P_v is increased, the airflow will be increased. With a high pressure, the flow tends to become nearly constant throughout the inflation cycle. However, there is great danger if high alveolar pressure results. For example, pulmonary vascular resistance will markedly increase. The blood flow to the left ventricle will decrease; cardiac output and blood pressure will fall. It is well to remember that pulmonary artery pressure is typically $25/10$ mmHg or $34/13.6$ cm H_2O. Alveolar pressures that approach these values for an appreciable time will impede blood flow through the lungs. Although intermittent high airway pressures are occasionally used to open collapsed alveoli, great caution is exercised, and high pressures should be used only when necessary because of the added danger of mechanical trauma to the alveoli. Figure 8 illustrates the reduction in blood pressure with the application of positive airway pressure.

If a leak develops in the tubing connecting the trachea to the ventilator or around the cuffed endotracheal tube, the ventilator will continue to deliver gas until the preset level of mouth pressure is reached or until the ventilator is unable to supply any more gas. Therefore an airtight system is needed for proper operation of the pressure-cycled ventilator.

If an obstruction, e.g., kink, occurs in the tube that delivers gas from the ventilator to the patient, the pressure delivered by the ventilator will rise to a high value, seeking to reach the preset triggering pressure where it is sensed at the mouth. Accordingly, a pressure alarm is required to identify the presence of such a fault.

Volume-Cycled Ventilator

In the volume-cycled ventilator (Fig. 9) lung inflation is arrested when a preset volume of gas has been delivered to the lungs. Figure 9a illustrates the relationships among pressure, volume, and flow with the volume-cycled ventilator set to deliver 0.5 L to a normal subject. Again, a relatively high pressure P_v is developed in the

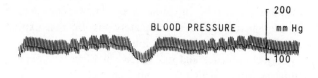

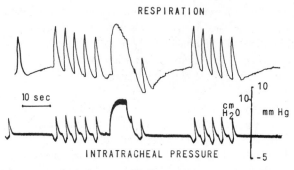

Figure 8 Blood pressure, impedance respiration, and intratracheal pressure. In the center of the record, positive pressure (9 cmH$_2$O) was transiently applied to the trachea. Note the transient decrease in blood pressure resulting from the decrease in venous return to the left heart due to the transient increase in pulmonary vascular resistance.

ventilator [Fig. 9a(1)]. Note that in Fig. 9a(3), when a preset volume has been delivered the gas pressure is reduced to zero [Fig. 9a(1)], and the expiratory phase takes place. The duration of inspiration depends on the applied pressure, the volume setting on the ventilator, and the lung-circuit resistance and compliance. The next inflation cycle occurs at a time corresponding to the rate setting on the ventilator.

Volume cycling can be accomplished by driving a piston or bellows through a preset distance. Another method involves the use of a pneumotachograph, which provides a flow-velocity signal. Integration of this signal yields volume information that can be used to arrest inflation. It should be noted, however, that with only a volume-dependent signal to inflate the lungs, a dangerously high airway pressure could be developed, especially in a low compliance situation [Fig. 9b(4)]. Pressure sensing at the mouth is often used to limit inflation to prevent the development of a high alveolar pressure.

A change in compliance or resistance can affect the operation of a volume-cycled ventilator. Consider first that the airway resistance remains the same and the compliance has been halved, i.e., the lungs have become stiffer. As shown in Fig. 9b, a much higher mouth pressure is reached [Fig. 9b(4)] when the same tidal volume has been delivered. The lung inflation time is slightly prolonged.

If the compliance is normal and the airway resistance is doubled, as shown in Fig. 9c, it will take slightly longer to deliver the preset volume. The pressure at the mouth will be slightly higher [Fig. 9c(4)] than with a normal resistance.

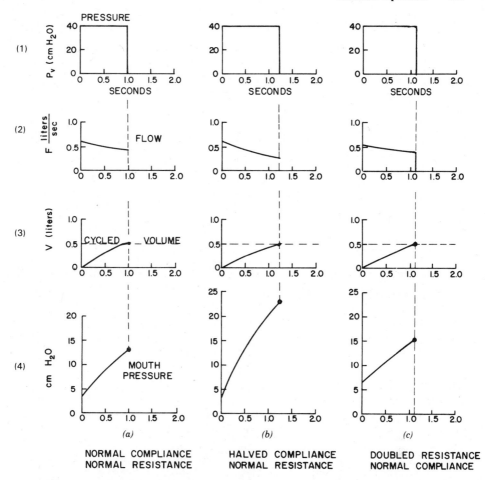

Figure 9 Operating conditions for the volume-cycled ventilator (*a*) with normal airway compliance and resistance, (*b*) with halved compliance and normal resistance, and (*c*) with doubled resistance and normal compliance. P_v is the ventilator pressure.

Time-Cycled Ventilator

In the time-cycled ventilator (Fig. 10), the duration of lung inflation is preset. The volume of gas delivered depends on the ventilator pressure P_v and airway resistance and compliance. Electronic, mechanical, or pneumatic circuits can be used to control timing of the inspiratory phase.

Fig. 10*a* illustrates the normal operation of a time-cycled ventilator that delivers gas for the preset time (e.g., 1 sec). The volume delivered is determined by the inflation duration, the ventilator pressure P_v and total circuit resistance and compliance. When this preset time has elapsed, the inflation pressure is reduced to zero and expiration begins [Fig. 10*a*(1)].

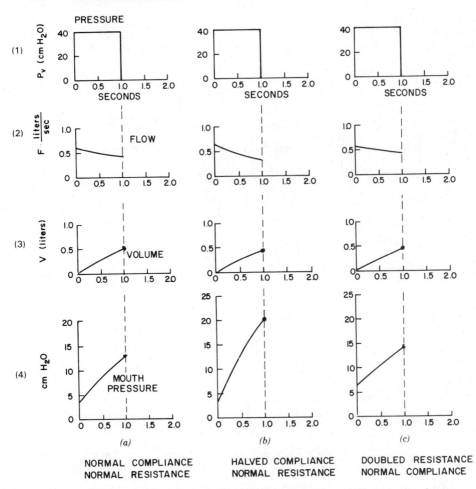

Figure 10 The time-cycled ventilator (*a*) with normal airway compliance and resistance, (*b*) with halved compliance and normal resistance, and (*c*) with doubled resistance and normal compliance. Only the lung-inflation phase is illustrated. P_v is the ventilator pressure.

Changes in lung compliance and resistance alter the performance of a time-cycled ventilator. Suppose that compliance is reduced by half without a change in airway resistance (Fig. 10*b*). The volume delivered to the lungs will be decreased. [Fig. 10*b*(3)]. The pressure measured at the mouth [Fig. 10*b*(4)] will be increased considerably.

The effect of an increase in resistance with normal compliance is shown in Fig. 10*c*. The flow will be decreased; therefore the inflation volume will be decreased slightly and the pressure at the mouth will be increased [Fig. 10*c*(4)] compared to normal.

With a time-cycled ventilator, the volume of gas delivered can be increased by increasing the ventilator pressure P_v and prolonging the duration of inflation. A leak will reduce the tidal volume.

Flow-Cycled Ventilator

In the flow-cycled ventilator, lung inflation is arrested when flow into the trachea ceases. This changeover is effected by using a flow sensor (e.g., pneumotacho-graph) in the airway. When its output falls to zero, the pressure source is removed and the expiratory phase begins. The volume of gas delivered depends on the pressure, resistance, and compliance of the airway circuit. The next lung inflation occurs in response to the rate setting on the ventilator.

In a typical flow-cycled ventilator, the changeover from lung inflation to defla-tion really occurs when flow of gas has fallen to a low value, which is near zero. The time taken for flow to fall to zero depends on the applied pressure and the airway resistance and compliance. Note that when the flow becomes zero, the alveolar pressure is the ventilator pressure P_v; therefore, care must be exercised in setting the pressure with this type of ventilator. To deliver a given tidal volume in the presence of a high resistance and low compliance, the duration of inflation may be long.

Patient-Cycled Ventilator

By sensing a spontaneous inspiratory negative pressure at the mouth, it is pos-sible to cause the patient to trigger the ventilator to deliver gas to the lungs. The use of such a ventilator requires that the patient exhibit spontaneous respiration. The ventilator then assists lung inflation. In this particular application, the venti-latory rate is controlled by the patient's respiratory center, which is in turn con-trolled by the arterial pCO_2, pO_2, and pH. When this type of ventilator is used, the patient's condition must be monitored carefully to avoid missing respiratory arrest. It is possible to set a basal rate in some patient-triggered ventilators so that ventilation is automatically provided in the event of respiratory arrest. In such a case, the device is a demand ventilator.

Mixed Cycling

Not all ventilators can be placed in one of the categories just described. Some ventilators permit selection of one or more of the cycling modalities. Others use a combination of pressure and volume cycling. For example, with the volume-cycled ventilator, if the mouth pressure exceeds a preset value inflation will be arrested and the tidal volume will be reduced. Thus the expiratory phase can begin after a predetermined volume or pressure has been attained. Likewise, volume cycling can be combined with time cycling. If a desired tidal volume is delivered in less time than is set, the expiratory phase can be initiated. A few ventilators respond to changes in airway compliance and resistance to provide a constant minute vol-ume.

CHEST COMPRESSORS AND VENTILATORS

Airway ventilators combined with chest compressors are used in cardiopulmonary resuscitation (CPR). These devices compress the chest five times and then provide positive-pressure oxygen to the airway. One popular model, called the Thumper (Michigan Instruments, Grand Rapids, MI), is shown in Fig. 11. A pneumatically driven piston presses the sternum toward the spinal column with a frequency of 60 strokes/min and a duty cycle of 50%. Figure 11 also illustrates the location of the chest compressor on a subject. With each chest compression, blood is squeezed from the heart and thorax and a small amount of air is forced from the lungs. The Thumper's piston is driven by gas from a standard oxygen cylinder, and after every five chest compressions, oxygen is delivered to the lungs via a face mask or cuffed endotracheal tube. Thus both circulatory and respiratory support are provided.

The compression force available at the chest pad on the piston is 0–145 lb. In

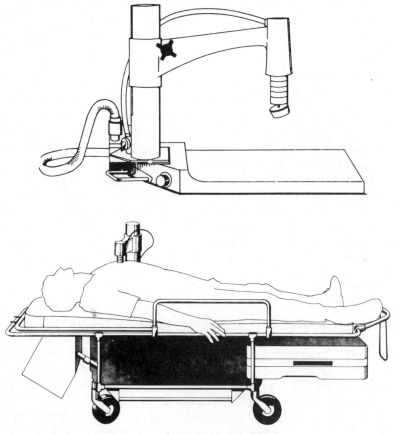

Figure 11 The Thumper, a compressor/ventilator used in cardiopulmonary resuscitation produced by Michigan Instruments, Grand Rapids, Michigan.

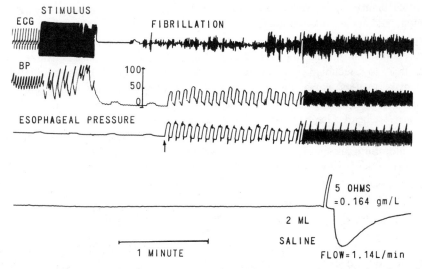

Figure 12 Recordings of the ECG, blood pressure, and esophageal pressure in a dog prior to, during, and after precipitation of ventricular fibrillation. At the arrow, the Thumper (see Fig. 11) was used to compress the chest rhythmically. The bottom channel displays a dilution wave obtained during CPR; 2 mL of 5% saline was injected into the left ventricle and detected in the aorta.

a typical application the sternum is compressed up to $3\frac{1}{2}$ in. The positive pressure that inflates the lungs can be adjusted from 5 to 60 cm H_2O.

Figure 12 is a recording obtained on a dog following precipitation of ventricular fibrillation and the use of the Thumper to provide CPR. The top channel displays the ECG; the second, blood pressure; and the third, intraesophageal pressure. The bottom channel shows a dilution curve obtained by injecting 2 mL of 5% saline into the left ventricle and detecting it in the aorta; in this case the flow was 1.14 L/min (Geddes and Babbs, 1980). Note the pulsatile blood pressure with each chest compression. Animal studies by Silver et al. (1981) reveal that the maximum blood flow with the Thumper used on dogs with ventricular fabrillation can reach about 40% of that produced when the heart was beating normally.

ELECTRICALLY INDUCED INSPIRATION

Contraction of the diaphragm and intercostal muscles produces inspiration. Contraction of the diaphragm produces by far the largest volume of inspired air. Delivery of an appropriate train of stimuli to the nerves supplying these muscles (or to the muscles directly) can produce inspiration. The various methods used to achieve this goal will be described.

Electrically induced inspiration is not new. In the latter part of the nineteenth century, the favorite anesthetic was chloroform, probably because it provided a smooth induction. However, in common with all anesthetics, it depresses respiration, and it has another undesirable side effect—it is vagotonic. Respiratory depression and arrest, as well as cardiac arrest, were not uncommon in surgical procedures, and the anesthetist had to be vigilant. Chloroform also sensitizes the ventricles to catecholamines, which can result in arrhythmias including fibrillation. To make matters worse, the resuscitation procedures then were at best limited. Thus, it was not surprising that electric current was used to restart respiration and the arrested heart. Green (1872), a British surgeon, reported successful resuscitation of five of seven patients who had ceased breathing, some becoming pulseless during the chloroform anesthesia procedure. Green applied one electrode to the neck and another to the left lower border of the rib cage. He used a battery (up to 300 V), and with each application of the electrodes, the patient's muscles twitched. It is very likely that he twitched the diaphragm and induced an ectopic heart beat. He advocated that the galvanic battery be ''at the ready'' at all times in the operating room.

To treat chloroform syncope, it was common to use the intermittent application of induction-coil shocks to electrodes on the neck or thorax. Such current is capable of producing a tetanic contraction of the inspiratory muscles. The method of applying intermittent tetanizing current to electrodes across the neck to stimulate the phrenic nerves and contract the diaphragm was first used by von Ziemssen (1857) on a 27-year-old servant girl who had been asphyxiated by coal-gas fumes; the girl was revived and survived. Friedberg (1859) used the same method to resuscitate a 4-year-old boy who experienced respiratory arrest due to chloroform anesthesia. In the second edition of his book on medical electricity, von Ziemssen (1864) reported further use of the same technique to resuscitate many cases of respiratory arrest due to carburetted hydrogen gas (methane) and freezing after alcohol intoxication. In the United Kingdom, Hardie (1871) reported similar successful resuscitations of an old woman and a 10-year-old boy, both of whom had experienced respiratory arrest due to chloroform anesthesia. The diaphragm was tetanized intermittently by using induction-coil shocks applied to transthoracic electrodes. The technique of inducing inspiration by phrenic nerve stimulation to contract the diaphragm became quite common; Duchenne (1872), Althaus (1873) and Beard and Rockwell (1891) all devoted substantial coverage to the technique in their textbooks. Duchenne (1872) wrote:

''Artificial respiration produced by electric contraction of the diaphragm develops considerable movement of air; increasing the vertical diameter of the thorax, and the inferior half of the transverse diameter. Moreover, electric excitation of the phrenic nerves, which provide contraction of the diaphragm, can also provide noisy respiration in the cadaver sometime after death.''

This remarkable procedure was both lifesaving and noninvasive, since the train of short-duration induction-coil pulses was applied to body-surface electrodes.

The use of electric current to stimulate the inspiratory muscles disappeared by the dawn of the twentieth century, probably because better anesthetics and mechanical ventilators began to appear. The reviver of direct electrophrenic stimulation was Waud (1937), who, in a short note in *Nature*, descibed its use in animals. He applied electrodes to the exposed cervical phrenics bilaterally and used two synchronized induction coils as stimulators. He found that with only one phrenic nerve stimulated he could produce a tidal volume much in excess of that exhibited with normal respiration. More important, he reported that phrenic nerve respiration "obviates the changes in circulation which result when the increased tracheal pressure method of artificial respiration is used." It was not until 1948, when Sarnoff and his colleagues revived it, that phrenic nerve stimulation became an accepted method of producing inspiration.

Respiration

Respiration is controlled by the respiratory center, which is a cluster of neurons located in the medulla that lies atop the spinal cord and at the base of the skull. The respiratory neurons originate rhythmic trains of action potentials that are carried by motor nerves to the muscles of inspiration, the diaphragm and the external intercostals. Figure 13 presents a highly simplified diagram of the respiratory system.

The diaphragm is innervated by the two phrenic nerves, which leave the cervical spinal cord at three levels (C3, C4, C5), enter the thorax, pass along the pericardium, and then spread laterally to innervate the left and right diaphragm. The external intercostal muscles are innervated by thoracic nerves; some are innervated by the long thoracic nerve, which runs laterally along the sides of the chest. In

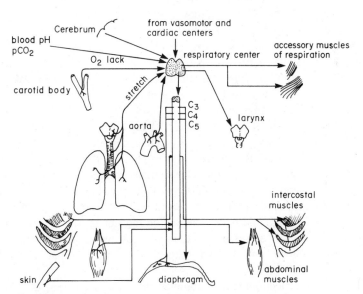

Figure 13   Simplified diagram of the respiratory system, showing the medullary respiratory center and the nerve connections to the diaphragm and the intercostal, abdominal, and accessory muscles.

quiet breathing, about three-quarters of the volume change of the thorax is provided by contraction of the diaphragm. If the spinal cord is transected below C5, breathing will continue. If the cord is cut above C3, respiration will cease.

It is obvious that if trains of stimuli are delivered to the nerves that innervate the inspiratory muscles, inspiration will result. Cessation of delivery of the stimuli will result in expiration due to elastic recoil of the rib cage. Note that inspiration is produced by negative intrathoracic pressure, as in normal respiration.

The respiratory system is far more complex than is shown in Fig. 13. In addition to the diaphragm and external intercostal muscles, inspiration can be assisted by contraction of the accessory muscles (scalene and sternocleidomastoid). In exercise, expiration is forced and involves contraction of the internal intercostals and abdominal muscles.

In addition to being spontaneously rhythmic, the respiratory center is controlled in many ways, the most obvious being by the cortex to enable vocalization. The respiratory center is stimulated by an increase in pCO_2 and receives information on pO_2 from the carotid bodies. It is also closely linked with the cardiac and temperature centers, as well as receiving inputs from sensory and stretch receptors in the airway.

Phrenic Nerve Stimulation

Sarnoff and his associates (1948) described the rhythmic application of bursts of stimuli (2-msec, 60/sec) to electrodes on one or both cervical phrenic nerves of cats, rabbits, dogs, and monkeys. They found that a tidal volume greater than normal could be produced easily. Moreover, spontaneous respiration was inhibited during phrenic nerve stimulation. The first application of this technique to humans appears to be due to Whittenberger et al. (1949), who implanted an electrode against the right phrenic nerve of a patient; an indifferent electrode on the wrist completed the circuit. When bursts of stimuli (2-msec, 60/sec) were delivered, a tidal volume in excess of normal was easily obtained; the volume of air moved was measured with a pneumotachograph.

After many more animal studies, Sarnoff et al. (1950) applied the method to nine poliomyelitis patients with respiratory center depression. A 4-mm-diameter cloth-covered (saline-soaked) electrode was applied to the neck, paired with a distant indifferent electrode. Using similar stimulus parameters (2-msec, 40/sec) and a pneumotachograph to measure tidal volume, they showed that effective ventilation could be produced. They also pointed out that the negative intrathoracic pressure produced by phrenic nerve stimulation did not impair the circulation, a response seen with positive-pressure ventilation. They also recommended that electrophrenic respiration be applied only by experienced personnel, but the experience was easily acquired.

Desiring to make electrophrenic respiration more easily applied, Daggett et al. (1966, 1970) developed the technique of stimulating the right phrenic nerve using a bipolar catheter electrode advanced into position via the superior vena cava. Acute and chronic studies were carried out in dogs using bursts of 2-msec stimuli at

60/sec. The intensity ranged from 2 to 6 V, which provided a tidal volume in excess of that produced by normal breathing. In the latter study, they used a linearly rising stimulus train to provide a smooth inspiration.

The event that made electrophrenic stimulation a therapeutic procedure was the development of a passive implantable stimulus receiver by Glenn et al. (1964). The implant consisted of a tuned circuit (receiver) and demodulator that recovered the stimulus telemetered from an external transmitter (see Chap. 10 for details). Designed primarily for cardiac pacing, it was soon used to deliver trains of stimuli to the phrenic nerves. Judson and Glenn (1968) described its use on patients with chronic ventilatory insufficiency. Calling the method "diaphragm pacing," Glenn et al. (1978a) reported that it had been applied to 180 patients and had been used successfully in patients with chronic underventilation (Glenn, 1978a, b).

Implantable stimulus receivers for exciting the phrenic (and other) nerves are available commercially from many suppliers. The more recent devices contain batteries to drive the pulse-generating circuit. In using such stimulators, several important facts should be recognized. For example, stimulation of a single phrenic nerve can provide more than adequate tidal volume. Moreover, electrophrenic respiration is like normal breathing, in that it produces a negative intrathoracic pressure and consequently does not impair the circulatory system. Fatigue of the diaphragm must be guarded against. Finally, it is not necessary to humidify the air with electrophrenic respiration, as is needed with mechanical ventilators connected to the airway.

An interesting type of transcutaneous phrenic nerve stimulator was described by Batrow and Batrow (1963). It consisted of an induction coil driven by a thyratron and delivered high-voltage, short-duration (70-μsec) pulses to a capacitive (glow-lamp) electrode placed lateral to the xiphoid process or on the lower rib cage at the level of the diaphragm. The indifferent electrode was placed on the feet or buttocks. It was found that when a train of these short-duration stimuli was delivered, the lower phrenic nerves were stimulated and the diaphragm contracted, producing inspiration.

Although the Batrow stimulator was used on humans for a few years, the results were variable and the device was withdrawn from the market. However, it had some unique features. For example, the choice of a short-duration pulse minimized skin sensation (see Chap. 10). The use of a capacitive electrode, with its more even current-density distribution, also favored minimizing skin sensation.

Electroventilation

Electroventilation is the term used by Geddes (Geddes et al., 1985) for the technique that employs the intermittent application of trains of short-duration current pulses to chest-surface electrodes to stimulate the inspiratory nerves. Depending on the location of the chest electrodes, inspiratory (I) and expiratory (X) and both inspiratory and expiratory, i.e., paradoxical (P), respiratory movements can be produced. Figure 14a illustrates these regions on the chest of a dog with the

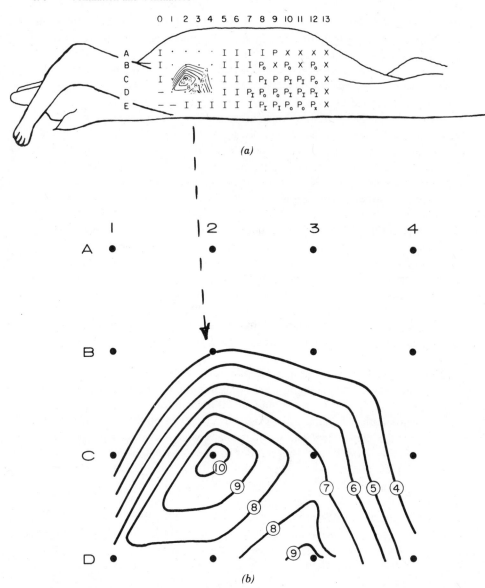

Figure 14 (*a*) Sites on the dog chest where inspiration (I), expiration (X) and paradoxical (P) respiratory movements were obtained. (*b*) A contour map that indicates the milliliters of air inspired per milliampere of current. [Redrawn in part from L. A. Geddes et al., *Am. J. Emerg. Med.* **3**(4):337–339 (1985).]

forelimbs tied headward. The obvious goal is to locate the electrodes so that only the inspiratory muscles are contracted, thereby providing an electrical means of providing artificial respiration. It has been found that the optimum site in the dog is just caudal and anterior to the axillae. It is about here where the lateral thoracic nerve branches. Figure 14*b* illustrates the volume–current contours for this site.

In recent studies on the dog and baboon, it has been found that inspiration can be produced with electrodes placed bilaterally on the lower chest at the level of the xiphoid process (in the regions marked P in Fig. 14). With such a stimulus, all the phrenic nerve fibers are excited and the diaphragm is contracted maximally. However, the volume of air inspired is less than with upper chest electrodes. With the lower chest electrodes, contraction of the abdominal muscles restricts expansion of the abdomen when it pushes the internal organs downward, thereby limiting the inspired volume (Geddes et al., 1989).

The type of stimulus required for electroventilation merits special consideration. To minimize cutaneous receptor and myocardial stimulation, very short-duration (10–50-μsec) pulses are required. To produce a smooth tetanic contraction in the inspiratory muscles, a frequency of about 20–40/sec is adequate. The use of a higher frequency will produce early fatigue. The period of inspiration is determined by the duration of this train, typically 0.3–0.7 sec. The ventilation rate (breaths per minute) is determined by the number of times per minute the train of stimuli is repeated; delivery every 4 sec provides an artificial respiration rate of 15 breaths/min.

Figure 15 illustrates the relationship between inspired volume and current with electrodes at the optimum site on the upper chest of a dog. Arrest of spontaneous breathing was created easily by stimulating the afferent fibers in the vagus nerve. These fibers carry the Hering-Breuer stretch-receptor information (which signals inspiration). Thus, by ligating the vagus nerve distally and stimulating in the cranial direction, respiratory arrest was easily produced with no cardiac effects.

In Fig. 15, no inspiratory effort is obtained until a threshold current is reached; beyond this point the inspired volume increases with increasing current. When the

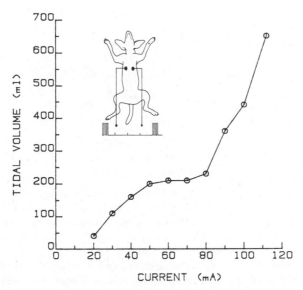

Figure 15 Volume of air moved versus stimulating current with transaxillary electrodes as shown. [Redrawn from L. A. Geddes et al., *Am. J. Emerg. Med.* **3**(4):337–339 (1985).]

current is increased further, the phrenic nerves are stimulated and the inspired volume increases dramatically.

To demonstrate the ability of electroventilation to provide adequate ventilation in the dog, oxygen saturation and blood pressure were recorded from a femoral artery. A flow-through oximeter was placed in an arteriovenous shunt to record O_2 saturation continuously. A spirometer was connected to the endotracheal tube to record the volume of air moved. With respiratory arrest produced by afferent vagal stimulation, the oxygen saturation was allowed to fall as shown in Fig. 16. After about a 20% fall in saturation (the tongue was cyanotic), electroventilation was applied, i.e., the trains of stimuli were applied to the respiratory nerves and muscles via the transchest electrodes; Fig. 16 illustrates the result. Oxygen saturation returned to control value within about 10 sec of electroventilation. After 15 electroventilation breaths, the vagal afferent stimulation and the electroventilation were turned off, and the animal resumed spontaneous respiration with no change in oxygen saturation.

To understand the mechanism underlying electroventilation, the thoracic skin

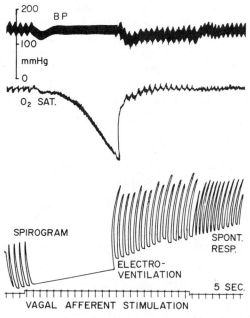

Figure 16 Blood pressure (BP), oxygen saturation (O_2 sat.), and volume of air breathed (spirogram) from a dog with transchest electrodes applied to stimulate the muscles of inspiration. On the left, the animal was breathing spontaneously; in the center, respiration was arrested by stimulating vagal afferent fibers. The oxygen saturation was allowed to fall, and electroventilation was applied to restore oxygen saturation. After 12 sec of electroventilation, the vagal afferent stimulation and electroventilation were discontinued, allowing spontaneous respiration to resume with no change in oxygen saturation. [Redrawn from L. A. Geddes et al., *Am. J. Emerg. Med.* **2**(4):20–24 (1984).]

from one recently expired and one deeply anesthetized animal was dissected, and local stimulation was applied to individual motor nerves and muscle groups. There are four muscles that when stimulated produced motion of the thorax similar to that produced by electroventilation: (1) the cranial fibers of pectoralis major, (2) the caudal fibers of pectoralis major, (3) the serratus ventralis (serratus anterior in humans) innervated by the long thoracic nerve, and (4) the individual intercostal muscles. Therefore, stimulation of each of these muscle groups may be a plausible mechanism for generating inspiration during electroventilation. The effectiveness of contraction of the cranial and caudal fibers of pectoralis in producing inspiration requires that the forelimbs of the animal be tied, in this case, in which the humerus is fixed, contraction of the muscle draws the rib cage outward. Importantly, inspiration caused by stimulation of serratus and intercostal muscles was not dependent upon tethering of the forelimbs, and it was these muscles that seemed to be most effective in producing inspiration with the lower current.

Research on electroventilation in humans is ongoing. As an emergency procedure for providing ventilation, it has many attractive features. By using a train of very short duration stimuli and locating the electrodes high on the lateral thorax, the risk of producing cardiac arrhythmias is minimal. Such arrhythmias have never been seen in the dog or baboon studies. Of course, the optimum sites for the electrodes for humans are yet to be determined. In closing, it is well to remember that electroventilation is like natural breathing in that air is brought into the lungs by negative intrathoracic pressure. One additional point sould be recognized— electroventilation requires functional myoneural junctions. In a limited number of studies with complete circulatory arrest, electroventilation continued for several minutes. After about 5 min of circulatory arrest, the myoneural junctions were so hypoxic that electroventilation was relatively ineffective. Therefore, electroventilation will see its maximum effectiveness in acute respiratory arrest.

REFERENCES

Adamson, J. P., I. Lewis, S. Leandro, and J. D. Steen. 1959. Application of abdominal pressure for artificial respiration. *JAMA* **169**:1613.

Althaus, J. A. 1873. *Treatise on Medical Electricity.* Presley Blakiston, Philadelphia, PA, 729 pp.

Batrow, J., and P. Batrow. 1963. Electrophysiotherapy apparatus. U.S. Patent 3,077,884, February 10.

Beard, G. M., and A. D. Rockwell. 1891. *On the Medical and Surgical Uses of Electricity*, 8th ed. G. Wood & Co., New York, 788 pp.

Collier, C. R., and J. E. Affeldt. 1954. Ventilatory efficiency of the cuirass respirator in totally paralyzed chronic poliomyelitis patients. *J. Appl. Physiol.* **6**:531–538.

Daggett, W. M., J. C. Piccinini, and W. G. Austen. 1966. Intracaval electrophrenic stimulation. *J. Thorac. Cardiovasc. Surg.* **51**(5):676–684.

Daggett, W. M., A. S. Shanahan, H. Kazemi, A. P. Morgan, and W. G. Austen. 1970. Intracaval electrophrenic stimulation. *J. Thorac. Cardiovasc. Surg.* **60**(1):98–107.

Duchenne, G. B., 1872. *L'électrisation localisée.* Bailliere, Paris, 1120 pp.

Emerson, J. 1979. Personal communication.

Fisher, H. E. 1947. Resuscitation. In *Medical Physics*, Vol. 1. O. Glasser (ed.), Year Book Publishers, Chicago, IL., 1744 pp.

Friedberg, H. 1859. Chloroformasphyxie. *Virchows Arch. Pathol. Anat. Physiol.* **16:**527–564.

Geddes, L. A., and C. F. Babbs. 1980. A new technique for repeated measurement of cardiac output during CPR. *CRC Crit. Care Med.* **8:**131–133.

Geddes, L. A., W. Voorhees, and C. F. Babbs. 1985. Electroventilation. *Am. J. Emerg. Med.* **3**(4):337–339.

Geddes, L. A., W. D. Voorhees, R. Lagler, C. Riscili, K. S. Foster, and J. D. Bourland. 1989. Electrically produced artificial ventilation. *Med. Instr.* **22**(5):263–271.

Glenn, W. W. L. 1978a. Diaphragm pacing: Present status. *Pace* **1:**357–370.

Glenn, W. W. L. 1978b. Diaphragm pacing. *J. Thorac. Cardiovasc. Surg.* **75**(2):273–283.

Glenn, W. W. L., J. H. Hageman, A. Mauro, L. Eisenberg, S. Flanagan, and M. Harvard. 1964. Electrical stimulation of excitable tissue. *Ann. Surg.* **160:**338–350.

Good, J. M. 1836. *The Study of Medicine*. Harper, New York, 733 pp.

Green, T. 1872. On death from chloroform; prevention by galvanism. *Br. Med. J.* **1:**551–553.

Hardie, J. 1871. Two cases of recovery from chloroform anesthesia. *Lancet* April 27:574–576.

Judson, J. P., and W. W. L. Glenn. 1968. Radiofrequency electrophrenic respiration. *JAMA* **203:**1033.

Mushin, W. M., L. R. Baker, P. W. Thompson, and W. W. Mapelson. 1969. *Automatic Ventilation of the Lungs*. Davis, Philadelphia, PA, 841 pp.

Sarnoff, S. J., E. Hardenbergh, and J. L. Whittenberger. 1948. Electrophrenic respiration. *Am. J. Physiol.* **155:**1–9.

Sarnoff, S. J., J. V. Maloney, L. C. Sarnoff, B. G. Ferris, and J. L. Whittenberger. 1950. Electrophrenic respiration in acute poliomyelitis. *JAMA* **143:**1383–1390.

Sauerbruch, I. 1904. Zur Pathologic des offenen Pneumothorax. *Mitt. Grenzgeb. Med. Chir.* **13:**388–477.

Silver, D. I., K. J. Murphy, C. F. Babbs, and L. A. Geddes. 1981. Cardiac output during CPR. *CRC Crit. Care Med.* **9**(5):419–420.

von Ziemssen, H. 1857. *Die Electricita in der Medicin*, 1st ed. Hirschwald, Berlin, 82 pp.

von Ziemssen, H. 1864. *Die Electricita in der Medicin*, 2nd ed. Hirschwald, Berlin, 169 pp.

Waud, R. A. 1937. Production of aritifical respiration by rhythmic stimulation of the phrenic nerve. *Nature* **140:**849.

Whittenberger, J. L., S. J. Sarnoff, and E. Hardenbergh. 1949. Electrophrenic respiration. *J. Clin. Invest.* **28:**124–128.

15

Anesthesia and Anesthesia Equipment

GENERAL ANESTHESIA

Anesthesia is a state of the central nervous system in which the responses to noxious stimuli are suppressed reversibly. Few surgical procedures could be carried out without general anesthesia. Despite the fact that chemical agents are used to produce anesthesia in a well-controlled manner, there is no single theory that can account for the actions of all substances that produce anesthesia. The word "anesthesia" originated with Oliver Wendell Holmes, who suggested its use to describe the state produced when ether vapor was first administered to a human patient about to undergo surgery (October 16, 1846; J. C. Warren, surgeon, at the Massachusetts General Hospital; the anesthetic was administered by William Morton). Although this was not the first use of an anesthetic substance for surgery, this demonstration attracted attention to the pain-killing properties of certain inhaled substances and to the ability to control the duration and depth of the anesthetic state. An excellent history of anesthesia was presented by Hoff (1937).

Anesthesia can be produced by the ingestion of substances; by subcutaneous, intramuscular, intraperitoneal, and intravenous injection; by rectal administration; and by the inhalation of anesthetic gases or vapors. In all cases the agent must reach a critical concentration in the bloodstream to produce anesthesia.

Table 1 presents the approximate concentrations required in inspired air to achieve surgical anesthesia using typical anesthetic agents in the absence of premedication. The unique feature of inhaled anesthetic substances is their easy and rapid controllability. By removing the substance from the inspired air, the anesthetic is soon washed out of the bloodstream by continued respiration; restoration of conciousness is rapid and can be caused to occur at any desired time. Conversely, it is easy to deepen the anesthetic state by increasing the concentration of the anesthetic substance in the inspired air. Ingested and injected anesthetic agents are less controllable, and the duration of the anesthetic state depends on the characteristics of the particular agent used. Rapid restoration of consciousness from anesthesia due to ingested and injected substances requires the administration of a central nervous system stimulant.

TABLE 1   Inspiratory Concentrations for General Anesthesia

Anesthetic	Flammability[a]	Concentration (vol %)
Liquids		
Halothane	NF	1–2
Diethyl ether	F	5–10
Chloroform	NF	0.5–1.6
Trichlorethylene[b]	NF	0.2–0.8
Methoxyflurane	NF	0.25–1.0
Gases		
Nitrous oxide	NF	90% N_2O + 10% O_2
Cyclopropane	F	10–20

[a]F, flammable; NF, nonflammable.
[b]Must not be used with soda-lime CO_2 absorber.

VOLATILE ANESTHETICS

Although many liquids and gases (see Table 1) have anesthetic properties, the substances used for surgical anesthesia are usually volatile liquids. It is the biochemical properties of a volatile liquid that determine its candidacy as an anesthetic. However, it is its physical properties that determine the practicality of the substance as an anesthetic agent. Of all the physical properties, the most important is the vapor pressure, which is a measure of the tendency for a liquid to evaporate. A substance with a high vapor pressure at room temperature is one that evaporates readily and forms a gas of high concentration. Vapor pressure is temperature-dependent, and perhaps the best way of illustrating the phenomenon is to point out that the vapor pressure of water at 37°C is 47 mmHg and at 100°C the vapor pressure is 760 mmHg; i.e., water exists only as a gas at 100°C. The higher the vapor pressure of a liquid at room temperature (e.g., 20°C), the higher the degree of evaporation and the higher the concentration of its gas in the space above the liquid. Hill (1976) composed an illustration that shows the vapor pressure and concentration in air of various volatile liquid anesthetic agents; Fig. 1 presents this information. Note that ether, the first surgical anesthetic, vaporizes readily and attains a high concentration in air at room temperature. The concentration of ether in the inspiratory air required to produce anesthesia is 5–10% (Table 1). It can be seen that it is not difficult to attain an adequate concentration of ether in the airway for anesthesia. It was probably this fact that made it a very practical first anesthetic agent.

DEPTH OF ANESTHESIA

Despite the widely different anesthetic agents that are in use, it is possible to identify signs that indicate the depth of anesthesia. The estimation of depth rests on a variety of physical signs, which include the responses to stimuli. One of the first to organize this spectrum was A. E. Guedel, who, facing the task of training

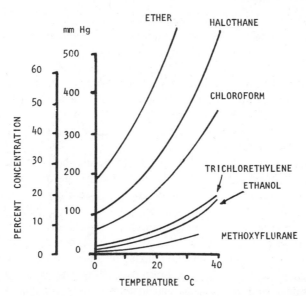

Figure 1   Vapor pressures and concentrations of various volatile anesthetic liquids. (Redrawn from D. W. Hill, *Physics Applied to Anaesthesia.* Butterworth, London, 1976.)

a large number of people to administer anesthetics during World War I (1914–1918), created a classification system that forms the basis of present-day techniques for estimating depth. Perhaps the best two generalizing statements that can be made relative to the depth of anesthesia are: (1) The central nervous system depression increases progressively from the highest centers (e.g., cortex) to the lowest (e.g., spinal cord) and (2) respiration (which is also a phenomenon of the central nervous system) is progressively depressed. Thus, general anesthesia extends from a depression of the sensitivity to painful stimuli to respiratory arrest.

The signs used to identify the depth of anesthesia are type and rate of respiration, pupillary size and response to light, eyeball movements, corneal reflex, muscle tone, and often the patellar tendon reflex. Inspiration is achieved by contraction of the muscles of the rib cage and diaphragm; expiration results from the relaxation of these muscles and the elastic recoil of the lungs and thorax. Thus, respiration has two components, thoracic and diaphragmatic. Contraction of the dome-shaped diaphragm causes the abdomen to move outward. Therefore the two signs of respiration are thoracic and abdominal movements. With progressively increasing depth of anesthesia, respiratory rate decreases, followed by a delay between the thoracic and abdominal components. With deeper anesthesia, the thoracic component becomes more depressed and ultimately disappears, leaving only the abdominal component. Finally, with very deep anesthesia, the abdominal component disappears when the respiratory center is paralyzed.

The eyes provide several types of useful information relative to the depth of anesthesia. The pupil is constricted by parasympathetic activity and dilated by sympathetic activity. In addition, pupillary constriction in response to light is a reflex. Since deepening anesthesia depresses reflexes, the absence of this light reflex is often used as an indicator of depth of anesthesia. It is important to note that profound hypoxia also causes wide dilation of the pupils; however, this state is easily differentiated from increased sympathetic activity by noting the other signs of anesthesia. In some species, and with many anesthetics, the eyeballs oscillate with light anesthesia. Perhaps the most frequently used eye sign is the corneal reflex. If the cornea is tapped very lightly, the eyelid blinks; this protective reflex is fairly resistant to anesthesia.

Muscle tone, which is characteristically altered by anesthesia, is one of the most difficult of the physical signs to describe; it is made more difficult because few have had the opportunity of feeling the flaccidity of a recently denervated muscle, which is without tone. Interestingly enough, a muscle at rest feels quite different from a denervated (paralyzed) muscle. In normal subjects, even when a muscle is at rest, there is an unmistakable firmness when it is squeezed. At rest, there is a slow repetitive "tonic" contracting and relaxing of some of the muscle fibers. This activity, which gives a muscle its characteristic feeling of firmness or tone, is effected by spinal cord reflex areas and a more or less continuous outflow of impulses from higher brain centers; anesthesia depresses this outflow.

When a member is passively moved, there is a slight resistance to its movement, which also describes the tone of its muscles. The amount of passive resistance depends on the integrity of the innervation, the spinal cord reflexes, and the influences from higher centers just described. If these higher and spinal cord influences are inhibited, as they are by anesthetics, the muscle loses its feeling of firmness and its resistance to passive movement. Therefore, these two effects, feeling of firmness and resistance to passive movement, underlie what is described as muscle tone. Under very deep anesthesia a muscle can feel as flaccid as it is when denervated.

Another sign of general anesthesia is a progressive lowering of body temperature due to depression of the hypothalamic temperature-regulation center. The decrease in temperature is related to the depth and duration of anesthesia. For this reason, special care must be taken to prevent excessive heat loss from subjects who are under anesthesia for prolonged periods.

Although the signs and responses just described are all used to estimate the depth of anesthesia, no single sign can be relied on, since different anesthetics often have slightly different effects and may enhance or attenuate the various signs and responses. In addition, preanesthetic medication often enhances or abolishes some of the signs. It is customary to use premedication to obtain a smooth induction and remove the side effects of some anesthetics.

Stages and Planes of Anesthesia

On the basis of his experience with ether and some of the early inhalation anesthetics, Guedel (1937, 1951) recognized four anesthesia stages: analgesia, delirium, surgical anesthesia, and respiratory paralysis. Guedel also subdivided the surgical anesthesia stage into four planes. There is no sharp division between the individual stages and planes, although each has its own characteristics. They have been organized into charts to facilitate identification of the depth of anesthesia. One of the most complete charts was presented by Goodman and Gilman (1955). The most important signs of anesthesia from these and other sources are presented in Fig. 2. With an increase in the amount of anesthetic, the signs develop from the top to the bottom of the chart.

In stage 1, analgesia, there is a progressive loss of pain sensation, following

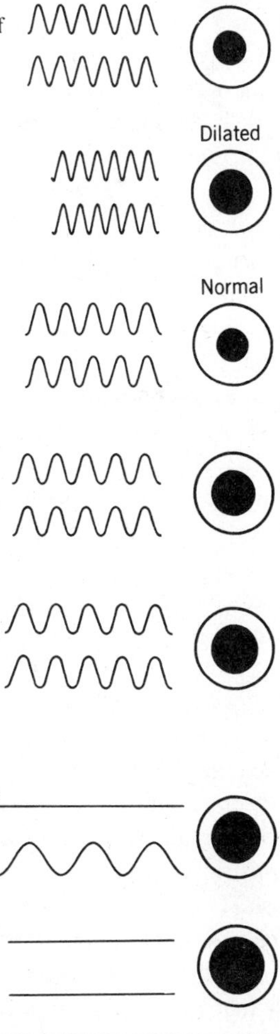

Description	Respiration	Pupil Size	Corneal Reflex	Response to Light	Muscle Tone
Stage 1: Analgesia Loss of pain sensation; loss of consciousness		Normal	Present	Present	Normal
Stage 2: Delirium Elevated heart rate of blood pressure; exaggerated responses		Dilated	Present	Present	Increased with motor activity
Stage 3: Surgical Anesthesia Plane 1 Normal respiration and blood pressure; eyes roll		Normal	Present	Present	Light muscular relaxation
Plane 2 Blood pressure and respiration reduced slightly			Present ___ Absent	Present	Moderate muscular relaxation
Plane 3 Blood pressure and respiration reduced			Absent	Sluggish to strong light	Marked muscular relaxation
Plane 4 Low blood pressure and heart rate; respiration reduced markedly			Absent	Absent	Marked muscular flaccidity
Stage 4: Medullary Paralysis Very low blood pressure and heart rate; no respiration			Absent	Absent	Extreme muscular flaccidity

Figure 2   The stages and planes of anesthesia.

which consciousness is lost. The pupils are normal and respond to light; they begin to dilate as stage 2 is approached. Respiration is normal.

In stage 2, delirium, the higher cerebral centers are depressed, leaving lower brain systems unchecked. Often there is considerable involuntary muscular activity. Responses to stimuli are usually exaggerated and often inappropriate. Noises and gentle contact with the subject can provoke a considerable muscular response, often to the point of injuring the subject. Respiration is frequently increased and irregular; often shivering accompanies inspiration. There is increased activity of the autonomic nervous system, with predominance of the sympathetic division. The heart rate is rapid, blood pressure is elevated, and the pupils are widely dilated. The eyeballs often oscillate laterally. Swallowing and vomiting occasionally occur. With some of the early anesthetics, the irritability of the heart was increased, and the increased sympathetic activity resulted in extrasystoles, tachycardia, and even ventricular fibrillation. Many of the early sudden anesthetic deaths with chloroform were due to ventricular fibrillation. An excellent account of death due to ventricular fibrillation associated with anesthesia was presented by Beecher (1938). Fortunately, the newer anesthetics are less irritating to the heart. Moreover, there are adequate antiarrhythmic drugs, and the danger of ventricular fibrillation is virtually nonexistent now.

As the concentration of anesthetic in the bloodstream increases, the delirium or excitement stage abates and the subject passes into stage 3, in which the vital signs are near normal; the subject is completely unconscious, and there is no response to painful stimuli. The technique of induction is designed to bring the subject through stage 2 as rapidly as possible.

The delirium stage often appears to a lesser degree when emerging from surgical anesthesia. For this reason, recovery from anesthesia should be monitored carefully.

Stage 3, or the stage of surgical anesthesia, is heralded by an abatement of delirium and excitement. The pupils become normal in size, and eyeball movements often persist. Respiration is slow and deep, and the heart rate and blood pressure are essentially normal with most anesthetics. Stage 3 is subdivided into four planes, which are characterized by the presence or absence of several signs and reflexes. The end of stage 3 is identified by a profound depression of respiration. Just beyond this point, spontaneous respiration ceases, which identifies that the subject has entered stage 4. If this point is reached, artificial respiration is essential.

The four planes of stage 3, surgical anesthesia, are distinguished as follows.

Plane 1 is characterized by slow deep respiration with both thoracic and abdominal components present. The eyeballs may oscillate in a lateral direction. The pupils are normal in diameter and constrict in response to illumination of the retina. The corneal reflex is present and brisk. There is fair muscular relaxation. The blood pressure and heart rate are essentially normal. Plane 1 of surgical anesthesia is used for surgery of the head, neck, and thorax and in obstetrics.

Plane 2 differs from plane 1 in that the eyeball movements are absent. The pupils still respond to light, and the corneal reflex is present in the upper part of the plane and disappears in the lower part. The rate and depth of respiration are reduced, and there is moderate muscle relaxation. Blood pressure is normal or reduced slightly. Plane 2 is used for most abdominal operations and procedures on the joints, tonsils, and larynx.

Plane 3 is ushered in by delayed thoracic respiration. The pupils are dilated and respond only sluggishly to strong light. The corneal reflex is absent, and there is marked muscular relaxation. Blood pressure is reduced, and respiratory support may be required. Plane 3 is occasionally used for some abdominal procedures and for breech extraction in obstetrics.

Plane 4 is characterized by the presence of abdominal respiration only. The pupils are markedly dilated and do not respond to light. The corneal reflex is absent. Skeletal muscles are flaccid, and blood pressure and heart rate are low. There are few, if any, uses for plane 4 in surgery.

Stage 4 is one of paralysis of the respiratory center; therefore there is respiratory arrest. Artificial respiration is mandatory. Blood pressure and heart rate are low. The pupils are widely dilated and fixed. There is no response to light or tapping the cornea. The muscles are extremely flaccid. Stage 4 is never reached by intent; it therefore has no use in surgery. Cessation of delivery of anesthetic, the prompt application of artificial respiration, with or without cardiac compression, and often the administration of stimulants can lighten the depth of anesthesia to the point of restoration of respiration and, ultimately, consciousness.

Veterinary anesthesiologists use a simple maneuver to estimate the degree of peripheral vasoconstriction. Called the filling-time test, it is applied by pressing a finger firmly against the surface of a gum just above the tooth line. The force is maintained for many seconds and squeezes the blood out of the underlying capillary bed. The finger is suddenly removed, and the compressed and surrounding normal tissue beds are viewed as blood returns to the previously compressed area. The time taken for the previously compressed region to resemble the adjacent tissue is known as the filling time. If there is considerable vasoconstriction, the filling time is very long, alerting the anesthesiologist to seek the cause for the unusual vaso-constriction.

A reflex frequently used by veterinarians to evaluate the depth of anesthesia in some animals is the anal pucker. With light anesthesia, a gentle tap on the anus causes it to contract briefly and withdraw slightly. With deeper anesthesia, the reflex is very weak, and with deep anesthesia it disappears.

Anesthesia Monitoring

Although the Guedel chart allows assessment of the depth of anesthesia, there is increasing awareness that better evidence is needed to evaluate the depth of anesthesia and to indicate a change, and in which direction. At present in the United States there are 20 million anesthetic procedures annually, and it is estimated that there are 5000 cases of brain damage associated with them. Most anesthesiologists believe that appropriate instrumental aids could reduce this number by 85% and would allow better management of all anesthetic procedures. The number of anesthetic mishaps that result in neurological deficit is unknown.

Because anesthesia is a phenomenon of controlled depression of the central nervous system (brain and spinal cord), it is logical to seek methods that provide information on the status of that system during anesthesia. Although the electroencephalogram (EEG) has been studied during anesthesia (see Chap. 12), it is not a reliable indicator of the depth of anesthesia because the most prominent changes occur with deep anesthesia. The most sensitive indicators of the status of the central nervous system are the signs shown in the Guedel chart (Fig. 2). Nonetheless, electrical monitoring of the nervous system is used in some circumstances. For example, during spinal surgery, sensory evoked potentials (SEPs) are sometimes monitored, as are motor evoked potentials (MEPs); these techniques are described in Chapter 12.

Monitoring of bioelectric events is difficult in the operating room because of its electrically noisy environment and frequent use of the electrosurgical unit. Thus monitoring the EEG, SEP, or MEP is difficult at best. However, the electrocardiogram (ECG) is often monitored to identify the heart rate and occasionally to detect arrhythmias. It must be recognized that every ventricular excitation signaled by an R wave does not necessarily mean that a forceful mechanical beat occurred. Nonetheless, a change in R-wave rate is an alerting signal to the anesthesiologist.

Perhaps the most routinely monitored quantity is blood pressure. Although blood pressure can be measured noninvasively with the auscultatory method, the operating room is usually noisy and the Korotkoff sounds are often difficult to hear, especially if the blood pressure is low. More frequently, the oscillometric method is employed in which the amplitude of cuff pressure oscillations is used to identify systolic, diastolic, and mean pressure as well as heart rate. Heart rate can be determined accurately in this way. Moreover, the oscillometric method performs well in situations of low blood pressure. However, blood pressure is not a sensitive indicator of the status of the cardiovascular system, because it reflects the product of cardiac output and peripheral resistance. Peripheral resistance can decrease and cardiac output increase, and the blood pressure will give no evidence of these events. In anesthesia, a decrease in peripheral resistance is not uncommon and is a sign that things are changing. At present, peripheral resistance is not determined, because cardiac output is not measured during anesthesia.

The respiratory system is assessed by the number of breaths per minute (as shown by the breathing bag) and the color of the lips, gums, or nailbeds. Although there may be adequate delivery of oxygen to the airway by the anesthesia machine, the uptake (milliliters per minute) is never measured; its measurement would require an airway flowmeter and a rapidly responding gaseous oxygen sensor. The uptake per breath is the volume per breath multiplied by the difference between inspired and expired oxygen concentrations. Current technology does not enable us to make this all-important measurement on line.

The oxygen uptake is assessed indirectly by the oxygen saturation measured by an oximeter (see Chap. 5). However, an oximeter indicates percent saturation, not content ($mL\ O_2/100\ mL$ blood). Nonetheless, a reduction in saturation is an alerting signal for the anesthesiologist to investigate the cause.

Measurement of the concentration of end-expired carbon dioxide concentration provides indirect assessment of arterial pCO_2, which is a sensitive indicator of the function of the cardiorespiratory system. Recording the concentration of expired carbon dioxide is called capnography (*capnos* = smoke). This technique is quite common in Europe and is beginning to be used in the United States.

It is noteworthy that if the minute volume of expired carbon dioxide is measured, this quantity relates to cardiac output, being the numerator in the Fick equation (see Chap. 8). However, to obtain this information, a flowmeter as well as a carbon dioxide analyzer must be applied to the airway. Both devices are available but have not yet been combined into a practical system for routine use.

Transcutaneous pO_2 and pCO_2 are occasionally measured (see Chap. 8). The need to arterialize the tissue bed requires that time be allowed for this to occur. During anesthesia, if generalized vasoconstriction occurs, the transcutaneous pO_2 and pCO_2 values become unreliable. However, a simple device that identifies vasoconstriction—the inexpensive photoplethysmograph (see Chap. 5)—is rarely used and could provide beneficial but not quantitative information.

Constant vigilance is the key factor for a successful anesthetic procedure. The clinical signs of anesthesia are supplemented by information from monitoring devices. Some provide historical information—the display is available after the event occurred or after it was measured; digital displays fall into this category. Analog displays report on contemporary events and provide temporal information having a predictive value.

An anesthetic agent is a drug, and the depth of anesthesia is related to the uptake per minute. Despite the fact that the concentration of an anesthetic presented to the airway is known, the uptake is not. The uptake per breath is equal to the difference between inspired and expired concentrations multiplied by the tidal volume. The uptake per minute is this product multiplied by the respiratory rate (breaths/minute). There are few, if any, breath-by-breath responding transducers for the anesthetic gases, although there are low-resistance flowmeters (e.g., the pneumotachograph). The combination of these devices to indicate anesthetic uptake per minute is in the future.

There have been many attempts to create a system that will automatically control the depth of anesthesia. These efforts have not resulted in the creation of a practical and dependable closed-loop system that will perform in all circumstances. The reason for the failure is that there is no physiological event that identifies the depth of anesthesia. The information in the Guedel chart still offers the best means for assessing the depth of anesthesia.

As one experienced anesthesiologist put it, managing the depth of anesthesia is like flying an airplane: The pilot responds to all the cues that permit a smooth flight, but an unexpected storm can occur, and the pilot must rely on instrumental aids to ensure a safe flight and happy landing.

ADMINISTRATION OF ANESTHESIA

Volatile and gaseous anesthetics are usually delivered by an anesthesia machine. The use of such devices dates only from the turn of the twentieth century. Epstein and Hunter (1968) presented an interesting pictorial history of anesthesia machines.

Prior to their use, and occasionally today in veterinary medicine, volatile anesthetics were introduced directly into the airway by inhalation of anesthetic vapors evaporating from a cloth; this technique is called the open-drop method. In modern practice anesthesia is first induced by a short-acting anesthetic that is injected intravenously. Then a cuffed endotracheal tube is installed to provide a patent airway for connection to the anesthesia machine.

ANESTHESIA MACHINE

The anesthesia machine must provide a metered amount of the anesthetic gases and oxygen, remove the expired carbon dioxide, and include a low-resistance path to a collapsible reservoir to permit easy inhalation of the gas mixture. Because most modern anesthetics are volatile liquids, a vaporizer is used to evaporate the liquid. The inspiratory reservoir is a collapsible bag that can be compressed rhythmically to apply artificial respiration. Valves are included in the circuit to ensure unidirectional flow of the gas mixture.

Closed-Circuit (Circle) Anesthesia Machine

The closed-circuit (circle) system diagramed in Fig. 3 is widely used for general anesthesia. It consists of a vaporizer (Vap) to evaporate the volatile anesthetic agent, a manifold of flowmeters and valves to control the flow of oxygen (and other gases) which pass through the vaporizer and into the circle circuit, which

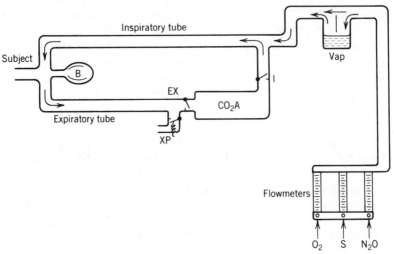

Figure 3   The closed-circuit (circle) anesthesia machine with the vaporizer (Vap) outside the circle. B, bag; S, supplemental gas; XP, excess pressure valve; EX, expiratory valve; I, inspiratory valve; CO_2A, CO_2 absorber.

contains a carbon dioxide absorber (CO_2A), breathing bag (B), and valves arranged so that the flow of gas is in one direction only. The flow of oxygen and other gases such as N_2O (which is an analgesic agent) passing through the vaporizer picks up the desired concentration of the volatile anesthetic. The gas mixture then passes into the inspiratory tube. The subject inhales this gas mixture and exhales some of it along with CO_2 into the CO_2 absorber (soda lime). The expired gas is prevented from flowing back into the inspiratory tube by the inspiratory valve (I).

In the absorber, CO_2 is converted to a solid. In this chemical reaction, heat is liberated and the soda lime changes color in proportion to the amount of CO_2 it traps. The color intensity indicates when the absorber is exhausted and should be replaced. After passing through the CO_2 absorber, the gas mixture is forced to return to the inspiratory tube via the expiratory valve (EX).

The breathing bag on the inspiratory side of the circuit serves several important functions. Because the system is closed, the flow of oxygen and other gases into the system must equal the amount absorbed by the subject plus the small amount due to any leak. The inflow of gases is constant and occurs slowly. Inspiration requires a relatively large volume of gas in a short time; the breathing bag acts as a reservoir to accommodate the demand of inspiration. If there is a slight net excess inflow of gas over uptake by the subject, the breathing bag acts as an elastic reservoir and will expand to accommodate this excess. However, with excessive inflow, the pressure in the circuit will continue to rise and the excess pressure valve (XP) will automatically open to reduce the pressure. The uptake of oxygen is about 300 mL/min, and the inflow is set at a value slightly above that to accommodate the small leakage from the circuit.

The breathing bag also acts as an indicator of spontaneous respiration, collapsing slightly during inspiration. Even more important, it affords a means for assisting respiration. Squeezing the bag forces gas into the lungs; releasing the bag allows the elastic recoil of the lungs and rib cage to effect expiration. The resistance offered to lung inflation informs the anesthetist about the airway compliance.

Mechanically assisted respiration is achieved by surrounding the breathing bag with a chamber to which intermittent positive gas pressure is applied. Some anesthesia machines provide a means of detecting an inspiratory effort and using it to trigger the delivery of gas to the airway.

It is obvious that the vaporizer (Vap) can be located within the circle as shown in Fig. 4. In this situation, the gas flowing through the vaporizer is at a higher temperature than when the vaporizer is outside the circle. Since evaporation is profoundly increased by an increase in temperature, locating the vaporizer within the circle will allow the use of less volatile anesthetic liquids. However, great care must be exercised with an in-circle vaporizer, because the temperature increases steadily after the breathing circuit is connected to the subject.

Vaporizer

The task of the vaporizer is to provide a controlled quantity of gas to be produced from the anesthetic liquid. To appreciate the task performed by the vaporizer, it is

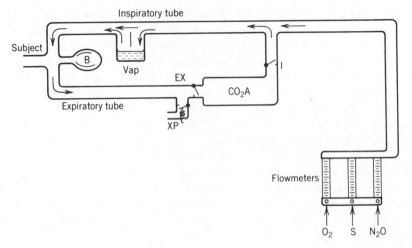

Figure 4   The closed-circuit (circle) anesthesia machine with the vaporizer inside the circle. For definition of symbols, see legend to Fig. 3.

important to understand the factors that affect the process of evaporation. The amount of liquid that evaporates to become a gas depends on its vapor pressure and temperature, the area available for evaporation, and the velocity of the gas passing over the liquid. Liquids with a low vapor pressure at room temperature do not evaporate readily. For example, water at 20°C has a vapor pressure of 40 mmHg. At 100°C the vapor pressure is 760 mmHg; water boils and exists as a gas at this temperature. Ether at 20°C has a vapor pressure of 460 mmHg; therefore, at room temperature ether vaporizes much more readily than water. Liquids with low boiling points have high vapor pressures at room temperature and vaporize readily.

When a liquid evaporates to produce a gas, the surface of the liquid is cooled. Conduction and convection in the liquid cause bulk cooling. Because the vapor pressure decreases as the liquid cools, the amount that evaporates decreases. Therefore it is necessary to provide heat to maintain the same evaporation rate. The amount of heat required depends on the latent heat of the liquid, which is the number of calories required to change 1 g of liquid to a gas at the same temperature. For example, it requires 94.4 cal/(g-°C) to convert 1 g of ether to a gas at 20°C, so the latent heat of ether is 94.4 cal.

Evaporative cooling plagued the early developers of vaporizers in which the anesthetic liquid was contained in a glass jar, which provided excellent thermal insulation. In most modern vaporizers the anesthetic liquid is contained in a metal vessel, which permits easy conduction of heat from the environment. Thus, environmental temperature becomes a factor in the operation of a vaporizer.

For the evaporative process to continue at a uniform rate, the gas above the anesthetic liquid must be removed. Therefore the flow of gas through the evaporating chamber is a factor in the concentration of the emergent gas.

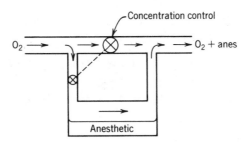

Figure 5   Principle employed in vaporizers.

The principle employed in nearly all vaporizers is illustrated in Fig. 5. The anesthetic liquid is contained in a vessel where evaporation takes place. A controlled amount of oxygen is passed through the evaporation chamber, while the remaining oxygen bypasses it. The concentration of the gas mixture emerging from the vaporizer is dependent on the proportion of flow through the evaporation chamber and that which bypasses it. It is the manner in which this basic principle is employed that distinguishes the different types of vaporizers. From the discussion of the factors that govern evaporation, it can be recognized that the simple vaporizer illustrated in Fig. 5 would have many practical defects.

Beyond the individual differences in vaporizers, there are two general types. One type offers a low resistance to gas flow, and only a portion of the subject's inspired air is drawn through the vaporizer. The other, more common, type has a high flow resistance, and oxygen and nitrous oxide from cylinders of compressed gas flow through the vaporizer. Although there are many vaporizers of each type, the goal of each is to provide a selectable concentration of anesthetic gas, despite changes in flow and temperature.

In many vaporizers, wicks or sponges are used to enhance evaporation by providing a large surface area. In some vaporizers, the carrier gas (oxygen and nitrous oxide) is bubbled through the anesthetic liquid. In one model, the "copper kettle" (Morris, 1952; Morris and Feldman, 1958), the carrier gas is passed through a porous disk of Porex that is well below the surface of the anesthetic liquid. In this way, a very large number of small gas bubbles are formed and rise to the surface of the liquid carrying the anesthetic gas with them. Bubbling air (or a gas) through a liquid increases the area available for evaporation because the evaporative surface then becomes the total surface area of all the bubbles. A large number of small bubbles provides more evaporative surface than the same number of large bubbles, because the surface-to-volume ratio for spheres is $3/r$, where r is the radius.

Many of the earlier vaporizers employed a glass container to allow visualization of the level of anesthetic liquid. Glass is an excellent thermal insulator, and the temperature of the anesthetic liquid decreased with continued use. A thermometer was provided to indicate the temperature and allow resetting of the concentration control. Usually, the concentration control has several scales corresponding to different temperatures. Modern vaporizers employ metallic containers and a large thermal mass consisting of a copper block that draws heat from the environment and tends to maintain the temperature constant. Often the copper block is bolted to the metal top of the anesthetic cart to provide additional thermal stability. A sight gauge is provided to identify the level of anesthetic liquid. A few of the earlier vaporizers used a water jacket to provide the latent heat of vaporization. A few used the heat provided by a chemical reaction; some used a thermostatically controlled water bath.

In some vaporizers, thermal control is automatically applied to the portion of gas flowing through the evaporation chamber. Bimetallic strips and metal bellows connected to valves provide this automatic type of temperature compensation for gas flow.

An important consideration in the use of a vaporizer relates to the resistance it offers to gas flow. Most vaporizers designed for use with a carrier gas (oxygen and nitrous oxide) exhibit a high resistance to gas flow. Therefore, they cannot be used in the draw-over mode of operation in which the subject's inspiration draws gas through the vaporizer. In draw-over operation, a vaporizer with a low resistance to flow must be used.

PRESSURE REGULATOR

Oxygen and nitrous oxide (and other gases) are obtained from cylinders in which the gas is stored under very high pressure. In order to deliver these gases at the flow rates required for anesthetic procedures, the pressure must be reduced by a pressure regulator. Figure 6 illustrates the principle underlying the operation of such devices. The high-pressure gas enters and passes through a valve into a chamber that is terminated by a spring-loaded diaphragm, which is connected to the valve. The valve opening, and hence the flow out of this chamber, is dependent on the force exerted on the diaphragm and the spring tension. An increase in gas pressure will tend to close the valve and reduce the flow at the low-pressure output. Likewise, an increase to outflow resistance will cause the valve to close slightly

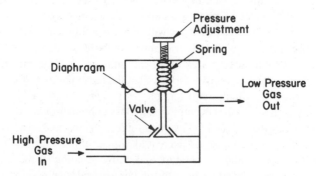

Figure 6   Principle employed in the pressure regulator.

and reduce the input of high-pressure gas. Therefore, the output flow and pressure can be controlled by adjusting the spring tension applied to the diaphragm.

CONCLUSION

It is appropriate to close this chapter by noting that the anesthesia machine in use today is not very different from the first ones developed in 1914 by Gwathmey in the United States, which employed a face mask and a gas mixture consisting of ether, nitrous oxide, and oxygen. Boyle (1917), in the United Kingdom, improved the machine but used the same gas mixture. Neither machine contained a CO_2 absorber, which was added by Waters (1924), thereby allowing closed-circuit breathing. The first such machine was described by Jackson (1927). Sword (1930) described the first practical model; pressure regulators and flowmeters had been added by this time. By the early 1930s the anesthesia machine had reached its present form. In this day of high technology, one might wonder why the anesthesia machine has not changed dramatically. The reason is simple. It is dependable, and it does not require electricity; therefore it is immune from power failure and electrical hazards. In the hands of an experienced anesthesiologist it performs very well.

Notwithstanding the attributes just described, steps are underway to add measuring facilities to the anesthesia machine. As stated in the section on anesthesia monitoring in this chapter, efforts are being made to provide transducers to measure the inspired volume and the inspired and expired concentrations of oxygen and the anesthetic gases, from which uptake can be determined. The availability of such data will allow the anesthesiologist to pilot the course of anesthesia with more confidence. There have been several attempts to apply closed-loop control to anesthesia; however, the results have not been spectacular because it is difficult to identify a physiological event that reflects the depth of anesthesia under all circumstances.

REFERENCES

Bleecher, H. K. 1938. *The Physiology of Anesthesia*. Oxford Univ. Press, London and New York.

Boyle, H. E. G. 1917. The use of nitrous oxide and oxygen with rebreathing in military surgery. *Br. Med. J.* **2:**653–655.

Epstein, H. G., and A. R. Hunter. 1968. Anesthetic apparatus; a pictorial review of the development of the modern anesthetic machine. *Br. J. Anaesth.* **40:**636–647.

Goodman, L. S., and A. Gilman (eds.). 1955. *The Pharmacological Basis of Therapeutics*, 2nd ed. Macmillan, New York.

Guedel, A. E. 1937. *Inhalation Anesthesia*. Macmillan, New York.

Guedel, A. E., 1951. *Inhalation Anesthesia*. Macmillan, New York.

Gwathmey, J. T. 1914. *Anesthesia*. Appleton, New York, 945 pp.

Hill, D. W. 1976. *Physics Applied to Anesthesia*. Butterworth, London, 411 pp.

Hoff, H. E. 1937. Ether versus chloroform. *N. Engl. J. Med.* **217:**579–592.

Jackson, D. E. 1927. A universal artificial respiration and closed anesthesia machine. *J. Lab. Clin. Med.* **12:**998–1002.

Morris, L. E. 1952. New vaporizer for liquid anesthetic agents. *Anesthesiology* **13:**587–593.

Morris, L. E., and S. A. Feldman. 1958. Condensations in the design and function of anesthetic vaporizers. *Anesthesiology* **19:**642–649.

Sword, B. C. 1930. The closed-circuit method of administration of gas anesthesia. *Anesth. Analg.* **9:**198–202.

Waters, R. M. 1924. Clinical scope and utility of carbon-dioxide filtration in inhalation anesthesia. *Anesth. Analg.* **3:**20–23.

16

Criteria for the Faithful Reproduction of an Event

ANALOG SYSTEMS

Introduction

For the familiar three-part system (transducer, processor, and reproducer) used to measure the time course of a physiological event, it is possible to set forth general conditions that, if satisfied, will guarantee faithful reproduction of the event. It is necessary either to appropriately impose the same conditions on the three parts of the channel or to incorporate any necessary compensation so that the overall system will meet the criteria if the individual parts do not. In such a system three criteria must be fulfilled. Because of the extreme importance of these criteria, their meaning must be clearly understood. Even though many of the underlying factors are of necessity technical and complex, simple examples can be chosen to illustrate their importance.

Any system designed for the faithful reproduction of an event must possess these characteristics:

1. Amplitude linearity.
2. Adequate bandwidth.
3. Phase linearity.

The first requisite, amplitude linearity, calls for the input–output characteristic to be linear in the working range. If, for example, the input is doubled in the positive direction, the output indication must also be doubled. If the operating range extends into the reverse direction, negative inputs must be reproduced by a linear output indication in the negative direction.

Fourier Series

Before the second and third criteria can be discussed, it is necessary to establish the relationship between sine waves and waves of nonsinusoidal form. All periodic nonsinusoidal waves are designated complex waves. By the use of the Fourier series it is possible to show that any periodic complex wave can be dissected into a series of sine and cosine waves that when added will reproduce the original complex wave. The sine or cosine wave that has the same frequency as the complex wave constitutes the fundamental or first harmonic. Those having twice and three times the frequency constitute the second and third harmonics, and so on. This can be restated by saying that a periodic complex wave can be represented by an infinite series consisting of a constant plus harmonically related sine and cosine waves. Expressed mathematically, the series for the function $F(t)$ can be written as follows:

$$F(t) = \frac{a_0}{2} + a_1 \cos \omega t + a_2 \cos 2\omega t + a_3 \cos 3\omega t + \cdots + a_n \cos n\omega t$$

$$+ \; b_1 \sin \omega t + b_2 \sin 2\omega t + b_3 \sin 3\omega t + \cdots + b_n \sin n\omega t,$$

where

$$a_n = \frac{1}{\pi} \int_0^{2\pi} F(t) \cos n\omega t \, dt,$$

$$b_n = \frac{1}{\pi} \int_0^{2\pi} F(t) \sin n\omega t \, dt,$$

and

$$\omega = 2\pi f$$

(where f is the fundamental frequency of the complex wave in hertz).

To use the series to describe a waveform, it is necessary to calculate the coefficients $a_0, \ldots, a_n$ and $b_0, \ldots, b_n$, some of which may be zero. However, for purposes of this study it is neither necessary nor profitable to perform the calculations to demonstrate the validity of the series. Many waves have been analyzed and the coefficients published. Figure 1 presents data for a few of the familiar waves. Two examples, the square wave and a blood pressure waveform, will suffice to show the value of the concept.

One of the most difficult waveforms to reproduce is the square (rectangular) wave (Fig. 2a), which instantaneously changes its value from zero to a fixed value, maintains this value for a time before reversing itself below zero by the same amount and for the same time, and returns abruptly to zero again. When this wave is analyzed for its harmonic content, some of the coefficients are zero, and the series reduces to the fundamental and an infinite series of odd harmonics in which the amplitudes of the higher-frequency components decrease; that is, these components contribute less to the resynthesis of the original wave.

In Fig. 2b, the first and the third harmonic components have been summed to yield the curve labeled 1 + 3. In this case, even with only two components, the beginnings of the square wave are apparent. When the first, third, and fifth components are summed (Fig. 2c), a better representation of the original wave is

WAVEFORM TYPE	HARMONIC NUMBER								MULTIPLY EACH BY
	0	1	2	3	4	5	6	7	
SQUARE WAVE	0	1 (sin)	0	1/3 (sin)	0	1/5 (sin)	0	1/7 (sin)	$4E/\pi$
SAW TOOTH	0	1 (sin)	-1/2 (sin)	1/3 (sin)	-1/4 (sin)	1/5 (sin)	-1/6 (sin)	1/7 (sin)	$2E/\pi$
TRIANGULAR	0	1 (cos)	0	1/9 (cos)	0	1/25 (cos)	0	1/49 (cos)	$8E/\pi^2$
HALF WAVE RECTIFIER	1	$\pi/2$ (cos)	2/3 (cos)	0	-2/15 (cos)	0	2/35 (cos)	0	E/π
SQUARE PULSE	k	$\frac{2}{\pi}\left(\frac{1}{n}\sin(k\pi n)\cdot\cos(n)\right)$							E

Figure 1   Summary of analyzed waveforms. Conclusions: (1) Symmetry about x axis results in $a_0 = 0$ (no d.c. component). Asymmetry about x axis gives $a_0 \neq 0$. (2) Amplitudes of harmonics decrease with increasing harmonic numbers. (3) The more abrupt transitions, the greater the number of harmonics present. The square pulse has the most components.

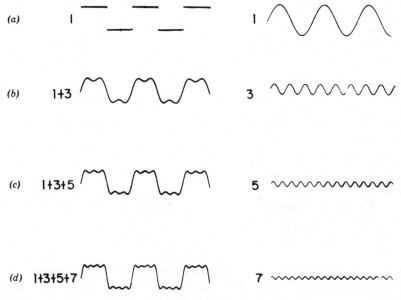

(a)   1

(b)   1+3

(c)   1+3+5

(d)   1+3+5+7

3

5

7

Figure 2   Synthesis of a square wave.

obtained $(1 + 3 + 5)$. By adding the first, third, fifth, and seventh components, an even better likeness of the original wave (Fig. 2d) is obtained $(1 + 3 + 5 + 7)$. The addition of more and more harmonics would further improve the reproduction; the addition of an infinite number of the ever-diminishing-amplitude high-frequency components would reconstitute the original wave.

The arterial pressure pulse provides a good example of the utilitarian value of harmonic analysis. Hansen (1949), using a high-fidelity system, recorded the arterial pulse wave and applied harmonic analysis to it. His data, redrawn and plotted in Fig. 3a, show the degree of fidelity obtainable by summing the first six harmonics. The arterial pressure waveform is designated a, and the waveform resulting

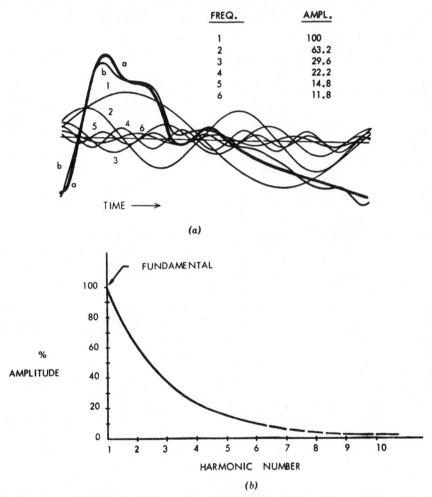

FREQ.	AMPL.
1	100
2	63.2
3	29.6
4	22.2
5	14.8
6	11.8

(a)

(b)

Figure 3 (a) Fourier analysis of a blood pressure curve; (b) harmonic amplitudes of components of a blood pressure pulse. (From data obtained by A. T. Hansen. *Pressure Measurement in the Human Organism*. Technisk Forlag, Copenhagen, 1949. By permission.)

from summing the first six harmonics is labeled b. The amplitudes of the higher-frequency components are progressively smaller with increasing harmonic numbers, the sixth being present with an amplitude of slightly more than 10%. Figure 3*b* illustrates this point.

To obtain a more faithful reproduction, addition of many more of the smaller-and-smaller-amplitude high-frequency components would be necessary. Thus the frequency response required is closely related to the degree of fidelity desired.

From these relatively simple examples, two very important conclusions can be drawn. The first is that the frequency of the periodic complex wave determines the frequency of the fundamental component. The second is that the fidelity of reproduction of the quickly changing parts of the wave is determined by the number of high-frequency components added. Thus, the flat portion of the sinusoidal frequency–response curve required for reproduction of the two waves analyzed must extend from the fundamental frequency of the complex wave to the highest harmonic deemed important for reproduction of the sharpest portions of the complex wave.

In the two examples cited, the waves chosen were symmetrical about the time axis. If they were not, the analysis would have shown the same components with one notable exception: The constant a_0 would have a value other than zero, for a_0 is the average amplitude over a complete period. It is easily proved mathematically, and indeed is obvious, that a train of unidirectional pulses must have an average value other than zero. In the case of the arterial pressure wave, a_0 would be the mean pressure. Therefore, to reproduce a train of unidirectional pulses, it is necessary to provide a uniform frequency response extending from 0 Hz to a value high enough for full reproduction of the highest harmonic deemed important. In practice, the high-frequency response is made to include the tenth harmonic and sometimes higher harmonics.

Amplitude and Phase Distortion

Perhaps of more importance than the cases in which the criteria are satisfied are those in which some criteria are not. The following examples illustrate some of the possible types of distortion. Because the square wave is one of the most difficult to reproduce, it is useful to examine the effects of alteration of the amplitudes of the harmonics on the reproduction of this waveform. Terman (1943) showed that if only the low-frequency components are attenuated, the square wave will have a concave top, as sketched in Fig. 4*a*. On the other hand, if the low-frequency components are enhanced, the top of the square wave will be convex, as in Fig. 4*b*.

If the harmonics are present in their proper amplitudes but displaced in time, a characteristic type of distortion occurs. Time displacement is not customarily expressed in seconds; it is usually stated in angular measure (radians or degrees) as a phase lag or lead. For example, if the time displacement for a given frequency f is t, since the period T corresponds to 360 degrees, the phase lag or lead ϕ in degrees is $(t/T) \times 360$ degrees. Since $T = 1/f$, one can express the phase lag or

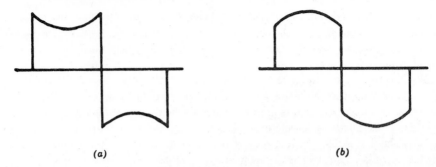

(a)   (b)

Figure 4 Amplitude distortion: (*a*) loss of low-frequency response (no phase distortion); (*b*) increased amplification of low frequencies (no phase distortion). (From F. E. Terman, *Radio Engineers Handbook*, 1st ed. McGraw-Hill, New York, 1943. By permission.)

lead in terms of frequency; that is, $\phi = tf \times 360$ degrees. Thus with equal time displacements for all frequency components ($t = k$), $\phi = kf$; that is, the phase shift must be linear with frequency. It is also possible to state this requirement by specifying that in relation to some reference (e.g., the fundamental), the components must be transmitted through the system such that they bear exactly the same time relationship to one another at the output as existed at the input.

Figure 5 illustrates the effect of phase distortion on the reproduction of the square wave. The harmonic components are present in their correct amplitudes, but time displacements have been caused to occur. In Fig. 5*a* the fundamental leads the higher harmonics, and in Fig. 5*b* the reverse condition exists. In each case the resulting reproduction is indicated by dashed lines.

Phase distortion can be present when only minimal loss of amplitude response occurs. Terman (1943) called attention to the fact that in many networks, such as those used to couple amplifier stages, when the low-frequency sine wave response is 99.94%, a 2-degree phase-shift error is encountered, which results in a 10% tilt to the top of the square wave of the same frequency.

Because phase shift and loss of amplitude response are usually inseparable, it is often difficult to appreciate the effect of each of these types of distortion. To

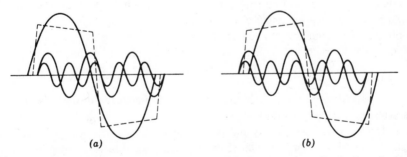

(a)   (b)

Figure 5 Phase distortion: (*a*) phase leads at low frequency (no amplitude distortion); (*b*) phase lags at low frequency (no amplitude distortion).

demonstrate the practical importance of this fact, Geddes (1951) constructed a variable-frequency oscillator that produced a sine wave having a notch at its peak positive amplitude. The location of the notch (square pulse) was fixed, but the frequency of the complex wave was variable. This wave was used to test electroencephalographs to estimate their ability to reproduce faithfully the familiar spike-and-wave complex found in recordings from patients with petit mal epilepsy.

The wave was applied to one of several EEG machines meeting existing standards; the frequency was varied, and the output was recorded. Figure 6a is a sketch of the input waveform. The other sections of the figure represent the reproduction achieved at various frequencies. In Fig. 6b, recorded at 1 Hz, it is obvious that there is a 45-degree phase shift. Increasing the frequency to 2 and 3 Hz (Figs. 6c and 6d) places the spike more nearly in its correct position, where it appears when the frequency is 6 Hz. However, although the phase distortion is minimal at 6 Hz, the amplitude of the spike has decreased (Fig. 6e), because the system had inadequate high-frequency response to pass the high-frequency components contained in the spike.

The practical significance of phase distortion was demonstrated by Saunders and Jell (1959), who recorded the effect in a unique way by using two identical channels of an EEG machine. The output of the first channel was attenuated and fed into the second; the output of both channels appeared on the same record. They first tested the system for phase distortion, using a 3-Hz sine wave. On a typical EEG machine in which a 3-Hz sine wave was attenuated insignificantly, they recorded a time delay between channels amounting to 51.3 msec or 55.4 degrees. This testing technique demonstrated the phase shift in the second channel only. Next,

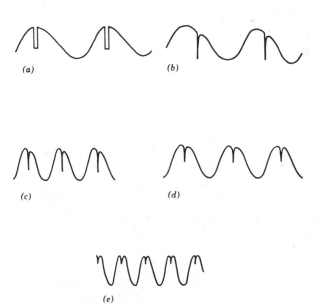

Figure 6   Amplitude and phase distortion.

in a practical study, stimulus–response waves, eye-blink artifacts, and spike-and-wave patterns were observed to exhibit time distortions when the recordings from the two channels were compared. A time separation of 75 msec between the spike and wave recorded on the first channel was reduced to 63 msec after passing through the second channel.

From the examples given, it is apparent that three criteria—amplitude linearity, frequency response, and phase linearity—must be satisfied to guarantee the faithful reproduction of an event. Amplitude linearity occurs when output and input are proportional. Frequency response is usually described in terms of bandwidth, which is designated as the frequency range between the lowest and highest sine wave frequencies at which a satisfactory amplitude response is obtained. It is also frequently designated as the spectrum between the two frequencies at which the output amplitude has fallen to 70% of the midfrequency response. In some instances the 50, 90, or 95% points are specified.

The Step Function

For practical testing of a system, the step function is of considerable value. It is a waveform that changes abruptly from one level to another and is employed as a calibration signal in many bioelectric recording instruments. Since the sine wave frequency–response curves of most devices are given by equipment manufacturers, it is illuminating to apply the step function to systems with known frequency-response curves to determine the relationship between sinusoidal and step-function responses.

If the step function shown in Fig. 7a is applied to a simple system that does not possess a sine wave frequency response extending to 0 Hz (Fig. 7b) but has an infinite high-frequency response, the reproduced wave is of exponential form (see Fig. 7c). The decay time is described as the time taken for the amplitude to fall from 100% to 37%. This time, measured in seconds, is called the time constant. The time constant is related to the sine wave frequency response by the relationship

$$T = \frac{1}{2\pi f_{L}},$$

where T is the time constant in seconds and f_{L} is the frequency on the sine wave curve at which the response is 70%.

Often in the recording of physiological and bioelectric events, as a result of the intermittent activity of a variety of cells and organs, short-duration asymmetrical (with respect to the time axis) or completely monophasic pulses are presented to the reproducing apparatus. A harmonic analysis of such waveforms reveals the presence of a first term (a_0) in the Fourier series. Therefore, faithful reproduction of such events requires the use of a system with a frequency response extending to 0 Hz, that is, a dc response. Frequently it is not practical to meet this requirement. Under many circumstances a reasonable reproduction of the event can be obtained with a processing system having a time constant that is very long with

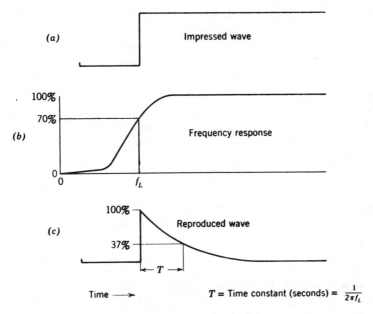

(a)   Impressed wave

100%
70%
(b)   Frequency response
0
0   f_L

100%
(c)   Reproduced wave
37%
$\leftarrow T \rightarrow$

Time $\longrightarrow$ $T = $ Time constant (seconds) $= \frac{1}{2\pi f_L}$

Figure 7 Relationship between time constant and low-frequency response.

respect to the duration of the event. This technique is employed in the instruments that record many of the bioelectric events such as the ECG, EEG, and EMG.

The effect of time constant on the reproduction of a single monophasic flat-topped pulse is illustrated in Fig. 8. The percentage drop (tilt) on the top of the reproduced wave is compared with the ratio of the duration of the pulse to the time

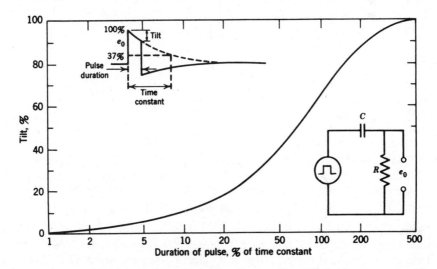

Figure 8 Rectangular pulse response of an *RC* circuit.

constant of the circuit passing it. For simplicity of illustration, the calculations were based on a single-section *RC* circuit.

It is readily apparent that a 10% tilt is encountered if the duration of the rectangular pulse is approximately one-tenth of the time constant of the circuit. Increasing the time constant of the circuit or decreasing the pulse duration would reduce the percentage tilt.

There is also an undershoot following the rectangular pulse, the magnitude of which is equal to the amount of tilt. If the pulse duration is many times greater than the time constant, the familiar biphasic condenser charge and discharge current wave is seen.

To further improve the reproduction of short-duration rectangular pulses when using amplifiers without dc response, investigators often add phase- and amplitude-compensating networks designed to flatten the top of the rectangular pulse. This technique is employed in most ECG amplifiers. A good treatment of this subject is given by Valley and Wallman (1948).

The undershoot just described can be seen in recording the electrocardiogram when the time constant is too short. This point was well recognized by Schwarzschild and Kissin (1934–1935) when the use of a coupling capacitor was proposed to eliminate the effect of electrode offset potentials when recording the ECG with the string galvanometer, which is a direct-coupled recorder. Figure 9 shows a record of the ECG obtained with a standard 3.2-sec (diagnostic) time constant. Also shown in Fig. 9 are ECG recordings obtained with time constants of 0.5, 0.17, 0.017,

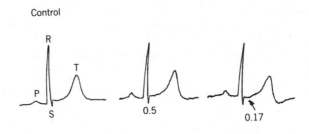

Figure 9 The control ECG recorded with a 3.2-sec time constant and recordings obtained with shorter time constants. Note the S-T segment displacement (arrows) when the time constant is 0.17 sec and shorter. The presence of an S-T segment displacement when using a 3.2-sec time constant would indicate reduced blood flow to the ventricles.

and 0.005 sec. Note the appearance of an S-T segment depression (at the arrows) with a time constant of 0.17 sec and the prominent S-T depression with a time constant of 0.05 sec. When such an S-T segment displacement is seen with the standard 3.2-sec time constant, it signals reduced blood supply (ischemia) to the ventricles. Note also in Fig. 9 that the ECG becomes differentiated as the time constant is reduced, a technique that removes the low-frequency components of the signal. When it is desired to obtain a triggering signal from the ECG, this technique is employed.

A reduction in the low-frequency response is often used in electrocardiography to eliminate low-frequency variations in the baseline of the recording, usually due to respiratory-induced electrode artifacts. Figure 10a illustrates the ECG recorded with the conventional 3.2-sec time constant ($f_L = 0.05$ Hz). Figure 10b illustrates the simultaneously recorded ECG with the monitoring time constant of 0.2 sec ($f_L = 0.8$ Hz). Note that the low-frequency oscillation in the baseline is almost eliminated. Note also that there is a slight displacement of the S-T segment.

If the step function (Fig. 7a) is impressed on a simple system having a low-frequency response extending to 0 Hz and a high-frequency response not extending to an infinitely high frequency (Fig. 11b) the type of response shown in Fig. 11c is encountered. It can be seen that the reproduced wave does not attain its final value instantly but takes a finite time to reach it. This rise or response time is frequently described as the time in seconds for the amplitude to rise from 10 to 90% of its final value. The rise time is related to the high-frequency sine wave response by the expression

$$t = \frac{1}{kf_h},$$

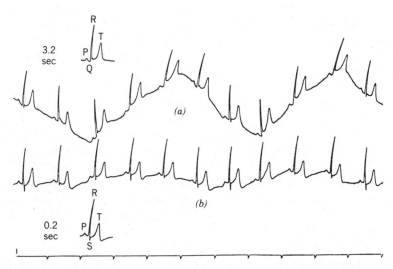

Figure 10 The ECG recorded with a sine wave frequency extending (a) to 0.05 Hz and (b) to 0.8 Hz.

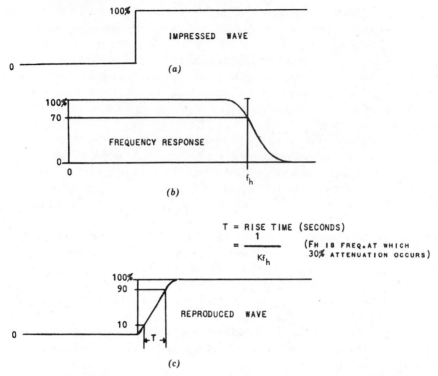

Figure 11   The effect of high-frequency response on the reproduction of a step function.

where t is rise time (10 to 90%) in seconds; f_h is frequency on the sine wave response curve where the response has fallen to 70%; and k depends on the circuit configuration, hence the rate at which the high-frequency response decreases with increasing frequency (high-frequency rolloff). In many circuits, k varies between 2 and 3. From this it is obvious that increasing f_h—that is, improving the high-frequency response—shortens the rise time. Figure 12 summarizes how low-frequency and high-frequency responses affect the reproduction of a step function.

From this discussion it is readily apparent that the sharp portions of a complex wave dictate the high-frequency response required for its faithful reproduction. The required low-frequency response is determined by the fundamental frequency of the complex wave and by the presence or absence of an average value. If the complex waveform possesses an average value, the required low-frequency response must extend to 0 Hz (i.e., the system must provide dc response) if baseline information is to be retained. However, in bioelectric recorders, a time constant many times longer than the width of the widest pulse is used instead of providing a frequency response to 0 Hz.

Damped Resonant Systems

The phenomenon of resonance is frequently encountered in the course of measuring physiological events. Basic to this phenomenon is the presence of at least

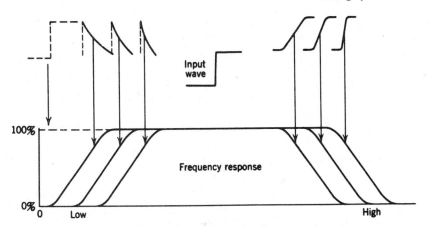

Figure 12   The effect of low- and high-frequency response on the reproduction of a step function.

two real or apparent energy-storage elements between which energy is continuously transferred. In the case of electrical components, capacitance and inductance are the real storage elements. It is also possible for the resonance phenomenon to exist in amplifier circuits that contain no inductive elements. Systems of this type show "ringing," or a tendency toward oscillation at a frequency for which there is a component of positive feedback around all or part of the circuit.

Resonance can also be purely mechanical, as in the case of devices possessing elasticity and mass. Two examples of such mechanical devices are blood pressure manometers, in which an elastic diaphragm or Bourdon tube is distorted by pressure, and moving-coil recorders, in which a torsion rod or spring returns the movement to its baseline when the signal is removed. The actual motion of the moving element (hence its capabilities as a transducer or reproducer) depends on three factors—inertia, elasticity or stiffness, and damping—and is described in mathematical terms by the interrelationship between them. *Inertia* is a measure of the force required to set the mass in motion or to alter its direction once it is in motion. *Stiffness* describes the rigidity of the system. It is defined in terms of the force required to deflect the moving member unit distance from its position of equilibrium. *Damping* is a measure of the frictional force acting on the mass. The frictional force is directed opposite to the direction of displacement of the mass. It is usually assumed that the magnitude of the frictional force varies directly with velocity; that is, the damping is viscous. Damping may be present as fluid resistance, or it may exist as an electrically induced force.

Simple mechanical systems can be described in terms of one-to-one electrical analogs because the behavior of both systems is expressed by the same mathematical equations. Inertia, damping, and stiffness determine the behavior of mechanical systems. In a series electrical circuit, these quantities correspond to inductance, resistance, and capacitance, respectively.

Because the dynamic behavior of mechanical systems is so important in physiological measurements, the interrelationship between inertia, damping, and stiffness must be appreciated to understand how the characteristics of a given system can be altered under various conditions of measurement. Many devices can be well represented by a simple system involving only one degree of freedom (i.e., a system that can be completely characterized in terms of a single variable). Two simple mechanical models can be used to illustrate the behavior of most of these devices under the influence of a unit step of force and a constant-amplitude variable-frequency sinusoidal force.

Consider a mass M free to move on a frictionless horizontal surface coupled to a fixed support by a spring. Connected to the mass is a rod terminated by a vane dipping into a reservoir of fluid, providing viscous damping. Figure 13a is a sketch of such a system in which the mass M is free to move in a left- or right-hand direction only. If a force is applied to move the weight from its position of equilibrium and then is removed, the mass will return to its original position slowly or rapidly and may overshoot and oscillate about the position of equilibrium several times before coming to rest, as shown. The type of motion executed depends on the relationship between the mass, stiffness, and damping.

Another simple example of the same phenomenon (Fig. 13b) illustrates the essential components of a recording pen or galvanometer having a mass with a given moment of inertia coupled to an elastic torsion rod. If a deflecting torque is applied to cause rotation and is then removed, the system will return to its position

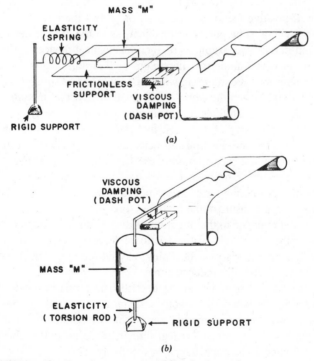

Figure 13   Transient response of lightly damped systems.

of equilibrium slowly or rapdily, as in the previous case, depending on the relationship between the same three quantities. The example of Fig. 13a deals with translation and describes the operation of blood pressure transducers and similar devices; that of Fig. 13b illustrates devices such as recording galvanometers in which rotary motion exists. Nonetheless, if the mass, stiffness, and coefficient of damping are time-invariant, the displacement in both cases is described by a linear differential equation of the second order and first degree. The following expressions describe the resultant motion:

Translation:

$$M\frac{d^2x}{dt^2} + K_1\frac{dx}{dt} + K_2x = \text{sum of applied forces.}$$

Rotation:

$$I\frac{d^2\phi}{dt^2} + K_1\frac{d\phi}{dt} + K_2\phi = \text{sum of applied torques.}$$

In these equations M and I are the mass-inertial components—M is the mass and I is the moment of inertia; K_1 is the viscous damping force; K_2 is the stiffness or restoring force (usually represented by a spring constant); x is the linear displacement; ϕ is the angular displacement; and t is time.

Note the similarity between the two expressions just given and the following equation, which represents the sum of the voltage drops across an inductance L, resistance R, and capacitance C in a series circuit:

$$L\frac{d^2q}{dt^2} + R\frac{dq}{dt} + \frac{q}{C} = \text{applied voltage,}$$

where q is the charge; dq/dt is the rate of change of charge, which is current i; and $d^2q/dt^2 = di/dt$.

Because the behavior of the mechanical systems is described by the same form of mathematical expression as that representing the electrical circuit, the electrical circuit is called an analog of either mechanical system. Thus the behavior of these simple mechanical systems, and of others more complicated, can be investigated by the use of simple electrical components. The inertial components (M and I) are represented by the inductance L, the damping force K_1 by resistance R, and the stiffness of the mechanical systems K_2 by the reciprocal of capacitance. The displacement (x or ϕ) has as its analog the charge q. Hence in the electrical simulation, the voltage across the capacitance describes x or ϕ.

Because these equations are of similar form, the solutions are the same except for the letter designation of terms. A mathematical solution to the equations may be difficult to carry out, depending on the time function required to describe the applied force. A graphic solution, however, is easily obtained from the electrical analog if the desired forcing function can be generated. The electrical analog also provides a convenient means of changing parameters, thus permitting the behavior of such systems under a variety of conditions to be demonstrated easily. Hence the mathematical ability necessary to solve the equations directly is not essential for an appreciation of the importance of the individual circuit elements in determining the response of the system to many different inputs. A description of the response to two different applied forces—(1) a step function and (2) a variable-frequency sine wave—will enable the reader to understand the behavior of a simple system under a variety of operating conditions.

The first and probably most important condition is the particular interrelationship between the quantities that provide just enough damping to render the motion nonoscillatory when a step force is applied or removed; that is, the moving element deflects or returns to its position of equilibrium as rapidly as possible without overshoot. Such a condition is called critical damping. Less damping results in a more rapid motion with overshoot. If the damping is reduced to zero, an oscillatory condition is produced. Although in practice it is never possible to achieve zero damping, a lightly damped system will oscillate for a long time before coming to rest. The frequency of force-free oscillation is called the natural frequency of the system.

When damping is made greater than critical, there is no overshoot, but the time taken to reach the position of equilibrium is considerably longer. The types of response encountered with critical damping and damping less than critical are summarized in Fig. 14a. With a step force applied or removed instantly, the response (curve a) is nonoscillatory for critical damping ($D = 1$). With light damping ($D = 0.2$), the response (curve b) is partially oscillatory. Increasing the damping to 0.5 (curve c) results in an overshoot of approximately 15% followed by a heavily damped oscillation.

The time axis of Fig. 14a is in percent of undamped period T_0 (equal to the reciprocal of the resonant frequency with zero damping, i.e., the natural frequency). The resonant frequency with zero damping (f_0) is dependent on the relationship between the inertial component M or I and the stiffness K_2. It can easily be shown that for the translational case,

$$f_0 = \frac{1}{2\pi} \sqrt{\frac{K_2}{M}},$$

for the rotational case,

$$f_0 = \frac{1}{2\pi} \sqrt{\frac{K_2}{I}},$$

and for the electrical case,

$$f_0 = \frac{1}{2\pi} \sqrt{\frac{1/C}{L}}.$$

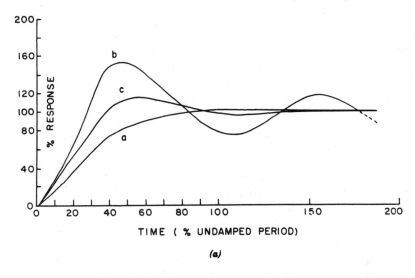

(a)

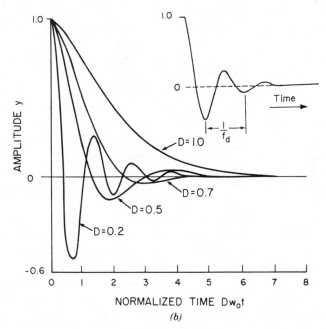

NORMALIZED TIME $Dw_0 t$

(b)

Figure 14 (*a*) Transient response for various damping coefficients D for the application of a deflecting force. (*b*) Normalized response for critically damped and underdamped systems for the sudden removal of unit deflecting force. The natural resonant frequency $f_0 = \omega_0/2\pi$; f_d is the damped resonant frequency $= f_0 \sqrt{1 - D^2}$;

$$y = e^{-D\omega_0 t}\left[\cos \omega_0 \sqrt{1 - D^2}\, t + \frac{D}{\sqrt{1 - D^2}} \sin \omega_0 \sqrt{1 - D^2}\, t\right].$$

Thus, specifying the system constants permits calculation of values for the abscissa of Fig. 14a. As the damping is decreased, the time for the system to rise from 0 to 100% becomes shorter and the overshoot is greater. Accordingly, the cost of elimination of transient overshoot is the prolongation of rise time. Therefore, to obtain a more rapid response without excessive overshoot, it is necessary to use a stiffer or lighter system, that is, one with a higher natural resonant frequency. Thus the undamped resonant frequency of a system, along with the coefficient of damping, determines the rise time.

It is frequently easier to demonstrate the dynamic response of a system by suddenly removing the deflecting force. For critically damped and underdamped systems, the normalized response for the sudden removal of unit deflecting force is shown in Fig. 14b; the legend includes the equation of motion in terms of the damping coefficient D.

Intimately associated with the response to a step input is the behavior of such systems when subjected to sinusoidal forces. Figure 15a illustrates the normalized response A_f/A_k when tested with a constant-amplitude, variable-frequency sine wave of amplitude A_f; A_k is the zero frequency amplitude. With critical damping ($D = 1$), the frequency–response curve has a characteristic form, falling progressively as the frequency is increased. With decreasing damping, the amplitude of motion increases and becomes larger and larger as the natural resonant frequency is approached. At the natural resonant frequency f_0, with $D = 0$, the amplitude approaches infinity. With driving frequencies above the natural resonant frequency, the amplitude is reduced; as the frequency is increased, the amplitude soon becomes immeasurably small. This condition (dashed curve in Fig. 15a) represents the boundary under which all operating characteristics are to be found.

If the same procedure is carried out with various degrees of damping between zero and approximately 0.7, the amplitude increases slightly at first, rises to a peak, and then falls rapidly as the frequency increases. The cases of $D = 0.2$ and $D = 0.5$ (Fig. 15a) illustrate this point. The interesting behavior when $D = 0.7$ is discussed later.

From Fig. 15 it is apparent that with critical damping ($D = 1$), the system can respond fully only to sine wave frequencies up to a few percent of the natural resonant frequency. With light damping ($D = 0.2$) there is a pronounced rise in the frequency–response curve at approximately 95% of the undamped natural resonant frequency. When the damping is increased to 0.5, the frequency–response curve is more uniform and exhibits a less pronounced resonant rise. The frequency at a resonant rise is less than that for the undamped condition. In both cases, as the frequency is increased beyond the maximum response, the amplitude falls progressively.

The foregoing discussion shows that by assigning various values to the damping coefficient, a family of amplitude-versus-frequency curves is determined. Those of most interest fall between zero and critical damping and assume a contour appropriate for their proximity to either of these curves. When a sine wave of force is presented to such systems, there is a time lag between the displacement of the mass and the applied force. This time lag is expressed in terms of degrees of a full cycle

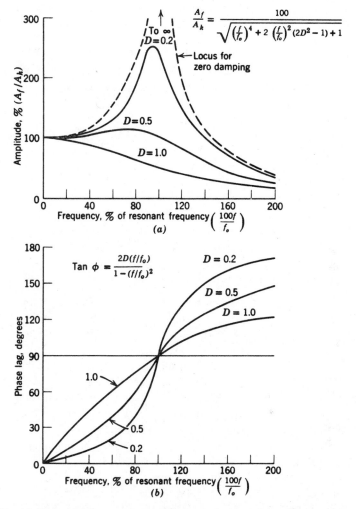

Figure 15 (a) Sinusoidal frequency and (b) phase response of damped resonant systems.

and is designated a phase shift. Damping has a pronounced effect on the phase characteristic of such systems. This relationship is presented in Fig. 15b. It is apparent from inspection of this figure that with some damping between 0.5 and 1.0, the phase shift can be nearly linear with frequency up to the natural resonant frequency f_0.

In deciding what degree of damping should be specified to obtain the best phase characteristic, it is useful to recall the three criteria for the faithful reproduction of an event: linearity of amplitude, adequate bandwidth of sine wave frequency response, and linearity of phase shift. Because amplitude linearity is usually easy to achieve, the following discussion deals with the effect of damping on the sine wave frequency and phase response.

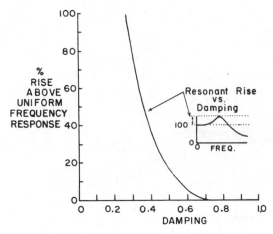

Figure 16 The effect of damping on the uniformity of the sine wave frequency response.

Figure 16 shows the amplitude of the resonant rise in the sine wave frequency-response curve as damping is increased. On the basis of uniform sine wave frequency response, a damping of 0.7 results in no resonant peak in the curve. Not shown in Fig. 16 but certainly indicated by Fig. 15b, it can be stated that this degree of damping provides a linear phase shift up to and slightly beyond the undamped resonant frequency. It is logical, then, to conclude that this degree of damping fulfills the requirements for faithful reproduction of an event. Although this is true, it must be remembered that the reproduction of a step input by a system having these constants is slightly compromised. Under these conditions the rise time (0 to 100%) is approximately half the undamped period. Moreover, a 5% overshoot is present. It is to be recalled that decreasing the damping shortens the rise time at the expense of overshoot. Since with 0.7 damping, some overshoot must exist, it is logical to investigate the improvement in rise time as damping is further decreased to obtain a more rapid response from the system. Just what degree of damping is to be specified usually depends on the penalty that can be paid in terms of overshoot and rise time for a step function, along with the loss produced in the sine wave frequency response.

From Fig. 17, which relates rise time and overshoot to the various degrees of damping, it is seen that if the damping is reduced from 0.7 to 0.65, the response time shortens by about 3% to 47% of the undamped period, while the overshoot increases by 2%, giving a total overshoot of 7%. Under these conditions, sine wave characteristics are not excessively compromised, since for 0.65 damping the resonant rise in the frequency–response curve is slightly more than 1% and the phase error is approximately 4 degrees.

If a larger overshoot to the step function can be tolerated, a further decrease in rise time can be attained. At 0.6 damping, the rise time is shortened to approximately 45% of the undamped period, but the overshoot is increased to about 10%. Under these conditions the resonant rise in the sine wave curve is approximately 5%.

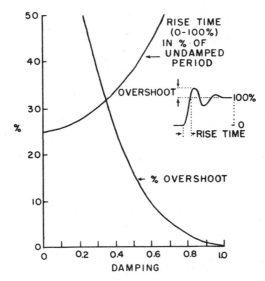

Figure 17 The effect of damping on rise time and overshoot in terms of the response to a step function.

Thus it is apparent that with devices in which resonance can occur, a shorter response time can be attained if a small degree of overshoot can be tolerated when a step input is applied. The improvement in rise time simulates to some extent the characteristics of a stiffer system, that is, one with a higher natural resonant frequency. With knowledge of the undamped resonant frequency and the degree of damping, the entire behavior of a system having one degree of freedom can be predicted. When the response to a step function (rise time and overshoot) is known, the sine wave frequency and phase characteristics can be deduced. Conversely, knowledge of the sine wave frequency and phase–response characteristics makes it possible to predict the response to a step function or a square wave.

In practice, to obtain a good compromise among all the factors discussed, the damping of dynamic systems is usually adjusted to about 0.65. The characteristics of a system with one degree of freedom and this damping coefficient are given in Table 1.

TABLE 1   Characteristics of a Resonant System with 0.65 Damping: Undamped Resonant Frequency = f_0

Step Function	
Rise time (0 to 100% of terminal amplitude)	$1/2.1\,f_0$ sec
Overshoot (% over terminal amplitude)	7%
Sine Wave	
Bandwidth (to 70% of uniform amplitude response)	$(0\text{--}108\%)\,f_0$
Resonant peak (above uniform response)	1.3%
Maximum phase error over $(0\text{--}100\%)\,f_0$ range	4%

Electrical Analog of Damped Resonant Systems

The behavior of a large number of damped resonant systems such as blood pressure transducers and graphic recorders can be simulated electrically and their properties investigated experimentally. Figure 18 shows the electrical analog of these and other damped resonant systems. The inductance L simulates the mass or inertia; the resistance R is equivalent to the viscous drag or frictional resistance; and the capacitance C represents the stiffness of the system. The input voltage E can be a sine wave or step function from a voltage source. The displacement, or output, is described by the voltage across the capacitor (C). By choosing values for L and C and varying R, the behavior of underdamped, critically damped, and overdamped systems can be investigated. For critical damping ($D = 1$), the resistance R_c is given by

$$R_c = 2\sqrt{L/C}.$$

For any value of R, the damping D is given by

$$D = \frac{R}{2}\sqrt{\frac{C}{L}},$$

and the natural resonant frequency f_0 is given by

$$f_0 = \frac{1}{2\pi\sqrt{LC}}.$$

The damped resonant frequency f_r is given by

$$f_r = f_0\sqrt{1 - D^2}.$$

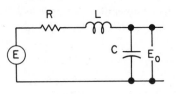

Figure 18 Electrical analog of a damped resonant system. E is voltage (source) input and E_0 is the output, which is the analog of displacement. The resistance R represents the total resistance in the circuit.

E = Constant voltage function generator
R = Resistance
L = Inductance
C = Capacitance
f_r = Resonant frequency = $1/2\pi\sqrt{LC}$
Damping coefficient = $R/2\sqrt{L/C}$

As stated previously, the voltage across the capacitor (E_0) represents displacement, which can be displayed for any type of voltage source (E) applied to the input terminals of the *RLC* circuit.

Conclusion

It is apparent that for a system to reproduce a complex waveform faithfully, consideration must be given to the harmonic spectrum of the waveform. Then the sine wave frequency and phase characteristics of the reproducing system must be examined for their suitability for reproduction of all the components of the complex wave. From such an investigation it is possible to determine the degree of fidelity of reproduction that can be expected.

ELEMENTARY SIGNAL PROCESSING

To conclude this chapter, it is appropriate to present a few elementary concepts relevant to the digital processing and display of physiological data. The starting point is, of course, the transducer, which converts the physiological event to an electrical signal. Transducers are sometimes called sensors or biosensors; the principles of many transducers are described elsewhere in this book. Having the physiological event in the form of an electrical signal permits the use of a wide variety of processing and display techniques.

Figure 19 illustrates a typical analog recording system in which the transducer signal is processed in a manner suitable for the reproducer or display device, which is often a recording pen or oscilloscope screen. The processor is sometimes called a signal conditioner and often provides linear amplification. In this case, the three criteria for the faithful reproduction of the event must be satisfied. Frequently, the physiological event is recorded on magnetic tape for later replay and study. Again, the overall performance of the tape recorder/playback system must obey the three criteria for faithful reproduction of the event. Alternatively, the processor may manipulate the signal to provide the desired type of display. For example, the processor may deliver a signal that represents the maximum or minimum value of the event, its rate of change, or the interval between components of the incoming signal. All of these and other manipulations can be made using analog techniques.

Analog Tape

Before discussing digital systems, it is useful to recognize the characteristics of analog tape recording systems. Although there are many techniques for recording data on magnetic tape, the overall performance can be described in terms of the sinusoidal frequency response. Conventional audiotape recorders, such as reel-to-reel and cassette types that are used for speech and music reproduction, do not provide a low-frequency response extending to 0 Hz; such recorders seldom have low-frequency response extending much below 50 Hz; direct-recording is the term

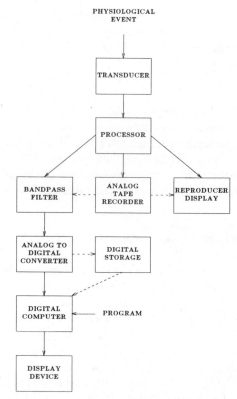

Figure 19 Analog recording and display of physiological data (upper) and the technique for conversion to digital form (lower).

used to describe this mode of operation. When it is desired to have a low-frequency response extending to 0 Hz, the information to be recorded is caused to modulate a carrier; usually frequency modulation (FM) is used. A variety of other techniques, such as pulse-width or pulse-position modulation, can also be employed. However, the most common technique employs a continuous wave carrier, the frequency of which is modulated by the information to be recorded. The frequency deviation is typically ±40%. Table 2 presents the center frequencies used with different tape speeds.

TABLE 2 Typical FM Analog Tape Recording Characteristics

Tape Speed (in./sec)	Center Frequency (Hz)	Bandwidth (±0.1 dB)	Signal-to-Noise Ratio (dB)
$\frac{15}{16}$	843.75	0–313	45
$1\frac{7}{8}$	1,687.5	0–625	46
$3\frac{3}{4}$	3,375	0–1,250	48
$7\frac{1}{2}$	6,750	0–2,500	48
15	13,500	0–5,000	48
30	27,000	0–10,000	48
60	54,000	0–20,000	48

The use of a carrier to record the desired data on magnetic tape permits the low-frequency response to extend to 0 Hz, i.e., direct current. The high-frequency limit of tape recording depends on the tape speed (in addition to design of the recording and playback heads); the higher the tape speed, the higher the high-frequency capability. Table 2 shows the high-frequency response capabilities of a typical FM tape recording system.

When data are recorded on magnetic tape, noise is introduced. Three types of noise are associated with analog tape systems—flutter, wow, and tape noise. Flutter is produced by oscillations in tape speed; wow is a slight change in tape speed. These two types of noise are small in a well-designed FM tape recorder. With inexpensive cassette and reel-to-reel direct-recording machines, these types of noise can be recognized when a sustained tone is being replayed, appearing as a change in frequency.

In a well-designed and well-constructed FM tape recorder, tape noise imposes a limit to the resolution of a signal. The term signal-to-noise (S/N) ratio is used to specify the amount of this type of noise in relation to the signal amplitude. The signal-to-noise ratio is dependent on tape speed; Table 2 presents S/N ratios for a typical FM analog tape recorder.

The concept of signal-to-noise (S/N) ratio is important to understand. It is conventionally expressed in decibels, i.e., a ratio defined as

$$S/N = 20 \log (A_s/A_n),$$

where A_s and A_n are the amplitudes of the signal and noise, respectively.

For a tape speed of 3.75 in./sec, a typical S/N ratio is 48 dB; this represents a ratio of signal amplitude to noise amplitude of 250/1. In other words, the noise added by the tape recorder is 1/250 of the dynamic range of the channel, providing a resolution of 0.4%. If the signal occupies only one-fifth of the dynamic range, then the noise added by the tape recorder is 1/50 of the signal; in this case, the resolution in the data cannot be greater than 2%. Note that with a speed of $\frac{15}{16}$ in./sec, the S/N ratio is 45 dB, which represents an amplitude ratio of 178/1, corresponding to a resolution of 0.56%. In a typical display system, noise is perceptible when the S/N ratio is 1/200 or less. Therefore, in addition to deciding on a tape speed for an adequate high-frequency response, attention must be paid to the S/N ratio desired.

The dynamic range of the tape recorder is typically selectable by a multiposition switch on the face of the recorder. The ranges available may include ±0.2, 0.5, 1, 2, 5, 10, and 20 V, and choice of the proper range is a balance between maximizing the S/N ratio and allowing sufficient range so that even with baseline drift the peaks in the signal amplitude will remain within the linear dynamic range. In the upcoming discussion of digital sampling, further considerations in the selection of the dynamic range will be presented. Regardless of the input range selected, the output range of the recorder is fixed, for example ±1 V. Therefore, the recorder must be considered not only as a storage device but also as an amplifier.

Before the availability of digital computers, recorded physiological data were analyzed for their information content by direct measurement of a graphic record or a photograph of a waveform on an oscilloscope screen. Numerical data from this source were processed manually to generate tables or graphs. The advent of the digital computer has greatly reduced the need for manual measurement of recordings. The price paid is conversion of the signal into a digital form and provision of a program to process the digitized data.

Digital Systems

To reap the many benefits of a digital computer for processing physiological data, it is necessary to have the event of interest in the form of an electrical signal. Therefore many elements of the analog system just described are necessary. Figure 19 illustrates a typical method used in signal processing with a digital computer. The electrical signal, representing the physiological event, is first passed through a bandpass filter having a bandwidth appropriate for the desired Fourier components of the physiological event. This step is necessary to eliminate noise or unwanted components from the signal and thereby prevent the generation of spurious signals (aliasing) due to the sampling process to be described subsequently. An alternative method employs replaying the signal recorded on analog tape into the bandpass filter.

Because the currency of a digital computer is zeros and ones, it is necessary to convert the analog signal into digital form by means of an analog-to-digital (A/D) converter. The signal, now in digital form, can be read by the digital computer. The type of processing that is accomplished and the type of display desired, depend on the type of computer and the instructions given to it in the form of a program. If the incoming signal is digitized and processed while the physiological event is occurring, the technique is called on-line processing. The digitized signal can be stored in any one of several different digital storage media, such as digital tape, floppy, hard, or compact disk. Such stored digital information can be replayed into the digital computer for processing at a later time; this technique is called off-line processing. Figure 19 summarizes the steps just described.

When converting an analog signal to digital form, there are two important considerations; the first is choice of an adequately high sampling rate that permits identification of all of the desired details in the waveform. The second consideration relates to the desired amplitude resolution for each sampled data point. The following simple examples can serve to establish the importance of these two considerations.

Figure 20A shows a waveform that exhibits a rapid (a), then a slower rise (b) to a flat top (c), followed by a slow decrease (d) in amplitude, the total duration of the wave being 1 sec. When this waveform is time-sampled, enough data points are needed to retain its details. Neglecting amplitude resolution for the moment, and starting the sampling at the onset of the wave, the effect of sampling rate can be demonstrated. It should be recognized also that the sampling can start at any time before or during the wave, which would result in a different set of data points. Figure 20B illustrates the amplitude of each sample using a sampling rate of 5 samples/sec, and Fig. 20C illustrates the result for 10 samples/sec. Note that this latter sampling rate is too infrequent to identify the transition in the a-b-c region

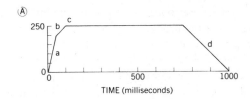

TIME (milliseconds)

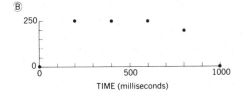

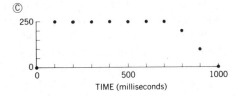

E. Data Content of D

Sample Time (msec)	Decimal Amplitude	8-Bit Binary Representation
0	0	00000000
50	200	11001000
100	250	11111010
150	250	11111010
200	250	11111010
250	250	11111010
300	250	11111010
350	250	11111010
400	250	11111010
450	250	11111010
500	250	11111010
550	250	11111010
600	250	11111010
650	250	11111010
700	250	11111010
750	250	11111010
800	200	11001000
850	150	10010110
900	100	01100100
950	50	00110010
1000	0	00000000

Figure 20 (*A*) Original waveform and (*B–D*) data points obtained by sampling at 5, 10, and 20 samples/sec. (*E*) Decimal and binary values for the amplitudes for each 50-msec sample of the record in *D*.

of the wave. Figure 20*D* illustrates the case for a sampling rate of 20/sec; observe that the a-b-c segment details are now identifiable. Obviously, the sampling rate must be selected to provide enough data points to identify the desired details in the most rapidly changing part of the sampled waveform. The Nyquist criterion for sampling requires that a minimum of two samples be obtained for the highest frequency harmonic considered to be necessary for faithful reproduction of the waveform. Sampling with a frequency below this rate results in the appearance of, in the output, the higher harmonics that were sampled less than twice per cycle, but translated to a lower frequency; this is called aliasing. Aliasing is spectral overlapping, which represents the introduction of noise. Aliasing can be prevented either by increasing the sampling rate or by limiting the bandwidth before sampling by using a low-pass filter to ensure that the Nyquist criterion is met.

In the foregoing simple example, it was assumed that the amplitudes of the sampled waveform were the actual values at the instants of sampling. However, when using digital techniques, it is necessary to represent the sampled amplitudes in binary form, the basis of which represents numbers in terms of two raised to a power. Because a digital computer recognizes numbers in terms of ones and zeros, the binary system is used, and ones and zeros represent the presence or absence of two raised to a power. For example, the eight-bit representation for the numbers from 1 to 5 are shown in Table 3.

Thus, the number 5 represents $2^2 + 0 + 2^0$ or, in eight-bit form, 00000101. Likewise, the largest number that can be represented by eight bits is 11111111, or 255. The number 50,000 is 11000011,01010000 which requires 16 bits or two bytes. The largest number that can be represented by 16 bits is 65,535 or 11111111,11111111.

With this information as a background, it is easy to illustrate the concept of amplitude resolution, which is determined by the number of bits used to represent an amplitude. Amplitude resolution is the smallest difference that can be distinguished between two values.

Figure 20E presents the binary representation for each sampled amplitude of the waveform in Fig. 20D. For illustrative purposes, 8 bits were chosen to represent the 0–250 units (maximum amplitude).

It must be recognized that when specifying the number of bits to represent an amplitude in a practical situation, it is necessary to be aware of the linear dynamic amplitude range of the system, which is represented by the number of bits selected. For example, if a dynamic range of 10 V is represented by 8 bits, the amplitude range corresponds to 255 levels, and the amplitude resolution is 1/255 or 0.39% of the full dynamic range, or 39 mV. If the signal being sampled occupies less than the full dynamic range, the amplitude resolution will be less. Therefore, when specifying the number of bits to represent a desired dynamic range, the amplitude

TABLE 3   Eight-Bit Binary Representation

2^7	2^6	2^5	2^4	2^3	2^2	2^1	2^0	Decimal number
0	0	0	0	0	0	0	0	0
0	0	0	0	0	0	0	1	1
0	0	0	0	0	0	1	0	2
0	0	0	0	0	0	1	1	3
0	0	0	0	0	1	0	0	4
0	0	0	0	0	1	0	1	5

is divided by the desired signal resolution. The number of levels represented by n bits is $2^n - 1$. Use of this expression permits easy calculation of the number of bits required. For example, if the dynamic range is 1 V (1000 mV) and the desired amplitude resolution is 1 mV, the number of levels is 1000 mV$/$1 mV = 1000. Ten bits provides 1023 levels, which would be adequate for the desired resolution.

Figure 21 illustrates a practical example of the process just described in which the ECG is derived from a subject. Assuming no Q and S waves, the peak of the R wave reaches its 1 mV peak value in 0.08 sec. Therefore, the slew rate is $1 \times 10^{-3}/0.08 = 0.0125$ V$/$sec, or 12,500 μV$/$sec. Assuming that a 20-μV resolution is desired, the sampling rate is $12,500/20 = 625/$sec. This sampling rate provides a resolution for the R wave of $(20 \ \mu$V$/1000 \ \mu$V$)100 = 2\%$ of the R-wave amplitude (for this slew rate).

The ECG has a peak amplitude of 1 mV. To accommodate R waves from other subjects, who may have larger or inverted R waves, the dynamic range of the channel may be made ± 2.5 mV or a total range of 5 mV. If the desired amplitude resolution is 20 μV, then the number of levels required is 5 mV$/20 \ \mu$V = 250 levels. If this range is represented by 8 bits (255 levels), each level represent 5 mV$/255$ levels = 19.6 μV. Therefore, the error due to sampling (called the quantization error) is $(19.6 \ \mu$V$/1$ mV$) \times 100 = 1.96\%$ of the signal.

If the ECG is passed through a preamplifier (gain = 200) and a unity-gain bandpass filter, the previous exercise can be repeated with similar results. The corresponding resolution after a gain of 200 would be 4 mV. The number of levels required to give a 4 mV resolution with a dynamic range of 1000 mV is 1000 mV$/4$ mV = 250. The quantization error is $(3.92$ mV$/200) \times 100 = 1.96\%$ of

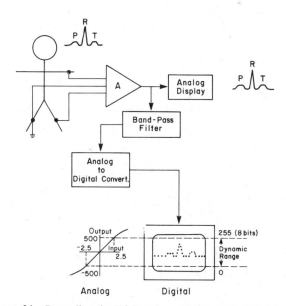

Figure 21   Recording the ECG and converting it to digital form.

the signal amplitude. If this range is represented by 8 bits (255 levels), each level represents $1000/255 = 3.92$ mV. Therefore the quantization error due to sampling the R wave is $(3.92/200)\,100 = 1.96\%$ of the R-wave amplitude.

An exaggerated representation of the digitized ECG is shown in Figure 21 (lower right). A slow sampling rate was chosen to illustrate the fact that with digital sampling the analog record is formed of a series of discrete amplitudes.

From the foregoing, and from an examination of Fig. 21E, it can be seen that increasing the number of bits used to represent an amplitude increases the amount of binary information that must be stored. If the sampling time is prolonged, or if an excessively high sampling rate is used, an enormous amount of data will be collected that must be stored somewhere. Although storage devices are being developed with increased capacity and shorter access and retrieval times, careful consideration should be given to the storage requirements resulting from a given sampling rate and bit selection. At present floppy disks store 0.3–1 Mbyte, hard disks 10–200 Mbytes, digital tape about 256 Mbytes, compact disks about 300 Mbytes, and cassette tape about 15 Mbytes.

REFERENCES

Geddes, L. A. 1951. A note on phase distortion. *EEG Clin. Neurophysiol.* **3**:517–518.

Hansen, A. T. 1949. *Pressure Measurement in the Human Organism.* Technisk Forlag, Copenhagen.

Saunders, M. G., and R. M. Jell. 1959. Time distortion in electroencephalograph amplifiers. *EEG Clin. Neurophysiol.* **11**:814–816.

Schwarzschild, M., and M. Kissin. 1934–1935. The effect of condensers in the electro/cardiograph. *Am. Heart. J.* **9**:517–525.

Terman, F. E. 1943. *Radio Engineers Handbook.* McGraw-Hill, New York.

Valley, G. E., and H. Wallman. 1948. *Vacuum Tube Amplifiers.* McGraw-Hill, New York.

Index

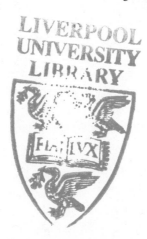